Clinical Nursing Skills

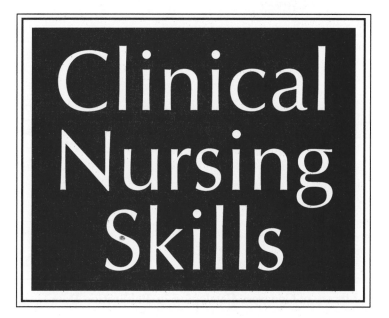

Clinical Nursing Skills

Carol Barnett Lammon, RN, MSN

Assistant Professor of Nursing
Capstone College of Nursing
University of Alabama
Tuscaloosa, Alabama

Anne W. Foote, RN, DSN

Associate Professor
University of Alabama School of Nursing
University of Alabama at Birmingham
Birmingham, Alabama

Patricia G. Leli, RN, MSN

Instructor
University of Central Florida
Orlando, Florida

Janice Ingle, RN, DSN

Chair, Department of Nursing
Southern Union State Junior College
Valley, Alabama

Marsha H. Adams, RN, DSN

Assistant Professor
Capstone College of Nursing
University of Alabama
Tuscaloosa, Alabama

W.B. Saunders Company
A Division of Harcourt Brace & Company

Philadelphia   London   Toronto   Montreal   Sydney   Tokyo

W.B. SAUNDERS COMPANY
A Division of
Harcourt Brace & Company

The Curtis Center
Independence Square West
Philadelphia, Pennsylvania 19106

Library of Congress Cataloging-in-Publication Data

Clinical nursing skills / edited by Carol Lammon . . . [et al.].

p.   cm.

ISBN 0–7216–6680–9

1. Nursing.

[DNLM: 1. Nursing Process.   WY 100 C6413 1995]

RT41.C67 1995

610.73—dc20

DNLM/DLC   93–44872

CLINICAL NURSING SKILLS   ISBN 0–7216–6680–9

Printed in the United States of America.

Last digit is the print number: 9   8   7   6   5   4   3   2   1

PREFACE

It has been said that nursing is both a science and an art. The nurse must utilize a vast body of knowledge to perform nursing care in a variety of clinical situations. The nurse must be able to provide nursing care in a safe, efficient, caring manner. The professional nurse must understand the rationale behind each action that is taken and the potential outcome for the client.

The marriage of knowledge and practice and its application in the clinical situation are often difficult concepts for the beginning learner to grasp. As nursing students begin their program of study, they are frequently overwhelmed by the volume of material that must be read, learned, and put into practice. With these concerns in mind, *Clinical Nursing Skills* was developed. *Clinical Nursing Skills* was designed to accompany and complement a basic nursing or fundamentals of nursing textbook. Information that would commonly be found in any basic nursing textbook is not repeated in *Clinical Nursing Skills*. Rather, students are led to use their knowledge as they carry out psychomotor skills in a safe and efficient manner. *Clinical Nursing Skills* would be a particularly effective companion to *Sorensen and Luckmann's Basic Nursing*, third edition (W.B. Saunders, 1994), some of the content of which forms the basis for portions of this book.

The skills presented in this textbook are basic psychomotor skills commonly performed in both primary and secondary care settings. Cognitive procedures (such as interviewing a client or admitting a client to a hospital), which are commonly discussed in a fundamentals of nursing textbook, are omitted to avoid repetition of content. The authors recognize differences among nursing curricula and have included selected skills that may be considered intermediate in some nursing programs. To facilitate the students' knowledge of assessment, twenty-five guidelines are included in the Appendix, *Guidelines for Health History and Physical Assessment*, following Chapter 21. These guidelines present a systematic head-to-toe approach to physical assessment and history-taking.

Organization

Each chapter in *Clinical Nursing Skills* begins with a brief discussion of the principles underlying the skills presented and the nurse's responsibilities to the client and family. This introduction is followed by a list of the skills in the chapter along with page numbers to facilitate quick location of the skills.

The professional nurse's practice should be guided by research findings whenever possible. Therefore, when applicable, a section entitled *Overview of Related Research* is presented at the beginning of each section of skills. Research findings have also been incorporated in the actions and rationales of the skill presentation.

Each skill begins with a brief overview entitled *Clinical Situations in Which You May Encounter This Skill*. These overviews support and extend the chapter introduction in setting the context for the skills being discussed. Bulleted lists of *Anticipated Responses* and *Adverse Responses* also precede each skill, as does a *Materials List*. These lists give students a preview of what to expect and enable them to gather the materials necessary to perform the skill.

Incorporating the Nursing Process

Performing nursing skills in the clinical setting involves the use of the nursing process. Within the steps of a skill, the student is led to make pertinent *assessments* of the client's health status. The student is instructed to *plan* for the skill by gathering necessary materials and making necessary preparations before beginning to perform the procedure.

Implementation of the skill is described in a numbered step-by-step format with a rationale given for each action. Carefully planned drawings and photographs illustrate the skills to enhance the student's understanding of the procedure. Boxes highlighted in red within the skill steps call the student's attention to precautionary notes, warnings, and nursing tips.

The final steps of each skill aid the student in *evaluating* the client's response to the procedure. The *Anticipated Responses* as well as possible *Adverse Responses* listed at the beginning of each skill guide the student in evaluating client outcomes.

Documentation, Teaching Tips, and Home Care Variations

Examples of Documentation are provided at the end of each skill, along with *Teaching Tips* and *Home Care Variations*. These help reinforce the student's sense of professional responsibility, awareness of the increasing importance of health teaching as a nursing role, and flexibility in addressing care settings outside the hospital.

The nurse must be particularly mindful of the need for documentation. Documentation serves two purposes. First, documentation is necessary to communicate to other health professionals about the client's health status and the care that has been given, an important consideration in an increasingly collaborative and interdisciplinary delivery system. Second, documentation establishes a legal record of the client's status and care that has been received. *Clinical Nursing Skills* provides short examples of narrative notes as well as graphic style charting to aid the student in devloping documentation skills.

When performing a skill, the nurse should always teach the client about the procedure that is to be performed and what to expect both during and after the procedure. Also, this is often a good time to teach the client about his or her body and how to take preventive health care measures. In the *Teaching Tips* section of each skill, the student is offered some ideas regarding timely teaching subjects.

More and more often, nursing care is being given in the client's home. The *Home Care Variations* following each skill discuss any changes that may need to be made in the performance of a skill in the home setting.

Standard Steps for Nursing Procedures

A series of steps that should be carried out when performing any skill is presented below. These steps are not repeated for each skill presented in this textbook; when learning a new skill, refer back to this section as necessary. (These steps also appear on the inside cover of this book.

▼ ACTION	▼ RATIONALE
1. Check the physician's order.	1. Many of the skills presented in this textbook are interdependent functions of nursing and require a physician's order. The physician's order may give guidance or identify limitations for carrying out the skill.
2. Wash hands before and after the procedure.	2. Handwashing is the single most effective measure to decrease the transmission of microorganisms from one person to another.
3. Assemble equipment.	3. Assemble equipment before entering the client's room in order to perform the skill in an efficient and organized manner.
4. Identify the client by checking the arm band and bed tag, and by asking the client to state his or her name.	4. Prevents the error of performing the skill on the wrong client.

▼ *ACTION*   ▼ *RATIONALE*

5. Introduce yourself to the client.

6. Explain the procedure to the client using developmentally appropriate language and technique. Be sensitive to cultural differences.

7. Use universal precautions at all times when providing care to a client.

8. Refer to this textbook for the steps of the skill you are performing.

9. If abnormal responses are noted, notify your instructor, charge nurse, and physician.

10. Document the skill.

5. Identifies you to the client and helps to establish rapport with the client.

6. Prepares the client for the procedure, decreases client anxiety, and elicits client cooperation and assistance.

7. Universal precautions protect you from contact with blood or body fluids. Universal precautions are described on the inside back cover of this book.

9. Abnormal responses may warrant further nursing or medical intervention, or both.

10. Documentation provides a way to communicate with other members of the health care team and provides a legal record of care given to the client.

Individualizing Skills

When using any textbook that describes nursing care, it is important to understand that agency policies or the client's condition may necessitate variations in the method of performing a skill. The steps in any skill should always be incorporated with the agency guidelines and individualized to each client's situation and needs.

Performance Checklists

Performance checklists are available in a separate book to aid students in evaluating their level of proficiency with a particular skill. These checklists do not simply repeat the steps of a skill but identify the critical behaviors that would be evaluated to determine safe and proficient execution of the skill.

Summary

Clinical Nursing Skills offers the student concisely written and abundantly illustrated guidelines for performing basic psychomotor skills in a variety of settings. The text leads the student to apply knowledge to perform nursing procedures, and not just to perform set activities by rote. The text avoids unnecessary repetition of content commonly found in basic nursing textbooks. We believe and hope that students will both appreciate and benefit from this approach to learning the performance of psychomotor skills.

CAROL BARNETT LAMMON, RN, MSN
ANNE W. FOOTE, RN, DSN
PATRICIA G. LELI, RN, MSN
JANICE INGLE, RN, DSN
MARSHA H. ADAMS, RN, DSN

CONTENTS

ix

UNIT II

ASSESSMENT SKILLS

CHAPTER 4

ASSESSING VITAL SIGNS
57
—

CHAPTER 5

HEALTH ASSESSMENT
99
___

CHAPTER 6

ASSISTING WITH DIAGNOSTIC PROCEDURES AND SCREENING TESTS
155
___

UNIT III

THERAPEUTIC SKILLS

CHAPTER 7

MEETING MOBILITY NEEDS
205

CHAPTER 8

PREVENTING COMPLICATIONS OF IMMOBILITY
249

CHAPTER 9

PROVIDING PHYSICAL PROTECTION AND BODILY SUPPORT
287
—

CHAPTER 10

PROMOTING HYGIENE
295
—

CHAPTER 15

MEETING BOWEL ELIMINATION NEEDS
443
—

CHAPTER 16

MEETING URINARY ELIMINATION NEEDS
473
—

CHAPTER 17

MEETING RESPIRATORY NEEDS
503
—

CHAPTER 18

ADMINISTERING MEDICATIONS
571
—

CHAPTER 21

POSTMORTEM CARE
717
—

APPENDIX
GUIDELINES FOR HEALTH HISTORY AND PHYSICAL ASSESSMENT
723
—

INDEX
773
—

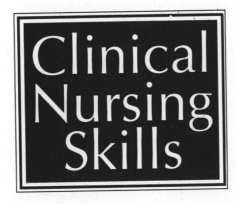

Clinical Nursing Skills

UNIT I

SKILLS REQUIRED FOR SAFE PRACTICE

CHAPTER 1

Infection Control

Preventing the spread of infectious microorganisms when providing nursing care is vitally important to the health of both you and the client. Nosocomial, or hospital-acquired, infections result in needless illness and death and contribute to the high cost of providing health care. Preventing the spread of microorganisms requires an understanding of both the mode of transmission of major infectious agents and the principles of medical and surgical asepsis.

Medical asepsis, or clean technique, refers to procedures that reduce the number of microorganisms and limit their growth and transmission from one person to another. *Surgical asepsis*, or sterile technique, refers to procedures that destroy all microorganisms and their spores. Surgical asepsis includes techniques to keep an area or object free of all microorganisms.

When providing nursing care to clients, you should always follow universal blood and body fluid precautions, which are sometimes called universal precautions. Universal precautions are a set of guidelines developed by the Centers for Disease Control and Prevention (CDC) for preventing contact with potentially infectious blood or body fluids that may harbor diseases such as hepatitis B or human immunodeficiency virus (HIV). The CDC universal precautions are described inside the back cover of this textbook for easy reference.

OVERVIEW OF RELATED RESEARCH

INFECTION CONTROL

Brown, D. G., et al. (1985). Sterile water and saline solution: Potential reservoirs of nosocomial infection. *American Journal of Infection Control*, 13(1), 35–39.

Large volume (250–1,000 ml) screw-capped bottles of sterile water, saline, and other solutions frequently are used in patient care and represent a significant hazard to patient safety if they are contaminated. In this study, 212 samples of opened sterile water and saline were analyzed for contamination. Thirty-seven (17.5%, or 1 in every 5) were positive for microbial contaminants. Although dating, timing, and discarding open solutions after 24 hours was a policy of the hospital, only 25% of the samples were dated and timed. Of these 53 dated bottles, 41.5% had been in use longer than 24 hours.

Cultures and sensitivities of the contaminants revealed highly resistant *Staphylococcus* and *enterococcus* group D as well as *Candida*, *Aspergillus*, and *Trichophyton*. Results indicated that health care professionals are not complying with written infection control policies and are not applying basic aseptic principles. It was suggested that sterile water and saline bottles no larger than 500 ml be used, that bottles be dated, and that policies be enforced to discard bottles 24 hours after opening.

Korniewicz, D. M., et al. (1989). Integrity of vinyl and latex procedure gloves. *Nursing Research*, 38, 144–146.

The purpose of this study was to examine the integrity of vinyl and latex pro-

cedure gloves for watertightness, bacterial penetration, and dye exclusion. Three hundred and fifteen vinyl and 330 latex gloves were examined for visual defects, and the watertight method was used to detect pinhole leaks. Visible defects were evident in 4.1% of the vinyl and 2.7% of the latex gloves. A significant difference was found between the two types in relation to dye permeability. The vinyl gloves (53%) were more permeable to dye. Only 3.3% of the latex gloves were permeable to dye. No significant difference in rate of permeability between the latex and the vinyl gloves was found. Both latex and vinyl gloves allowed bacterial penetration through puncture sites. The latex gloves performed better than the vinyl in relation to watertightness, bacterial penetration, and dye exclusion.

HANDWASHING

Ansari, S. A., et al. (1991). Comparison of cloth, paper, and warm air drying in eliminating viruses and bacteria from washed hands. *American Journal of Infection Control*, 19(5), 243–249.

Proper handwashing is regarded as the single most important step in infection control. This study compared the efficacy of paper, cloth, and electric warm air drying in eliminating rotaviruses and *Escherichia coli* remaining on finger pads washed with either 70% isopropanol, medicated liquid soap, or tap water. Results indicated that regardless of the handwashing agent used, electric air drying produced the highest reduction in the numbers of both test organisms and cloth drying produced the lowest. These findings indicate the importance of selecting the right means for drying washed hands, particularly when less effective handwashing agents are used.

Larson, E., Mayur, K., and Laughon, B. A. (1989). Influence of handwashing frequencies on reduction in colonizing flora with three handwashing products used by health care personnel. *American Journal of Infection Control*, 17(2), 83–88.

Handwashing products, including 2% chlorhexidine gluconate, 0.6% parachlorometaxylenol, 0.3% triclosan, and a nonantimicrobial control at two handwashing frequencies (6 or 18 times per day) were compared with regard to their effectiveness in reducing colonizing hand flora. Eighty adult volunteers were assigned by block randomization to one of the four products and one of the two frequency schedules (n = 10/group) and washed their hands under supervision for 5 consecutive days. There were no significant differences between products, nor were there significant differences in products after 5 days among subjects

washing 6 times per day. For those who washed 18 times per day, the effectiveness of all three antimicrobial soaps was significantly better than that of the control soap. Chlorhexidine gluconate produced significantly greater reductions than triclosan or parachlorometaxylenol, which were not significantly different from each other. On the basis of these findings, an antimicrobial soap is recommended when handwashing frequency is high and a long-term reduction in colonizing flora is desirable. When handwashing frequency is low (6 times/day), there appears to be less advantage of one product over another, although the use of chlorhexidine gluconate resulted in greater reductions at both high and low handwashing frequencies.

SKILL 1–1   HANDWASHING

Clinical Situations in Which You May Encounter This Skill

Handwashing is essential before and after any contact with a client or with supplies or equipment that have had contact with a client. Handwashing is also necessary before and after assisting with or performing any procedure; whenever gloves are worn; when handling blood, body fluids, secretions, or excretions; or when there will be contact with mucous membranes. Wash your hands after urinary and bowel eliminations and before eating to prevent transferring or acquiring microorganisms from the client.

Anticipated Responses

▼ The client does not develop a nosocomial infection.
▼ You do not acquire an infection from the client or transmit the infection to another client.

Adverse Responses

▼ The client develops a nosocomial infection.
▼ You acquire an infection from the client or transmit the infection to another client.

Materials List

Gather these materials before beginning the skill:

▼ Sink with hot and cold running water
▼ Soap dispenser
▼ Paper towels
▼ Trash can with foot pedal for lid removal (or trash can without lid)
▼ Nail brush or nail cleaner

▼ *A C T I O N*

1. Visually inspect your hands for obvious dirt or contamination.

2. Remove your jewelry (a plain wedding band does not have to be removed).

3. Pin your watch to your uniform, or wear it 1 to 2 inches above your upper wrist.

4. Standing away from the sink, use a paper towel to turn on the water to a lukewarm temperature and a moderate stream.

5. Wet your hands while holding them lower than your elbows.

6. Place approximately 1 teaspoon of soap on each of your hands.

7. Lather your hands thoroughly. Rub them together vigorously for at least 10 seconds.

8. Wash each of your wrists by rubbing the opposite hand in a circular motion around the wrist (Fig. 1–1).

▼ *R A T I O N A L E*

1. Dirt should be removed to decrease the transmission of microorganisms.

2. Total bacterial counts, especially gram-negative bacteria, are higher when rings are worn. Microorganisms accumulate in ring settings.

3. Prevents spread of microorganisms to your lower arm.

4. Standing away from the sink protects your uniform from splashes. A towel protects the faucet from contamination. Water is comfortable at a lukewarm temperature.

5. Water should flow from the least contaminated area to the most contaminated area.

6. Soap helps to emulsify body secretions, oils, or greases that harbor microorganisms and promotes their removal.

7. A topical antimicrobial product must be in contact with the skin for 10 seconds to have the desired effect. Friction helps to loosen and remove any dirt or secretions that harbor microorganisms.

8. Friction helps loosen dirt and microorganisms.

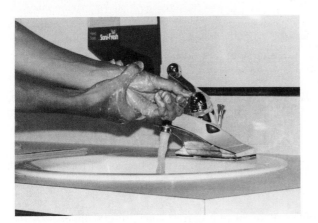

▼ **FIGURE 1–1.** Washing wrists.

▼ *A C T I O N* ▼ *R A T I O N A L E*

9. Interlace your thumbs and fingers and rub them back and forth (Fig. 1–2).

9. Helps loosen dirt and microorganisms between the thumb and fingers.

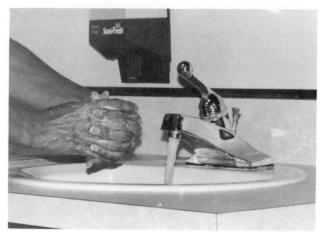

▼ **FIGURE 1–2.** Interlacing fingers.

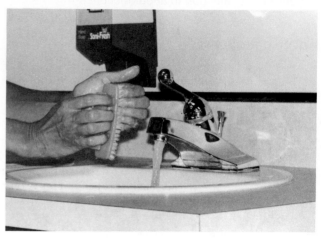

▼ **FIGURE 1–3.** Cleaning under fingernails.

10. Use a small brush to clean the subungual region (beneath the fingernails) (Fig. 1–3).

10. Microbes can lodge in the subungual region.

11. Thoroughly rinse each of your hands from the wrist to fingertips (Fig. 1–4). If your hands are very soiled, repeat Steps 6 through 11.

11. Running water rinses dirt, microorganisms, and soap residue into the sink.

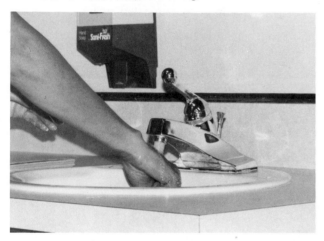

▼ **FIGURE 1–4.** Rinsing hands.

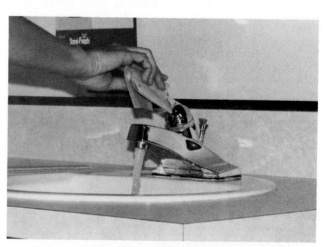

▼ **FIGURE 1–5.** Using paper towel to turn off faucet.

12. Keeping your hands at an angle with the fingertips higher than the elbow, dry them with disposable towels, wiping from the fingertips to the wrist and above.

12. Your hands are now the least contaminated area. Thorough drying prevents chapping and irritation.

13. Discard the towels in a trash can using your foot to open the lid, or drop them into an open trash can.

13. By using a foot pedal or an open trash can, contamination of clean hands is avoided.

14. Take a fresh paper towel and turn off the water faucets (Fig. 1–5). Discard the towel as before.

14. A towel is a barrier that protects the hands from contact with a soiled surface such as a faucet.

15. Visually inspect your hands for remaining dirt or soap.

15. The procedure may need to be repeated.

Example of Documentation

Documenting handwashing is not done routinely but may be required under special circumstances when infection exists.

DATE	*TIME*	*NOTES*
10/18/93	0800	Hands washed before and after assisting the client with mouth care.
		S. Williams, RN

Teaching Tips

As you wash your hands, use the opportunity to teach the client how to wash his or her hands properly. This is often the first step in many types of self-care.

Home Care Variations

Substitute bar soap. Rinse the bar of soap before and after using to remove any superficial microorganisms. Use disposable paper towels instead of cloth towels so that you will not transmit microorganisms from or to the towels. Place used paper towels into an open wastebasket after you have dried your hands.

SKILL 1–2   DONNING AND REMOVING A PROTECTIVE GOWN

Clinical Situations in Which You May Encounter This Skill

Protective gowns are worn to prevent contamination by a client's bodily secretions or microorganisms. For example, if the client has infected stool or copious secretions, a clean disposable gown will protect your uniform. Proctective gowns also may be used to protect the client from organisms on your uniform.

Protective gowns may be either paper or cloth and may be disposed of or discarded with the contaminated laundry after use. Gowns should be used only once and then discarded. The gown should not be worn during subsequent contact with other clients to prevent the transmission of infectious agents.

If the gown tears or becomes moist, remove the contaminated gown and replace it with another clean gown.

Anticipated Responses

▼ Infection is not spread via contamination of your uniform.
▼ The client is protected from infections.

Adverse Responses

▼ The disposable gown tears or becomes moist or saturated from the client's secretions.

Materials List

Gather these materials before beginning the skill:

▼ Paper or cloth gown

▼ *ACTION*

1. Review the physician's orders, medical diagnosis, and hospital infection control manual to determine if a gown is needed.

2. Pick up the gown and allow it to unfold without touching your uniform or the floor.

▼ *RATIONALE*

1. The type of infection will determine the type of protective clothing that should be worn.

2. Prevents contamination of the gown.

▼ *A C T I O N*	▼ *R A T I O N A L E*
3. Hold the inside of the gown in front of you. (Hold it so that the opening of the gown will be in the back when you put the gown on.)	**3.** Will allow for easy donning of the gown.
4. Place one arm at a time into the sleeves (Fig. 1–6).	**4.** Will allow for easy donning of the gown.

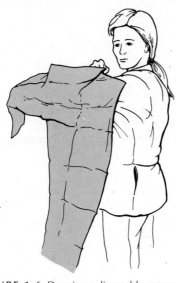

▼ **FIGURE 1–6.** Donning a disposable paper gown.

5. Tie the strings in back, making sure to overlap gown edges as much as possible.	**5.** Will provide maximum protection of your uniform.

Removing the Gown

6. Untie the strings in back of the gown.	**6.** Will allow the gown to be removed.
7. Remove the gown, folding it inside out to cover the outside of the gown.	**7.** The outside of the gown is considered contaminated. Do not allow it to touch your clothing.
8. If the gown is disposable, place it in a receptacle for the gown. If the gown is cloth, place it in a designated laundry bag.	**8.** Multiple use of gowns should be avoided to prevent spread of microorganisms.
9. Remove your gloves, if they were worn. (See Skill 1–8 for glove removal.)	**9.** Gloves are considered contaminated.
10. Wash your hands.	**10.** Prevents possible transmission of microorganisms.
11. Record the isolation precautions maintained.	**11.** Communicates to the other members of the health care team and contributes to the legal record by documenting the care given to the client.

Example of Documentation

DATE	TIME	NOTES
10/19/93	0900	Dressing change completed. Wound drainage purulent, yellow, foul-smelling. Protective clothing worn.
		S. Williams, RN

Home Care Variations

Use only disposable gowns. Place the used gown in a red plastic bag, seal, and remove it from the client's residence. Dispose of contaminated material according to your agency policy.

SKILL 1–3 DONNING AND REMOVING A PROTECTIVE FACE MASK AND EYEWEAR

Clinical Situations in Which You May Encounter This Skill

Face masks and eye goggles are used to protect your eyes, nose, and mouth from splashes of the client's body secretions. Face masks also may be required as a part of isolation precautions when caring for a client with a disease that is spread by the airborne route. Face masks vary in their permeability to airborne particles, however, and a face mask will not filter out all airborne pathogens. For this reason susceptible individuals should not care for clients who have diseases that are spread by the airborne route. Caregivers who are immune to the disease in question can safely provide care to these individuals.

Anticipated Responses

▼ Your eyes, nose, and mouth are protected from contamination by splashes of the client's body fluids.

Adverse Responses

▼ The mask becomes moist and allows the transmission of particles to and from the client.
▼ The eyewear does not fit well and allows the transmission of particles from the client.

Materials List

Gather these materials before beginning the skill:

▼ Disposable clean face mask
▼ Protective eye goggles or eye glasses

▼ ACTION

1. To determine if a mask is necessary, check the client's diagnosis and the physician's orders, and review the infection control manual.

2. Explain to the client the reason for the mask and goggles.

3. Put on eye protection.

4. Pick up the mask by the strings that are located by the metal strip.

5. Place the mask over the bridge of your nose.

6. Tie the upper strings behind the back of your head.

7. Tie the lower strings at the nape of your neck.

▼ RATIONALE

1. It may be necessary to reduce client contact with airborne microorganisms or to protect you and others entering the room from the client's body secretions.

2. Explanation will help reduce the client's apprehension.

3. Protects your eyes from contamination with splashes of the client's body fluids.

4. Avoids contamination of the mask.

5. By covering your nose, any contact with body secretions is avoided.

6. Prevents the mask from slipping down.

7. The mask will completely cover the nose and mouth and will prevent contact with body secretions.

▼ *A C T I O N*   ▼ *R A T I O N A L E*

8. Adjust the metal strip to fit comfortably over your nose. If you are wearing glasses, adjust the edge of the mask to fit securely under the glasses (Fig. 1–7).

8. Prevents escape of microorganisms from around the edges of the mask and prevents fogging of your glasses.

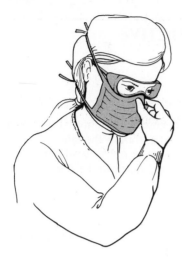

▼ **FIGURE 1–7.** Adjusting edge of mask to fit under glasses.

Removing the Mask

9. Untie the lower strings first and then the upper strings.

9. Prevents the mask from falling forward and contaminating your clothing.

10. Discard the mask, touching only the strings.

10. Only the strings are considered clean.

11. Remove eye protection, touching only the rear of the goggles. Discard in appropriate containers.

11. Only the back is considered clean.

12. Wash your hands.

12. Decreases the transfer of microorganisms.

13. Record the procedure, noting that isolation precautions were followed.

13. Communicates to the health care team and contributes to the legal record by documenting the care given to the client.

Example of Documentation

DATE	TIME	NOTES
10/3/93	0800	Isolation procedure followed to take vital signs.
		S. Williams, RN

Teaching Tips

This is an appropriate time to discuss routes of infection and infection control measures with the client.

SKILL 1–4   DONNING AND REMOVING DISPOSABLE EXAMINATION GLOVES

Clinical Situations in Which You May Encounter This Skill

Examination gloves serve as a protective barrier for your hands whenever they come in contact with a client's blood or body fluids. These gloves should be worn when you perform client care that requires medical asepsis. Procedures that require sterile technique require the use of sterile gloves. Carry a pair of examination gloves in your pocket at all times to ensure that they will be readily available when needed.

Examination gloves may be made of vinyl or latex. Refer to the "Overview of Related Research" at the beginning of this chapter for a comparison of vinyl and latex examination gloves.

Anticipated Responses

▼ You do not come in contact with the client's blood or body fluids.

Adverse Responses

▼ The examination gloves leak, thus failing to protect your hands from contamination with blood and body fluids.

Materials List

Gather these materials before beginning the skill:

▼ One pair of examination gloves

▼ ACTION	▼ RATIONALE
1. Wash your hands.	1. Decreases the transmission of microorganisms.
2. Slip your hands into the gloves.	2. There is no special technique for putting on examination gloves, since they are not sterile and provide a barrier only.

Removing Soiled Gloves

3. With your nondominant gloved hand, grasp the outside of the cuff of the other glove and remove the glove, turning it inside out as you pull it off your hand (Fig. 1–8). Continue to hold the just-removed glove with your remaining gloved hand.	3. Prevents skin contact with a contaminated glove and turns the soiled glove surface to the inside of the glove.

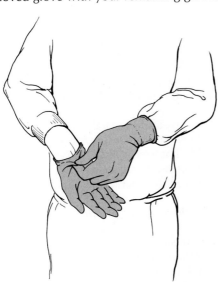

▼ FIGURE 1–8. Removing first glove.

▼ *ACTION*   ▼ *RATIONALE*

4. Slide your ungloved fingers under the cuff of the other soiled glove, and pull the glove off, turning it inside out (Fig. 1–9) and pulling it over the glove you continue to hold in your hand (Fig. 1–10).

4. Placing your fingers under the cuff protects them from contact with the soiled surface of the glove. Turning the glove inside out puts the soiled surface on the inside of the glove, providing a protective barrier from contamination within.

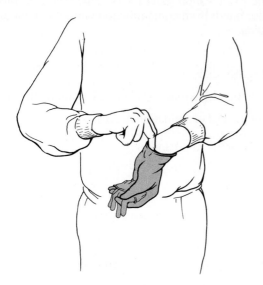

▼ **FIGURE 1–9.** Removing second glove.

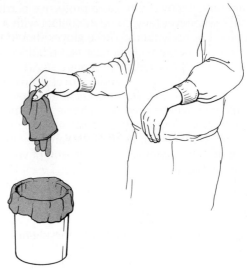

▼ **FIGURE 1–10.** Discarding soiled gloves.

5. Discard the soiled gloves in the appropriate receptacle.

5. Decreases the transmission of microorganisms.

6. Wash your hands.

6. Decreases the transmission of microorganisms.

Example of Documentation

Use of examination gloves usually is not documented.

PRINCIPLES OF STERILE TECHNIQUE

When performing procedures that require surgical asepsis, you should adhere to sterile technique. Use these principles as guidelines whenever sterile technique is required.

1. Keep sterile objects in your line of vision at all times to prevent their accidental contamination. Never turn your back on a sterile field. Do not leave the sterile field uncovered.
2. Keep sterile objects above table-level or waist-level at all times to avoid accidental contamination. If an object is held below these borders, it is considered contaminated.
3. Avoid speaking, coughing, laughing, or sneezing over a sterile field. The sterile field may become contaminated by airborne droplets containing microorganisms. Wearing a mask when preparing a sterile field may be required in certain areas such as the operating room.
4. Avoid holding nonsterile objects over a sterile field to prevent accidental contamination by microorganisms that may fall onto the field.
5. A sterile object becomes contaminated whenever it is touched by a nonsterile object.
6. Do not allow the sterile field to become wet. Moisture will draw microorganisms from the surface under the sterile field into the sterile field by capillary action. Use caution when pouring liquids to avoid splashing and splattering. If the field becomes wet, it is considered contaminated.

7. A 1-inch margin around the edge of the sterile field is considered contaminated. When putting items into the sterile field, be sure to place them inside this 1-inch border.

8. Do not allow contaminated fluids to flow back into a sterile area and contaminate it. Fluid flows by gravity. Always hold instruments with the contaminated end down and the clean end up.

9. If there is any doubt that sterile technique was compromised when gloving, gowning, setting up a sterile field, or passing sterile instruments or other objects, consider the object to be contaminated and obtain fresh sterile supplies.

SKILL 1–5 DONNING AND REMOVING SHOE COVERS, CAP, AND SURGICAL MASK

Clinical Situations in Which You May Encounter This Skill

A cap and mask are used to decrease the transmission of microorganisms. The cap and mask should be worn in the operating suite or delivery room and may be required for certain sterile procedures. The cap and mask are not sterile. Shoe coverings also are required in the operating suite or delivery room to decrease transmission of microorganisms (Fig. 1–11).

The hair harbors microorganisms. For a man with facial hair, the cap may not completely cover the hair. If you have a full beard, a special hood may be worn instead of a cap. The hood covers the head as well as the bearded facial area (Fig. 1–12).

If the cap or mask becomes moist or wet, airborne microorganisms may be transferred. A new cap or mask should be donned.

Anticipated Responses

▼ The cap completely covers your hair.
▼ The mask remains dry and covers your nose and mouth.

Adverse Responses

▼ The cap does not completely cover your hair.
▼ The mask becomes moist.

Materials List

Gather these materials before beginning the skill:

▼ Protective cap
▼ Protective mask
▼ Shoe covers

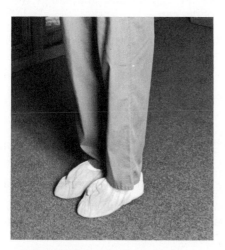

▼ FIGURE 1–11. Shoe coverings.

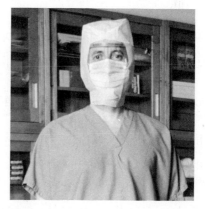

▼ FIGURE 1–12. Hood covers head and facial hair.

▼ *ACTION*	▼ *RATIONALE*
1. Determine if a cap, mask, and shoe covers are necessary for the procedure by checking the procedure manual.	**1.** Isolation and some sterile procedures require this protective wear.

▼ *A C T I O N* ▼ *R A T I O N A L E*

2. Put on your shoe covers.	**2.** Decreases transmission of microorganisms.
3. If your hair is long, secure it away from your face.	**3.** Prevents your hair from falling down below your cap. Hair is considered contaminated.
4. Place the cap on your head so that it completely covers your hair.	**4.** Prevents loose hair from falling into the sterile area.
5. If the cap has string ties, position it with the strings at the back of your head and secure the ties in a knot or bow.	**5.** Secures cap snugly to your head and protects your hair from exposure.
6. Pick up the mask by the strings that are located by the metal strip.	**6.** Avoids contamination of the mask.
7. Place the mask over the bridge of your nose.	**7.** By covering your nose, any transfer of airborne microorganisms is avoided.
8. Tie the upper strings behind the back of your head.	**8.** Prevents your mask from slipping down.
9. Tie the lower strings at the nape of your neck.	**9.** The mask will completely cover your nose and mouth and will decrease the transfer of microorganisms.
10. Adjust the metal strip to fit comfortably over your nose. If you are wearing glasses, adjust the edge of the mask to fit securely under the glasses.	**10.** Prevents escape of microorganisms from around the edges of the mask and prevents fogging of your glasses.

Removing Cap, Mask, and Shoe Covers

11. After removing the gown and gloves, remove the mask.	**11.** The gloves and gown are considered contaminated.
12. Untie the lower strings first and then the upper strings.	**12.** Prevents the mask from falling forward and contaminating your clothing. The mask is removed before the cap because the strings were tied on top of the cap.
13. Discard the mask, touching only the strings.	**13.** Decreases the transmission of microorganisms. The strings are considered clean.
14. Remove the cap and discard it in the proper receptacle. Paper caps can be deposited in a trash can and cloth caps can be deposited in a laundry hamper.	**14.** Decreases the transmission of microorganisms.
15. Remove the shoe covers and discard them in the proper receptacle.	**15.** Decreases the transmission of microorganisms.
16. Wash your hands.	**16.** Decreases the transmission of microorganisms.
17. Record the procedure, noting that sterile technique was followed.	**17.** Communicates to health care team and contributes to the legal record by documenting the care given to the client.

Example of Documentation

Use of shoe covers, cap, and mask usually is not documented.

SKILL 1–6   PERFORMING A SURGICAL HAND SCRUB

Clinical Situations in Which You May Encounter This Skill

Although skin cannot be sterilized, the purpose of a surgical hand scrub is to render the skin as free of microorganisms as possible. A surgical hand scrub is likely to be required when you are working in the operating room, delivery room, burn units, and invasive diagnostic areas of the hospital. Agency policy may require scrubbing each area of the hands and forearms a specific number of times. This is called a counted stroke scrub. Other agencies may use a timed scrub, during which each area of the hands and forearms is scrubbed for a specific number of minutes. A surgical hand scrub usually takes from 5 to 10 minutes with either method.

Anticipated Responses

▼ Your hands are rendered as free of microorganisms as possible.

Adverse Responses

▼ You are unable to complete the scrub due to skin irritation, cuts, or abrasions on the skin surface.

Materials List

Gather these materials before beginning the skill:

▼ Surgical cap
▼ Surgical mask
▼ Nail cleaner
▼ Antimicrobial soap and plain scrub brush or scrub brush impregnated with povidone-iodine (Betadine).
▼ Sink with foot, knee, or elbow control; deep bowl; and high faucet
▼ Sterile towels

▼ ACTION

1. Remove all jewelry, including your watch.

2. Trim your nails if needed. No nail polish or artificial nails should be worn.

3. Apply a cap and surgical mask. (See Skill 1–5.)

4. Obtain a brush and place the opened package containing the brush near the sink.

5. Turn on the water and adjust it to a lukewarm temperature (Fig. 1–13).

▼ RATIONALE

1. Jewelry harbors microorganisms.

2. Microorganisms collect in chipped nail polish and under artificial or long fingernails.

3. Provides a barrier to reduce the spread of microorganisms from the hair or respiratory tract.

4. The outside of the package is contaminated and you should not touch it once you have begun the surgical scrub.

5. Warm water is more comfortable and less irritating to the skin than cold water.

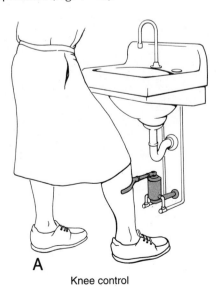

A
Knee control

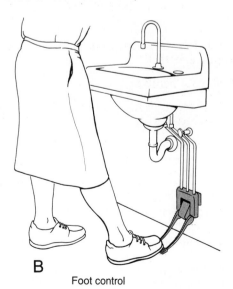

B
Foot control

▼ **FIGURE 1–13.** Turning on water.

▼ *ACTION*

▼ *RATIONALE*

6. Holding your hands above your elbows, wet the skin from your fingertips to elbows (Fig. 1–14).

6. Since your hands will be the cleanest area once the scrub is completed, follow the principle of allowing water to flow from the cleanest area to the most contaminated area.

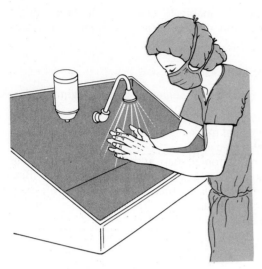

▼ **FIGURE 1–14.** Hands higher than elbows.

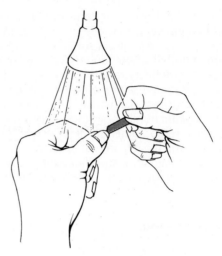

▼ **FIGURE 1–15.** Cleaning under fingernails.

7. Apply 1 teaspoon of antimicrobial soap to your hands or stroke your fingertips with a Betadine-saturated sponge.

7. Soap emulsifies skin oils and contaminants and facilitates their removal.

8. Using a nail cleaner, clean under each fingernail (Fig. 1–15). Discard the nail cleaner.

8. Removes bacteria-harboring contamination from under the fingernails.

9. Scrub all skin surfaces of your fingers, thumbs, hands, and forearms for the prescribed number of strokes or the prescribed amount of time (Fig. 1–16).

9. The scrubbing action loosens bacteria and contamination, thus facilitating their removal.

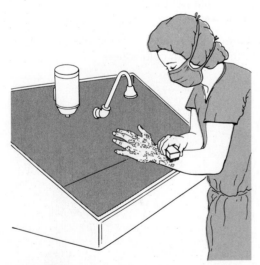

▼ **FIGURE 1–16.** Scrubbing hands and forearms.

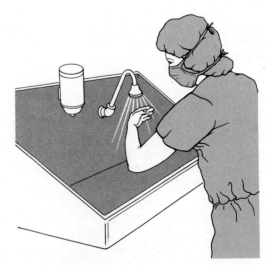

▼ **FIGURE 1–17.** Rinsing hands and arms.

10. Discard the brush.

10. Scrubbing is completed.

11. Rinse the soap from your skin, allowing the water to run from your fingertips to elbows. Keep your hands above your elbows at all times (Fig. 1–17).

11. Water should run from the area of least contamination to the area of most contamination.

▼ _A C T I O N_	▼ _R A T I O N A L E_
12. Turn off the water.	**12.** Use foot, knee, or elbow control to avoid contamination of your hands.
13. Dry each hand and arm with opposite ends of a sterile towel, working from the fingertips toward the elbows.	**13.** Drying prevents irritation of the skin. Dry from the cleanest area to the most contaminated area.
14. Discard the towels.	**14.** Drying is completed.
15. Keep your hands above your waist at all times.	**15.** Keeps your hands in your line of vision to prevent contamination.

Example of Documentation

Surgical hand scrubs usually are not documented.

SKILL 1–7 DONNING AND REMOVING A STERILE GOWN

Clinical Situations in Which You May Encounter This Skill

A sterile gown is used to provide a microbial-free barrier between your uniform and the client. The sterile gown prevents nosocomial infections in the client and protects you from exposure to the client's microorganisms.

An assistant is needed to tie the gown. A sterile gown may be either paper (disposable) or cloth (reusable).

If the gown becomes contaminated or contamination is suspected, don another sterile gown. If the gown becomes wet, replace the contaminated gown with another sterile gown.

Anticipated Responses

▼ The client is not exposed to microorganisms from your uniform, and the client does not experience a nosocomial infection.

▼ You are not exposed to bodily secretions from the client.

Adverse Responses

▼ The sterile gown becomes contaminated before the procedure is completed.

Materials List

Gather these materials before beginning the skill:

▼ Sterile gown

▼ _A C T I O N_	▼ _R A T I O N A L E_
1. Ask an assistant to be available to tie your gown.	**1.** The gown ties in the back. Reaching around would contaminate your hands and gown.
2. Examine the package containing the gown for signs of contamination or tears.	**2.** If the package is soiled, torn, or moist, microorganisms may have been transmitted to the contents.
3. Place the gown package waist-high on a clean, flat, dry surface.	**3.** Maintains sterility of the gown inside the package. Moisture increases the transmission of microorganisms.
4. Don a hair cover and mask, if indicated.	**4.** Apply anything nonsterile first.

▼ *ACTION* _____   ▼ *RATIONALE* _____

5. Complete the surgical scrub of your hands. (See Skill 1–6.)

6. Open the outer wrapper of the gown:

   a. Open the top fold of the wrapper away from you.
   b. Fold back the sides of the wrapper.
   c. Open the last fold of the wrapper toward you (Fig. 1–18).

5. A surgical scrub is more effective in removing microorganisms than simply washing your hands.

   a. If you reach across the sterile field, your gown is considered to be contaminated.

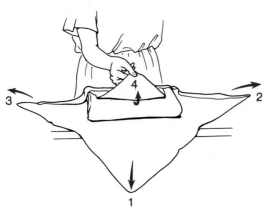

▼ FIGURE 1–18. Opening outer wrapper.

7. Pick up the gown by the folded edges inside the neck of the gown.

8. Touch only the side of the gown that will be next to your uniform when the gown is tied.

9. Pick up the gown, step back from the sterile field, and allow the gown to unfold away from other objects. Do not allow the gown to touch your uniform (Fig. 1–19).

10. Place your arms, one at a time, into the sleeves of the gown (Fig. 1–20).

7. Maintains sterility of the outside of the gown.

8. This side is considered to be contaminated.

9. Maintains sterility of the gown.

10. Maintains sterility of the gown.

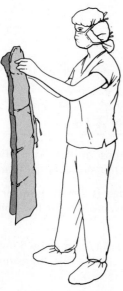

▼ FIGURE 1–19. Allowing gown to unfold.

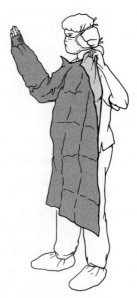

▼ FIGURE 1–20. Placing arms into sleeves.

▼ _ACTION_ _ _ _ _ _ _ _ _ _ _ _ _ _ _ _ ▼ _RATIONALE_ _ _ _ _ _ _ _ _ _ _ _ _ _

11. Have an assistant adjust the sleeves by reaching inside the sleeves.

11. If the outside of the sleeves is touched, the gown is considered to be contaminated.

12. Have an assistant tie the gown in the back (Fig. 1–21).

12. The back of the gown is not considered to be sterile. Tying the gown would contaminate your hands, which already have been surgically scrubbed.

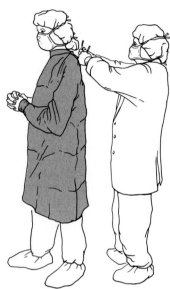

▼ **FIGURE 1–21.** Assistant tying gown.

13. Don sterile gloves. (See Skill 1–8.)

13. Sterile gloves usually are indicated if a sterile gown is needed.

Removing the Soiled Gown

14. Untie the strings in back of the gown.

14. Allows the gown to be removed.

15. Remove the gown, folding it inside out to cover the outside of the gown.

15. The outside of the gown is considered contaminated. Do not allow it to touch your clothing.

16. Dispose of the gown properly. Discard paper gowns into a designated trash receptacle and cloth gowns into a designated laundry bag.

16. The gown is contaminated and may not be reused.

17. Remove your gloves. (See Skill 1–8.)

17. The gloves are contaminated and must be discarded.

18. Wash your hands.

18. Prevents the transmission of microorganisms.

19. Record the procedure, noting that sterile technique was used.

19. Communicates to the health care team and contributes to the legal record by documenting the care given to the client.

Example of Documentation

DATE	_TIME_	_NOTES_
10/19/93	1100	Dressing change completed using sterile technique.
		S. Williams, RN

Home Care Variations

The gown used in home health situations is usually made of paper. It will not unfold as easily as a cloth gown. When transporting the gown to the client's home, do not let the gown become punctured, torn, or moist. Inspect the outer wrapper carefully. Check the agency protocol for the procedure for disposing of a used gown. Usually it will be put into a waste receptacle unless it is very soiled. If this occurs, remove the gown from the client's home in a sealed red plastic bag at the completion of the home visit.

SKILL 1–8 DONNING AND REMOVING STERILE GLOVES

Clinical Situations in Which You May Encounter This Skill

Sterile gloving is necessary anytime a sterile procedure is conducted (catheterization, sterile dressing change, operation, or delivery). Sterile gloving protects the client from microorganisms that may cause infection.

Anticipated Responses

▼ The client is not introduced to any microorganisms and does not develop a nosocomial infection.
▼ You do not become infected with any microorganisms from the client.

Adverse Responses

▼ The gloves become contaminated.
▼ You are exposed to microorganisms from the client.
▼ The client develops an infection.

Materials List

Gather these materials before beginning the skill:

▼ Sterile gloves

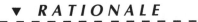

▼ *ACTION*	▼ *RATIONALE*
1. Determine if sterile gloving is necessary.	1. Sterile gloving is not necessary for every procedure. It may be safe for the client and cost-effective to use disposable, nonsterile gloves.
2. Thoroughly wash your hands.	2. Decreases the transmission of microorganisms.
3. Explain to the client that sterile gloving is necessary for protection against infection.	3. Explanations help to reduce the client's apprehension.
4. Place the unopened package of gloves on a clean and dry surface.	4. If the package becomes wet, it is no longer considered to be sterile.
5. Open the outside paper covering the sterile gloves by grasping the tabs on top of the package and peeling the paper open (Fig. 1–22).	5. Avoids contamination of the sterile gloves.

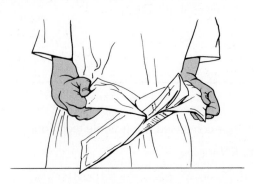

▼ **FIGURE 1–22.** Opening glove package.

▼ _A C T I O N_ ────── ── ── ── ─   ▼ _R A T I O N A L E_ ─── ── ── ── ─

6. Remove the outer wrapper and lay the exposed package of gloves on a clean, dry surface.

6. Provides for easy access to the gloves.

7. Open the inner package containing the sterile gloves by touching only the bottom of the package (Fig. 1–23).

7. Avoids contamination of the sterile gloves inside the wrapper.

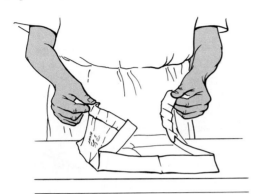

▼ **FIGURE 1–23.** Opening inner package.

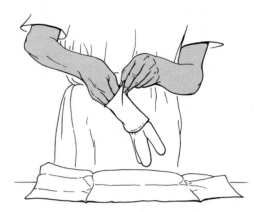

▼ **FIGURE 1–24.** Putting on first glove.

8. With the thumb and finger of one hand, grasp the cuffed portion of the opposite glove and lift the glove while holding your fingers down.

8. Contaminates only the inside of one glove.

9. Slide the glove onto your hand, taking care not to touch any portion of the glove except the cuffed portion (Fig. 1–24).

9. Avoids contamination of the outside of the glove. Your hand and the inside of the gloves are not sterile.

10. Using your gloved hand, slide your fingers under the cuffed portion of the other glove.

10. Avoids contamination of the second glove. Your gloved hand and the outside of the second glove are sterile.

11. Slide the second glove on your hand without touching your skin (Fig. 1–25).

11. Maintains sterility of the glove. Your skin is not sterile.

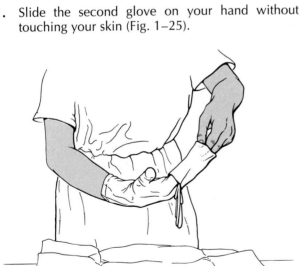

▼ **FIGURE 1–25.** Putting on second glove.

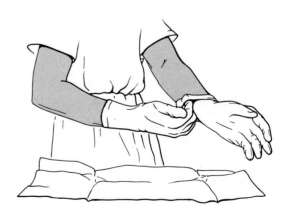

▼ **FIGURE 1–26.** Turning back cuffs.

12. Turn the cuff of the second glove onto your wrist without touching the inside of the cuff.

12. Maintains sterility of the gloves. The inside portion is not sterile.

13. Turn the cuff up on the other hand, taking care not to touch the inside of the cuff (Fig. 1–26).

13. The inside part of the cuff is contaminated.

▼ *ACTION*   ▼ *RATIONALE*

Removing the Soiled Gloves

14. Grasp the outside of one glove and pull it off, inside out (Fig. 1–27).

14. Prevents your hands from coming in contact with the outside contaminated portion.

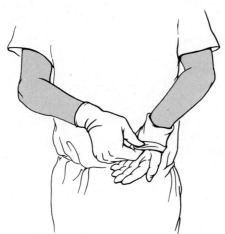

▼ **FIGURE 1–27.** Taking off first glove.

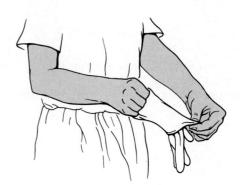

▼ **FIGURE 1–28.** Taking off second glove.

15. Slide your fingers under the remaining gloved hand and remove the glove inside out (Fig. 1–28).

15. You avoid touching the contaminated outside surface of the second glove and decrease the transmission of microorganisms.

16. Dispose of the gloves in a proper receptacle.

16. Decreases the transmission of microorganisms.

17. Wash your hands.

17. Decreases the transmission of microorganisms.

18. Record the procedure, noting the use of sterile technique.

18. Communicates to the health care team and contributes to the legal record by documenting the care given to the client.

Example of Documentation

DATE	TIME	NOTES
10/18/94	1000	Dressing changed using sterile technique.
		S. Williams, RN

Home Care Variations

Wash your hands thoroughly using bar soap. Use paper towels to dry your hands. Avoid touching any surfaces in the client's home after washing your hands. After the procedure, dispose of the gloves in a small plastic bag and remove them from the client's home before leaving.

SKILL 1–9 PREPARING AND MAINTAINING A STERILE FIELD

Clinical Situations in Which You May Encounter This Skill

A sterile field is necessary for sterile dressing changes, suturing, thoracentesis, paracentesis, or other sterile procedures at the client's bedside. Sterile fields are also used in the operating room and labor and delivery rooms. If a sterile field is prepared for the operating room or labor and delivery rooms, a hair covering and surgical mask to cover the nose and mouth must be worn.

Be sure to adhere to the principles of sterile technique (preceding Skill 1–5) when preparing a sterile field. If the sterile field becomes contaminated or if contamination is suspected, the sterile field and any items within the sterile field should be discarded and a new sterile field will be needed.

Anticipated Responses

▼ The field remains sterile.

Adverse Responses

▼ The field becomes contaminated.

Materials List

Gather these materials before beginning the skill:

▼ Prepackaged sterile tray
▼ Packages of sterile towels (2)
▼ Sterile basin
▼ Disposable sterile field
▼ Antiseptic solution
▼ Sterile gloves
▼ Other supplies (depends on the procedure)

▼ ACTION

1. Check the physician's order to determine the procedure to be performed.

2. Assess the client's understanding of sterile procedures.

3. Visually inspect the wrapping around packaged supplies to verify their sterility. Check the expiration date and look for tears in the wrapper or evidence that the wrapper has become wet (Fig. 1–29).

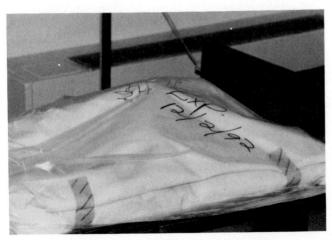

▼ FIGURE 1–29. Wrapping with expiration date.

4. Wash your hands.

▼ RATIONALE

1. Allows you to determine the supplies needed.

2. Client education reduces apprehension and gains the client's cooperation.

3. If the expiration date has passed or the wrapper has been damaged in any way, the contents are not considered sterile. Moisture enhances the transmission of microorganisms from a nonsterile area to a sterile area by capillary action.

4. Decreases the transmission of microorganisms.

▼ _ACTION_ _____ ▼ *RATIONALE* _____

5. Place the sterile tray in its wrapper or set up a sterile field on the bedside table and adjust the table to waist-height.

5. Provides a working surface that is waist-high. Articles must be kept above the waist and in the line of vision to be considered uncontaminated.

Setting Up a Prepackaged Sterile Tray

6. Remove the tape from the outer wrapper.

6. Provides easy access to the tray when needed.

7. Place the tray so that when you fold the first flap back you will be folding it away from you.

7. Once the sterile area is exposed, reaching over the area will contaminate it.

8. Fold back the first flap away from you.

8. Avoids reaching over the sterile field once all folds are open.

9. Using both hands, pull the two middle flaps open.

9. Avoids contaminating the tray.

10. Pull the remaining flap toward you, exposing the sterile tray (Fig. 1–30).

10. Avoids contaminating the tray.

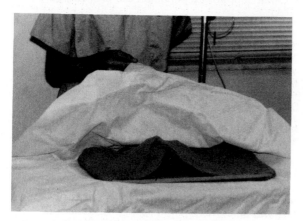

▼ **FIGURE 1–30.** Opening sterile tray.

Adding Wrapped Items to a Sterile Field

11. Standing away from the sterile tray, open the package and put it on the tray:
    a. Hold the package in one hand and remove the tape from the covering.
    b. While still holding the package, fold back the first flap away from you.

    c. Fold back the middle flaps one at a time, each with a different hand, so that you do not cross over the package.
    d. Unfold the last flap toward you, exposing the package contents.
    e. With your free hand, secure the outer wrapping away from your other hand to expose the contents of the package.

11. Avoids contaminating the sterile field and allows the package to be opened and sterility of the contents to be maintained.

    b. If this flap was not opened first, you would have to reach over to open it. Contamination occurs when you reach over a sterile object or field.
    c. Prevents contamination.

    d. Prevents contamination

    e. Avoids the outer wrapping falling into the sterile field and contaminating it. The inside of the package is sterile. By folding back the wrapping, your nonsterile hand is covered. Sterile will touch only sterile.

▼ ACTION _____   ▼ RATIONALE _____

   f. Drop the item onto the sterile field inside of a 1-inch border (Fig. 1–31).

      f. The outside 1 inch of the sterile field is considered to be contaminated.

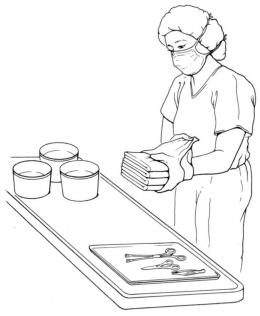

▼ **FIGURE 1–31.** Adding items to a sterile field.

Pouring a Solution into a Sterile Basin

12. Open and place a sterile container for antiseptic solution on a tray inside of the 1-inch border. (See Step 11.)

12. This procedure can be used to place another object within the sterile field.

13. Hold the antiseptic solution with the label in your palm.

13. When the solution is poured, it will not drip or run on the label.

14. Holding the bottle above the tray, carefully pour the solution into the sterile container without splashing or spilling the solution (Fig. 1–32).

14. The field is considered to be contaminated if the solution is spilled or splattered on it.

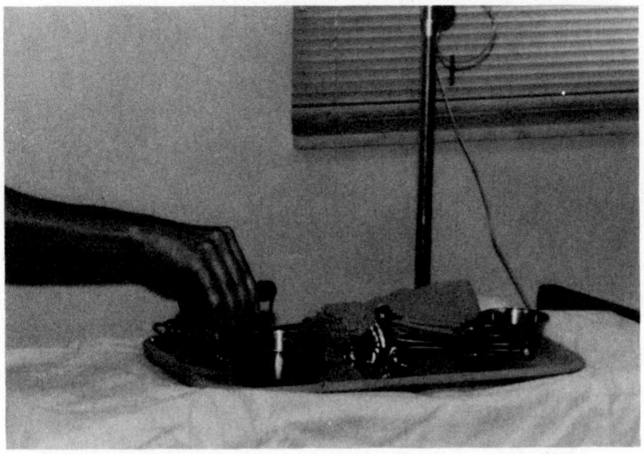

▼ FIGURE 1–32. Pouring a solution into a sterile basin.

Adding Prepackaged Items to a Sterile Field

15. Peel open the package at the site indicated on the wrapper.

15. Most prepackaged items include directions for opening the item.

▼ *ACTION*   ▼ *RATIONALE*

16. Drop the item inside the 1-inch barrier onto the sterile field. Keep your hands behind the wrapper while you drop the supplies onto the sterile field (Fig. 1–33).

16. A 1-inch border is considered contaminated. By keeping your hands behind the wrapper and the sterile side of the wrapper toward the sterile field you avoid placing a nonsterile object (your hand) directly over the sterile field.

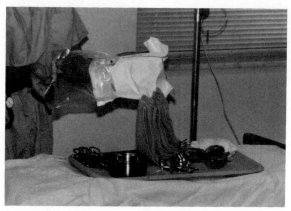

▼ **FIGURE 1–33.** Adding prepackaged items to a sterile field.

17. Open and place any other sterile supplies on the sterile tray.

17. The sterile tray should be completely ready for use.

Preparing a Sterile Field Using a Disposable Drape

18. Open the sterile field by peeling open the package containing the drape in the direction opposite from you (Fig. 1–34).

18. You are considered to be contaminated.

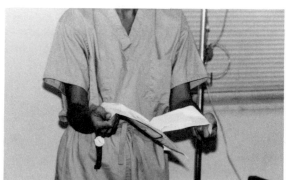

▼ **FIGURE 1–34.** Opening sterile drape.

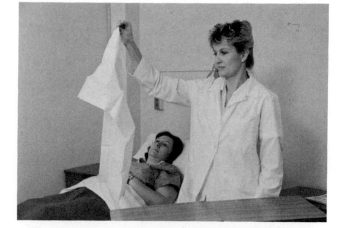

▼ **FIGURE 1–35.** Allowing sterile drape to unfold.

19. Remove the sterile drape from the package by the corner and allow it to unfold (Fig. 1–35).

19. The corners are within the 1-inch border and are considered contaminated.

▼ _ACTION_ _ _ _ _ _ _ _ _ _ _ _ _ _ _ _   ▼ _RATIONALE_ _ _ _ _ _ _ _ _ _ _ _ _ _ _

20. Place the sterile drape on the overbed table from back to front (Fig. 1–36). If the drape has a waterproof side, place it down.

21. Follow Steps 11 to 17 to place the remaining items within the sterile field.

20. You avoid reaching across the sterile field. Placing waterproof side down protects sterile field from contamination with moisture.

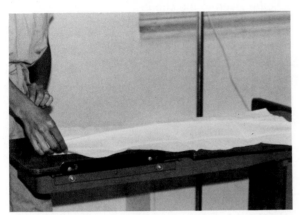

▼ **FIGURE 1–36.** Placing sterile drape on table.

Using Sterile Transfer Forceps

22. If the forceps were stored in disinfectant solution, hold them above waist-level with the tips lower than your wrist. If the forceps were packaged dry, carefully remove them without touching them to the sides of the package.

23. Do not allow the forceps tips to touch any non-sterile object.

24. Transfer the sterile items to the sterile field without touching moist forceps to the sterile field or allowing the moisture to contaminate the sterile field (Fig. 1–37).

22. Uses gravity to prevent the solution from flowing to the contaminated handles and then back to the tips of the forceps.

23. Prevents contamination of the forceps.

24. Moisture will contaminate the sterile field by capillary action.

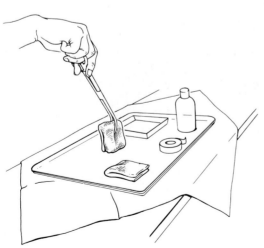

▼ **FIGURE 1–37.** Using sterile transfer forceps.

▼ ACTION	▼ RATIONALE
25. Discard the disposable forceps and return the reusable forceps to be decontaminated and repackaged.	**25.** Prevents the transmission of microorganisms.
26. Record the procedure.	**26.** Communicates to the health care team and contributes to the legal record by documenting the care given to the client.

Example of Documentation

DATE	TIME	NOTES
10/19/93	1300	Dressing changed using sterile procedure.
		S. Williams, RN

Home Care Variations

Examine sterile packages for tears or moisture damage that may have occurred in transport. Place sterile supplies on a clean surface that is waist-high. After the procedure, place all discardable supplies in a waterproof bag and remove the bag from the client's home.

References

Anasari, S. A., et al. (1991). Comparison of cloth, paper, and warm air drying in eliminating viruses and bacteria from washed hands. *American Journal of Infection Control*, 19 (5), 243–249.

Brown, D. G., et al. (1985). Sterile water and saline solution: Potential reservoirs of nosocomial infection. *American Journal of Infection Control*, 13 (1), 35–39.

Jackson, M. M., Lynch P. I., and Bolander, V. B. (1993). Infection control. In V. Bolander (Ed.), *Basic nursing* (3rd ed.). Philadelphia: W. B. Saunders.

Korniewicz, D. M., et al. (1989). Integrity of vinyl and latex procedure gloves. *Nursing Research*, 38, 144–146.

Larson, E., Mayur, K., and Laughon, B. A. (1989). Influence of handwashing frequencies on reduction in colonizing flora with three handwashing products used by health care personnel. *American Journal of Infection Control*, 17 (2), 83–88.

CHAPTER 2

Preventing Back Injury

Providing nursing care often requires you to lift, move, or carry heavy loads. By utilizing your knowledge of scientific principles from physics to correctly use your body, you can reduce the amount of work required, as well as protect your musculoskeletal system (especially your back) from injury. You should understand and work with the forces of motion, gravity, friction, and leverage.

Newton's first law of *motion* states that matter tends to remain at rest (if it is at rest) or in motion (if it is in motion) at a constant speed and in a straight line unless acted upon by an outside force. *Gravity* and *friction* are examples of forces that affect motion. Gravity is a force that pulls an object to the ground. When lifting a heavy object, you must exert sufficient force to overcome gravity. For this reason, it takes less force to push or pull an object than to lift it.

Friction is the resistance created when two objects are moved across each other. Even the movement of an object across a horizontal plane is affected by friction. Less friction is encountered when pulling an object than when pushing it.

Leverage is the use of the body as a simple machine to increase lifting power. Leverage involves the use of a lever (a rigid structure) and a fulcrum (a fixed point on which the lever moves) and the application of force to move a load. The three types of levers are shown in Figure 2–1.

You often use levers to increase lifting power when moving a heavy load. When moving heavy loads it is important to maintain proper body alignment. This will reduce strain on your musculoskeletal system and will aid in preventing back injuries. Your body should face the direction in which you plan to move the load. Your spine should be straight, with your head erect and your chin tucked in. Your arms should be held at your sides with your elbows slightly flexed in a position of comfort. Your abdominal muscles should be tightened and pulled up and in. Your gluteal muscles should be tightened and tucked in. Your knees should be slightly flexed and your feet should face forward.

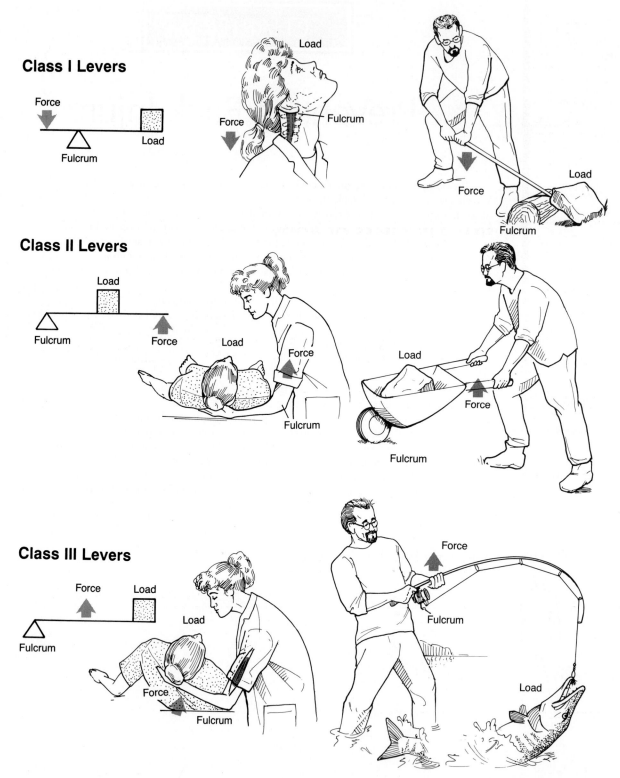

▼ **FIGURE 2–1.** Three classes of levers. Class I levers consist of a load on one end, a fulcrum in the middle, and downward force exerted on the opposite end of the lever (e.g., using a crowbar). The posterior cervical muscles contracting to lift the anterior head provide another example of class I levers. Class II levers consist of a fulcrum at one end, an upward or lifting effort at the other end, and the load in between (e.g., using a wheelbarrow). The use of the wrists as fulcra, the arms as levers, and an upward force on the arms to lift a helpless client provides another example of a class II lever. Class III levers consist of a fulcrum at one end, a load at the opposite end, and an upward or lifting force in the middle (e.g., a fisherman reeling in a fish). The contraction of the biceps muscles to apply a force between the elbows as fulcra and a load on the lower forearm is another example of a class III lever.

OVERVIEW OF RELATED RESEARCH

Wollenberg, S. P. (1989). A comparison of body mechanic usage in employees participating in three back injury prevention programs. *International Journal of Nursing Studies*, 26 (1), 43–52.

Data were collected from 58 individuals who participated in one of three different back injury prevention programs. The first group had two informational classes, exercise instruction, and mandatory participation in daily exercise. The second group received three informational classes and exercise instruction, and the third group received 1 hour of informational instruction and an exercise demonstration, rather than exercise instruction. All groups increased their use of proper body mechanics by 3 months, with the first and third groups having the greatest increase.

SKILL 2–1   GENERAL PRINCIPLES OF BODY MECHANICS

Clinical Situations in Which You May Encounter This Skill

Good body mechanics should be used anytime you lift or move a heavy object, a piece of equipment, or a client. Improper use of your body to lift or move a load may result in an injury to your musculoskeletal system. In addition, using correct body mechanics can give you more power. Your body should be kept in proper alignment at all times and you should maintain good posture. The following principles of body mechanics should always be followed.

▼ ACTION

Do

1. Evaluate the weight of the object you are trying to lift or move. Get help if necessary.

2. Stand with your feet apart and firmly planted to increase your stability (Fig. 2–2).

▼ RATIONALE

Do Not

1. Do not try to lift more than you can safely carry.

2. Do not assume a stance with your feet together. This weakens your base of support and makes it easier to topple over.

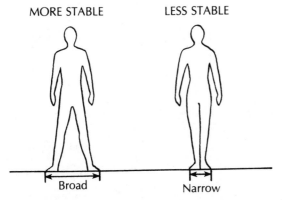

▼FIGURE 2–2.

▼ _A C T I O N_   ▼ _R A T I O N A L E_

Do

3. When moving a load, keep your center of gravity as low as possible and centered over your base of support (Fig. 2–3). This will increase your stability and balance (Fig. 2–4).

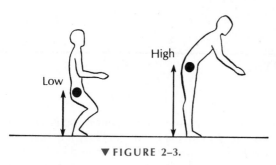

MORE STABLE   LESS STABLE

▼ FIGURE 2–3.

Do Not

3. Do not bend over at the waist or lean when moving a load. This moves your center of gravity away from your base of support and results in instability and back strain.

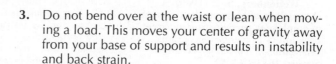

MORE STABLE   LESS STABLE

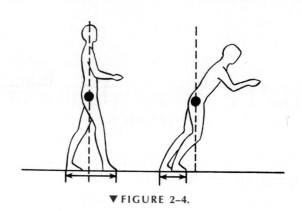

▼ FIGURE 2–4.

4. When lifting a load from the floor, flex your knees and stoop down (Fig. 2–5). Keep your back straight. Lift the object using your leg and hip muscles for power.

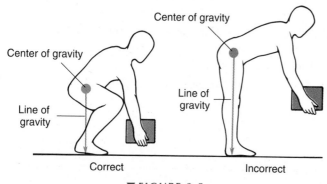

Center of gravity

Center of gravity

Line of gravity

Line of gravity

Correct   Incorrect

▼ FIGURE 2–5.

4. Do not lean over at the waist or use your back to lift the item.

5. Use smooth coordinated movements to lift and move a load. When working with others, count "one . . . two . . . three . . . lift." When lifting a heavy load, rocking the load back and forth before lifting may make the lifting easier.

5. Do not use jerky, uncoordinated, snatching movements to move a load.

6. Always face in the direction of intended movement when lifting or moving a load. This will maintain good spinal alignment.

6. Do not twist your spine when moving a load.

7. Push, pull, or slide an object when possible instead of lifting. These actions require less force and do not involve moving the load against gravity. If possible, pull a load rather than push it. There is less friction when pulling a load, and therefore the amount of force required will be less.

7. Do not lift a load when it can be pushed, pulled, or moved by sliding. You will have to exert more force when working against gravity.

▼ *ACTION* _   ▼ *RATIONALE* _ _ _ _ _ _ _ _ _ _ _

Do

Do Not

8. When carrying a load, hold it close to your body (Fig. 2–6). This keeps your center of gravity over your base of support and reduces the strain on your back muscles.

8. When carrying a load, do not hold it away from your body. This shifts your center of gravity from your base of support, reduces your stability, and stresses your back muscles.

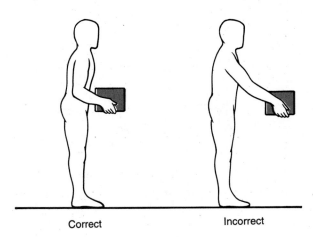

Correct   Incorrect

▼ FIGURE 2–6.

9. Use your entire hand rather than just your fingers when moving a load. The hand muscles are larger and stronger than the finger muscles.

9. Do not attempt to move a load without first grasping it with your entire hand.

10. Use your arms as mechanical levers to decrease the amount of force needed to move a load.

11. When moving a heavy load, protect your lower intervertebral discs by putting on an "internal girdle." To do this, tighten your abdominal muscles by pulling them in and upward. Tighten and lift your gluteal muscles.

Teaching Tips

It may be necessary for the family to lift or move the client in the home. The purpose and principles of using correct body mechanics should be explained. The correct technique should be demonstrated for the family and the family should be given an opportunity to demonstrate the technique prior to the client's discharge.

Home Care Variations

The same principles should be used in the home setting. If a family member will be providing care for the client in the home, these principles should be explained.

References

Bolander, V. B. (1993). Preventing back injury. In V. Bolander (Ed.), *Basic nursing* (3rd ed.). Philadelphia: W. B. Saunders.

Wollenberg, S. P. (1989). A comparison of body mechanic usage in employees participating in three back injury prevention programs. *International Journal of Nursing Studies*, 26 (1), 43–52.

CHAPTER 3

Cardiopulmonary Resuscitation

CPR stands for cardio- (heart) pulmonary (lungs) resuscitation (restoring life). CPR is indicated whenever a client suffers either cardiac arrest or respiratory arrest.

A cardiac arrest is defined as the cessation of cardiac function. Respiratory arrest occurs seconds after the heart ceases to function. Four to 6 minutes after a cardiopulmonary arrest, the lack of oxygen to the brain reaches critical levels and permanent extensive brain damage occurs.

Respiratory arrest is defined as the cessation of breathing. Cardiac arrest occurs soon after breathing ceases because of lack of oxygen to the heart muscle. Respiratory arrest may occur secondary to cardiac arrest or because of an obstructed airway or other causes. Respiratory arrest is the most common cause of cardiac arrest in infants and children.

CPR or basic cardiac life support (BCLS) consists of external cardiac compressions coupled with rescue breathing. BCLS measures are designed to support the client and maintain oxygenation to the brain and other vital organs until people trained in advanced cardiac life support (ACLS) measures can arrive. ACLS measures include establishment of an airway as with an endotracheal tube, insertion of an intravenous line, administration of cardioactive drugs, and defibrillation.

When a cardiopulmonary arrest occurs in a hospital setting, it is commonly called a *code*. Every institution has policies on how to respond to an arrest situation. You should become familiar with these policies and be able to respond quickly and efficiently should a client suffer an arrest. Hospital policies usually include the following sequence of events when a cardiopulmonary arrest occurs:

1. The person who discovers the client in cardiopulmonary arrest should notify the nurses' station that an arrest is in progress without leaving the client's bedside.
2. The person who discovered the client should lower the head of the client's bed to a level position, place a firm surface such as the headboard of the bed under the client's back, and begin CPR.
3. Most hospitals have a special team of physicians, nurses, respiratory therapists, and sometimes a pharmacist who respond to cardiopulmonary arrests. This group is called the *code team*.
4. Personnel at the nurses' station should announce the code over the hospital paging system to summon the code team.
5. After summoning the code team, personnel should bring the following equipment to the client's room: a bag-valve-mask device with oxygen setup, suction, an emergency drug box, a defibrillator, and equipment to start an intravenous line. Most institutions have all this equipment on a special cart called a *crash cart*.
6. Extra personnel should assist with CPR until the code team arrives. In most institutions, registered nurses may initiate an intravenous line with 5% dextrose in water (D_5W) and oxygen therapy.
7. When the code team arrives, the nurse who discovered the arrest usually provides information about the client to the code team and assists with recording the event as the resuscitation effort progresses.
8. Other personnel should notify the client's family members of the arrest and provide them with information and support during this crisis.

OVERVIEW OF RELATED RESEARCH

The volume of research on CPR is far too extensive to report in a skills handbook. The student is instead referred to the following article, which contains the guidelines with research support for all aspects of cardiopulmonary resuscitation:

(1992) Guidelines for cardiopulmonary resuscitation and emergency cardiac care. *Journal of the American Medical Association*, 286 (16), 2171–2302.

SKILL 3–1   PERFORMING CARDIOPULMONARY RESUSCITATION

Clinical Situations in Which You May Encounter This Skill

Cardiopulmonary resuscitation (CPR) is indicated in any situation in which either breathing or both breathing and heartbeat are absent. CPR must be initiated for all clients who do not have a "do not resuscitate" order. All settings have a procedure that is to be followed when a client is determined to be in respiratory or cardiopulmonary arrest, or both. This procedure must be reviewed prior to working in that setting.

Child CPR techniques are appropriate for children ages 1 to 7 years; however, these age guidelines are relative and you also should consider the size of the child when deciding whether to use adult CPR techniques or child CPR techniques. Infant CPR techniques are appropriate for infants up to 1 year of age.

Anticipated Responses

▼ The client experiences return of spontaneous breathing and heartbeat with brain function to the pre-arrest level.

Adverse Responses

▼ The client experiences irreversible brain death.
▼ The client experiences decreased brain function after return of breathing and heartbeat.

▼ Injuries from CPR include: aspiration of stomach contents; fractured ribs or sternum, or both; lacerated liver or spleen, or both; pneumothorax; hemothorax; or fat embolus.

Materials List

In general CPR is not a planned procedure and may be carried out without the benefit of any equipment. However, there are times when the need for CPR may be anticipated. In these cases you can have the equipment listed below available for quick access. At all times you should be prepared to initiate CPR if needed.

▼ Face shield or one-way valve pocket mask, or bag-valve-mask device (AMBU bag)
▼ Flat surface such as the cardiac board or headboard of many hospital beds
▼ Oxygen source if available
▼ Suction device if available

▼ *ACTION* ────────────────── ▼ *RATIONALE* ──────────────

Performing One-Person CPR

1. Assess for unresponsiveness by shaking the victim and asking "Are you OK?"

1. Determining unresponsiveness will help to prevent further injury from starting CPR if the client is just asleep.

▼ *A C T I O N*   ▼ *R A T I O N A L E*

> **NOTE:** Assess the victim for possible neck injury before moving him or her.
>
> Improper movement of the victim with a neck injury can cause paralysis.

2. If the client is unresponsive, activate the emergency medical system (EMS) if you are outside the hospital. Inside the hospital, initiate your agency policy for calling a code.

2. Provides early response by persons trained in advanced cardiac life support.

3. Position the victim on a firm, flat surface in a horizontal, supine position. Turn the victim by logrolling. If possible, place a small flat towel under the scapula of the infant.

3. A firm, flat surface facilitates proper compression of the heart. A supine position facilitates blood flow to the brain. Improper movement of a victim with a neck injury can cause paralysis. The towel aids in maintaining an open airway in the infant.

4. Open the airway.
   a. Use the head tilt–chin lift method if no neck injury is suspected (Fig. 3–1*C*)

4. An open airway is necessary for oxygenation.
   a. Provides for an open airway and moves the victim's tongue and epiglottis away from the back of the throat (Fig. 3–1*A* and *B*).

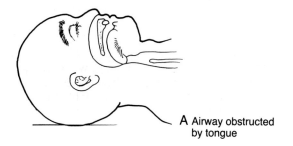

A Airway obstructed by tongue

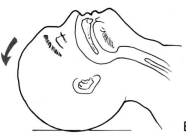

B Obstruction relieved by head tilt

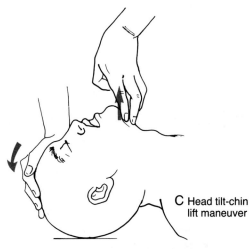

C Head tilt-chin lift maneuver

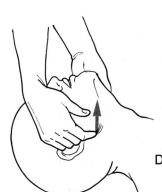

D Jaw thrust maneuver

▼ **FIGURE 3–1.** Opening the airway.

   i. Place your hand that is nearest the victim's head on the victim's forehead.
   ii. Apply firm, backward pressure with your palm. Do not overextend the victim's head.
   iii. Place the fingers of your other hand under the bony part of the victim's lower jaw near the chin.
   iv. Lift the victim's chin forward, bringing his or her teeth closer together.

   iii. Prevents your fingers from pressing on the soft tissue under the victim's chin. This soft tissue can obstruct the airway.
   iv. Opens airway by moving tongue and epiglottis away from back of throat.

▼ *A C T I O N* | ▼ *R A T I O N A L E*

b. Use the jaw thrust method if neck injury is suspected.
   i. Using both hands, grasp the angles of the victim's lower jaw.
   ii. Lift the victim's lower jaw forward (Fig. 3–1*D*).
   iii. If the jaw thrust alone is unsuccessful, slightly tilt the victim's head backward to open the airway. Protect the victim's neck from hyperextension or movement from side to side.

b. Provides for an open airway without extending the victim's neck.
   i. Allows you to move jaw forward.

   ii. Opens airway by moving tongue and epiglottis away from back of throat.
   iii. Minimizes the victim's neck movement.

5. Determine breathlessness by:
   a. Placing your ear over the victim's mouth and nose while maintaining the victim's open airway.
   b. Looking for the rise and fall of the victim's chest.
   c. Listening for exhaled air to escape the victim's airway.
   d. Feeling for the flow of exhaled air against your cheek.
   This assessment should take 3 to 5 seconds.

a–d. If the victim is breathing, giving breaths is unnecessary and could damage the victim's respiratory tract.

Minimizes the amount of time the victim is without oxygen.

6. If the victim is breathing effectively, maintain the victim's airway and continue to monitor his or her breathing. If no cervical trauma is suspected, the victim should be logrolled onto his or her side (recovery position). If injury is suspected, the victim should not be moved.

6. The victim's respiratory effort may worsen. Remain with the victim until help arrives. Sidelying position minimizes airway blockage by the tongue.

7. If the victim is breathless, prepare to initiate rescue breathing using one of the following:
   a. Mouth to mouth: Occlude the victim's nose by pinching his or her nostrils closed with your fingers while placing your mouth over the victim's mouth. If the victim is an infant, place your mouth over the infant's mouth and nose, making a tight seal (see Fig. 3–2).
   b. Mouth to stoma: Place your mouth over the victim's neck stoma, making a tight seal.
   c. Mouth to barrier device: Following the manufacturer's directions, place a face shield or face mask over the victim's mouth and nose. Place your mouth on the barrier device. Secure a tight seal when using a mask device to prevent air from leaking around the mask.
   d. Bag-valve-mask device: see Skill 3–2.

7. Rescue breathing is done to oxygenate client. A tight seal prevents loss of volume during ventilation. If possible, use a mouth-to-barrier device or a bag-valve-mask device to avoid contact with the client's body secretions.

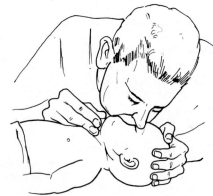

▼ **FIGURE 3–2.** Infant rescue breathing.

8. Ventilate the victim by giving two breaths that make the victim's chest rise and fall. Remove your mouth from the victim's mouth between breaths. Each breath should take 1.5 to 2 seconds for adults and 1 to 1.5 seconds for infants and children.
   a. Observe the rise and fall of the victim's chest.
   b. Hear and feel air escape during the victim's exhalation.

8. Provides for good chest expansion while decreasing the possibility of gastric distention.

   a. Indicates adequate ventilation.
   b. Indicates adequate ventilation.

▼ *ACTION*   ▼ *RATIONALE*

NOTE: If you cannot ventilate the victim, reposition his or her head and reattempt ventilation. If the victim still cannot be ventilated, the obstructed airway procedure (Skill 3–3) should be followed.

Improper head positioning is the most common cause of difficulty with ventilation. The victim's airway must be open for CPR to be successful.

---

9. In adults and children, palpate for the presence or absence of a carotid pulse. In infants, palpate the brachial pulse (Fig. 3–3). This should take from 5 to 10 seconds.

9. The carotid pulse is the most accessible and reliable pulse in adults and children. An infant's short neck makes the carotid pulse difficult to find. The brachial pulse is more accessible in infants.

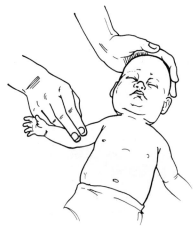

▼ **FIGURE 3–3.** Palpating brachial pulse in infant.

10. If there is a pulse, but no spontaneous breathing, then rescue breathing should be continued:
  a. Adult: Rescue breathing consists of giving one breath every 5 to 6 seconds (10–12 times per minute) until spontaneous breathing begins.
  b. Infant and child: Rescue breathing consists of giving one breath every 3 seconds (20 breaths per minute) until spontaneous breathing begins.

10. Performing CPR on a victim with a pulse can result in further problems.
  a–b. Without breathing, the victim is not being oxygenated and his or her heart will soon stop. The breathing rate is adequate for short-term oxygenation.

11. If there is no pulse, initiate external chest compressions:

11. Compressions provide circulation to the heart, lungs, brain, and the rest of the body at about 20 to 30% of normal cardiac output. The correct position allows for an overall increase in pressure within the thoracic cavity along with direct compression of the heart, and reduction of the chance of injury.

  a. First locate your correct hand position on the victim's chest:
    i. Adult
      • Locate the lower margin of the victim's rib cage on the side next to you (Fig. 3–4A).

Single-Rescuer Adult CPR

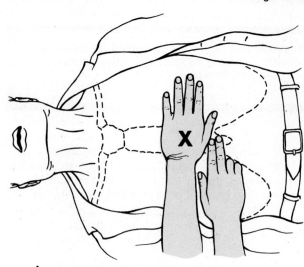

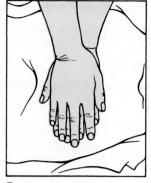

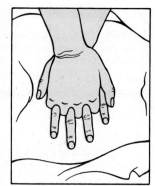

B Finger positions

A Hand positions for chest compression

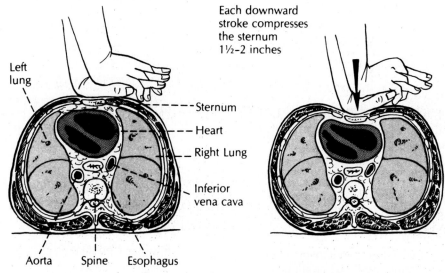

Each downward
stroke compresses
the sternum
1½–2 inches

Left
lung

Sternum

Heart

Right Lung

Inferior
vena cava

Aorta   Spine   Esophagus

C Cross section of thorax during CPR

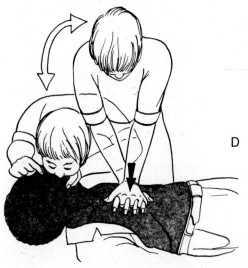

D Compressions alternate with ventilations at a ratio of 15
compressions to 2 ventilations per cycle. Reassess victim
after 4 cycles.

▼ **FIGURE 3–4.**

▼ *ACTION*   ▼ *RATIONALE*

- Run your fingers up the victim's rib cage to the point where the ribs meet the sternum.
- With your middle finger on this area, place your index finger next to your middle finger.
- Place the heel of your hand that is closest to the victim's head on the lower half of the victim's sternum, next to the fingers of your other hand. (The long axis of your hand should be placed on the long axis of the victim's sternum.)
- Remove your first hand from the victim's xiphoid process and place it on top of the hand on the victim's sternum, so that both hands are parallel and directed straight away from you.
- Your fingers may be interlaced or extended but must be kept off the victim's chest (Fig. 3–4*B*).
- Your arms should be straight with the elbows locked and your shoulders positioned directly over your hands (Fig. 3–4*D*).
- Compressions should be started at a rate of 80 to 100 per minute with a depth of 1.5 to 2 inches (Fig. 3–4*C*). Use of a counting mnemonic "one and two and three..." up to 15 will aid in timing the rate of compressions. You should generate a carotid or femoral pulse with each compression.
- At the end of each fifteenth compression, reopen airway and ventilate the victim 2 times. (Fig. 3–4*D*).
- Reassess the victim after 4 cycles of CPR (at a ratio of 15 compressions to 2 ventilations per cycle).

ii. Child (see Fig. 3–5).
- Using your middle and index fingers, locate the lower margin of the victim's rib cage on the side closest to you.
- Follow the child's rib cage to the point where the ribs meet the sternum.
- Place the heel of your hand next to your index finger, with the long axis of the heel parallel to the child's sternum (see Fig. 3–5, Step 6, right). Keep your fingers up and off the child's chest wall.
- Use your first hand to stabilize the child's head and maintain the child's airway.
- Compress the child's sternum to a depth of 1 to 1.5 inches at a rate of 100 times per minute. Use the same mnemonic as described above to aid in counting.

- Compressions over the xiphoid process can cause it to break and lead to internal injuries
- Allows hand placement on the part of the sternum closest to the victim's heart, but not over the xiphoid process. Allows the main line of the force of compression on the victim's sternum and decreases the risk of rib fracture.
- Allows for enough force to compress the victim's sternum 1.5 to 2 inches. Allows for the long axis of your hands to be on the long axis of the victim's sternum.

- Fingers on the victim's chest lead to an increased risk of rib fractures.

- Thrusts that are not straight down result in loss of force and less effective compressions.

- Allows for an optimal compression-to-ventilation ratio resulting in oxygenation with time for ventilation. Presence of pulse indicates optimal compression.

- Oxygenates the victim.

- Determines the need to continue CPR.

- Correct hand placement is essential to avoid injury to the victim.

- Allows for optimal compression-to-ventilation ratio, resulting in oxygenation with time for ventilation.

CPR for Infants and Children

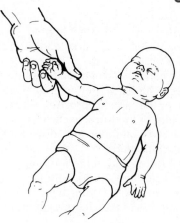

Step 1:
Determine responsiveness.

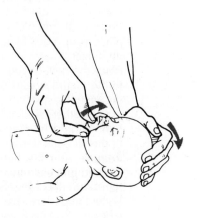

Step 2:
Chin lift-head tilt. Observe for spontaneous respiration.

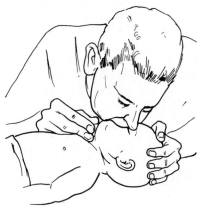

Step 3:
Begin rescue breathing by forming an airtight seal covering victim's mouth and nose with rescuer's mouth. Infants and children require a rescue breathing rate of 20 per minute.

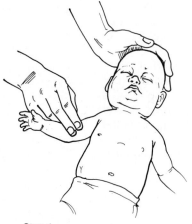

Step 4:
Palpate brachial pulse in infants; carotid pulse in children.

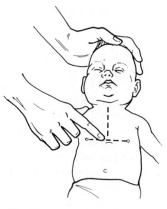

Step 5:
Locate correct landmarks for performing chest compressions in infants.

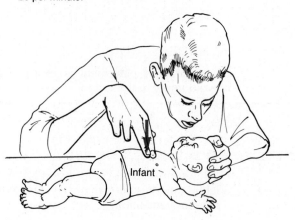

Infant

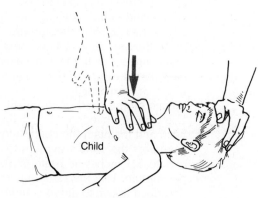

Child

Step 6:
Perform external chest compressions at a rate of 5:1 artificial breaths.
Use finger-pressure chest compression on infants; one hand on children.

▼ **FIGURE 3–5.**

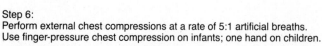

▼ *ACTION*

- At the end of each fifth compression, ventilate the child 1 time (1–1.5 seconds).
- Reassess the child after 20 cycles (at a ratio of 5 compressions to 1 ventilation per cycle).

iii. Infant (see Fig. 3–5)
  - Visualize an imaginary line between the infant's nipples that crosses over his or her sternum.
  - Place your index finger just under this imaginary line over the infant's sternum.

  - Using two fingers, compress the sternum 0.5 to 1 inch at a rate of at least 100 times per minute (Fig. 3–5, Step 6, left).
  - At the end of each fifth compression, ventilate the infant 1 time (1–1.5 seconds).
  Reassess the infant after 20 cycles of CPR (at a ratio of 5 compressions to 1 ventilation per cycle).

12. After the initial set of completed cycles, the victim should be assessed for circulatory and respiratory effort.
  a. Check for return of the victim's pulse. Take 3 to 5 seconds for this step.
    i. If the pulse is absent, resume CPR with 2 ventilations followed by the correct compression-ventilation cycles for the victim's age.
    ii. If the pulse is present, check for return of the victim's breathing.
  b. Return of the victim's breathing:
    i. If it is present, monitor the victim's breathing and pulse closely.
    ii. If the victim's breathing is absent, begin rescue breathing at the appropriate rate for the age of the victim. Monitor the victim's pulse closely.

▼ *RATIONALE*

- Oxygenates the victim.

- Determines the need to continue CPR.

- Correct hand placement is necessary to avoid injury to the victim. Do not place your fingers over the tip of the sternum.

- Oxygenates the victim.

- Determines the need to continue CPR.

12. Determines the current status of the victim and if further CPR is needed.

  i. Compressions are needed if there is no pulse.

  ii. Compressions are not needed if the pulse is present.

  i. The victim's breathing and pulse may cease again
  ii. Ventilation is needed if the victim's breathing is absent. Compressions should be started if the victim's pulse is absent.

NOTE: Do not interrupt CPR for more than 7 seconds except for special circumstances.

Interruption in CPR can lead to complications.

Performing Two-Person CPR

In two-person CPR, one person performs compressions while the second person maintains the victim's airway, delivers rescue breathing, and monitors the victim's pulse (Fig. 3–6). The ratio of compressions to ventilations for victims of all ages is 5:1 with a 1- to 1.5-second pause after each cycle of compressions to deliver a slow breath to the victim.

When the first rescuer becomes fatigued and signals the need for relief, the second rescuer delivers one breath, moves to the victim's chest, and locates the proper hand position for compressions. The first rescuer then moves to the victim's head, delivers a breath, checks the pulse, and signals for compressions to resume. The switch should be accomplished smoothly and quickly.

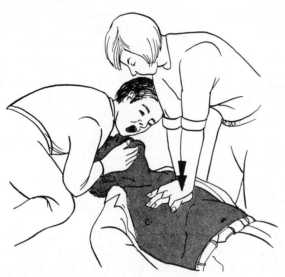

▼ **FIGURE 3–6.** Two-rescuer adult CPR.

Example of Documentation

DATE	TIME	NOTES
11/21/94	0800	Client found without breathing or pulse. CPR initiated. Code called. Dr. J. Jones notified. Spontaneous pulse and breathing returned within 5 minutes. Vital signs: AP = 104 irreg., RR = 28, BP = 136/92. Skin color flushed. Client awake, oriented to person and place, but not time. Client agitated and asks "What happened?" Client to be transferred to ICU. See code sheet for specific code information. *S. Smith, RN*

Teaching Tips

Explain the necessity for all adults to know CPR and encourage the client's family to take a basic CPR course such as those offered by the American Heart Association or the American Red Cross.

Home Care Variations

When a family member is at increased risk for experiencing a respiratory or cardiac arrest, family members should be trained in CPR and should be taught how to contact the emergency medical service (EMS) system in their area.

SKILL 3–2   USING A BAG-VALVE-MASK DEVICE (AMBU BAG)

Clinical Situations in Which You May Encounter This Skill

A manual resuscitation device such as an air mask bag unit (AMBU) is used to provide manual inflation of the lungs. The bag is attached to an adapter that connects the bag to either a face mask, endotracheal tube, or tracheostomy tube. The bag contains a one-way valve that allows for the client's exhalation away from the rescuer.

An AMBU bag is necessary in emergency situations when the client needs partial (during apneic episodes) or total assistance with breathing. It is kept at the bedside for clients receiving mechanical ventilation and is used during suctioning of these clients to provide hyperventilation of the lungs and during transport of ventilator-dependent clients.

Anticipated Responses

▼ The client receives adequate oxygenation of the brain and vital organs.
▼ The client's arterial blood gases are within normal limits.

Adverse Responses

▼ The client receives inadequate oxygenation of the brain and vital organs.
▼ The client exhibits signs and symptoms of alkalosis or acidosis.

Materials List

Gather these materials before beginning the skill:

▼ AMBU bag with mask or endotracheal tube or tracheostomy tube adapter
▼ Oral airway (may be needed)
▼ Oxygen setup (may be needed)
▼ Suctioning apparatus

▼ *ACTION*	▼ *RATIONALE*
1. Assess the client's need for the device.	1. Clients who do not have good air exchange (because of apnea or pulselessness, or during suctioning) may need this procedure.
2. Assess the client for a patent airway.	2. The airway must be open for air exchange to occur.
3. If it is not an emergency situation, wash your hands.	3. Handwashing decreases the transmission of microorganisms.
4. Open the client's airway using the head tilt–chin lift or jaw thrust maneuver (see Fig. 3–1). If neck injury is suspected, use the jaw thrust method and do not extend the client's head or rotate his or her neck. An oral airway can be inserted if necessary (see Skill 17–9).	4. The airway must be open for air exchange to occur. Manipulation of a neck-injured client can result in paralysis.
5. Maintain the client's head in this position while using one of your hands to tightly fit the mask firmly over the client's nose and mouth. If the client has an endotracheal tube or a tracheostomy, use the adapter to connect the bag to the artificial airway. Oxygen may be connected to the AMBU bag via a connecter on the bag. Oxygen flow rates vary between 15 and 30 liters per minute depending on client needs.	5. Maintains an open airway. An airtight seal over the client's nose and mouth is needed for adequate ventilation. Increases oxygen delivery to the client.

▼ *ACTION*   ▼ *RATIONALE*

6. As you hold the mask firmly in place, compress and release the bag portion with your other hand in a slow, controlled rhythmical motion at a rate of 12 to 20 respirations per minute (Fig. 3–7).

6. This motion allows for adequate ventilation without overinflating the client's lungs, which can lead to stomach distention and compromise of ventilation efforts.

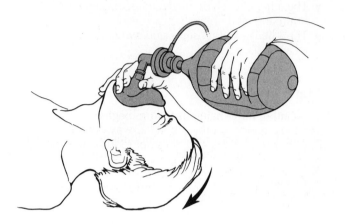

▼ **FIGURE 3–7.** Ventilating a client using an AMBU bag.

7. If chest compressions are being performed, the rate and rhythm of ventilation should be done according to CPR guidelines for two-person CPR.

7. Provides for effective ventilation and circulation.

8. Observe the rise and fall of the client's chest.

8. Shows that air is entering the client's lungs.

9. Observe the client for gastric distention.

9. An enlarged abdomen creates pressure on the diaphragm and can compromise the ability of the client's lungs to inflate.

10. Observe the client for the return of spontaneous breathing.

10. Breathing may resume at any time.

11. Chart the procedure, including the reason for using the AMBU bag, assessment and evaluation of the client's respiratory status, and the client's response.

11. Communicates to the other members of the health care team and contributes to the legal record by documenting the care given to the client.

Example of Documentation

DATE	TIME	NOTES
10/12/94	1030	Client found not breathing. Color cyanotic. Carotid pulse = 50, irreg. Respiratory arrest protocol initiated. Rescue breathing started with AMBU bag. RR = 24. Spontaneous breathing returned within 1 minute.
		C. Lane, RN

Further documentation of the client's condition should be done.

SKILL 3–3 MANAGING A FOREIGN BODY AIRWAY OBSTRUCTION

Clinical Situations in Which You May Encounter This Skill

Complete airway obstruction results when a foreign body such as a bolus of food or a small object (such as a coin or small toy) lodges in the victim's trachea and completely obstructs the passage of air. The victim with complete airway obstruction cannot cough or speak. If the obstruction is not cleared, a full cardiopulmonary arrest results.

If the victim has a partial airway obstruction with good air exchange and is coughing, do not attempt to clear the airway. You may only push the object farther down the trachea, resulting in a complete airway obstruction. Instead, remain with the victim and encourage vigorous coughing to clear the obstruction.

If the individual with a partial obstruction has poor air exchange, he or she will exhibit a weakening cough effort, dusky skin, a high-pitched crowing sound with respiration, and increasingly labored breathing. You should treat partial obstructions with poor air exchange in the same manner as a complete airway obstruction.

Materials List

Gather these materials before beginning the skill: Usually, clearing a foreign-body airway obstruction (FBAO) is unplanned and does not require any special equipment. If examination gloves are available, wear them when performing a finger sweep of the client's oral cavity to prevent contact with the client's body secretions.

▼ *ACTION*

Managing the Conscious Victim

1. If choking is suspected, ask the victim "Can you speak?"

2. If the victim is coughing effectively, stay with him or her but do not attempt to clear the obstruction manually.

3. Attempt to relieve the obstruction:

   a. Infant (up to age 1 yr): Position the infant with his or her head lower than the trunk and face down. Administer 5 back blows (Fig. 3–8*A*) followed by 5 chest thrusts (Fig. 3–8*B*).
   b. Adult or child over 1 year: apply 5 abdominal thrusts (Heimlich maneuver) (Fig. 3–9). Use chest thrusts as an alternative procedure when the client is very obese, or when trauma or complications might arise from abdominal thrusts (e.g., because of pregnancy).

▼ *RATIONALE*

1. Determines if FBAO is present and complete.

2. Attempting to remove the foreign body manually may only lodge it deeper in the trachea, resulting in a complete obstruction. Remain with the victim until the obstruction is cleared, since he or she may become fatigued and experience respiratory distress.

3. Abdominal thrusts displace the abdomen, forcing air from the lungs upward and creating an artificial cough.
   a. In the infant, chest thrusts are used instead of abdominal thrusts to avoid trauma to the abdominal organs.

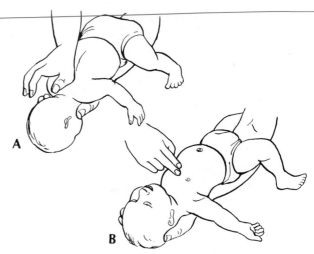

▼ **FIGURE 3–8.** Infant technique for removing an airway obstruction.

▼ _A C T I O N_ _ _ _ _ _ _ _ _ _ _ _ _ _ _ ▼ _R A T I O N A L E_ _ _ _ _ _

4. Repeat Step 3 as needed until the victim's airway
   is cleared or the victim becomes unconscious.

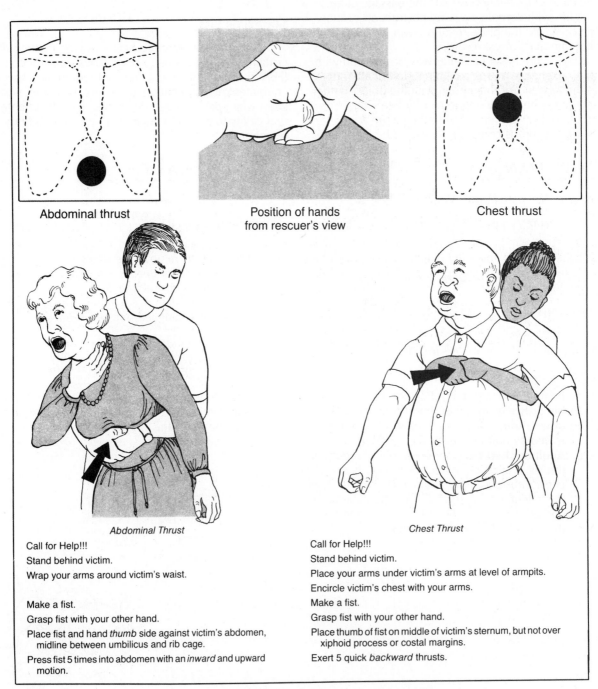

Abdominal thrust

Position of hands
from rescuer's view

Chest thrust

Abdominal Thrust

Call for Help!!!

Stand behind victim.

Wrap your arms around victim's waist.

Make a fist.

Grasp fist with your other hand.

Place fist and hand *thumb* side against victim's abdomen,
   midline between umbilicus and rib cage.

Press fist 5 times into abdomen with an *inward* and upward
   motion.

Chest Thrust

Call for Help!!!

Stand behind victim.

Place your arms under victim's arms at level of armpits.

Encircle victim's chest with your arms.

Make a fist.

Grasp fist with your other hand.

Place thumb of fist on middle of victim's sternum, but not over
   xiphoid process or costal margins.

Exert 5 quick *backward* thrusts.

▼ **FIGURE 3–9.** Thrust techniques for conscious victim (adult or child over 1 year).

▼ *ACTION*   ▼ *RATIONALE*

Managing the Conscious Victim Who Becomes Unconscious

5. Call for help. Activate the EMS or code system of your hospital.

   5. The victim may require more advanced life support measures.

6. Place the victim in the supine position and open the victim's airway using the head tilt–chin lift or jaw thrust method (see Fig. 3–1).

   6. Opening the victim's airway prevents obstruction by the victim's tongue and facilitates ventilation.

7. Attempt to ventilate the victim's lungs using mouth-to-mouth rescue breathing, a pocket mask (Fig. 3–10), or a bag-valve-mask device (see Skill 3–2).

   7. The victim will suffer cardiopulmonary arrest without adequate delivery of oxygen.

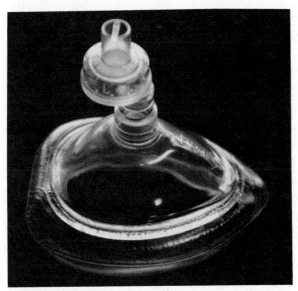

▼ **FIGURE 3–10.** Transparent, collapsible pocket mask for use in ventilation.

8. Place your face against the victim's mouth and look at the victim's chest. Look for the victim's chest to rise and fall, and listen and feel for air to escape from the victim's mouth.

   8. Allows you to evaluate whether or not your ventilation efforts were successful.

9. If you are unable to ventilate the victim, reposition the head and reattempt ventilation.

   9. Improper head position is the most common cause of inability to ventilate.

▼ *A C T I O N*   ▼ *R A T I O N A L E*

10. If you are still unable to ventilate the victim:
   a. Adult or child (aged 1–7 yrs): Position yourself astride the victim's thighs and apply 5 manual abdominal thrusts, or chest thrusts if abdominal thrusts are contraindicated (e.g., pregnancy) (Fig. 3–11).

a. Abdominal thrusts displace the abdomen, forcing air from the lungs upward, creating an artificial cough.

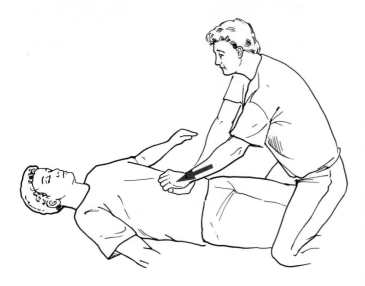

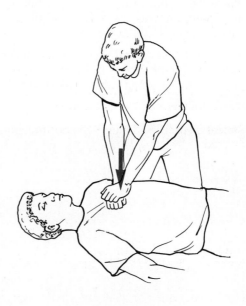

ABDOMINAL THRUST

Call for Help!!!

Position yourself either to victim's side (close to hips) or astride victim with legs over person's thighs.

Open victim's airway and turn head chin-up.

Place heel of one of your hands against victim's abdomen midline between umbilicus and rib cage.

Place heel of your second hand over the other.

Your shoulders should be directly over victim's abdomen.

Use heel of your hands to press into victim's abdomen with a fist.

Press into abdomen with five quick inward and upward thrusts.

DO NOT PRESS TO EITHER SIDE. PRESS IN DIRECTION OF CHEST AND HEAD.

CHEST THRUST

Call for Help!!!

Kneel to side of victim.

Open victim's airway and turn head chin-up.

Locate victim's rib border and follow it to xiphoid process.

Place two of your fingers over base of sternum just above xiphoid process.

Bring heel of your other hand alongside the two fingers.

Your shoulders should be directly over victim's chest, as if doing chest compressions.

Use heel of your hands to compress the sternum. Rescuer may either make a fist or use heel of hand with fingers held away from chest.

Apply five quick downward thrusts to compress chest cavity.

▼ **FIGURE 3–11.** Adult thrust techniques for a choking victim who becomes unconscious.

▼ *ACTION*	▼ *RATIONALE*
b. Infant (up to 1 yr): Apply 5 back blows followed by 5 chest thrusts (see Fig. 3–8).	b. For the infant, chest thrusts are done to avoid trauma to the abdominal organs.
11. Open the victim's mouth by grasping the victim's tongue and lower jaw (mandible) between your thumb and fingers. Look to see if the obstructing object can be visualized. If the object is at the level of the epiglottis or higher, use the first two fingers of your other hand to sweep the victim's mouth and remove the object. Wear examination gloves if available to perform the finger sweep.	**11.** Drawing the victim's tongue forward may partially relieve the obstruction. Objects lower than the epiglottis should not be manipulated, to prevent pushing then back down the trachea. Gloves protect you from exposure to the victim's body secretions.
12. Reposition the victim's head, open the victim's airway, and attempt to ventilate the victim.	**12.** The victim will suffer cardiopulmonary arrest without adequate ventilation.
13. Repeat Steps 10 to 12 until the obstruction is cleared.	

Managing the Unconscious Victim (Undetermined Cause)

1. Confirm unresponsiveness by shaking the victim and asking "Are you OK?"	**1.** CPR procedures should not be performed on a sleeping person.
2. Activate the EMS system.	**2.** The victim may require more advanced life support measures.
3. Logroll the victim into the supine position. Keep the victim's head and neck stable if neck injury is suspected. Open the victim's airway using the head tilt–chin lift method or the jaw thrust method. If a neck injury is suspected, use the jaw thrust method (see Fig. 3–1).	**3.** The supine position facilitates ventilation. Opening the airway prevents the victim's tongue from obstructing the flow of air. Stabilizing the victim's neck prevents injury to the spinal cord that could result in possible paralysis.
4. Look, listen, and feel for air movement.	**4.** Allows you to assess for presence and effectiveness of ventilation.
5. Attempt to ventilate the victim. If you are unable to ventilate the victim, follow Steps 8 to 13 for "Managing the Conscious Victim Who Becomes Unconscious."	**5.** The victim will suffer cardiopulmonary arrest without adequate delivery of oxygen.

Example of Documentation

DATE	TIME	NOTES
6/19/94		Client choked on a piece of meat while eating. Unable to speak or cough. Abdominal thrusts performed and foreign body was dislodged. Spontaneous respirations resumed after procedure. VS: BP = 136/88, R = 20, P = 92. Dr. May notified of incident. *C. Lemmon, RN*

Teaching Tips

Since choking can occur without warning at any time, all individuals should know how to respond appropriately. Classes are available through the American Heart Association and the American Red Cross to teach the public how to manage an obstructed airway.

When a person is choking, he or she cannot call out for help. All persons should learn the universal sign for choking (Fig. 3–12) to facilitate rapid communication of the need for help.

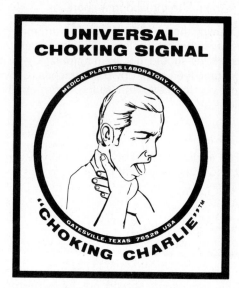

▼ **FIGURE 3–12.** Universal sign language for choking.

Home Care Variations

No alterations in the procedure are needed in the home. If a person is alone and chokes, he or she can perform abdominal thrusts using the hands as shown in Figure 3–9 or by striking the abdomen halfway between the rib cage and umbilicus forcefully against the back of a chair, a table edge, or a porch railing. The maneuver should be repeated until the airway is cleared.

References

(1992). Guidelines for cardiopulmonary resuscitation and emergency cardiac care. *Journal of the American Medical Association,* 268 (16), 2171–2197.

American Heart Association. (1990). *Health care provider's manual.* Dallas: AHA Office of Communications.

Straub, C. C. (1993). Cardiopulmonary resuscitation. In V. Bolander (Ed.) *Basic nursing* (3rd ed.). Philadelphia: W. B. Saunders.

UNIT II

UNIT II

ASSESSMENT SKILLS

CHAPTER 4

Assessing Vital Signs

- -

Assessing vital signs is a common but extremely important nursing skill. Vital signs, sometimes referred to as cardinal signs, include temperature, pulse, respirations, and blood pressure. Fluctuations in the vital signs can indicate changes in the client's physical or emotional well-being.

When a client first enters a clinic or hospital seeking care, vital signs are assessed. This initial reading serves as a baseline assessment against which subsequent measurements are evaluated for change.

The frequency of vital sign measurement is based on the client's condition. Clients with unstable illnesses require constant assessment of vital signs, whereas stable clients may need vital sign assessment only every 4 to 8 hours. Whenever a client's condition appears to be changing, you should assess his or her vital signs and report the assessment to the physician when appropriate.

In certain situations, additional assessments are made to determine the client's condition. For example, clients with neurologic conditions require a neurologic assessment in addition to an assessment of temperature, pulse, respirations, and blood pressure. This assessment is commonly called a "neuro check." Clients with the potential for circulatory impairment require an assessment of the circulatory system. These common assessment skills are discussed in this chapter.

- -

- -

OVERVIEW OF RELATED RESEARCH

ASSESSING VITAL SIGNS

Dairs, M. J., and Nomura, L. A. (1990). Vital signs of Class I surgical patients. *Western Journal of Nursing Research*, 12 (1), 28–41.

This retrospective, descriptive study was conducted to determine the frequency of abnormal vital signs or other abnormal signs and symptoms in Class I postoperative clients. Data were gathered on a total of 32 possible abnormal events. A Class I surgical client, according to the American Society of Anesthesiologists, is one who has no organic, physiologic,

biochemical, or psychiatric disturbance. These data could be used to determine appropriate assessment protocols for such surgical clients. The sample consisted of 250 Class I surgical clients who had one of five procedures: inguinal hernia repair, hemorrhoidectomy, arthroscopy, myomectomy, or tonsillectomy. The findings revealed that 40.8% of the clients had abnormal vital signs and 48% had abnormal signs and symptoms after surgery. Only one-half (50.9%) of the clients with abnormal vital signs experienced these only in the surgical unit. The occurrence of

abnormal vital signs was highest during the first postoperative hour in the surgical unit (11.6%) and decreased to an incidence of 1.2% by the fourth postoperative hour in the unit. As a result of these findings, the assessment protocol for vital signs in Class I surgical clients at this hospital was changed from every 15 minutes times 4, then every one-half hour times 2, then every hour times 1, and then every 4 hours times 4, to every 15 minutes times 1, every 30 minutes times 2, every 1 hour times 1, and then every 4 hours times 4.

MEASURING TEMPERATURE

Abrams, L., et al. (1989). Effect of peripheral IV infusion on neonatal axillary temperature measurement. *Pediatric Nursing*, 15, 630–632.

Axillary temperature measurements were taken without and with a peripheral intravenous infusion to determine if the measurements were significantly different. Temperature measurements were taken of 29 infants who had a gestational age of 27 to 32 weeks, 33 to 37 weeks, or 38 to 42 weeks. A digital probe thermometer was used to measure temperature. The results indicated no statistically significant difference in temperature readings between the two sites. Furthermore, there was no significant relationship between gestational age and temperature difference.

Baker, N., et al. (1984). The effect of type of thermometer and length of time inserted on oral temperature measurements of afebrile subjects. *Nursing Research*, 33, 109–111.

This study examined the effect of type of thermometer (glass as opposed to electronic) and length of time inserted (2 minutes as opposed to 4 minutes) on oral temperature measurements. Data were obtained from 24 female afebrile subjects. There was a statistically significant difference between 2- and 4-minute readings. The study demonstrated no difference between temperatures taken with glass and electronic thermometers.

Barber, N., and Kilmon, C. A. (1989). Reactions to tympanic temperature measurement in an ambulatory setting. *Pediatric Nursing*, 15, 477–481.

The purpose of this study was to compare children's reactions to tempera-

ture measurement by the rectal or oral route with temperature measurement by the tympanic route. Reactions were observed by the adult accompanying the child and the nurse as to whether the child resisted, seemed afraid, ignored the procedure, or complied cheerfully. There were 129 children in the control group whose temperatures were taken by either the oral or rectal route. The experimental group consisted of 255 children whose temperatures were measured by the tympanic route. The accompanying adults indicated that 32% of the children complied cheerfully, 31% resisted, 28% ignored the procedure, and 17% were fearful of the oral or rectal measurement. In response to tympanic temperature measurement, the adults indicated that 42% of the children complied cheerfully, 36% ignored the procedure, 15% resisted, and 8% seemed afraid. The nurses indicated that 43% complied cheerfully, 39% complied cheerfully, 13% ignored the procedure, and 13% seemed fearful of oral or rectal temperature measurements. The reactions to tympanic measurement reported by the nurses were similar to those of the accompanying adults. Tympanic temperature measurement is timesaving and helps to enhance nurse-child rapport.

Bliss-Holtz, J. (1989). Comparison of rectal, axillary, and inguinal temperatures in full-term newborn infants. *Nursing Research*, 38, 85–87.

Data were collected from 120 (62 female and 58 male) full-term infants during their first 12 to 48 hours of life to compare temperature measurements at the rectal, axillary, and inguinal sites. Temperature measurements were significantly different for all three sites. The largest variation in temperature readings (0.8° F) was between the rectal and in-

guinal sites. However, the highest correlation of readings was between the rectal and inguinal sites. The infants reached their maximum inguinal temperature in 3 minutes, their maximum axillary temperature in 5 minutes, and their maximum rectal temperature in 3 minutes.

Durham, M. L., Swanson, B., and Paulford, N. (1986). Effect of tachypnea on oral temperature estimation: A replication. *Nursing Research*, 35, 211–214.

This descriptive study assessed the effect of respiratory rate (normal as opposed to tachypnea) on temperature measurement (oral and rectal) in 53 clients. The same IVAC 811A electronic thermometer was used to obtain all temperature measurements. The sample consisted of 20 individuals without tachypnea and 33 individuals with tachypnea. A statistically significant difference was found between the two groups. The difference between rectal and oral temperature was greater in the individuals with tachypnea.

Erickson, R. (1980). Oral temperature differences in relation to thermometer and technique. *Nursing Research*, 29, 157–159.

Fifty febrile and 50 afebrile subjects were assessed to determine differences in oral temperature measurements using electronic and mercury thermometers in three sublingual sites and to determine if the method of probe insertion (slow slide as opposed to direct placement) would result in different measurements. The findings suggest that the posterior sublingual pocket should be used as the site for oral temperature measurement. The technique of thermometer insertion was not clinically significant.

Erickson, R. S., and Yount, S. T. (1991). Comparison of tympanic and oral temperatures in surgical patients. *Nursing Research, 40, 90–93.*

Oral and tympanic temperatures were measured in 60 adults who had major abdominal operations. The temperature measurements were taken at four specified times during the perioperative period. There was a moderately high correlation between temperature measurements at the two sites for each measurement time. Temperature ranges were greater for the oral site. The tympanic measurement was higher in 99% of the measurements. The investigators concluded that both sites provide a satisfactory measurement of body temperature. They recommend that temperature be measured consistently at the same site.

Graves, R. D., and Markarian, M. F. (1980). Three-minute time interval when using an oral mercury-in-glass thermometer with or without J-Temp Sheaths. *Nursing Research, 29, 323–324.*

This study compared oral temperature measurements using sheathed and unsheathed thermometers at 3-, 5-, 8-, and 12-minute intervals. Unsheathed thermometers consistently registered higher measurements. However, the differences were not clinically significant. Since the 3-minute readings were consistent with the 5-, 8-, and 12-minute readings, the findings of this study suggest that a 3-minute interval for assessing oral temperature is adequate when using sheathed or unsheathed thermometers.

Hasler, M. E., and Cohen, J. A. (1982). The effect of oxygen administration on oral temperature assessment. *Nursing Research, 31, 265–268.*

Hasler and Cohen investigated the effect of oxygen administration (aerosol mask, Venturi mask, and nasal prongs) on oral temperature. Data were collected from 40 healthy male and female clients. The findings indicated no difference in the oral temperature measurement before and during oxygen administration.

Heidrenreich, T., and Giuffre, M. (1990). Postoperative temperature measurement. *Nursing Research, 39, 153–155.*

Data were collected from 18 postoperative adult clients to determine the va-lidity of axillary temperature measurements. Electronic axillary, mercury axillary, mercury rectal, and core body temperature measurements were taken on the clients' admission to the intensive care unit from the operating room. The majority of the axillary measurements were lower than the core measurements, with the mercury axillary readings being the least different. The highest correlation between sites was between the rectal and core readings, and the rectal site was the best predictor of core body temperature.

Heinz, J. (1985). Validation of sublingual temperatures in patients with nasogastric tubes. *Heart and Lung: Journal of Critical Care, 14, 128–130.*

This study was conducted to determine if the presence of a nasogastric tube affected temperature measurement at the sublingual site. Temperature measurements were taken from 20 clients with nasogastric tubes. Rectal temperatures were measured simultaneously as reference points for comparison. The results of this study demonstrated that sublingual temperature is not affected by the presence of a nasogastric tube.

Kunnel, M. T., et al. (1988). Comparisons of rectal, femoral, axillary, and skin-to-mattress temperatures in stable neonates. *Nursing Research, 37, 162–164.*

This study compared four sites for measurement of temperature in neonates (n = 99). The temperatures were taken simultaneously at the four sites. Measurements of temperature across the four sites were not significantly different. However, statistically significant differences were found relative to the amount of time necessary to register the highest temperature. Rectal measurements required less time (approximately 2.66 minutes) to register the highest temperature than measurements at the other three sites. The skin-to-mattress measurement required the most time (approximately 8.52 minutes).

Lanuza, D. M., et al. (1989). Body temperature and heart rate rhythms in acutely head-injured patients. *Applied Nursing Research, 2 (3), 135–139.*

This descriptive study investigated the effect an acute head injury had on circadian rhythms of heart rate and body temperature, and the relationship between these physiologic variables. Data were collected from a convenience sample of 10 clients. Results revealed that only 1 patient demonstrated normal circadian rhythms for body temperature and heart rate. Three additional patients demonstrated rhythms for these variables, but the rhythms were abnormal. For example, the cycles were less than 24 hours in length with peaks in heart rate and temperature at inappropriate times.

Mown, J. E., et al. (1987). Axillary versus rectal temperatures in preterm infants under radiant warmers. *Journal of Obstetric, Gynecologic, and Neonatal Nursing, 16, 348–352.*

This descriptive study compared axillary and rectal temperatures in 25 preterm infants under radiant warmers. No statistically significant difference was found.

Neff, J., et al. (1989). Effect of respiratory rate, respiratory depth, and open- versus closed-mouth breathing on sublingual temperature. *Research in Nursing and Health, 12, 195–202.*

Data were collected from 78 healthy adults to determine the "effect of open mouth breathing, tachypnea, and hyperpnea, either alone or in combination, on sublingual and tympanic membrane temperature" (p. 195). The results indicated that mouth breathing was the only variable that significantly affected sublingual temperature.

Samples, J., et al. (1985). Circadian rhythms: Basis for screening for fever. *Nursing Research, 34, 377–379.*

The findings of this study indicate that one daily routine temperature recording at the peak of the circadian thermal rhythm (5 P.M.–7 P.M.) is adequate to screen for fever in adult hospitalized clients. Body temperature may be measured more often based on professional nursing judgments about the status of the clients.

Yonkman, C. A. (1982). Cool and heated aerosol and the measurement of oral temperature. *Nursing Research, 31, 354–357.*

This study assessed the effects of cool and heated aerosol therapy on oral temperature measurements in 30 subjects. A baseline temperature was recorded for each subject, the therapy was administered, and the temperature was measured again at 1- and 5-minute intervals after treatment. A statistically significant difference was found in oral temperatures after therapy. However, the clinical significance is relatively little.   ■

MEASURING PULSE

Hollerbach, A. D., and Sneed, N. (1990). Accuracy of radial pulse assessment by length of counting interval. *Heart & Lung,* 19, 258–264.

Resting and rapid (greater than or equal to 100 beats per minute) pulse rates were counted at 15-, 30-, and 60-second intervals in 103 adults. Fifteen-second rates were multiplied by 4 and 30-second rates were multiplied by 2. A significant difference was found between rapid and resting rates, with the rapid rate being less accurate. There was a significant difference between the 15-second rapid count and all of the resting counts. The 30-second count was the most accurate for rapid rates and the 60-second count was the most accurate for resting rates.

MEASURING BLOOD PRESSURE

Byra-Cook, C. J., Dracup, K. A., and Lazik, A. J. (1990). Direct and indirect blood pressure in critical care patients. *Nursing Research,* 39, 285–288.

Direct intraarterial blood pressure readings and indirect blood pressure readings with the bell and the diaphragm of a stethoscope were taken from 50 clients. Readings using both the bell and the diaphragm were taken over the antecubital fossa and the brachial artery. Direct blood pressure readings were correlated with indirect blood pressure measurements at both sites. When systolic indirect measurements were compared with direct measurements, the bell of the stethoscope over the antecubital fossa provided the most accurate reading. The diaphragm over the antecubital fossa provided the most accurate diastolic reading when the four measurement techniques were compared to direct measurements. The systolic pressure was lower on auscultation than on direct measurement and the diastolic pressure reading was higher on auscultation than on direct measurement for all four techniques.

Clochesy, J. M. (1986). Systemic blood pressure in various lateral recumbent positions: A pilot study. *Heart and Lung: Journal of Critical Care,* 15, 593–594.

This was a quasi-experimental study to determine the effect of lateral positions on the blood pressure of 5 female and 5 male adults. Blood pressure measurements were recorded with the clients in the supine position and four lateral positions: 45 degrees left, 35 degrees left, 35 degrees right, and 45 degrees right. The findings of the study indicate that pressures obtained in the arm opposite to the position differ from supine readings to the point of clinical significance. It therefore is recommended that blood pressure be measured from the "down" arm when the client is in a lateral recumbent position.

Hellman, R., and Grimm, S. A. (1984). The influence of talking on diastolic blood pressure readings. *Research in Nursing and Health,* 7, 253–256.

To investigate the effect of talking on diastolic blood pressure, 48 subjects with one previous diastolic reading of 90 mmHg or more and who were not taking antihypertensive medications had their blood pressures measured under three conditions. The conditions included not talking, talking during cuff inflation only, and talking during blood pressure measurement. Diastolic measurements increased significantly during both talking conditions.

Mauro, A. M. (1988). Effects of bell versus diaphragm on indirect blood pressure measurement. *Heart and Lung: Journal of Critical Care,* 17, 489–494.

This experimental study examined the effects of the use of the bell as opposed to the diaphragm of the stethoscope on the indirect measurement of blood pressure in 255 female nursing students. The findings revealed that the use of the bell produced a higher systolic value and a statistically significant lower diastolic value when the stethoscope was placed over the brachial artery site. Comparison of these findings to those of an earlier study suggested that the position of the stethoscope may significantly affect the values obtained by the two methods.

Norman, E., Gadaleta, D., and Clayton, C. C. (1991). An evaluation of three blood pressure methods in a stabilized acute trauma population. *Nursing Research,* 40, 86–89.

Data were collected from 16 male and 14 female clients with a mean age of 55.6 years who had sustained trauma. A direct blood pressure measurement was obtained via a radial arterial catheter and an indirect measurement was made using the bell and the diaphragm of the stethoscope over the brachial artery. A statistically significant difference was found between the bell and the diaphragm in K1 (systolic) measurements. No significant differences were found between the bell and the diaphragm for the K4 (fourth phase diastolic) and K5 (fifth phase diastolic) measurements. No significant differences were found among the three methods for K1, K4, or K5 measurements.

Rebenson-Piano, M., et al. (1989). An evaluation of two indirect methods of blood pressure measurement in ill patients. *Nursing Research,* 38, 42–45.

Direct and indirect blood pressure measurements were compared in 32 clients. Direct measurements were determined using 10-second radial arterial catheter strip recordings. Indirect measurements were made using a mercury sphygmomanometer and an automatic blood pressure machine. No differences were found among the three measurements of normotensive diastolic blood pressure. However, a significant difference was found in the measurement of systolic blood pressure using the automatic blood pressure machine. Significant differences also were found between direct and indirect systolic blood pressure readings in the hypertensive clients. The direct measurement was greater than the two indirect measurements. The results indicate that the automatic blood pressure machine can be safely substituted for direct blood pressure measurements in normotensive individuals.

Tachovsky, B. J. (1985). Indirect auscultatory blood pressure measurement at two sites in the arm. *Research in Nursing and Health,* 8, 125–129.

The study by Tachovsky compared the results of indirect auscultatory blood pressure measurement at the forearm site with values obtained at the traditional upper arm site. The forearm site has been suggested as an alternative site for more accurate measurement of blood pressure in obese clients. The findings of this study revealed statistically significant differences between the upper arm and forearm sites. Forearm values tend to be lower systolically and higher diastolically than upper arm values; therefore, the forearm technique is inadvisable in cases in which accuracy is imperative for clinical decision making.

ASSESSING NEUROLOGIC STATUS

Lord-Feroli, K., and Maguire-McGinty, M. (1985). Toward a more objective approach to pupil assessment. *Journal of Neurosurgical Nursing, 17,* 309–312.

The purpose of this study was to compare interrater reliability between nurses using a printed millimeter scale and nurses using a hand-held tongue depressor pupil gauge. Usable data were collected from 42 pairs of nurses: 14 pairs who used the printed millimeter scale and 28 pairs who used the tongue depressor pupil gauge. Correlations ranged from 0.33 to 0.53 for nurses using the millimeter scale to 0.68 to 0.69 for nurses using the tongue depressor pupil gauge. However, this was not a statistically significant difference.

Wilson, S. F., et al. (1988). Determining interrater reliability of nurses' assessments of pupillary size and reaction. *Journal of Neuroscience Nursing, 20* (3), 189–192.

This study was conducted to determine if nurses (68 pairs) rated pupil size the same with and without an objective measure (penlight gauge or observation) and if the same descriptor was selected for pupillary reaction to light. No significant difference was found in relation to the assessment of pupil size. However, agreement on the descriptor selected for pupillary reaction was poor to good.

TEMPERATURE

The human body continually produces heat as a by-product of metabolic processes. Body temperature reflects the balance between heat production and heat loss. The human body loses heat by radiation, conduction, convection, and evaporation.

Body temperature can be measured with a tympanic thermometer, an electronic thermometer, or a mercury-in-glass thermometer. The four sites commonly used to measure temperature are the oral cavity, the rectum, the axilla, and the ear canal (see Figs. 4–1, 4–2, and 4–3).

Body temperature is measured in degrees using either of two scales, the centigrade (Celsius) scale or the Fahrenheit scale (see Fig. 4–3). Occasionally, you may need to convert a temperature from one scale to the other. Use the following formulas to make this conversion:

To convert from centigrade to Fahrenheit:

$$F = (\text{temperature in centigrade} \times 9/5) + 32$$

To convert from Fahrenheit to centigrade:

$$C = (\text{temperature in Fahrenheit} - 32) \times 5/9$$

Charting Temperature and Other Vital Signs

Most hospitals and clinics use a graphic style of charting to record vital signs (see Fig. 4–9).

SKILL 4–1 MEASURING TYMPANIC TEMPERATURE

Clinical Situations in Which You May Encounter This Skill

Temperature is measured to obtain baseline data and to detect the presence of infection, increased intracranial pressure, hypothermia, or other changes in the client's physical condition. Temperature may be measured by the tympanic route using an electronic tympanic thermometer (Fig. 4–1). Tympanic thermometry is used for adults as well as for infants and children.

Anticipated Responses

▼ The client's temperature is between 36.5 and 37.5° Celsius (C) or between 97.6 and 99.4° Fahrenheit (F).
▼ You are able to seal the client's ear canal with the tympanic thermometer probe.

Adverse Responses

▼ You have difficulty sealing the client's ear canal with the tympanic thermometer probe.
▼ The client has hypothermia or hyperthermia.

Materials List

Gather these materials before beginning the skill:

▼ Electronic tympanic thermometer with charger
▼ Disposable probe cover

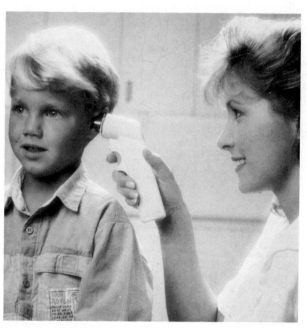

▼ **FIGURE 4–1.** Tympanic thermometer. (Courtesy of IVAC Corporation, San Diego, CA.)

▼ _ACTION_

1. Check the chart and determine the client's temperature readings over the last 24 hours.

2. Check the chart for the client's medical problems and temperature notification parameters.

3. Remove the probe from the base unit and note the lighted display.

4. Be sure that the machine is in tympanic mode.

5. Place the disposable cover on the probe tip.

6. Press the scan button while inserting the probe tip into and sealing the client's ear canal.

7. Release the scan button.

8. Remove the probe when you hear a signal that indicates that the thermometer has registered.

9. Read the temperature on the display and record it on a notepad.

10. Press the release button to discard the probe cover into a waste receptacle.

▼ _RATIONALE_

1. Provides baseline data from which to make comparisons.

2. Alerts you to any possible problems that may cause hypothermia or hyperthermia. Most physicians ask to be notified when a client's temperature is above 38.2° C or 101 to 102° F.

3. The display indicates that the thermometer is charged.

4. Some machines also measure surface temperature.

5. Protects the client from cross-contamination.

6. The outer opening of the ear canal must be sealed to measure the temperature accurately.

7. Activates the machine.

8. Indicates that the temperature measurement is completed.

9. The temperature is recorded in degrees on the Celsius or the Fahrenheit scale. The notepad prevents you from relying on memory.

10. Probe covers are disposable.

▼ _ACTION_	▼ _RATIONALE_
11. Return the probe to the charger.	11. Ensures that the probe will be ready for the next use.
12. Explain the results to the client if appropriate.	12. Keeps the client informed of his or her health status and allows the client to actively participate in his or her care.
13. Wash your hands.	13. Decreases the transmission of microorganisms.
14. Assess the results and notify your instructor or charge nurse, or both, of abnormal results.	14. Abnormal temperature measurements may indicate the need for further nursing intervention.
15. Record the results.	15. Communicates the findings to the other members of the health care team and contributes to the legal record by documenting the care given to the client.

Example of Documentation

See Figure 4–9.

Teaching Tips

While you measure the client's temperature, teach the client or his or her parents appropriate measures for fever control.

Home Care Variations

The tympanic thermometer usually is not used in the home. If the client is unable to read a mercury-in-glass thermometer, a digital thermometer may be purchased for home use.

SKILL 4–2   MEASURING ORAL TEMPERATURE

Clinical Situations in Which You May Encounter This Skill

Temperature is measured to obtain baseline data and to detect the presence of infection, increased intracranial pressure, hypothermia, or other changes in the client's physical condition. Temperature may be measured by the oral route when the client is old enough to safely hold the thermometer in his or her mouth (age 4 or 5 yr) and when not contraindicated by conditions such as coma or seizures or by oral surgery. You may use an electronic (see Fig. 4–2) or glass thermometer (see Fig. 4–3).

If the client has just eaten, smoked, or consumed a hot or cold liquid, you should wait 15 minutes to measure his or her temperature by the oral route.

The client's body temperature may not be accurately measured by an oral thermometer if the client has excessively dry mucous membranes or cannot hold the thermometer under the tongue with his or her lips closed. An axillary or rectal, or tympanic, temperature should then be taken.

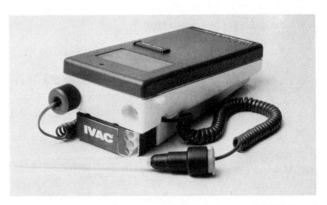

▼ **FIGURE 4–2.** Electronic thermometer. (Courtesy of IVAC Corporation, San Diego, CA.)

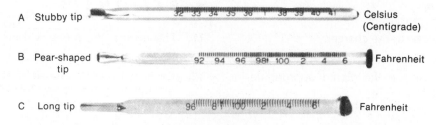

▼ **FIGURE 4–3.** Mercury thermometers. Those with stubby and pear-shaped tips (A and B) can be used as rectal and axillary thermometers. Long-tipped thermometers (C) are intended for oral use only. All designs are available in the Celsius (centigrade) and Fahrenheit scales. (Courtesy of Becton, Dickinson and Co., Rutherford, NJ 07070.)

Anticipated Responses

▼ The client's temperature is between 36.5 and 37.5° Celsius (C) or between 97.6 and 99.4° Fahrenheit (F).
▼ The client is able to hold the thermometer in his or her mouth without difficulty.

Adverse Responses

▼ The client has difficulty holding the thermometer in his or her mouth.
▼ The client has hypothermia or hyperthermia.

Materials List

Gather these materials before beginning the skill:

When Using a Glass Thermometer

▼ Glass thermometer in disinfectant
▼ Cleaning supplies or thermometer sheath
▼ Facial tissues

When Using an Electronic Thermometer

▼ Electronic thermometer
▼ Charger
▼ Probe covers

▼ *ACTION*

1. Check the chart to determine the person's temperature readings over the last 24 hours.

2. Check the chart for the client's medical problems and temperature notification parameters.

Using a Glass Thermometer

3. a. Hold the thermometer at the end opposite from the bulb and remove the disinfectant from the clean oral thermometer by rinsing the thermometer in cold water. Dry it with facial tissue, wiping from the bulb to the stem using a firm twisting motion.
   b. Shake down the mercury in the thermometer to 35° C or 95° F using a snapping wrist motion (Fig. 4–4).
   c. If you are using a thermometer sheath, insert the thermometer into the cover and remove the paper (Fig. 4–5).

▼ *RATIONALE*

1. Provides baseline data from which to make comparisons.

2. Alerts you to any possible problems that may cause hypothermia or hyperthermia. Most physicians ask to be notified when a client's temperature is above 38.2° C or 101 to 102° F.

3. a. Disinfectant can irritate the client's oral tissues and can taste bad. The direction of the flow of fluids and cleansing always should proceed from the area of least contamination to the area of most contamination.

   b. Lowers the mercury to a level usually below the client's body temperature.

   c. Prevents the thermometer from becoming contaminated with the client's oral secretions.

▼ _ACTION_ _ _ _ _ _ _ _ _ _ _ _ _ ▼ _RATIONALE_ _ _ _ _ _ _ _ _

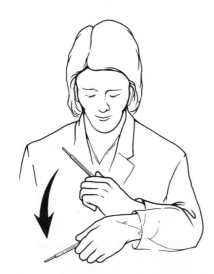

▼ **FIGURE 4–4.** Shaking down a thermometer.

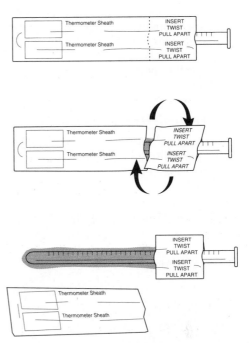

▼ **FIGURE 4–5.** Using a thermometer sheath.

d. Place the thermometer in the client's posterior sublingual pocket (Fig. 4–6) for 3 to 4 minutes if the client is afebrile, and up to 8 minutes if the client is febrile. Terminate insertion time when the temperature stabilizes and is no longer rising.

d. Research has shown the posterior sublingual pocket to be the optimal site for temperature taking (Erickson, 1980). Research has demonstrated that oral thermometers provide an accurate reading in 3 to 4 minutes for afebrile persons (Baker et al., 1984; Graves and Markarian, 1980), but may require up to 8 minutes to fully register in febrile clients.

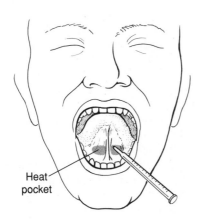

Heat pocket

▼ **FIGURE 4–6.** Oral thermometer placement.

e. Remind the client to keep his or her lips closed.

e. The thermometer will not give an accurate reading if the client's lips are open.

f. Remove the thermometer from the client's mouth. If you are using a thermometer sheath, remove it to read the thermometer. If you are not using a thermometer sheath, remove any secretions from the thermometer by wiping from the stem to the bulb.

f. Removal of the sheath or wiping away secretions enables you to read the thermometer clearly.

g. Read the thermometer by holding it at eye-level and rotating the stem until the mercury is seen clearly. Record the findings on a notepad.

g. The temperature may be recorded in degrees on the Celsius or Fahrenheit scale. A notepad prevents you from relying on memory.

▼ *ACTION*

▼ *RATIONALE*

h. If you did not use a thermometer sheath, clean the thermometer by holding it with the bulb in a downward direction and wiping it with soap and water.
i. Return the thermometer to the disinfectant solution.

Using an Electronic Thermometer

3. a. Remove the electronic thermometer from the charger and note the lighted display.
　　b. Be sure that the blue probe is attached.

　　c. Place the probe cover on the probe (Fig. 4–7).

h. Thermometers contaminated with oral secretions provide a growth medium for microorganisms.

i. Reduces the number of microorganisms on the thermometer.

3. a. The display indicates that the thermometer is charged.
　　b. Electronic thermometers have interchangeable probes: blue is for oral use and red is for rectal use.
　　c. Protects the client from cross-contamination.

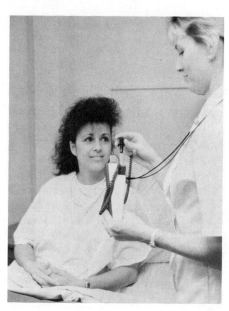

▼ **FIGURE 4–7.** Placing the probe cover on the probe.

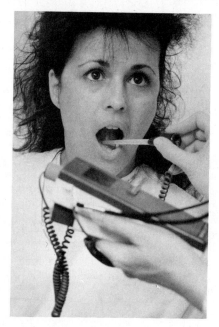

▼ **FIGURE 4–8.** Inserting the probe of the electronic thermometer.

　　d. Place the probe with the cover in the client's posterior sublingual pocket (Fig. 4–8).
　　e. Instruct the client to keep his or her lips closed.

　　f. Observe the digital display until it becomes stable and the machine emits a tone.
　　g. Read the results from the display and record them on a notepad.

　　h. Discard the probe cover.

4. Explain the results to the client if appropriate.

5. Wash your hands.

6. Assess the results and notify your instructor or charge nurse, or both, of abnormal results.

7. Record the results.

　　d. Facilitates accurate measurement of the client's temperature.
　　e. The thermometer will not give an accurate reading if the client's lips are open.
　　f. Indicates that the temperature measurement is completed.
　　g. The temperature is recorded in degrees on the Celsius or Fahrenheit scale. The notepad prevents you from relying on memory.
　　h. Probe covers are disposable.

4. Keeps the client informed of his or her health status and allows the client to actively participate in his or her care.

5. Decreases the transmission of microorganisms.

6. Abnormal temperature measurements may indicate the need for further nursing intervention.

7. Communicates the findings to the other members of the health care team and contributes to the legal record by documenting the care given to the client.

Example of Documentation

See Figure 4–9.

GRAPHIC CHART

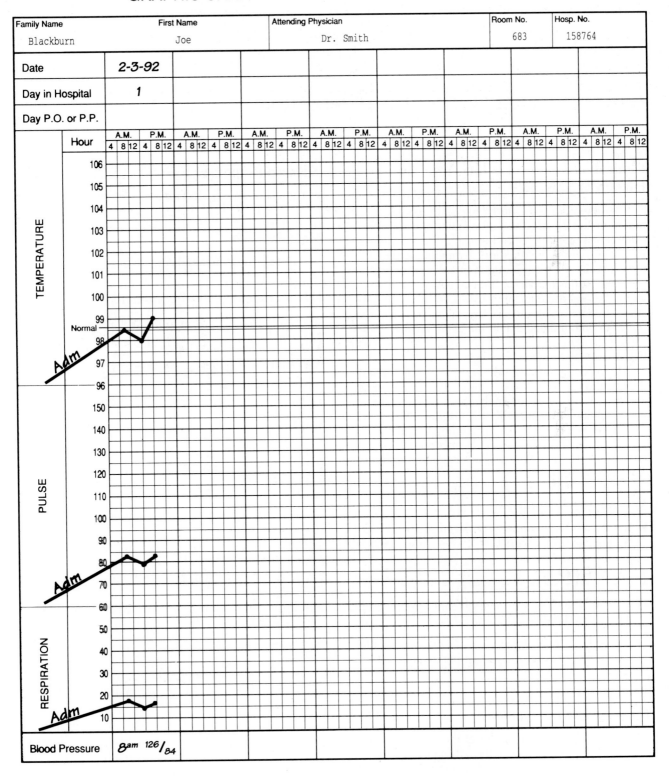

▼ FIGURE 4–9. Graphic chart for recording vital signs.

Teaching Tips

While you measure the client's temperature, teach the client or his or her parents how to use a thermometer and appropriate measures for fever control.

Home Care Variations

If the client is unable to read a mercury-in-glass thermometer, a digital thermometer may be purchased for home use.

SKILL 4–3   MEASURING RECTAL TEMPERATURE

Clinical Situations in Which You May Encounter This Skill

Temperature is measured to obtain baseline data and to detect the presence of infection, increased intracranial pressure, hypothermia, or other changes in the client's physical condition. Temperature may be measured by the rectal route in infants and young children. Adults may have a rectal temperature taken when the oral route is contraindicated by conditions such as coma or seizures, or by oral surgery. The rectal route is contraindicated after the client has had rectal surgery. Electronic (see Fig. 4–2) or glass thermometers (Fig. 4–3) may be used.

Insertion of a rectal thermometer may be difficult if the client has hemorrhoids. Visualization of the anus and generous lubrication of the thermometer with a water-soluble lubricant will ease insertion. You also may insert your gloved, lubricated finger gently into the client's anus, and ease the thermometer in beside your finger. Then withdraw your finger and hold the thermometer in place.

Anticipated Responses

▼ The client's temperature is between 37.0 and 38.0° C or between 98.6 and 100.4° F.

Adverse Responses

▼ The client has hypothermia or hyperthermia.

Materials List

Gather these materials before beginning the skill:

When Using a Glass Thermometer

▼ Cleaning supplies or thermometer sheaths
▼ Facial tissues
▼ Water-soluble lubricant
▼ Examination gloves

When Using an Electronic Thermometer

▼ Charger
▼ Probe covers
▼ Facial tissues
▼ Water-soluble lubricant
▼ Examination gloves

▼ ACTION

1. Check the chart and determine the client's temperature readings over the last 24 hours.

2. Check the chart for the client's medical problems and temperature notification parameters.

Using a Glass Thermometer

3. a. Hold the thermometer at the end opposite the bulb and remove the disinfectant from the clean thermometer by rinsing it in cold water. Dry it with a facial tissue, wiping from the bulb to the stem using a firm twisting motion.

▼ RATIONALE

1. Provides baseline data from which to make comparisons.

2. Alerts you to any possible problems that may cause hypothermia or hyperthermia. Most physicians ask to be notified when a client's temperature is above 38.2° C or 101 or 102° F.

3. a. The direction of the flow of fluids and cleansing should proceed from the area of least contamination to the area of most contamination.

▼ _A C T I O N_ _____   ▼ _R A T I O N A L E_ _____

b. Close the door and draw the curtains around the bed. Raise the bed to working height.

c. Position the client. Adult or child: Lateral or Sims' position (Fig. 4–10). Infant: Prone over your lap (Fig. 4–11).

b. Provides privacy. Raising bed provides for proper body mechanics.

c. Facilitates ease of thermometer insertion.

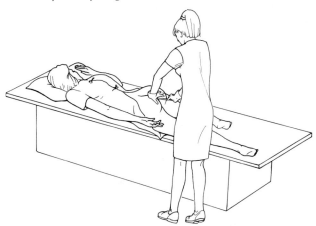

▼ **FIGURE 4–10.** Client in Sims' position for rectal temperature measurement.

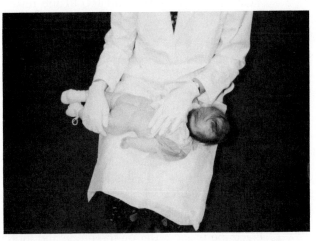

▼ **FIGURE 4–11.** Position an infant over your lap for rectal temperature measurement.

d. Put on examination gloves.

e. Shake down the thermometer to 36° C or 95° F using a snapping wrist motion (see Fig. 4–4).

f. If you are using a thermometer sheath, insert the thermometer in the cover and remove the paper (see Fig. 4–5).

g. If you are using an uncovered thermometer, lubricate the tip with a water-soluble jelly.

h. Spread the client's buttocks and gently insert the bulb of the thermometer into the anus in the direction of the client's umbilicus to a depth of 0.5 inch for an infant, up to 1 inch for a child, and 1.0 to 1.5 inches for an adult. Keep the bulb of the thermometer in contact with the client's rectal wall.

i. Hold the client's buttocks closed with one hand while holding the thermometer with the other hand for 2 to 4 minutes (Fig. 4–12). *Never* leave a client alone with a rectal thermometer in place.

d. Decreases the transmission of microorganisms.

e. Lowers the mercury to a level usually below the client's body temperature.

f. Prevents the thermometer from being contaminated with feces.

g. Eases insertion and prevents trauma to the client's rectal mucosa.

h. Inserting the thermometer too deeply or forcefully can cause trauma to the client's rectal mucosa. The direction of the thermometer insertion conforms to the normal rectal anatomy. Keeping the thermometer in contact with the client's rectal wall ensures measurement of the client's body temperature rather than the temperature of the feces.

i. Prevents expulsion of the thermometer.

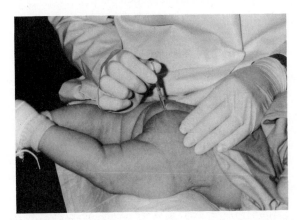

▼ **FIGURE 4–12.** Hold the buttocks closed during temperature measurement.

▼ *A C T I O N* ▼ *R A T I O N A L E*

j. Remove the thermometer and slide off the sheath, if used. If you did not use a cover, remove the secretions from the thermometer by wiping from the stem to the bulb.

k. Read the thermometer and record the results on a notepad.

l. If you did not use a thermometer sheath, clean the thermometer by holding it with the bulb in a downward direction and wiping with soap and water from the stem of the thermometer to the bulb.

j. Removing the sheath or wiping away secretions enables you to read the thermometer clearly.

k. The temperature may be recorded in degrees on the Celsius or Fahrenheit scale. The notepad prevents you from relying on memory.

l. The direction of the flow of fluids and cleansing should proceed from the area of least contamination to the area of most contamination.

Using an Electronic Thermometer

3. a. Remove the electronic thermometer from the charger and note the lighted display.
   b. Attach the red probe.

   c. Place the probe cover on the probe and lubricate the tip using a water-soluble jelly.

   d. Position the client: Adult or child: Lateral or Sims' position (see Fig. 4–10). Infant: Prone over your lap (see Fig. 4–11).
   e. Spread the client's buttocks and insert the probe tip 0.5 inch for an infant, up to 1 inch for a child, and 1.0 to 1.5 inches for an adult. Remain with the client and hold the probe in place.
   f. Hold the client's buttocks closed with one hand while holding the probe with the other hand. *Never* leave a client alone with a rectal probe in place.
   g. Observe the changing temperature display until it stabilizes and the machine emits a tone.
   h. Read the results from the display and record them on a notepad.

   i. Discard the used probe cover.

3. a. The display indicates that the thermometer is charged.
   b. Electronic thermometers have interchangeable probes: red is for rectal use and blue is for oral use.
   c. The cover protects the client from cross-contamination. The lubricant eases insertion and prevents trauma to the client's rectal mucosa.
   d. Facilitates ease of probe insertion.

   e. Inserting the probe too deeply can cause trauma to the client's rectal mucosa.

   f. Prevents expulsion of the probe.

   g. Indicates that the temperature measurement is completed.
   h. The temperature will be recorded in degrees on the Celsius or Fahrenheit scale. The notepad prevents you from relying on memory.
   i. Probe covers are disposable.

4. Explain the results to the client if appropriate.

4. Keeps the client informed of his or her health status and allows the client to actively participate in his or her care.

5. Cleanse the client's anal area to remove the lubricant and assist the client to a position of comfort. Lower the bed.

5. Promotes the client's comfort. Lowering the bed promotes safety.

6. Wash your hands.

6. Decreases the transmission of microorganisms.

7. Assess the results and notify your instructor or charge nurse, or both, of abnormal results.

7. Abnormal temperature measurements may indicate the need for further nursing intervention.

8. Record results.

8. Communicates the findings to the other members of the health care team and contributes to the legal record by documenting the care given to the client.

Example of Documentation

See Figure 4–9.

Teaching Tips

While you measure the client's temperature, teach the client or his or her parent how to use a thermometer and appropriate measures for fever control.

Home Care Variations

If the client is unable to read a mercury-in-glass thermometer, a digital thermometer may be purchased for home use.

SKILL 4–4 MEASURING AXILLARY TEMPERATURE

Clinical Situations in Which You May Encounter This Skill

Temperature is measured to obtain baseline data and to detect the presence of infection or hypothermia or other changes in the client's physical condition. Temperature may be measured by the axillary route in adults when oral and rectal routes are contraindicated. The axillary route is often used in infants and children. An electronic thermometer (see Fig. 4–2) or glass thermometer (see Fig. 4–3) with a stubby or pear-shaped tip may be used to measure an axillary temperature. If the client has difficulty holding the thermometer in place, you should hold the thermometer in the client's axilla with the client's arm firmly at his or her side.

Anticipated Responses

▼ The client's temperature is between 36.0 and 37.0° C or between 96 6 and 98.4° F.

Adverse Responses

▼ The client has difficulty holding the thermometer in his or her axilla for 10 minutes.
▼ The client has hypothermia or hyperthermia.

Materials List

Gather these materials before beginning the skill:

When Using a Glass Thermometer

▼ Oral glass thermometer
▼ Cleaning supplies

When Using an Electronic Thermometer

▼ Electronic thermometer
▼ Charger
▼ Probe covers

▼ ACTION	▼ RATIONALE
1. Check the chart to determine the client's temperature readings over the last 24 hours.	1. Provides baseline data from which to make comparisons.
2. Check the chart for the client's medical problems and temperature notification parameters.	2. Alerts you to any possible problems that may cause hypothermia or hyperthermia. Most physicians ask to be notified when a client's temperature is above 101 or 102° F.
Using a Glass Thermometer	
3. a. Remove disinfectant from a clean thermometer by wiping from the bulb to the stem using a firm twisting motion, while holding the thermometer in an upward direction.	3. a. The direction of the flow of fluids and cleansing should proceed from the area of least contamination to the area of most contamination.

▼ *ACTION*   ▼ *RATIONALE*

b. Shake down the mercury in the thermometer to 36° C or 95° F using a snapping wrist motion.

c. Raise bed to working height and position the client. The adult should be in a supine or semi-Fowler's position. The infant or child should be in a supine position.

d. Place the bulb of the thermometer in the client's clean, dry axilla and have the client hold his or her arm firmly to his or her side with the elbow flexed and the hand in contact with the chest (Fig. 4–13).

b. Lowers the mercury to a level usually below the client's body temperature.

c. Raising bed promotes proper body mechanics. Facilitates placement of the thermometer in the client's axillary area.

d. Aids in accurate measurement of the client's body temperature.

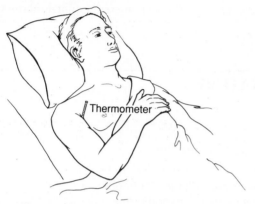

▼ **FIGURE 4–13.** Placement of thermometer for axillary temperature measurement.

e. Wait 5 to 7 minutes, then remove the thermometer.

f. Read the thermometer by holding it at eye-level and rotating the stem until the mercury is clearly seen. Record the findings on a notepad.

g. Clean the thermometer by holding it with the bulb in a downward direction and wiping it with soap and water from the stem to the bulb.

h. Return the thermometer to the disinfectant solution.

i. Wash your hands.

e. Allows adequate time for the thermometer to register the client's body temperature.

f. Temperature may be recorded in degrees on the Celsius or Fahrenheit scale. The notepad prevents you from relying on memory.

g. Thermometers contaminated with bodily secretions provide a growth medium for microorganisms.

h. Reduces the growth of microorganisms on the thermometer.

i. Decreases the transmission of microorganisms.

Using an Electronic Thermometer

3. a. Follow the same procedure as for oral temperature (see Skill 4–2), except place the covered probe in the client's axilla with the client's arm held firmly to his or her side. The client should flex the elbow and keep his or her hand in contact with his or her chest to hold the thermometer snugly in the axillary area.

b. Read the thermometer when the digital display stabilizes and the machine emits a tone, and record the findings on a notepad.

4. Explain the results to the client.

3. a. See Skill 4–2 for measuring oral temperature with an electronic thermometer.

b. The tone indicates that the measurement is completed. The notepad prevents you from relying on memory.

4. Keeps the client informed of his or her own care and allows the client to actively participate in his or her care.

▼ _ACTION_	▼ _RATIONALE_
5. Lower the bed.	**5.** Promotes client safety.
6. Wash your hands.	**6.** Decreases the transmission of microorganisms.
7. Assess the results and notify your instructor or charge nurse, or both, of abnormal results.	**7.** Abnormal temperature measurements may indicate the need for further nursing intervention.
8. Record the results.	**8.** Communicates the findings to the other members of the health care team and contributes to the legal record by documenting the care given to the client.

Example of Documentation

See Figure 4–9.

Teaching Tips

While you measure the client's temperature, teach the client or his or her parent how to use a thermometer and appropriate measures for fever control.

Home Care Variations

If the client is unable to read a mercury-in-glass thermometer, a digital thermometer may be purchased for home use.

PULSE

The pulse is a rhythmical throbbing that results from a wave of blood passing through an artery as the heart contracts. You can palpate the client's peripheral pulse by gently compressing an artery against a bone or other firm surface with your fingers. You can auscultate an apical pulse by listening to the client's heart with a stethoscope. You may assess the pulse at any one of nine sites as shown in Figure 4–14. The apical and radial sites are most commonly used when counting a heart rate. When assessing the client's pulse, note the rate, rhythm, and volume of the pulse.

1. *Temporal site:* Palpate between the client's eye and hairline above the cheekbone (the zygomatic arch).
2. *Femoral site:* Palpate halfway between the client's anterior iliac spine and the symphysis pubis in the groin area.
3. *Popliteal site:* Palpate the back of the client's knee along the outer side of the medial tendon. Having the client flex his or her knee will facilitate location of this pulse.
4. *Posterior tibial site:* Palpate behind the client's inner ankle bone (medial malleolus).
5. *Carotid site:* Palpate the client's neck between the trachea and the sternocleidomastoid muscle. You should palpate only one side of the neck at a time and avoid vigorous stimulation when palpating to prevent stimulation of the carotid sinus, which may result in bradycardia.
6. *Brachial site:* Palpate between the client's biceps and triceps muscles above the elbow or medially in the antecubital fossa.
7. *Radial site:* Palpate along the client's radial bone on the inner wrist.
8. *Dorsalis pedis site:* Palpate along the top of the client's foot lateral to the extensor tendon of the great toe.
9. *Apical site:* Auscultate the apex of the client's heart. Location of the apex will vary with age (Fig. 4–15).

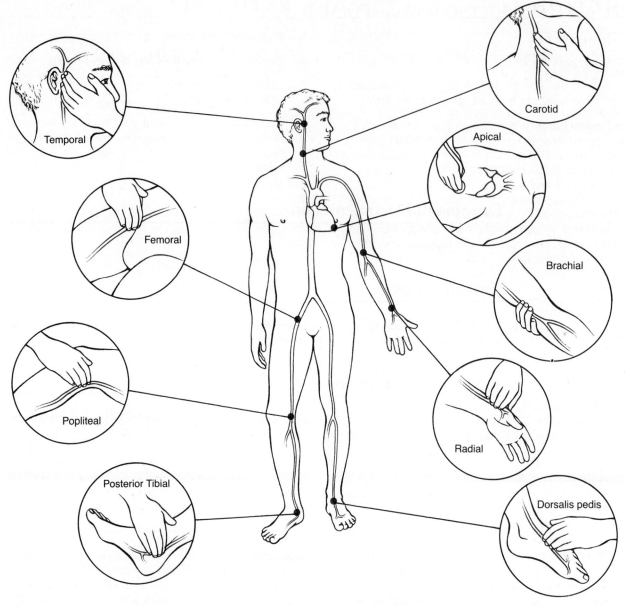

▼ **FIGURE 4–14.** Pulse sites.

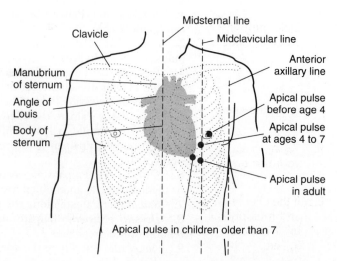

▼ **FIGURE 4–15.** Locating the apical pulse.

SKILL 4–5   MEASURING RADIAL PULSE

Clinical Situations in Which You May Encounter This Skill

Pulse may be measured to obtain baseline data and to detect the presence of arrhythmias or inadequate circulation or other changes in the client's physical condition. The normal rate for adults is between 60 and 100 beats per minute although a well-conditioned athlete may have a normal resting pulse rate between 50 and 60 beats per minute. Table 4–1 shows the normal resting pulse rates across age groups.

The client may have bradycardia (heart rate less than the norm) or tachycardia (heart rate greater than the norm). Heart rates that are too rapid or slow may result in poor perfusion to the body's organs.

Anticipated Responses

▼ The client's pulse is regular and full.
▼ The client's pulse is within normal limits.

Adverse Responses

▼ The client's pulse is irregular and thready.
▼ The client has bradycardia.
▼ The client has tachycardia.

Materials List

Gather these materials before beginning the skill:

▼ Watch with a second hand or digital readout

TABLE 4–1. Normal Resting Pulse Rates–Across Age Groups

Age	Average (Beats per Minute)	Normal Limits
Neonate	120	70–190
1 year	120	80–160
2 years	110	80–130
4 years	100	80–120
6 years	100	75–115
8 years	90	70–110
10 years	90	70–110
12 years		
Female	90	70–110
Male	85	65–105
14 years		
Female	85	65–105
Male	80	60–100
16 years		
Female	80	60–100
Male	75	55–95
18 years		
Female	75	55–95
Male	70	50–90
Well-conditioned athlete	May be 50–60	50–100
Adult		60–100
Aging		60–100

From Jarvis, C. (1992). Physical examination and health assessment. Philadelphia: W. B. Saunders.

▼ ACTION

1. Examine the client's previous pulse rate recordings.

2. Ascertain the client's medical diagnosis and any prior history of arrhythmias.

3. Determine if the client is taking any medications that may affect his or her pulse rate.

4. Assist the client to a position of comfort.

5. Locate the client's radial pulse and palpate with your first three fingers (see Fig. 4–14).

6. If the client's pulse is regular, count for 30 seconds and multiply by 2. If the pulse is irregular, count for 1 minute. Start your count with 0, then "1, 2, 3," etc.

▼ RATIONALE

1. Provides a basis from which to make comparisons.

2. Alerts you to any possible problems or drug use that may cause an irregular pulse or an unusually fast or slow pulse.

3. Drugs such as digoxin slow the pulse and drugs such as antihistamines and theophylline can cause tachycardia. Tricyclic antidepressants, phenothiazines, lithium, and theophylline can cause dysrhythmias.

4. The client's pulse should be measured when the client is at rest.

5. Your thumb should not be used to palpate the client's pulse, as your thumb has a pulse and it may be confused with the client's.

6. The pulse rate is recorded in beats per minute. Irregular pulses should be counted for a full minute to ensure an accurate measurement. Zero begins the time interval and must be included to get an accurate count.

▼ *ACTION*	▼ *RATIONALE*
7. Note the rhythm and volume of the client's pulse.	**7.** Assessing the client's pulse involves more than just counting the rate. The pulse should be described as having a regular or irregular rhythm and should be graded on a four-point scale to describe the volume: 0 = absent; 1+ = weak, thready; 2+ = normal; and 3+ = full, bounding (Jarvis, 1992).
8. Discuss the findings with the client unless inappropriate.	**8.** Keeps the client informed of his or her health status and allows the client to actively participate in his or her care.
9. Wash your hands.	**9.** Decreases the transmission of microorganisms.
10. Record the results.	**10.** Communicates the findings to the other members of the health care team and contributes to the legal record by documenting the care given to the client.

Example of Documentation

See Figure 4–9.

Teaching Tips

When you assess the client's heart rate, teach him or her to check his or her own pulse.

Home Care Variations

Clients may be taught to assess their own pulse using the carotid site. Advantages of this site include easy access and ease of location of the pulse point.

SKILL 4–6   MEASURING APICAL PULSE

Clinical Situations in Which You May Encounter This Skill

The client's heart rate may be assessed by the apical method when the peripheral pulse is weak or irregular, or both. The apical heart rate is commonly assessed before administering medications such as digitalis preparations. The method of choice for obtaining the heart rate of infants and children is by auscultating the apical pulse. See Table 4–1 in Skill 4–5 for information on normal heart rates across age groups.

Anticipated Responses

▼ The client's pulse is regular and the rate is within normal limits.

Adverse Responses

▼ The client's pulse is irregular.
▼ There is bradycardia (pulse less than the norm) or tachycardia (pulse greater than the norm).

Materials List

Gather these materials before beginning the skill:

▼ Stethoscope
▼ Watch with second hand
▼ Alcohol wipes

▼ *A C T I O N* _ _ _ _ _ _ _ _ _ _ _ _ _ _ _ _ _ _   ▼ *R A T I O N A L E* _ _ _ _ _ _ _ _ _ _ _ _ _ _ _

1. Examine the client's previous pulse rate recordings.

2. Ascertain the client's medical diagnosis and any prior history of arrhythmias.

3. Determine if the client is taking any medications that may affect his or her pulse rate.

4. Assist the client to a position of comfort.

5. Locate the apical impulse (see Fig. 4–15):

   For adults: Fourth–Sixth intercostal space, left midclavicular line.
   For children (aged 1 mo–4 yr): Fourth intercostal space, lateral of the left midclavicular line.
   For children (aged 4–7 yr): Fourth intercostal space, left midclavicular line.
   For children (older than 7 yr): Fifth intercostal space, medial to the left midclavicular line.

6. Cleanse the stethoscope chest piece and earpieces with an alcohol wipe before and after the procedure.

7. Warm the endpiece of the stethoscope first by rubbing it in the palm of your hand. Insert the earpieces in your ears with the tips bent forward toward your nose. Place the stethoscope over the apex of the client's heart and count for 1 minute (Fig. 4–16). Start your count with zero, then one, two, three, etc.

1. Provides a basis from which to make comparisons.

2. Alerts you to any possible problems that may cause an irregular pulse or an unusually fast or slow pulse.

3. Drugs such as digoxin slow the pulse and drugs such as antihistamine preparations and theophylline can cause tachycardia. Tricyclic antidepressants, phenothiazines, lithium, and theophylline can cause dysrhythmias.

4. A resting apical pulse is the most accurate.

5. The apical pulse is auscultated best at the apex of the heart.

6. Reduces the transmission of microorganisms.

7. A cold stethoscope can cause discomfort to the client. Earpiece placement conforms to the normal anatomy of the ear canal. Counting for a full minute helps you to obtain an accurate rate. Zero begins the time interval and must be included to get an accurate count.

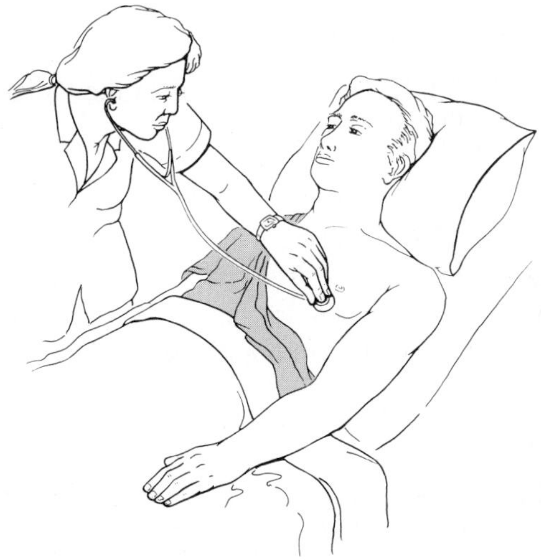

▼ FIGURE 4–16. Auscultating the apical pulse.

8. Note the rhythm.

8. Irregular rhythms should be noted in the client's record.

▼ ACTION	▼ RATIONALE
9. Discuss the findings with the client if appropriate.	9. Keeps the client informed of his or her health status and allows the client to actively participate in his or her care.
10. Wash your hands.	10. Decreases the transmission of microorganisms.
11. Record the results.	11. Communicates the findings to the other members of the health care team and contributes to the legal record by documenting the care given to the client.

Example of Documentation

DATE	TIME	NOTES
1/1/94	0900	Apical heart rate is 64/minute and regular. Digoxin 0.25 mg. P.O. given.
		C. Lammon, RN

Teaching Tips

While you assess the client's heart rate, teach the client to check his or her own pulse.

Home Care Variations

Clients may be taught to assess their own pulse using the carotid site. Advantages of this site include easy access and ease of location of the pulse point.

SKILL 4–7 MEASURING RADIAL-APICAL PULSE

Clinical Situations in Which You May Encounter This Skill

The client's radial-apical pulse is measured when you suspect the presence of a pulse deficit. A pulse deficit is a condition in which the radial pulse rate is less than the apical pulse rate. It indicates that some cardiac impulses are not producing adequate cardiac output to result in a peripheral pulse.

Anticipated Responses

▼ The radial pulse rate is equal to the apical pulse rate.

Adverse Responses

▼ The apical pulse rate is greater than the radial pulse rate, resulting in a pulse deficit.

Materials List

Gather these materials before beginning the skill:

▼ Stethoscope
▼ Watch with second hand or digital display
▼ Alcohol wipes

▼ ACTION	▼ RATIONALE
1. Find an assistant. If a second person is unavailable, an alternate technique is to take serial pulse measurements by assessing the client's radial pulse for 60 seconds followed by the apical pulse for 60 seconds. Then compare the findings.	1. This procedure requires 2 nurses.
2. Examine the client's previous pulse rate recordings.	2. Provides a basis from which to make comparisons.

▼ A C T I O N	▼ R A T I O N A L E

3. Ascertain the client's medical diagnosis and any history of problems that may affect his or her peripheral pulse rate.

3. Alerts you to any possible problem with assessing a radial-apical pulse.

4. Assist the client to a position of comfort.

4. Aids in assessing the apical rate.

First Nurse

5. Clean the earpieces and diaphragm of the stethoscope with alcohol wipes.

5. Prevents the transmission of microorganisms.

6. Locate the client's apical impulse on his or her chest wall.

6. The apical heartbeat is heard best in this position.

7. Warm the endpiece of the stethoscope first by rubbing it in the palm of your hand. Place the diaphragm of the stethoscope over the site of the apical pulse and signal the second nurse that you are ready to count.

7. A cold stethoscope can be uncomfortable for the client. Both nurses must begin and end counting at the same time.

Second Nurse

8. Locate the client's radial pulse using your fingertips and not your thumb. Begin your count.

8. You may feel your own pulse in your thumb.

9. Signal the first nurse that you are ready and both nurses should begin counting the heart rate simultaneously for 1 minute (Fig. 4–17). Start your count with zero, then one, two, three, etc.

9. To obtain an accurate assessment for the presence of a pulse deficit, radial and apical measurements must be taken at the same time. Zero begins the time interval and must be included to get an accurate count.

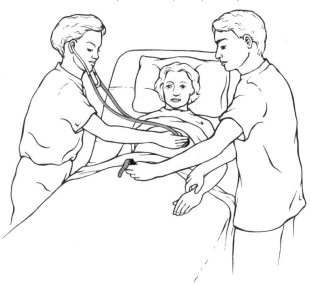

▼ **FIGURE 4–17.** Assessing the apical-radial pulse to identify a pulse deficit.

10. Signal the first nurse to stop counting after 1 minute.

10. To obtain an accurate measurement, the pulse is counted for 1 minute.

Both Nurses

11. Compare the findings.

11. The apical and radial measurements should be the same. If the apical measurement is larger, a pulse deficit exists. If the radial measurement is larger, an error was made and the apical-radial pulse should be reassessed.

▼ *ACTION*	▼ *RATIONALE*
12. Wash your hands.	**12.** Decreases the transmission of microorganisms.
13. Record the results.	**13.** Communicates the findings to the other members of the health care team and contributes to the legal record by documenting the care given to the client.

Example of Documentation

DATE	TIME	NOTES
1/1/94	0800	Peripheral pulse 74/minute, irregular, and thready. Apical pulse 80/minute, irregular. Pulse deficit 6/minute. Occasional PVCs noted on the monitor. BP 110/70. Dr. Smith notified.
		C. Lammon, RN

Teaching Tips

The purpose of and procedure for assessing the radial-apical pulse should be explained to the client or his or her family, or both.

Home Care Variations

A radial-apical pulse measurement usually is not taken in the home setting.

RESPIRATIONS

Normal respiration consists of regular effortless inspiration followed by expiration. Oxygen is inhaled and exchanged in the alveoli for carbon dioxide, which is exhaled.

When you assess respirations, observe their rate and depth. You also should note the character of the respirations. Effortless respiration is called eupnea. Deviations from the norm include dyspnea, orthopnea, wheezing, crackles, and stridor. The rhythm of respirations is also important. Normal respirations are regular. Abnormal breathing patterns include Cheyne-Stokes, Biot's, and Kussmaul's respirations. When you note abnormal respiration patterns, observe for the use of accessory muscles such as the sternocleidomastoid muscle, trapezius muscle, and intercostal muscles; the presence of nasal flaring; a change in the client's level of consciousness; and the presence of pallor or cyanosis. Disturbances in respirations may result in acid-base imbalances. Evaluate the results of an arterial blood gas analysis to determine the presence of acidosis or alkalosis.

SKILL 4–8   MEASURING RESPIRATIONS

Clinical Situations in Which You May Encounter This Skill

Respirations may be measured to obtain baseline data and to detect the presence of respiratory depression or respiratory distress, or other changes in the client's physical condition. Respirations should be moderate to deep in depth, regular, with no use of accessory muscles. There should be no cyanosis of the client's skin, mucous membranes, or nail beds. The adult respiratory rate is 10 to 20 breaths per minute. Table 4–2 shows normal respiration rates across the age groups.

Bradypnea occurs when respirations are less than the norm, tachypnea occurs when respirations are greater than the norm, and dyspnea occurs when respirations are labored or difficult. Apnea is the absence of respirations.

When counting the client's respiratory rate, observe for any signs of respiratory distress such as the use of accessory muscles; cyanosis; retraction of the intercostal muscles and sternum; or nasal flaring. Respiratory distress and apnea are medical emergencies.

Anticipated Responses

▼ The client's respiratory rate is normal.
▼ There are no signs of respiratory distress.
▼ The client's mucous membranes and nail beds are pink.
▼ The client is not using accessory muscles.

Adverse Responses

▼ The client is experiencing bradypnea, tachypnea, dyspnea, or apnea.

Materials List

Gather these materials before beginning the skill:

▼ Watch with second hand

TABLE 4–2. Normal Respiratory Rates

Age	Breaths per Minute
Neonate	30–40
1 year	20–40
2 years	25–32
4 years	23–30
6 years	21–26
8 years	20–26
10 years	20–26
12 years	18–22
14 years	18–22
16 years	16–20
18 years	12–20
Adult	10–20

From Jarvis, C. (1992). Physical examination and health assessment. Philadelphia: W. B. Saunders.

▼ ACTION

1. Examine the client's previous respiratory rate recordings.

2. Ascertain the client's medical diagnosis and any history of respiratory problems or difficulties.

3. Determine if the client is taking any medications that may affect his or her respiratory rate or depth.

4. Explain to the client that you are taking his or her vital signs. Do not specifically tell the client that you are counting respirations.

5. Observe the client's color, depth of respiration, presence of nasal flaring, retractions, use of accessory muscles, and rhythm of respirations. Also observe the body position he or she assumes to breathe.

6. If respirations are regular, count respirations that occur in 30 seconds and multiply by 2. If respiratory efforts are irregular, count the respirations for 1 minute. Count infant respirations for 1 full minute.

7. Note the depth and pattern of respirations.

8. If respiratory distress is noted, report it immediately to the appropriate health care professional.

9. Wash your hands.

10. Record the results.

▼ RATIONALE

1. Provides a basis from which to make comparisons.

2. Alerts you to possible respiratory problems.

3. Medications such as morphine can decrease the rate and depth of respirations.

4. Prevents the client from consciously controlling his or her respirations.

5. Assessing respirations involves more than just counting the client's respiratory rate. Abnormal findings in any of these areas indicate respiratory difficulty and a need for further assessment of the client.

6. Respiratory rate is recorded in breaths per minute. Counting for 15 seconds gives a result that can vary by plus or minus 4, which is significant when working with such small numbers. Irregular respirations should be counted for the full minute to ensure an accurate measurement. It is normal for infants to vary their respiratory rate and pattern.

7. Alerts you to respiratory distress.

8. The client may need immediate medical attention to prevent respiratory failure.

9. Decreases the transmission of microorganisms.

10. Communicates the findings to the other members of the health care team and contributes to the legal record by documenting the care given to the client.

Example of Documentation

See Figure 4–9.

DATE	TIME	NOTES
1/1/94	0800	Respirations 30 and labored. Client in orthopneic position. Use of accessory muscles (sternocleidomastoid and trapezius) noted. Experiencing difficulty speaking due to dyspnea. Nail beds and mucous membranes cyanotic. Skin diaphoretic. Bilateral breath sounds present with inspiratory wheezing noted. Dr. White notified of client's condition.
		C. Lammon, RN

Teaching Tips

While you are assessing the client's respirations, teach the client or his or her family, or both, how to assess respirations.

Home Care Variations

The same procedure is used to assess respirations in the home setting.

BLOOD PRESSURE

Blood pressure is the force exerted by the blood against the arterial wall as it moves through the circulatory system. The systolic pressure represents the maximum pressure exerted on the arteries as the left ventricle contracts. The diastolic pressure represents the amount of pressure always present on the arterial walls during diastole, when the heart is between contractions. The difference between the systolic and diastolic pressure is called the pulse pressure.

When auscultating a blood pressure, you hear a series of sounds called Korotkoff's sounds. These sounds are divided into five phases:

PHASE I: Clear tapping sounds that become more intense. The systolic blood pressure is recorded when you hear two consecutive tapping sounds (American Heart Association (AHA), 1980).

PHASE II: Swishing sounds.

PHASE III: Sounds increase in intensity.

PHASE IV: Sounds muffle to a soft blowing quality. Phase IV is recorded as the diastolic blood pressure in children (AHA, 1980).

PHASE V: Silence. This is recorded as the diastolic blood pressure in adults (AHA, 1980).

SKILL 4–9 MEASURING BLOOD PRESSURE

Clinical Situations in Which You May Encounter This Skill

Blood pressure may be measured to obtain baseline data and to detect changes in the client's physical condition that may lead to the development of hypertension or hypotension. Hypotension can result in inadequate perfusion to the body tissues and organs and prolonged hypertension can result in damage to target organs of the heart (increased risk of myocardial infarction), brain (increased risk of cerebrovascular accident), and kidneys (increased risk of renal disease).

Blood pressure is usually measured in the client's upper arm. Blood pressure may be measured in the thigh when the client's arms are in traction or casts, or when the client has undergone procedures such as an amputation or bilateral radical mastectomy, or has renal dialysis shunts in place.

The adult blood pressure should be between 90/60 and 140/90. An adult blood pressure below 95/60 represents hypotension but, in healthy adults, a persistent systolic pressure of 90 to 100 with no accompanying symptoms is not clinically significant.

Table 4–3 shows the average blood pressure values for children.

Anticipated Responses

▼ The client's blood pressure is within normal limits for the client's age.

Adverse Responses

▼ The client has hypotension (his or her blood pressure is less than the norm).
▼ The client has hypertension (his or her blood pressure is greater than the norm).

Materials List

Gather these materials before beginning the skill:

▼ Stethoscope (Fig. 4–18)
▼ Sphygmomanometer (mercury [Fig. 4–19A] or aneroid [Fig. 4–19B]) with appropriate-sized cuff
▼ Alcohol wipes

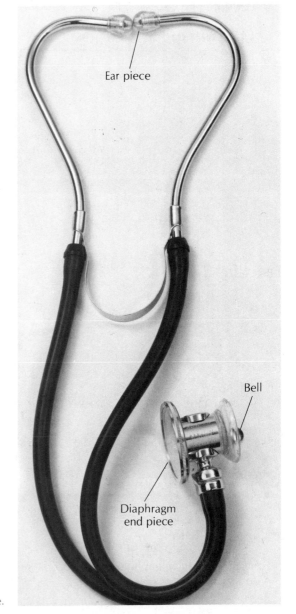

▼ FIGURE 4–18. Stethoscope.

TABLE 4–3. Blood Pressure Readings for Children

Age	Girls		Boys	
	Systolic Blood Pressure	*Diastolic Blood Pressure*	*Systolic Blood Pressure*	*Diastolic Blood Pressure*
6 mo	91	53	90	53
1 yr	91	54	90	56
2 yr	90	56	91	56
3 yr	91	56	92	55
4 yr	92	56	93	56
5 yr	94	56	95	56
6 yr	96	57	96	57
7 yr	97	58	97	58
8 yr	99	59	99	60
9 yr	100	61	101	61
10 yr	102	62	102	62
11 yr	105	64	105	63
12 yr	107	66	107	64
13 yr	109	64	109	63
14 yr	110	67	112	64
15 yr	111	67	114	65
16 yr	112	67	117	67
17 yr	112	66	119	69
18 yr	112	66	121	70

Adapted from the Second Task Force on Blood Pressure Control in Children. (1987). National Heart Lung and Blood Institute. Bethesda, MD: Tabular data (original) prepared by Dr. B. Rosner, 1987.

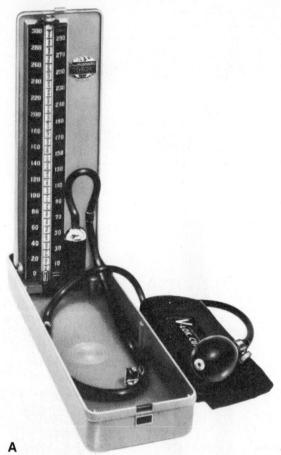

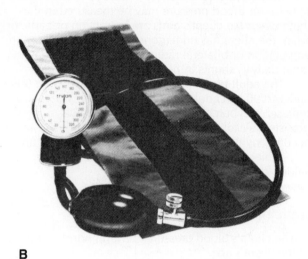

▼ **FIGURE 4–19.** Portable mercury (*A*) and aneroid (*B*) sphygmomanometers. (*A,* Courtesy of W. A. Baum Co., Inc., Copiague, NY 11726.)

▼ *ACTION*	▼ *RATIONALE*
1. Examine the client's previous blood pressure recordings.	1. Provides a basis from which to make comparisons.
2. Ascertain the client's medical diagnosis and any history of problems that may affect his or her blood pressure.	2. Alerts you to any possible problems or medications that may affect the blood pressure measurement.
3. Determine if the client is taking any medications that may affect his or her blood pressure.	3. Drugs such as phenothiazines or antihypertensives can decrease blood pressure.

▼ *ACTION*

▼ *RATIONALE*

4. Select the appropriate cuff size (Fig. 4–20).

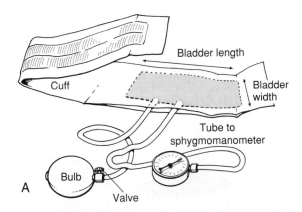

4. The width of the bladder of the blood pressure cuff should equal 40% of the circumference of the client's upper arm (Fig. 4–20C). The length of the bladder of the blood pressure cuff should equal 80% of the circumference of the client's upper arm (AHA, 1980). A cuff that is too narrow will give a false high reading. A false low reading will be obtained if the cuff is too wide.

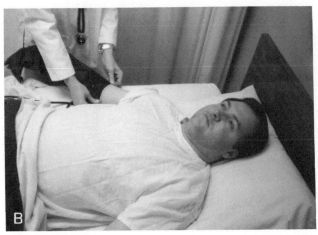
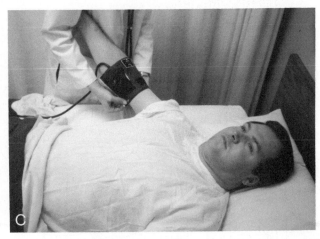

▼ **FIGURE 4–20.** (*A*) Blood pressure cuff with attachments. The cuff shows the bladder length and width. The width of the bladder should equal 40% of the circumference of the client's upper arm. (*B* and *C*) The length of the bladder should equal 80% of the circumference of the client's upper arm.

5. Position the client's arm at heart level with his or her palm up.

5. Placement of the arm below heart level causes false high readings. Placement of the arm above heart level causes false low readings.

6. Locate the brachial pulse.

6. Facilitates correct placement of the stethoscope so that you can hear Korotkoff's sounds.

7. Snugly apply the cuff with the center of the bladder over the client's brachial artery, 1 to 2 inches above the antecubital fossa. Do not apply the cuff over the client's clothes.

7. Facilitates equal compression of the brachial artery. Clothing interferes with correct cuff placement. A loose cuff may cause a false high reading (Thompson, 1981).

For a Palpatory Reading

8. a. Palpate the client's brachial artery as you inflate the cuff.
   b. Pump the cuff up 30 mmHg higher than the point at which you last felt the client's pulse.

   c. Slowly deflate the cuff and identify the point at which you feel the pulse return.

8. a. Checking the palpatory pressure aids in identifying the presence of an auscultatory gap.
   b. The pulse will disappear when the cuff pressure equals the systolic pressure. Pumping the cuff higher helps you to find the exact point at which the return of a palpable pulse will be felt.
   c. Record this value as the palpatory systolic reading.

▼ *ACTION*   ▼ *RATIONALE*

For an Auscultatory Reading

8. a. Clean the earpieces and the chest piece of the stethoscope with alcohol and insert the earpieces into your ears.

b. Apply the bell of the stethoscope firmly over the client's brachial artery.

c. To read a mercury scale, position yourself so the scale is at eye-level and at a distance of no more than 3 feet (Fig. 4–21A). To read an aneroid scale, look directly at the gauge (Fig. 4–21B).

8. a. Prevents the transmission of bacteria.

b. Korotkoff's sounds are of low frequency, and the bell is best for auscultating low-frequency sounds.

c. Ensures accurate visualization of the scale.

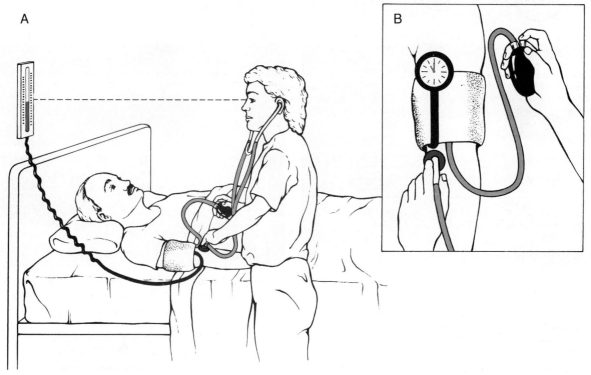

▼ **FIGURE 4–21.** (A) Reading a mercury scale. (B) Reading an aneroid scale.

d. Close the valve, and inflate the cuff rapidly about 20 to 30 mmHg above the point at which the artery pulsation is obliterated.

e. Deflate the cuff by slowly opening the valve at a rate of 2 to 3 mmHg per heartbeat.

f. Note when you hear the first beat.

g. Note a "muffling" sound. Note the last beat heard.

h. Completely deflate the cuff and remove it from the client's arm. Wait 30 to 60 seconds before taking the blood pressure again. If the sounds are faint, elevate the client's arm and inflate the cuff. Then lower the client's arm and assess the blood pressure as you deflate the cuff.

d. Rapid inflation causes Korotkoff's sounds to be louder. By inflating above the point at which pulsation is no longer felt, you avoid missing an auscultatory gap.

e. Ensures the accurate measurement of blood pressure.

f. The first beat corresponds with Phase I of Korotkoff's sounds. This represents the systolic pressure.

g. In children, the diastolic pressure corresponds best with Phase IV (muffling); in adults, Phase V (silence) best reflects diastolic pressure.

h. Continuous cuff inflation causes decreased arterial blood flow, numbness to the client's arm, and falsely elevated succeeding blood pressure readings. Arm elevation decreases venous pressure and makes the sounds louder.

▼ *A C T I O N*   ▼ *R A T I O N A L E*

For a Thigh Reading

8. a. Select the appropriate size cuff.

8. a. The width of the bladder of the blood pressure cuff should equal 40% of the circumference of the client's lower extremity. The length of the bladder of the blood pressure cuff should equal 80% of the circumference of the client's lower extremity (AHA, 1980).

b. Position the client in the prone position.

b. Facilitates access to the client's popliteal artery.

c. Locate the client's popliteal pulse. This pulse may be difficult to locate in many adults.

c. Facilitates the correct placement of the stethoscope so that you can hear Korotkoff's sounds.

d. Snugly apply the cuff with the center of the bladder over the artery, 1 to 2 inches above the bend of the client's knee (Fig. 4–22).

d. Facilitates equal compression of the popliteal artery.

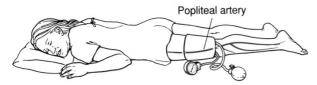

Popliteal artery

▼ **FIGURE 4–22.** Applying a blood pressure cuff for a thigh reading.

e. Apply the bell of the stethoscope directly over the popliteal pulse.

e. Facilitates optimal sound. When using the bell, lightly place it over the artery. If you are using the diaphragm, firmly place it over the artery.

f. To read an aneroid scale, look directly at the gauge. To read a mercury scale, position yourself so that the scale is at eye-level and at a distance of no more than 3 feet.

f. Ensures accurate visualization of the scale.

g. Close the valve and inflate the cuff rapidly 20 to 30 mmHg above the anticipated systolic reading.

g. Rapid inflation causes Korotkoff's sounds to be louder. By inflating above the systolic reading, you avoid missing an auscultatory gap.

h. Deflate the cuff by slowly opening the valve at a rate of 2 to 3 mmHg per second.

h. Ensures accurate measurement of the client's blood pressure.

i. Note when you hear the first beat.

i. The first beat corresponds with Phase I. This represents the systolic pressure.

j. Note when you hear the last beat.

j. The last beat corresponds with Phase IV for children and Phase V for adults.

k. Completely deflate the cuff and remove it from the client's leg.

k. Continuous cuff inflation causes decreased arterial blood flow and numbness to the client's leg.

9. Discuss the findings with the client if appropriate.

9. Keeps the client informed of his or her own health status and allows the client to actively participate in his or her own care.

10. Wash your hands.

10. Decreases the transmission of microorganisms.

11. Record the results.

11. Communicates the findings to the other members of the health care team and contributes to the legal record by documenting the care given to the client.

> **NOTE:** The systolic pressure may be 10 to 40 mmHg higher in the thigh than in the arms.

Diastolic pressure is the same in both sites.

Example of Documentation

See Figure 4–9.

Teaching Tips

When you assess the client's blood pressure, begin to teach the client good health practices to control or prevent hypertension, as well as how to check his or her own blood pressure at home.

Home Care Variations

If the client is unable to manipulate a standard sphygmomanometer, an electronic blood pressure machine may be useful for frequent monitoring of the client's blood pressure at home.

SKILL 4–10   MEASURING FETAL HEART TONES

Clinical Situations in Which You May Encounter This Skill

Fetal heart tones may be measured to obtain baseline data and to detect changes in the physical condition of the unborn child. The normal fetal heart tone rate is 120 to 160 beats per minute. Bradycardia is indicated by a heart rate of less than 120 beats per minute and tachycardia is indicated by a heart rate of more than 160 beats per minute.

You may be unable to auscultate fetal heart tones because of the position of the fetus in the mother's uterus. Assess for fetal movements to differentiate this situation from absent heart tones resulting from fetal demise. Alterations in the rate of fetal heart tones can indicate fetal distress.

Fetal heart tones are audible with a Doppler ultrasonic flow meter approximately 14 to 16 weeks after the woman's last menstrual period. Fetal heart tones can be auscultated with a fetoscope approximately 20 weeks after the woman's last menstrual period.

Anticipated Responses

▼ Fetal heart tones are present.

Adverse Responses

▼ The fetus has bradycardia or tachycardia.
▼ There are no fetal heart tones.

Materials List

Gather these materials before beginning the skill:

▼ Fetoscope and alcohol wipes
▼ Doppler ultrasonic flow meter and transmission gel for ultrasound

---

▼ ACTION	▼ RATIONALE
1. Examine the previous recording of the heart rate of the fetus.	1. Provides a basis from which to make comparisons.
2. Raise bed to working height. Help the client to lie down in the supine position.	2. Provides for proper bed mechanics. Enables you to palpate the mother's abdomen.

▼ *ACTION* _ ▼ *RATIONALE* _ _ _ _ _ _ _ _ _ _ _ _ _ _ _ _ _

3. Use Leopold's maneuvers to locate the position of the fetus in the client's abdomen by gently palpating the upper and lower borders of the uterus and the lateral borders of the uterus (Fig. 4–23).

3. Locating the fetal position is necessary to assess fetal heart tones since you must place your fetoscope or Doppler ultrasonic flow meter on the mother's abdomen overlying the baby's upper back.

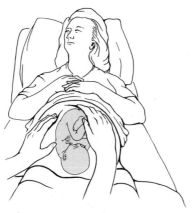

A First maneuver

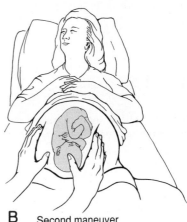

B Second maneuver

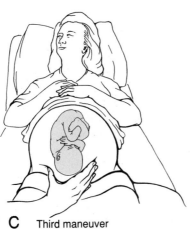

C Third maneuver

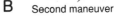

D Fourth maneuver

▼ **FIGURE 4–23.** Leopold's maneuvers.

Using a Fetoscope

4. a. Clean the earpieces and abdominal piece of the fetoscope with alcohol wipes and place the earpieces in your ears.
   b. Place the forehead rest of the fetoscope on your forehead.

4. a. Prevents the spread of bacteria.

   b. The fetoscope uses both air and bone conduction to enhance fetal heart tones.

▼ A C T I O N   ▼ R A T I O N A L E

c. Position the bell of the fetoscope on the mother's abdomen over the area where the back of the fetus was previously located (Fig. 4–24).

c. Fetal heart tones will be heard best here because there is less tissue between the baby's heart and your fetoscope.

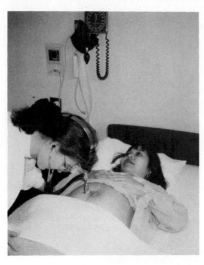

▼ FIGURE 4–24. Assessing fetal heart tones with the fetoscope.

d. Press the fetoscope bell firmly onto the mother's abdomen. You may need to relocate the fetus and fetoscope if no fetal heart tones are heard in this position.

e. Count the fetal heart rate for 1 minute.

f. Discuss the findings with the client if appropriate.

g. Lower the bed.
h. Wash your hands.
i. Record the results in the client's chart.

d. Facilitates the best sound. The baby may have moved.

e. Fetal heart tones are recorded in beats per minute.

f. Keeps the client informed of her health status and allows the client to actively participate in her own care.

g. Provides client safety.
h. Decreases the transmission of microorganisms.
i. Communicates the findings to the other members of the health care team and contributes to the legal record by documenting the care given to the client.

Using a Doppler Ultrasonic Flow Meter

4. a. Follow Steps 1 through 3 of the above procedure.
   b. Place a small amount of transmission gel over the mother's abdomen where the back of the fetus was previously located.

4. a. Facilitates the use of the Doppler ultrasonic flow meter.
   b. Facilitates the location of heart tones.

▼ *ACTION* _ _ _ _ _ _ _ _ _ _ _ _ _ _ _ _ ▼ *RATIONALE* _ _ _ _ _ _ _ _ _ _

c. Turn on the Doppler ultrasonic flow meter and gently move it along the skin of the mother's abdomen. Listen for the sound of blood flowing through the arteries (Fig. 4–25).

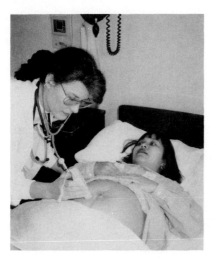

▼ **FIGURE 4–25.** Assessing fetal heart tones with the Doppler ultrasonic flow meter.

d. Follow Steps e through g (p. 90) of the above procedure.

5. Wash your hands.

6. Record the results.

5. Decreases the transmission of microorganisms.

6. Communicates the findings to the other members of the health care team and contributes to the legal record by documenting the care given to the client.

Example of Documentation

DATE	*TIME*	*NOTES*
4/5/94		First visit of this 23 y.o. primigravida. Weight 168 lb., BP 130/80. Estimated gestation 22 weeks. Fundal height 20 cm. FHT auscultated at 150/min. in maternal right upper quadrant of abdomen.
		C. Lammon, RN

Teaching Tips

While you assess fetal heart tones, talk with the client about normal fetal growth and development.

Home Care Variations

Fetal heart tones can be assessed in the client's home using the same technique.

SKILL 4–11   ASSESSING CIRCULATION

Clinical Situations in Which You May Encounter This Skill

You should assess a client's peripheral perfusion after a splint, cast, or traction has been applied to an extremity; after a vascular procedure or surgery on an extremity; or after other trauma to an extremity. See Figure 4–14 for locations of peripheral pulse sites.

Anticipated Responses

▼ There is satisfactory circulation to the client's extremity as indicated by warm skin and absence of pallor or cyanosis.
▼ There is an absence of numbness, pain, tingling, or other unusual sensations.
▼ The client is able to move the extremity.
▼ There is rapid capillary refill of the client's nail beds (1–3 sec).
▼ There is absence of edema.
▼ There is a palpable peripheral pulse.

Adverse Responses

▼ The client experiences diminished or absent circulation indicated by cool skin, pallor or cyanosis, numbness, pain, tingling, or other unusual sensations.
▼ The client is unable to move the extremity.
▼ There is delayed or absent capillary refill of the client's nail beds (greater than 3 sec).
▼ The client experiences edema.
▼ There is a weak thready or absent peripheral pulse.
▼ Diminished or absent circulation has resulted in tissue hypoxia that may lead to the death of tissues if not corrected rapidly.

Materials List

Gather these materials before beginning the skill:

▼ Doppler stethoscope (optional)
▼ Transmission gel (optional)
▼ Felt-tipped marker (optional)

▼ ACTION	▼ RATIONALE
1. Examine the client's previous circulation check recordings.	1. Provides a basis from which to make comparisons.
2. Ascertain whether the client has a medical condition or has had diagnostic testing that may have impaired his or her circulatory status.	2. Alerts you to the pulse points to be assessed.
3. Plan to assess the portion of the client's extremity distal to the point of the potential constriction of circulation.	3. Oxygenated blood flows proximal to distal in the arterial system.
4. Ask the client if he or she feels any numbness, pain, tingling, or other unusual sensations in the distal portion of the extremity.	4. Numbness, tingling, and loss of sensation indicate hypoxia caused by poor circulation.
5. Inspect the distal portion of the client's extremity for the color of the skin and nail beds; edema; and the client's ability to move.	5. A pale or cyanotic color of the skin or nail beds, cool or cold skin, or a decreased or absent ability to move the extremities indicates poor circulation.

▼ *ACTION* _ _ _ _ _ _ _ _ _ _ _ _ _ _ _   ▼ *RATIONALE* _ _ _ _ _ _ _ _ _ _ _ _ _ _

6. Inspect the client's nail beds for capillary refill by pressing on them and observing for blanching (Fig. 4–26). Note the refill time.

6. The capillary refill of nail beds should occur immediately after blanching.

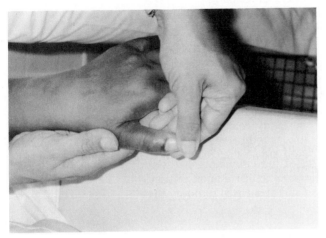

▼ **FIGURE 4–26.** Press on the nail bed to assess capillary refill.

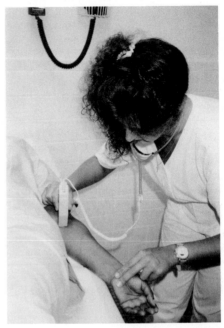

▼ **FIGURE 4–27.** Assessing circulation with a Doppler ultrasonic flow meter.

7. Use the backs of your fingers to feel both of the client's distal extremities in order to compare the temperature.

7. Cool or cold skin can indicate poor circulation. You will be better able to discriminate temperature differences if you use the dorsal aspects of your fingers.

8. Palpate the client's peripheral pulses below the area of potential circulation constriction for presence and volume. Grade the pulse volume using a scale approved by your institution (sample scale: 0 = absent; 1+ = weak, thready; 2+ = full; and 3+ = bounding).

8. Weak or absent pulses can indicate poor circulation.

9. If necessary, use a Doppler ultrasonic flow meter to locate faint or weak pulses by placing a small amount of transmission gel over the pulse site and slowly moving the Doppler over the area. Auscultate for the rhythmical sound of blood flowing through the artery (Fig. 4–27).

9. The Doppler ultrasonic flow meter amplifies the sound of blood flowing through the artery.

10. If the client's pulses are weak and thready, you may wish to mark the location of the pulse with a felt-tipped marker for future reference.

10. Assists in providing interrater reliability.

11. Wash your hands.

11. Decreases the transmission of microorganisms.

12. Notify the physician if your assessment indicates poor or deteriorating circulation.

12. Immediate medical care may be necessary to prevent loss of the client's extremity.

13. Chart your findings in the client's record.

13. Communicates the findings to the other members of the health care team and contributes to the legal record by documenting the care given to the client.

Example of Documentation

DATE	TIME	NOTES
1/1/94	0800	Cast intact on right leg. Pedal pulse 2 + . Toes warm, pink. No edema, pallor, or cyanosis noted. Denies pain, numbness, tingling, or unusual sensations in toes of right foot. Can move toes without difficulty. Capillary refill = 2 seconds.
		C. Lammon, RN

Teaching Tips

Explain the procedure and the purpose of the procedure to the client or his or her family, or both. If the client has a cast and needs to check his or her circulatory status at home, demonstrate the procedure and have the client perform a return demonstration. The client also should know the signs of decreased circulation and be advised to notify the physician if there are signs of decreased circulation.

Home Care Variations

The same procedure can be used to do circulatory checks in the client's home.

SKILL 4–12   ASSESSING NEUROLOGIC STATUS

Clinical Situations in Which You May Encounter This Skill

Neurologic checks are usually performed for clients with a suspected or known brain injury, intracranial bleed, intracranial tumor, or after the client has had cranial surgery. Neurologic checks are used to detect neurologic changes and to assess the client's neurologic status.

Anticipated Responses

▼ The client is alert and oriented.
▼ The client is able to follow commands.
▼ The client is able to open his or her eyes spontaneously.
▼ The client's pupils are equal, round, and reactive to light.
▼ There is a consensual light reflex.
▼ There is spontaneous movement of all of the client's extremities with equal strength.

Adverse Responses

▼ The client is no longer oriented to time, place, or person.
▼ The client is unable to follow commands or open his or her eyes spontaneously.
▼ The client's pupils are unequal, not round, sluggishly reactive, or nonreactive to light.
▼ A consensual light reflex is not present.
▼ There is absence of spontaneous movement, movement only to painful stimuli, or absence of movement to painful stimuli.
▼ The client has decorticate or decerebrate posturing.
▼ There is weakness or drift in an upper extremity.

Materials List

Gather these materials before beginning the skill:

▼ Penlight or flashlight
▼ Pen or pencil

▼ ACTION

1. Note the results of the client's last neurologic assessment.

2. Check the client's medical diagnosis and health history.

▼ RATIONALE

1. Provides baseline data with which to compare your results.

2. Alerts you to areas that may be affected by current or previous health problems.

▼ *ACTION*   ▼ *RATIONALE*

3. If the client is alert, explain that you will be asking some "easy" questions over and over and it may seem silly but it is important that he or she answer seriously each time.

3. A client may get upset at having to answer the same question over and over. An explanation will help the client to understand that this is necessary to determine if there has been a change in his or her neurologic status.

Assessing the Client's Level of Consciousness

4. Ask the client to:
  a. State his or her name.
  b. State where he or she is.
  c. Identify the year, month, date, and day of the week.

4. Determines the client's orientation to time, place, and person.

5. Ask the client to squeeze your hand.

5. Determines the client's ability to follow simple motor commands.

6. Ask the client to open his or her eyes. If the client does not open his or her eyes, apply pressure to the client's nail beds with your pen.

6. Determines if the client can open his or her eyes spontaneously to sound, pain, or not at all.

Assessing the Client's Pupillary Status

7. Inspect the position and shape of the client's pupils. It may be necessary to hold the client's eyelid open (Fig. 4–28).

7. Determines if the client's pupils are deviated from the midline and are of a normal shape. Abnormally shaped pupils may indicate damage to the central nervous system.

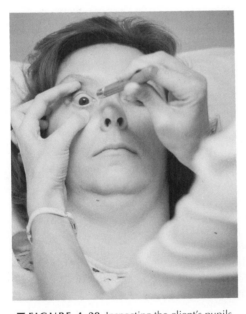

▼ **FIGURE 4–28.** Inspecting the client's pupils.

8. Darken the client's room and quickly bring the penlight or flashlight from behind the client's head to the side and into his or her eye and then back to the side. Note if the pupils react equally and briskly, sluggishly, or do not respond to light.

8. Determines if the client's pupils react to light. The range for the diameter of the pupil is 2 to 6 millimeters. A normal reaction is a brisk constriction of the pupil. Bilateral fixed and dilated pupils indicate increased intracranial pressure; this is an ominous sign. Anticholinergic drugs may dilate the pupils with a corresponding decrease in neurologic status. Bilateral pinpoint pupils can indicate damage to the pons or use of miotic medications or narcotics.

▼ *ACTION*	▼ *RATIONALE*

9. Bring the penlight or flashlight in laterally and shine it directly into one of the client's pupils. Note the reaction of the other pupil.

9. Tests for a consensual light reflex. Both pupils should constrict simultaneously. The lack of constriction of the opposite pupil can indicate damage to the third cranial nerve.

Assessing the Client's Motor Function

10. Observe all of the client's extremities.

   a. If the client is conscious, ask him or her to squeeze your hands. Both of the client's hands should be tested simultaneously. Also, have the client push against your hands with both feet.

   b. If the client is not conscious and no spontaneous movement is observed, apply pressure to the nail bed of each of his or her extremities with a pen or pencil. Observe whether the client localizes the pain (flexes the extremity and withdraws), assumes a decerebrate or decorticate posture (Fig. 4–29), or has no response.

10. Checks for any spontaneous movement.

   a. Checks the strength of the client's extremities. Motor strength diminishes or becomes absent with increased intracranial pressure.

   b. A painful stimulus may be necessary to elicit movement of the client's extremity. The client who exhibits decorticate posturing will hold his or her arms tight to the chest with the elbows, wrists, and fingers flexed. There will be extension and internal rotation of the legs with plantar flexion of the feet. The client who exhibits decerebrate posturing will adduct and stiffly extend the arms at the elbows. The forearm will be pronated with flexion of the fingers and wrists. There will be hyperextension of the neck and extension of the legs with plantar flexion of the feet.

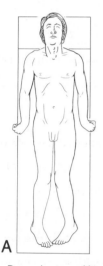
A
Decerebrate position

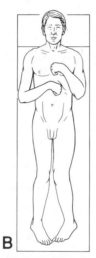
B
Decorticate position

▼ **FIGURE 4–29.**

11. Ask the client to close his or her eyes and extend both arms with the palms turned up and to keep his or her arms in that position for approximately 30 seconds. This may be done with the client in a sitting or standing position.

11. Tests the client's arm strength against gravity. If the client has a weak arm, it will drift downward and the palm will pronate; this could suggest a mild hemiparesis.

12. Wash your hands.

12. Decreases the transmission of microorganisms.

13. Notify the physician if your assessment indicates a deteriorating condition.

13. Immediate medical care may be necessary.

14. If the assessment revealed a deteriorating condition, reassess the client's neurologic status again in 15 to 30 minutes.

14. It is important to know if the client continues to deteriorate.

15. Chart the exact findings of each step of the examination.

15. Communicates the findings to the other members of the health care team and contributes to the legal record by documenting the care given to the client.

Example of Documentation

DATE	TIME	NOTES
10/25/94	0800	Alert and oriented ×3. Able to follow simple commands. Pupils 3.0 mm, in midposition, equal, round, and reactive to light. Consensual light reflex present. Moves and has equal strength in all of extremities.

L. White, RN

Teaching Tips

When you perform a neurologic assessment, talk with the client's family regarding his or her predisease state and teach the family about any deficits.

References

Abrams, L., et al. (1989). Effect of peripheral IV infusion on neonatal axillary temperature measurement. *Pediatric Nursing*, 15, 630–632.

American Heart Association. (1980). *Recommendations for human blood pressure determination by sphygmomanometers.* Dallas: The Association.

Anderson, M. S. (1984). Assessment under pressure: When your patient says, "My head hurts." *Nursing 84*, 14 (9), 34–41.

Baker, N., et al. (1984). The effect of type of thermometer and length of time inserted on oral temperature measurements of afebrile subjects. *Nursing Research*, 33, 109–111.

Barber, N., and Kilmon, C. A. (1989). Reactions to tympanic temperature measurement in an ambulatory setting. *Pediatric Nursing*, 15, 477–481.

Bliss-Holtz, J. (1989). Comparison of rectal, axillary, and inguinal temperatures in full-term newborn infants. *Nursing Research*, 38, 85–87.

Byra-Cook, C. J., Dracup, K. A., and Lazik, A. J. (1990). Direct and indirect blood pressure in critical care patients. *Nursing Research*, 39, 285–288.

Cahill, M. (1984). *Neurological disorders.* Springhouse, PA. Springhouse Corporation.

Clochesy, J. M. (1986). Systemic blood pressure in various lateral recumbent positions: A pilot study. *Heart and Lung: Journal of Critical Care*, 15, 593–594.

Dairs, M. J., and Nomura, L. A. (1990). Vital signs of Class I surgical patients. *Western Journal of Nursing Research*, 12 (1), 28–41.

Durham, M. L., Swanson, B., and Paulford, N. (1986). Effect of tachypnea on oral temperature estimation: A replication. *Nursing Research*, 35, 211–214.

Erickson, R. (1980). Oral temperature differences in relation to thermometer and technique. *Nursing Research*, 29, 157–159.

Erickson, R. S., and Yount, S. T. (1991). Comparison of tympanic and oral temperature in surgical patients. *Nursing Research*, 40, 90–93.

Graves, R. D., and Markarian, M. F. (1980). Three-minute time interval when using an oral mercury-in-glass thermometer with or without J-Temp Sheaths. *Nursing Research*, 29, 323–324.

Hasler, M. E., and Cohen, J. A. (1982). The effect of oxygen administration on oral temperature assessment. *Nursing Research*, 31, 265–268.

Heidrenreich, T., and Giuffre, M. (1990). Postoperative temperature measurement. *Nursing Research*, 39, 153–155.

Heinz, J. (1985). Validation of sublingual temperatures in patients with nasogastric tubes. *Heart & Lung: Journal of Critical Care*, 14, 128–130.

Hellman, R., and Grimm, S. A. (1984). The influence of talking on diastolic blood pressure readings. *Research in Nursing and Health*, 7, 253–256.

Hollerbach, A. D., and Sneed, N. (1990). Accuracy of radial pulse assessment by length of counting interval. *Heart & Lung*, 19, 258–264.

Holtz, J. B. (1989). Comparison of rectal, axillary, and inguinal temperatures in full-term newborn infants. *Nursing Research*, 38, 85–87.

Jarvis, C. (1992). *Physical examination and health assessment.* Philadelphia: W. B. Saunders.

Jarvis, C. M., and Heffernan, L. (1993). Assessing vital signs. In V. Bolander (Ed.), *Basic nursing* (3rd ed.). Philadelphia: W. B. Saunders.

Kunnel, M. T., et al. (1988). Comparisons of rectal, femoral, axillary, and skin-to-mattress temperatures in stable neonates. *Nursing Research*, 37, 162–164.

Lanuza, D. M., et al. (1989). Body temperature and heart rate rhythms in acutely head-injured patients. *Applied Nursing Research*, 2 (3), 135–139.

Lord-Feroli, K., and Maguire-McGinty, M. (1985). Toward a more objective approach to pupil assessment. *Journal of Neurosurgical Nursing*, 17, 309–312.

Mauro, A. M. (1988). Effects of bell versus diaphragm on indirect blood pressure measurement. *Heart and Lung: Journal of Critical Care*, 17, 489–494.

Mown, J. E., et al. (1987). Axillary versus rectal temperatures in preterm infants under radiant warmers. *Journal of Obstetric, Gynecologic, and Neonatal Nursing*, 16, 348–352.

Neff, J., et al. (1989). Effect of respiratory rate, respiratory depth, and open- versus closed-mouth breathing on sublingual temperature. *Research in Nursing and Health*, 12, 195–202.

Norman, E., Gadaleta, D., and Clayton, C. C. (1991). An evaluation of three blood pressure methods in a stabilized acute trauma population. *Nursing Research*, 40, 86–89.

Rebenson-Piano, M., et al. (1989). An evaluation of two indirect methods of blood pressure measurement in ill patients. *Nursing Research*, 38, 42–45.

Samples, J., et al. (1985). Circadian rhythms: Basis for screening for fever. *Nursing Research*, 34, 377–379.

Second Task Force on Blood Pressure Control in Children. (1987). Bethesda, MD: National Heart Lung and Blood Institute.

Tachovsky, B. J. (1985). Indirect auscultatory blood pressure measurement at two sites in the arm. *Research in Nursing and Health*, 8, 125–129.

Thompson, D. R. (1981). Recording patient's blood pressure: A review. *Journal of Advanced Nursing*, 6, 283.

Walleck, C. A. (1982). A neurologic assessment procedure that won't make you nervous. *Nursing 82*, 12 (12), 50–57.

Wilson, S. F., et al. (1988). Determining interrater reliability of nurses' assessments of pupillary size and reaction. *Journal of Neuroscience Nursing*, 20 (3), 189–192.

Yonkman, C. A. (1982). Cool and heated aerosol and the measurement of oral temperature. *Nursing Research*, 31, 354–357.

CHAPTER 5.

Health Assessment

You will participate as a member of the health care team in collecting health assessment data. You may measure vital signs (see Chapter 4), weigh and measure clients, and collect specimens of various body fluids for analysis. Universal precautions should always be followed when collecting specimens. Refer to the inner cover of this text for information on universal precautions.

OVERVIEW OF RELATED RESEARCH

COLLECTING A STOOL SPECIMEN

Yannelli, B., et al. (1988). Yield of stool cultures, ova and parasite tests, and *Clostridium difficile* determinations in nosocomial diarrheas. *American Journal of Infection Control*, 16, 246–249.

This retrospective study investigated the incidence of pathogens in nosocomial diarrhea. Stool cultures were obtained from clients with nosocomial diarrhea. A total of 452 stool cultures were obtained from 118 clients. None of the stools were positive for ova or parasites. One culture was positive for *Campylobacter jejuni* and 47 were positive for *Clostridium difficile*. The findings suggest that it may not be cost-effective to culture stools for ova and parasites in clients with nosocomial diarrhea.

SKILL 5–1   MEASURING THE HEIGHT AND WEIGHT OF THE AMBULATORY CLIENT

Clinical Situations in Which You May Encounter This Skill

Height and weight are measured to provide baseline data, determine drug dosages, monitor changes in physical status, and determine the effectiveness of treatments. Plot the infant's or child's height and weight on a growth chart. Compare the height and weight of an adult to standardized tables of height and weight by body frame size (Table 5–1). Also, consider the family and ethnic heritage of the individual before making the determination that the individual's growth and development are abnormal.

Anticipated Responses

▼ The client demonstrates normal growth and development for his or her age.

Adverse Responses

▼ The person is underweight (at least 10% less than the norm).
▼ The person is overweight (at least 10% more than the norm).
▼ The person is obese (at least 20 to 30% more than the norm).
▼ There has been a large shift in the person's weight since the day before (indicates fluid loss or retention).

Materials List

Gather these materials before beginning the skill:

▼ Platform balance scales
▼ Paper towel

▼ *ACTION*	▼ *RATIONALE*
1. Determine if the client is able to safely balance and stand on the scales.	1. If the client is unable to safely balance and stand, you should use the bed scales.
2. If available, assess the client's previous weight.	2. Enables you to detect changes in the client's weight.
3. Ask the client to remove his or her shoes.	3. Allows measurement of more accurate body weight.
4. Place a paper towel on the scale platform.	4. Prevents cross-contamination of microorganisms to the client's feet.
5. Calibrate the scale to 0.	5. Allows the scale to reflect the client's weight accurately.
6. Help the client to stand on the platform and face the balance beam. Toddlers may sit on the scale.	6. Prevents potential injury to the client.
7. Instruct the client to remain still while you weigh him or her.	7. Allows the beam to balance and measure the client's weight accurately.

TABLE 5–1. Height and Weight by Body Frame Size

To Make an Approximation of Your Frame Size...

Extend your arm and bend the forearm upward at a 90-degree angle. Keep fingers straight and turn the inside of your wrist toward your body. If you have a caliper, use it to measure the space between the two prominent bones on *either side* of your elbow. Without a caliper, place thumb and index finger of your other hand on these two bones. Measure the space between your fingers against a ruler or tape measure. Compare it with these tables that list elbow measurements for *medium-framed* men and women. Measurements lower than those listed indicate you have a small frame. Higher measurements indicate a large frame.

Height in 1″ heels Men	*Elbow* Breadth
5′2″–5′3″	2½″–2⅞″
5′4″–5′7″	2⅝″–2⅞″
5′8″–5′11″	2¾″–3″
6′0″–6′3″	2¾″–3⅛″
6′4″	2⅞″–3¼″

Women	
4′10″–4′11″	2¼″–2½″
5′0″–5′3″	2¼″–2½″
5′4″–5′7″	2⅜″–2⅝″
5′8″–5′11″	2⅜″–2⅝″
6′0″	2½″–2¾″

	Men					*Women*		
Height Feet	*Inches*	*Small* *Frame*	*Medium* *Frame*	*Large* *Frame*	*Height* Feet Inches	*Small* *Frame*	*Medium* *Frame*	*Large* *Frame*
5	2	128–134	131–141	138–150	4 10	102–111	109–121	118–131
5	3	130–136	133–143	140–153	4 11	103–113	111–123	120–134
5	4	132–138	135–145	142–156	5 0	104–115	113–126	122–137
5	5	134–140	137–148	144–160	5 1	106–118	115–129	125–140
5	6	136–142	139–151	146–164	5 2	108–121	118–132	128–143
5	7	138–145	142–154	149–168	5 3	111–124	121–135	131–147
5	8	140–148	145–157	152–172	5 4	114–127	124–138	134–151
5	9	142–151	148–160	155–176	5 5	117–130	127–141	137–155
5	10	144–154	151–163	158–180	5 6	120–133	130–144	140–159
5	11	146–157	154–166	161–184	5 7	123–136	133–147	143–163
6	0	149–160	157–170	164–188	5 8	126–139	136–150	146–167
6	1	152–164	160–174	168–192	5 9	129–142	139–153	149–170
6	2	155–168	164–178	172–197	5 10	132–145	142–156	152–173
6	3	158–172	167–182	176–202	5 11	135–148	145–159	155–176
6	4	162–176	171–187	181–207	6 0	138–151	148–162	158–179

Weights at ages 25 to 59 years based on lowest mortality. Weight in pounds according to frame (in indoor clothing weighing 5 lbs for men and 3 lbs for women; shoes with 1-inch heels).

(Source of basic data 1979 Build Study Society of Actuaries and Association of Life Insurance Medical Directors of America, 1980. Copyright 1983 Metropolitan Life Insurance Company.)

▼ *ACTION* ──────────── ▼ *RATIONALE* ──────────

8. Adjust the weights across the scale until the beam balances (Fig. 5–1).

    8. The scale will indicate the weight of the client.

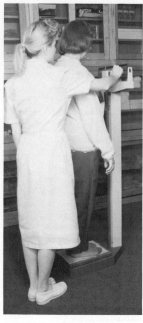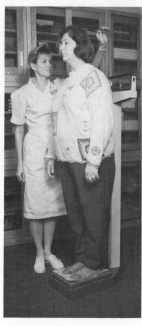

▼ **FIGURE 5–1.** Weighing and measuring the client.

9. Read the weight and record it on a notepad.

    9. Weight is measured in kilograms or pounds. The notepad prevents you from relying on memory.

10. Help the client to turn around with his or her back to the scale and instruct the client to stand up straight.

    10. Allows accurate measurement of the client's fully extended body.

11. Raise and extend the height rod over the client's head.

    11. Prevents potential injury to the client.

12. Lower the height rod to the top of the client's head (see Fig. 5–1).

    12. The scale will indicate the client's height.

13. Read and record the client's height on a notepad.

    13. Prevents you from relying on memory. Height is measured in centimeters or inches.

14. Discuss the findings with the client if appropriate.

    14. Keeps the client informed of his or her health status and allows the client to actively participate in his or her care.

15. Wash your hands.

    15. Decreases the transmission of microorganisms.

16. Record the client's height and weight on the client's chart.

    16. Communicates the findings to the other members of the health care team and contributes to the legal record by documenting the care given to the client.

Example of Documentation

DATE	10/9/93	10/10/93	10/11/93
Height	69″	69″	69″
Weight	175 lb	176 lb	176.5 lb

Teaching Tips

When you weigh and measure a client, you can initiate a discussion regarding weight reduction or special diet needs.

Home Care Variations

In the client's home, bathroom scales can be used to monitor the client's weight. Accuracy of the scales can be checked by weighing an object of known weight such as 5 pounds of sugar.

SKILL 5–2 MEASURING THE HEIGHT AND WEIGHT OF THE NONAMBULATORY CLIENT

Clinical Situations in Which You May Encounter This Skill

Height and weight are measured to provide baseline data, determine drug dosages, monitor changes in physical status, and determine the effectiveness of treatments. (See Skill 5–1 for a discussion of how "normal" growth and development are determined.)

Use proper body mechanics during the transfer of the client to bed scales to avoid injury to yourself. There are several types of scales that may be used. The two most commonly used are a bed scale and a hydraulic lift bed scale.

Anticipated Responses

▼ The client demonstrates normal growth and development for his or her age.
▼ The client is transferred from the bed to the bed scale without injury. The proper alignment of the client's body is maintained.

Adverse Responses

▼ The person is underweight (at least 10% less than the norm).
▼ The person is overweight (at least 10% more than the norm).
▼ The person is obese (at least 20–30% more than the norm).
▼ There has been a large shift in the client's weight since the day before.

Materials List

Gather these materials before beginning the skill:

▼ Bed scales
▼ Sheet

▼ ACTION

1. If available, assess the client's previous weight.

2. Determine if the client can assist in moving onto the bed scales.

Bed Scales

3. a. Roll the bed scales to the edge of the client's bed and lock the brakes.
   b. Raise the client's bed to the level of the scales and lock the bed brakes.
   c. Place a sheet over the top of the scale surface.

   d. Calibrate the scale to 0 with the sheet in place.

▼ RATIONALE

1. Enables you to detect changes in the client's weight.

2. If the client cannot assist you, obtain help from another nurse to transfer the client onto the scales.

3. a. Promotes easy transfer of the client to the scales and prevents potential injury.
   b. Promotes easy transfer of the client to the scales and prevents potential injury.
   c. Minimizes the client's discomfort and protects the client from cross-contamination with microorganisms.
   d. Allows the scale to reflect the client's weight accurately.

▼ *ACTION*　　　　　　　　　　　　　　　　▼ *RATIONALE*

   e. Using proper transfer technique and good body mechanics (see Chapter 2), move the client onto the scale.

   f. Instruct the client to be still.

   g. Weigh and measure the client and note the findings on a notepad.

   h. Return the client to the bed. Use proper transfer technique and make him or her comfortable.

   e. Prevents injury to the client or the nurses, or both.

   f. Allows the scale to measure the client's weight accurately.

   g. Weight is measured in kilograms or pounds. Height is measured in inches or centimeters. A notepad prevents you from relying on memory.

   h. Prevents injury to the client or to you.

Hydraulic Lift Bed Scales

4. a. Place the lifter seat under the client by logrolling the client from side to side (see Skill 7–6).

   b. Attach the hooks or straps of the scale to the lifter seat and elevate the client until his or her body is not in contact with the bed.

   c. Weigh the client and record the measurement (Fig. 5–2).

4. a. Prevents unnecessary stress on the client and maintains the client's good body alignment.

   b. The client must be free of contact with any surface except the scale lifter seat to ensure an accurate weight measurement.

   c. Weight is measured in kilograms or pounds. A notepad prevents you from relying on memory.

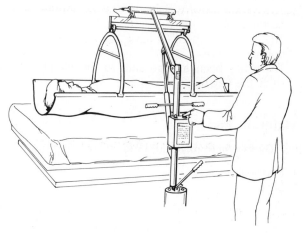

▼ **FIGURE 5–2.** Weighing the client using hydraulic lift bed scales.

   d. Slowly lower the client to the bed surface, logroll the client, and remove the lifter seat from under the client.

5. Discuss the findings with the client if appropriate.

6. Wash your hands.

7. Record the findings on the client's chart.

   d. Prevents unnecessary stress on the client and maintains the client's good body alignment.

5. Keeps the client informed of his or her health status and allows the client to actively participate in his or her care.

6. Decreases the transmission of microorganisms.

7. Communicates the findings to the other members of the health care team and contributes to the legal record by documenting the care given to the client.

> **NOTE:** If a hydraulic lift-type bed scale is used, it is not possible to obtain a height measurement.

Example of Documentation

DATE	TIME	NOTES
6/10/93	0700	Client weighed in hospital gown before breakfast. Wt. 184 lb. Has gained 2.5 lb since yesterday. —pitting edema noted in lower extremities.
		C. Lammon, RN

Teaching Tips

Discuss with the client or the client's family, or both, the purpose of determining the client's height and weight. Discuss the findings and any needed alterations in diet.

Home Care Variations

The nonambulatory client's weight is usually not measured in the home.

SKILL 5–3 MEASURING THE WEIGHT OF INFANTS

Clinical Situations in Which You May Encounter This Skill

The infant's weight may be measured at birth and at specified intervals of time to determine his or her rate of growth and development. The infant's weight also may be measured to determine total body surface area, drug dosages, and responsiveness to treatments. (See Skill 5–1 for a discussion of how "normal" growth and development is determined.) At 40 weeks' gestation, the weight of newborns may range between 5.5 and 9.5 lb. When weighing an infant, keep your hand over him or her at all times. Do not turn away from an infant on a scale.

Anticipated Responses

▼ The infant demonstrates normal growth and development for his or her age.
▼ The child is weighed on an infant scale without injury.

Adverse Responses

▼ The infant is underweight (less than the 10th percentile).
▼ The infant is obese (more than the 90th percentile).

Materials List

Gather these materials before beginning the skill:

▼ Infant scale
▼ Small sheet or paper drape

▼ ACTION	▼ RATIONALE
1. If available, assess the child's previous weight.	1. Enables you to detect any changes in the child's weight.
2. Place a small sheet or drape in the scale.	2. Provides comfort to the infant and prevents cross-contamination with microorganisms.
3. Undress the infant and place him or her on the scale.	3. Allows for accurate measurement of the infant's body weight.

▼ *ACTION* _ _ _ _ _ _ _ _ _ _ _ _ _ _ _ ▼ *RATIONALE* _ _ _ _ _ _ _ _ _ _ _

4. Hold your hand over the child's body while weighing him or her (Fig. 5–3).

4. Prevents falls and potential injury. To prevent potential injury, *never* leave an infant on any surface unattended.

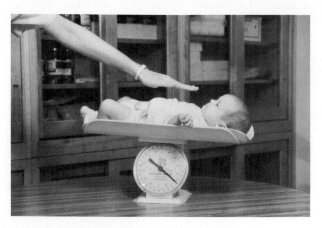

▼ **FIGURE 5–3.** Weighing an infant.

5. Read the child's weight and record it on a notepad.

5. Weight usually is recorded in kilograms. The notepad prevents you from relying on memory and provides a record for the child's parents or caretakers.

6. Discuss the findings with the child's parents or caretakers.

6. Keeps the parents or caretakers informed of the child's health status and allows the parents or caretakers to actively participate in the child's care.

7. Wash your hands.

7. Prevents the transmission of microorganisms.

8. Record the child's weight on the client's chart or a weight graph.

8. Communicates the findings to the other members of the health care team and contributes to the legal record by documenting the care given to the client.

Example of Documentation

See growth charts, Figure 5–6*A* through *D*.

Teaching Tips

When you weigh and measure an infant, you can initiate a discussion with the infant's parents or caretakers regarding normal infant growth and development and feeding schedules.

Home Care Variations

Infants can be weighed on ordinary bathroom scales. First the adult should weigh himself or herself while holding the infant. Then the adult should weigh himself or herself alone. Subtract the lesser number from the greater number and this value is the infant's weight.

SKILL 5–4 MEASURING THE LENGTH OF INFANTS

Clinical Situations in Which You May Encounter This Skill

An infant's length may be measured at birth and at specified intervals of time to determine his or her rate of growth and development. (See Skill 5–1 for a discussion of how "normal" growth and development are determined.) The newborn is approximately 51 cm at birth and by 6 weeks his or her length will increase 10%. Keep your hand on the infant at all times. Do not turn away from an infant on an examination table.

Anticipated Responses

▼ The infant demonstrates normal growth and development for his or her age.
▼ The infant is measured without injury.

Adverse Responses

▼ The infant shows retarded growth (less than the 10th percentile).
▼ The infant shows accelerated growth (more than the 90th percentile).

Materials List

Gather these materials before beginning the skill:

▼ Tape measure
▼ Towel

▼ *ACTION*	▼ *RATIONALE*
1. If available, assess the previous measurement of the child's length.	**1.** Allows you to determine changes in the child's length.
2. Place a clean towel on a firm surface.	**2.** Provides comfort to the child and prevents cross-contamination with microorganisms.
3. Lay the infant in a supine position on the towel and keep your hand on him or her at all times.	**3.** Enables you to fully extend the infant's body. To prevent potential injury, *never* leave an infant unattended on any surface.
4. Hold the child's head at the midline and gently extend his or her legs fully.	**4.** The infant's body must be fully extended to obtain an accurate measurement of length.
5. Stretch a tape measure from the crown of the child's head to the heel of his or her foot (Fig. 5–4).	**5.** Denotes the upper and lower measurement boundaries.

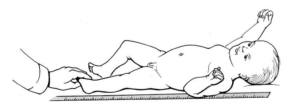

▼ FIGURE 5–4. Measuring an infant's length.

6. Read the measurement and record it on a notepad.	**6.** Length usually is recorded in centimeters. A notepad prevents you from relying on memory and also gives the child's parents or caretakers a record of his or her length.
7. Discuss the findings with the child's parents or caretakers if appropriate.	**7.** Keeps the parents or caretakers informed of the infant's health status and allows the parents to actively participate in the infant's care.
8. Wash your hands.	**8.** Prevents the transmission of microorganisms.
9. Record the results on the infant's chart or graphic sheet.	**9.** Communicates the findings to the other members of the health care team and contributes to the legal record by documenting the care given to the client.

Example of Documentation

See growth charts, Figure 5–6*A* and *C.*

Teaching Tips

When you weigh and measure an infant, you can initiate a discussion with the child's parents or caretakers regarding normal infant growth and development and feeding schedules.

Home Care Variations

An infant's length can be measured in the home using the same technique.

SKILL 5–5   MEASURING HEAD CIRCUMFERENCE

Clinical Situations in Which You May Encounter This Skill

Head circumference may be measured at birth and at specified intervals of time to determine a child's rate of growth and development. Head circumference measurement also may be performed as part of an assessment for specific conditions such as hydrocephalus, in which the head is larger than normal, or microcephaly, in which the head is smaller than normal. The head circumference of newborns is larger than the chest circumference. At birth, the head circumference is approximately 35 cm. It should increase approximately 3 cm in 6 weeks. The head and chest circumferences are usually equal at 1 year.

Anticipated Responses

▼ The child's cranium is found to have normal growth and development.

Adverse Responses

▼ The infant's head circumference is smaller or larger than normal for his or her age.

Materials List

Gather these materials before beginning the skill:

▼ Tape measure
▼ Towel or paper drape

▼ *ACTION*

▼ *RATIONALE*

1. If available, assess the child's previous head circumference measurement.

1. Enables you to detect changes in the child's head circumference.

2. Lay the infant in a supine position on a clean towel or drape. Keep your hand on the infant at all times.

2. This position facilitates cephalic measurement. The towel provides comfort to the infant and prevents cross-contamination of microorganisms. To prevent potential injury, *never* leave an infant unattended on any surface.

3. Place a tape measure around the fullest part of the infant's head over the brow (Fig. 5–5).

3. The measurement should be taken at the point of the largest head circumference.

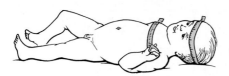

▼ **FIGURE 5–5.** Measuring an infant's head circumference and chest circumference.

4. Read the results and record them on a notepad.

4. The measurement usually is recorded in centimeters. The notepad prevents you from relying on memory and also provides a record for the child's parents or caretakers.

5. Discuss the findings with the child's caretakers.

5. Keeps the child's parents or caretakers informed of the infant's health status and allows the parents to actively participate in the infant's care.

6. Wash your hands.

6. Prevents the transmission of microorganisms.

7. Record the results on the client's chart or graphic sheet.

7. Communicates the findings to the other members of the health care team and contributes to the legal record by documenting the care given to the client.

Example of Documentation

See growth charts, Figure *5–6B* and *D.*

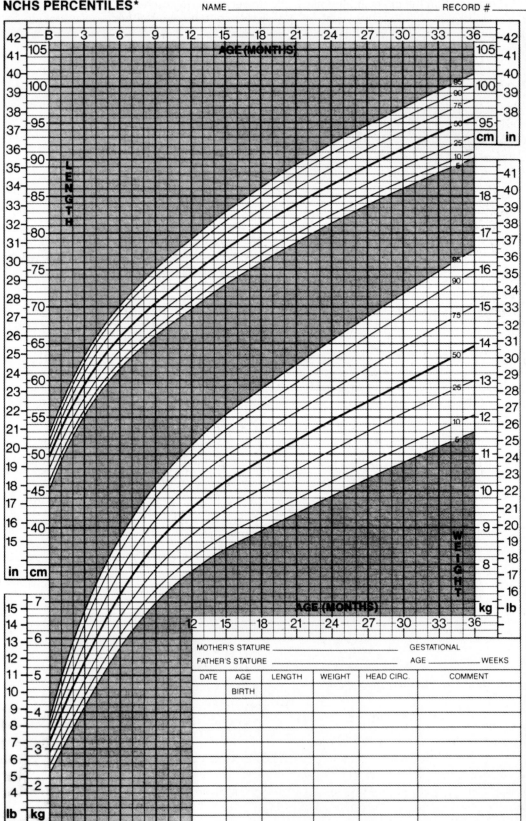

**GIRLS: BIRTH TO 36 MONTHS
PHYSICAL GROWTH
NCHS PERCENTILES***

NAME _____ RECORD # _____

Ross
Growth &
Development
Program

MOTHER'S STATURE _____ GESTATIONAL
FATHER'S STATURE _____ AGE _____ WEEKS

DATE	AGE	LENGTH	WEIGHT	HEAD CIRC.	COMMENT
	BIRTH				

* Adapted from: Hamill PVV, Drizd TA, Johnson CL, Reed RB, Roche AF, Moore WM: Physical growth: National Center for Health Statistics percentiles. AM J CLIN NUTR 32:607-629, 1979. Data from the Fels Longitudinal Study, Wright State University School of Medicine, Yellow Springs, Ohio.

© 1982 Ross Laboratories

A

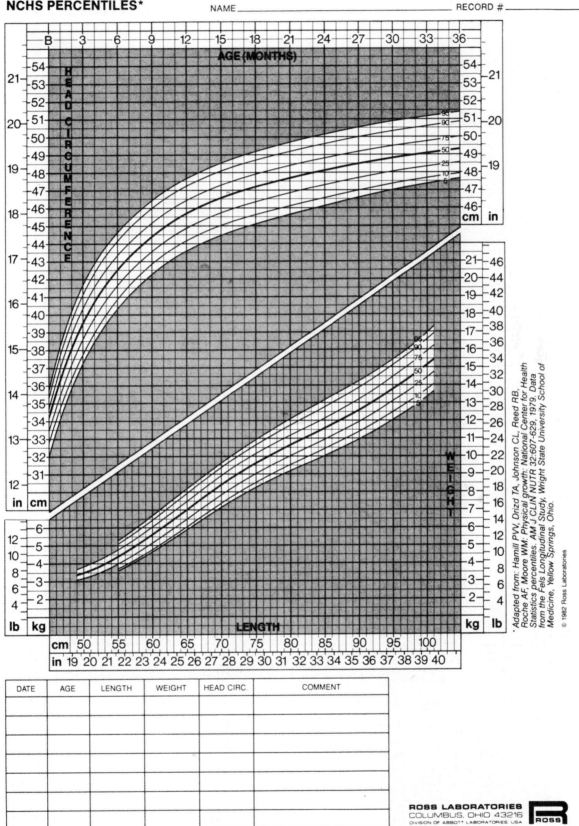

ROSS LABORATORIES
COLUMBUS, OHIO 43216
DIVISION OF ABBOTT LABORATORIES, USA

G106(0.05)/JANUARY 1986   LITHO IN USA

B

▼ **FIGURE 5–6.** *A,* Physical growth chart for girls, birth to 36 months, showing length and weight. (Courtesy of Ross Laboratories, Columbus, Ohio.) *B,* Physical growth chart for girls, birth to 36 months, showing head circumference and weight. (Courtesy of Ross Laboratories, Columbus, Ohio.)

Illustration continued on following page

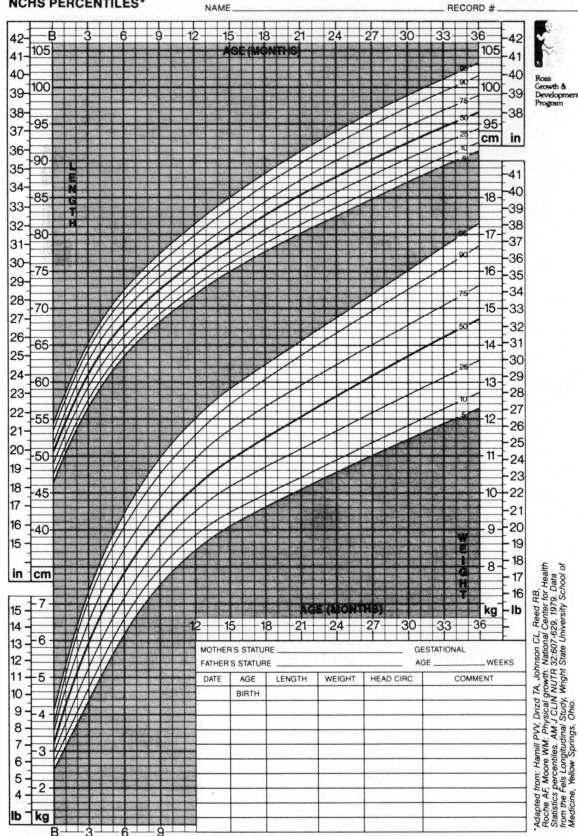

▼ **FIGURE 5–6.** *Continued C,* Physical growth chart for boys, birth to 36 months, showing length and weight. (Courtesy of Ross Laboratories, Columbus, Ohio.)

**BOYS: BIRTH TO 36 MONTHS
PHYSICAL GROWTH
NCHS PERCENTILES***

NAME _____

RECORD # _____

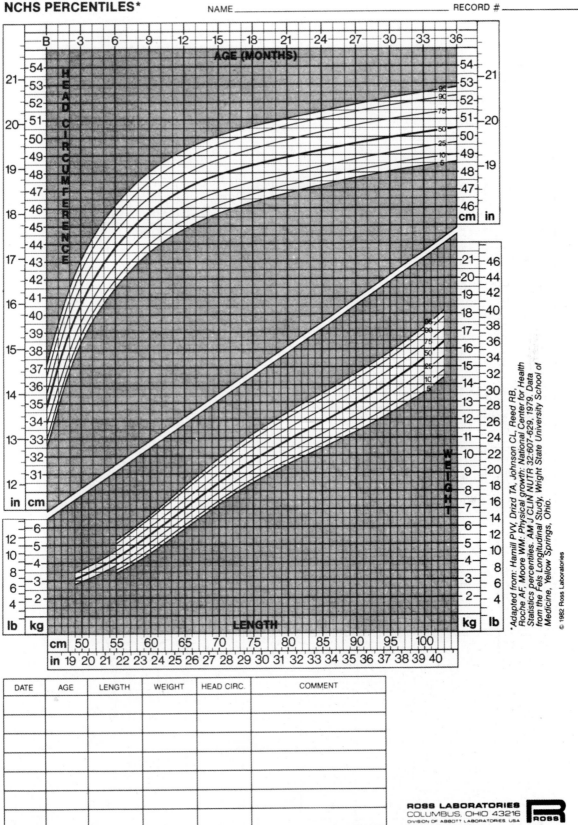

DATE	AGE	LENGTH	WEIGHT	HEAD CIRC.	COMMENT

*Adapted from: Hamill PVV, Drizd TA, Johnson CL, Reed RB, Roche AF, Moore WM: Physical growth: National Center for Health Statistics percentiles. AM J CLIN NUTR 32:607-629, 1979. Data from the Fels Longitudinal Study, Wright State University School of Medicine, Yellow Springs, Ohio.

© 1982 Ross Laboratories

ROSS LABORATORIES
COLUMBUS, OHIO 43216
DIVISION OF ABBOTT LABORATORIES USA

G105(0.05)/APRIL 1989   LITHO IN USA

D

▼ **FIGURE 5–6.** *Continued D,* Physical growth chart for boys, birth to 36 months, showing head circumference and weight. (Courtesy of Ross Laboratories, Columbus, Ohio.)

Illustration continued on following page

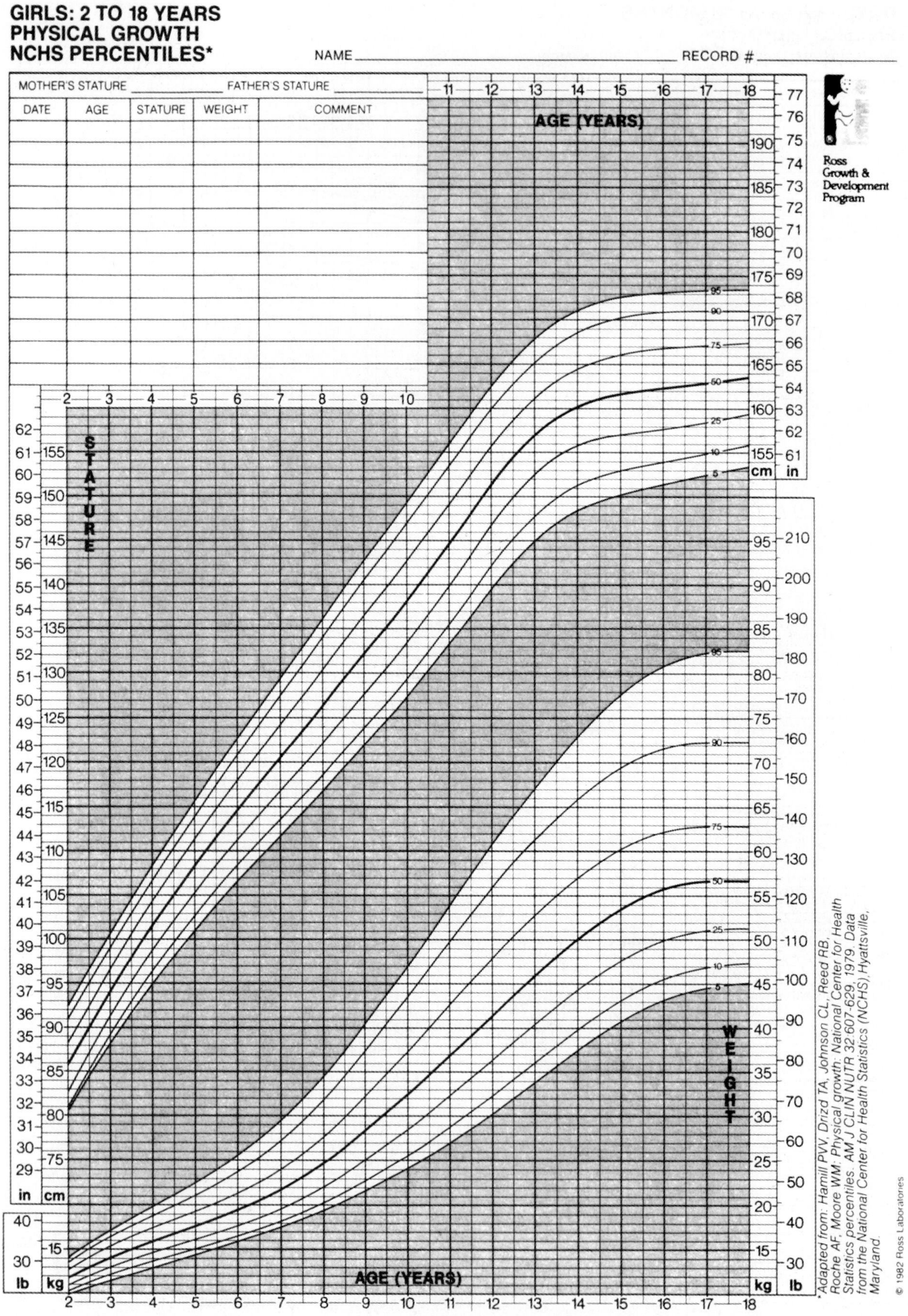

GIRLS: 2 TO 18 YEARS
PHYSICAL GROWTH
NCHS PERCENTILES*

NAME _____   RECORD # _____

▼ **FIGURE 5–6.** *Continued E,* Physical growth chart for girls, age 2 to 18 years, showing stature and weight. (Courtesy of Ross Laboratories, Columbus, Ohio.)

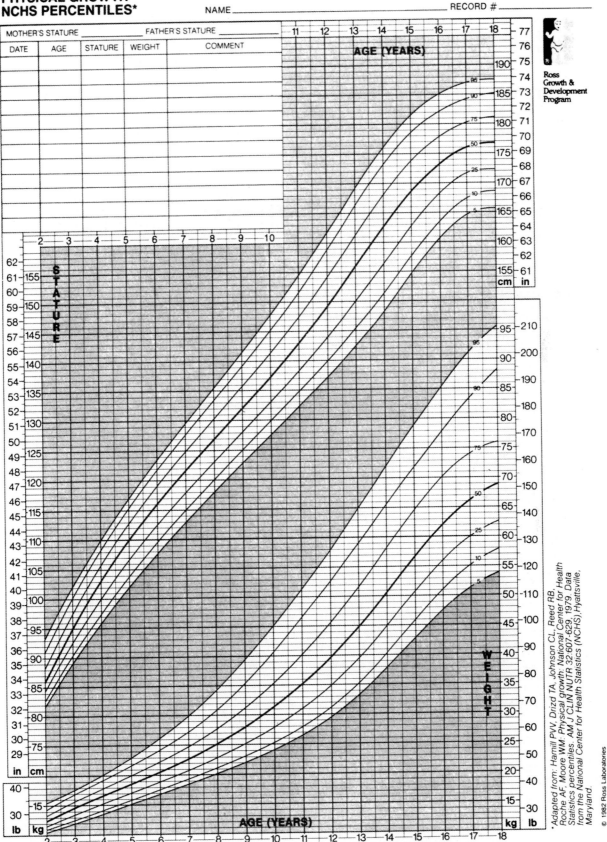

BOYS: 2 TO 18 YEARS
PHYSICAL GROWTH
NCHS PERCENTILES*

▼ **FIGURE 5–6.** *Continued F,* Physical growth chart for boys, age 2 to 18 years, showing stature and weight. (Courtesy of Ross Laboratories, Columbus, Ohio.)

Teaching Tips

When you measure an infant, you can initiate a discussion with the infant's parents or caretakers regarding normal growth and development. Explain the purpose of measuring the head circumference and the results to the child's parents or caretakers.

Home Care Variations

The client's head circumference can be measured in the home using the same procedure.

SKILL 5–6 MEASURING CHEST CIRCUMFERENCE

Clinical Situations in Which You May Encounter This Skill

A measurement of chest circumference is obtained at birth and at specified intervals of time to determine the child's rate of growth and development. At birth, the child's chest circumference is smaller than the head circumference. At 1 year of age, the head and chest circumferences are usually equal.

Anticipated Responses

▼ The child's thorax is found to have normal growth and development.

Adverse Responses

▼ The child is found to have excessive or retarded growth or deformities of the thorax.

Materials List

Gather these materials before beginning the skill:

▼ Tape measure
▼ Towel or paper drape

▼ ACTION	▼ RATIONALE
1. If available, assess the child's previous chest circumference measurement.	1. Enables you to detect changes in the child's chest circumference.
2. Lay the infant in the supine position on a clean towel or drape. Keep your hand on the infant at all times.	2. This position facilitates chest measurement. The towel provides comfort to the child and prevents cross-contamination of microorganisms. To prevent potential injury, *never* leave an infant unattended on any surface.
3. Place the tape measure around the infant's chest at the nipple line (see Fig. 5–5).	3. The measurement should be taken at the point of the largest chest circumference.
4. Read the results and record them on a notepad.	4. The measurement usually is recorded in centimeters. The notepad prevents you from relying on memory and provides a record for the child's parents or caretakers.
5. Discuss the findings with the child's parents or caretakers when appropriate.	5. Keeps the parents or caretakers informed of the infant's health status and allows the parents to actively participate in the infant's care.
6. Wash your hands.	6. Prevents the transmission of microorganisms.
7. Record the results on the infant's chart or graphic sheet.	7. Communicates the findings to the other members of the health care team and contributes to the legal record by documenting the care given to the client.

Example of Documentation

DATE	TIME	NOTES
6/19/93	1000	1-year-old female. Head circumference 47 cm. Chest circumference 47 cm. Height and weight 50th percentile.
		C. Lammon, RN

Teaching Tips

When you measure an infant, you can initiate a discussion with his or her parents or caretakers regarding normal growth and development.

Home Care Variations

The chest circumference can be measured in the child's home using the same procedure.

SKILL 5–7   MEASURING FUNDAL HEIGHT

Clinical Situations in Which You May Encounter This Skill

Fundal height is measured during the prenatal period to determine the growth and development of the fetus. Table 5–2 describes the normal fundal height for gestational age.

Excessive growth may indicate multiple gestation, a hydatidiform mole, or polyhydramnios. Retarded growth is indicative of intrauterine growth retardation. No growth may signal fetal demise.

Fundal height is determined during the postpartum period to determine the degree of uterine contraction and involution.

Anticipated Responses

▼ The client has a normal fundal height for the gestational age of the fetus.

Adverse Responses

▼ The measurement indicates excessive growth.
▼ The measurement indicates retarded growth.
▼ The measurement indicates no growth.

Materials List

Gather these materials before beginning the skill:

▼ Tape measure
▼ Drape

TABLE 5–2. Normal Fundal Height for Gestational Age

Gestational Age	Approximate Height of Fundus
8–10 weeks	Uterus is rising out of the pelvic cavity
16 weeks	Fundus is halfway between the umbilicus and the symphysis pubis
22 weeks	Fundal height is at the umbilicus

For the second and third trimester, use McDonald's rule: the height of the fundus (in centimeters) × 8/7 = duration of the pregnancy in weeks.

▼ _ A C T I O N _   ▼ R A T I O N A L E

1. Assess the client's previous fundal height measurement and weeks of gestation.

2. Assist the mother to lie down in a supine position and drape her, exposing only the abdomen.

3. Locate the symphysis pubis by gently palpating the lower abdominal area.

4. Locate the top of the fundus by gently palpating for the firm rounded top of the uterus.

5. Stretch a tape measure from the symphysis pubis to the top of the fundus (Fig. 5–7) and read the results. Record the data on a notepad.

1. Enables you to determine if the client's uterine growth is appropriate for the stage of pregnancy.

2. This position facilitates access to the client's abdomen. The drape protects the client's privacy and dignity.

3. Locates the lower landmark of the area to be measured.

4. Locates the upper landmark of the area to be measured.

5. This measurement usually is recorded in centimeters. Use of a notepad prevents you from relying on memory.

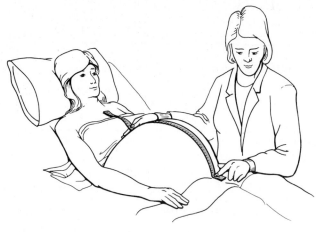

▼ FIGURE 5–7. Measuring the height of the fundus.

6. Discuss the findings with the client if appropriate.

7. Wash your hands.

8. Record the results on the client's record.

6. Keeps the client informed of her health status and allows the client to actively participate in her care.

7. Prevents the transmission of microorganisms.

8. Communicates the findings to the other members of the health care team and contributes to the legal record by documenting the care given to the client.

Example of Documentation

Patient's name ___Jane Whitehead___

Age _23_

Baby's physician ___Johnson___

Visit Date 19 93	Weight this visit	Blood pressure B/L /	Urine protein	Urine sugar	EST weeks gestation	Fundal height	Fetal heart rate/quadrant	Edema		
5/12	168	130/80	0	0	22 wks	20cm	* ⊕ 150 S&R	ng		First visit of 23 year old prima
/		/		/		⊕				gravida. No complaints when
/		/		/		⊕				questioned.

(Permission to reproduce this copyrighted material has been granted by the owner, Hollister Incorporated.)

Teaching Tips

When you measure fundal height, you can discuss fetal growth and development and the importance of good health practices during pregnancy (nutrition, not smoking, not drinking alcohol, and not taking medicine unless prescribed by the doctor) with the mother.

Home Care Variations

Fundal height can be measured in the client's home using the same skill.

SKILL 5–8   MEASURING ABDOMINAL GIRTH

Clinical Situations in Which You May Encounter This Skill

Abdominal girth is measured to determine the presence of and changes in volume of ascites, or fluid in the peritoneal cavity. Conditions that may contribute to ascites include liver diseases such as cirrhosis; cardiac disease that obstructs venous return; obstructed lymphatic drainage; electrolyte imbalances; and obstructed blood flow in the vena cava or the portal vein.

If the client has abdominal distention and it increases on a daily basis, an abdominal paracentesis may be performed by the physician. In this procedure, the physician obtains a sample of the ascitic fluid for laboratory testing to rule out intraabdominal hemorrhage or to relieve intraabdominal pressure caused by large volumes of ascitic fluid. Abdominal girth is measured before and after this procedure.

Anticipated Responses

▼ The abdominal girth is normal for the size of the individual.

Adverse Responses

▼ There has been a significant change in the client's abdominal size since the last measurement.

Materials List

Gather these materials before beginning the skill:

▼ Tape measure
▼ Felt-tipped marker

▼ ACTION

1. Assist the client to assume a supine position. If the client cannot lay supine, the abdominal girth can be measured while the client is in the semi-Fowler's position.

2. Assess the client's abdomen. Note distention, fluid wave, and skin turgor. Also note any difficulty with respirations.

▼ RATIONALE

1. Facilitates your evaluation of the client's abdomen. The supine position may cause respiratory difficulty for some clients.

2. Alerts you to factors that may be altering the client's abdominal girth.

▼ *ACTION*	▼ *RATIONALE*
3. Place a tape measure around the client's abdomen at the largest point and measure the abdominal girth (Fig. 5–8).	**3.** Measurement at the largest point gives the most accurate measure of the amount of distention present.

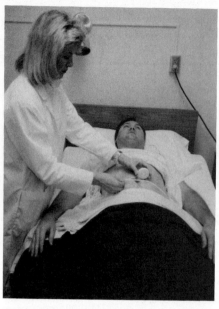

▼ **FIGURE 5–8.** Measuring abdominal girth.

4. Before removing the tape measure, use a pen to mark on the client's body where the measuring tape lies.	**4.** The measurement must be taken at the same point on the abdomen each time in order to make accurate comparisons between measurements.
5. Help the client to assume a position of comfort.	**5.** Assist the client to rest.
6. Wash your hands.	**6.** Decreases the transmission of microorganisms.
7. Record the results in the client's chart.	**7.** Communicates the findings to the other members of the health care team and contributes to the legal record by documenting the care given to the client.

Example of Documentation

DATE	TIME	NOTES
1/10/94	0830	Abdomen is distended and fluid wave noted. Skin over abdomen is shiny and taut. Respirations 24 and shallow. Abdominal girth measures 100 cm.
		S. Smith, RN

Teaching Tips

Explain the purpose of measuring the abdominal girth and the findings to the client or the client's family, or both.

Home Care Variations

The same skill can be used in the client's home to measure the client's abdominal girth.

SKILL 5–9 COLLECTING A ROUTINE VOIDED URINE SPECIMEN

Clinical Situations in Which You May Encounter This Skill

Routine voided specimens are collected for routine urinalysis to examine the urine for color, specific gravity, pH, protein, glucose, acetone, bilirubin, and blood. A routine voided specimen cannot be used to assess for the presence of bacteria in the urine. It is collected upon the client's admission to the hospital, before surgery, or during visits to the physician's office. If possible, collect the specimen at the client's first voiding in the morning, since such a specimen is more likely to reveal any abnormalities than later voidings.

Anticipated Responses

▼ Urine is collected.

Adverse Responses

▼ The client is unable to void.
▼ The urine contains toilet paper or feces.

Materials List

Gather these materials before beginning the skill:

▼ Urine specimen container
▼ Adhesive label or marker
▼ Bedpan, toilet specimen container, or infant collection device
▼ Examination gloves
▼ Biohazard bag or container to hold the specimen when transporting it to the laboratory

▼ ACTION

1. Assess the client's ability to follow directions and cooperate.

2. Put on examination gloves.

3. If a woman is menstruating, provide perineal care and place a tampon or 4- × 4-inch gauze pad in her vaginal orifice.

4. Have the client urinate in a clean bedpan or toilet specimen container. Instruct the client not to defecate with the specimen or contaminate the specimen with toilet paper.

   a. For an infant or a child who is not toilet trained: Wash and dry the perineum and attach a collection device to the infant (Fig. 5–9). If the child is a boy, place the penis and the scrotum in the bag. Stretch the device tautly on girls.

▼ RATIONALE

1. Alerts you to the amount of assistance that the client or the client's parent may need.

2. Gloves should be worn when there is a chance of coming in contact with any body fluid to prevent the possible transmission of microorganisms.

3. Menstrual blood will alter the results of the test. Therefore, the laboratory should be notified of the presence of menstrual blood.

4. Feces and toilet paper can alter the results.

   a. A special collection device is necessary. The perineum is cleansed so the adhesive surface of the device will stick.

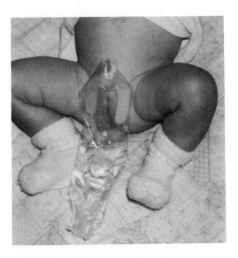

▼ **FIGURE 5–9.** Infant urine collection device.

▼ *ACTION*

▼ *RATIONALE*

5. Pour the fresh urine in the specimen container, put the lid on, label it, and place the specimen in a biohazard bag (Fig. 5–10). Send the specimen immediately to the laboratory.

5. The label identifies the source of the specimen. The biohazard bag protects workers from contact with body fluids. The urinalysis may be altered if the urine specimen is more than 1 hour old. Fresh urine is used because bacteria may enter urine that is allowed to sit and other components can break up and disintegrate.

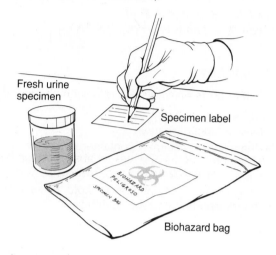

▼ **FIGURE 5–10.** Label and bag the urine specimen cup.

6. Remove the examination gloves and wash your hands.

6. Prevents the possible transmission of micro-organisms.

7. Assess the color and clarity of the urine and the presence of any sediment.

7. These data are necessary for charting and also alert you to the presence of potential problems such as a urinary tract infection.

8. Record the procedure and note the color, appearance, and odor of the urine.

8. Communicates the findings to the other members of the health care team and contributes to the legal record by documenting the care given to the client.

Example of Documentation

DATE	TIME	NOTES
10/23/93	1030	Voided 120 cc of clear, yellow urine in toilet specimen container. Urine for urinalysis collected and sent to lab.
		L. White, RN

Teaching Tips

Explain the purpose of the sample and the collection procedure to the client or the client's family member.

Home Care Variations

Transport the specimen in a cooler from the client's home to the laboratory.

SKILL 5–10   COLLECTING A CLEAN-CATCH (MIDSTREAM) URINE SPECIMEN

Clinical Situations in Which You May Encounter This Skill

A clean-catch urine specimen is collected when a urinary tract infection is suspected and uncontaminated urine is needed for a urine culture and sensitivity test. The client or the parent of a child may help to produce such a specimen after adequate explanation from you. If possible, collect the specimen at the time of the client's first voiding in the morning since bacterial counts are highest in this voiding.

Anticipated Responses

▼ The urine is collected without contamination.

Adverse Responses

▼ The client is unable to void.
▼ The client contaminates the specimen.

Materials List

Gather these materials before beginning the skill:

▼ Sterile specimen container
▼ Adhesive label or marker
▼ Sterile gloves
▼ Antimicrobial perineal wipes, swabs, or cotton balls
▼ Biohazard bag to hold the specimen while transporting it to the laboratory.
▼ 4 × 4 gauze pads or tampon if needed.

▼ ACTION

1. Determine the reason for the test.

2. Assess the client's ability to follow directions and cooperate.

3. Close the door and the curtains around the bed. If the specimen is being collected in the bathroom, close the door.

4. Remove the lid and place it inside up within easy reach on a clean surface.

5. Put on sterile gloves using sterile technique and clean around the client's urinary meatus with antimicrobial wipes.

   a. For a female client, spread the labia with your nondominant hand and clean from front to back using the antimicrobial wipes or cotton balls (Fig. 5–11). The labia must be kept separated after cleaning until after the specimen is obtained.

▼ RATIONALE

1. The reason for the test should be explained to the client.

2. Alerts you to the amount of assistance the client or his or her parent may need.

3. Provides privacy for the client.

4. Touching the inside of the lid will cause contamination.

5. Since the specimen is collected for a culture of any microorganisms, sterile technique should be used to prevent contamination of the specimen.

   a. The area around the meatus is cleansed to prevent contamination. If the labia are allowed to close, the area will be contaminated and should be cleansed again. Cleansing from front to back prevents fecal contamination.

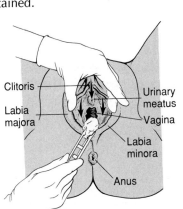

Clitoris
Labia majora
Urinary meatus
Vagina
Labia minora
Anus

▼ FIGURE 5–11. Cleaning the labia in preparation for a clean-catch urine specimen.

▼ *ACTION*   ▼ *RATIONALE*

   b. For a male client, clean around the meatus (Fig. 5–12). You should retact the client's foreskin before cleaning if he is not circumcised. Return the forskin to its normal position after the specimen has been collected.

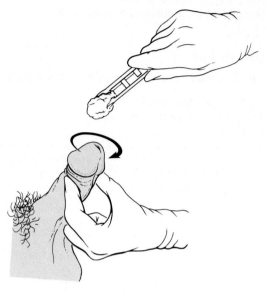

▼ **FIGURE 5–12.** Cleaning around the meatus in preparation for a clean-catch urine specimen.

6. If the woman is menstruating, place a tampon or a 4- × 4-inch gauze pad in her vaginal orific.

6. Menstrual blood may alter the test results. Record the possible presence of menstrual blood on the label of the specimen container.

7. Have the client void a small amount into the toilet or urinal.

7. Cleanses the meatus of any remaining bacteria.

8. Then have the client urinate 30 to 50 cc directly into a sterile specimen container. The client then can finish voiding in the toilet or urinal.

8. By urinating directly into the specimen container, the possibility of contaminating the specimen is decreased.

9. Put the lid on the container. Avoid touching the inside of the lid or container. Wipe off the outside of the container.

9. If the lid or inside of the container is touched, the specimen will be contaminated.

10. Assist the client with perineal hygiene.

10. Cleansing promotes the client's sense of well-being.

11. Remove your gloves and wash your hands.

11. Prevents the possible transmission of micro-organisms.

12. Label the specimen and send it to the laboratory immediately.

12. The results may be altered if the urine is allowed to sit. Bacteria may enter the urine and multiply. Urine also will become alkaline if it is allowed to sit.

13. Assess the color and clarity of the urine and the presence of any sediment.

13. These data are necessary for charting. They also alert you to possible problems such as a urinary tract infection.

14. Record the procedure and note the color, appearance, and odor of the urine.

14. Communicates the findings to the other members of the health care team and contributes to the legal record by documenting the care given to the client.

Example of Documentation

DATE	*TIME*	*NOTES*
10/26/93	1100	Clean-catch urine specimen obtained. Urine was cloudy, yellow, with sediment noted.
		S. Hill, RN

Teaching Tips

Explain the purpose of the sample and the collection procedure to the client or the client's family member.

Home Care Variations

Transport the specimen from the client's home to the laboratory in a cooler. Dispose of used equipment in a sealed plastic bag to decrease the transmission of microorganisms.

SKILL 5–11 COLLECTING A URINE SPECIMEN FROM AN INDWELLING CATHETER

Clinical Situations in Which You May Encounter This Skill

A urine specimen may be collected from an indwelling catheter for routine urinalysis, or to examine the urine for microorganisms, specific gravity, pH, glucose, acetone, and protein. The urine should not be taken from the collection bag since that urine is contaminated, and the components of the urine change when it has been sitting at room temperature. The urine should be obtained from the collection port on the catheter.

Anticipated Responses

▼ The urine specimen is obtained without contamination of the closed drainage system.

Adverse Responses

▼ The closed system is contaminated during the procedure.

Materials List

Gather these materials before beginning the skill:

▼ Clamp
▼ 5-ml syringe with a 21- to 25-gauge needle
▼ Specimen container (must be sterile if the specimen is collected for culture and sensitivity)
▼ Adhesive label or marker
▼ Antimicrobial wipes
▼ Biohazard bag for transporting the specimen to the laboratory

▼ *ACTION*

1. Determine the need for the urine specimen.

2. Close the door and the curtains around the bed.

3. Clamp the indwelling catheter just distal to the injection port for approximately 15 to 20 minutes.

4. Assess the color and clarity of the urine in the tubing.

5. Once urine has collected in the tubing, wipe the injection port with an antimicrobial wipe and allow it to dry.

▼ *RATIONALE*

1. The reason for the specimen should be explained to the client.

2. Provides privacy for the client.

3. Allows urine to collect in the drainage tubing. The amount of time necessary for urine to collect may vary in relation to the client's urine output.

4. It is important to note these characteristics. Cloudy urine can indicate a urinary tract infection.

5. The injection port is cleansed to reduce any contamination of the specimen and to reduce any contamination of the closed catheter system.

▼ *ACTION*   ▼ *RATIONALE*

6. Insert a 23- or 25-gauge needle into the port and aspirate the required amount of fresh urine into a sterile syringe (Fig. 5–13).

6. Aspirate 2 to 3 ml of urine for a culture. Thirty milliliters of urine will be needed for a urinalysis. Do not take the urine specimen from the collection bag. When the urine collects and remains in the bag at room temperature, the components of the urine change and alter the test results.

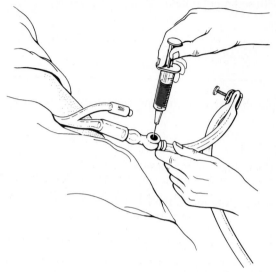

▼**FIGURE 5–13.** Using syringe to aspirate urine from collection port on catheter.

7. Withdraw the needle and inject the urine into the sterile specimen container.

7. Prevents contamination of the specimen by microorganisms.

8. Unclamp the tubing.

8. Urine will not flow into the drainage bag. Stasis of urine in the bladder can cause urinary tract infections.

9. Put the lid on the container, label it, place it in a biohazard bag, and send it to the laboratory immediately.

9. The results may be altered if the urine is allowed to sit.

10. Properly dispose of contaminated equipment.

10. Proper disposal prevents the transmission of microorganisms.

11. Wash your hands.

11. Decreases the transmission of microorganisms.

12. In the client's chart, record the procedure for and the purpose of obtaining the urine sample.

12. Communicates to the other members of the health care team and contributes to the legal record by documenting the care given to the client.

Example of Documentation

DATE	TIME	NOTES
10/25/93	0930	Urine obtained from catheter tubing for culture and sensitivity. Urine appeared cloudy. Specimen sent to the lab.
		S. Williams, RN

Teaching Tips

Explain the purpose of the specimen to the client and the client's family. Reinforce teaching or teach the client or the client's family member, or both, about catheter care.

Home Care Variations

Take a sealed bottle to dispose of the needle and syringe and remove the bottle from the client's home. Dispose of other used equipment in a sealed plastic bag. Transport the specimen from the client's home to the laboratory in a cooler.

SKILL 5–12 COLLECTING A URINE SPECIMEN WITH A STRAIGHT CATHETER

Clinical Situations in Which You May Encounter This Skill

A urine specimen is collected by means of a catheter when a urinary tract infection is suspected and a sterile urine specimen is needed for a urine culture and sensitivity test. Catheterization is also performed to assess the presence and amount of residual urine after voiding, to empty the bladder before surgery, and to relieve a distended bladder when the client is temporarily unable to void.

Anticipated Responses

▼ The nurse uses sterile technique and the catheter is inserted and the specimen is obtained without contamination or trauma.

Adverse Response

▼ The catheter meets an obstruction and cannot be inserted.
▼ There is no urine drainage from the catheter.

Materials List

Gather these materials before beginning the skill:

▼ Good light source (lamp or flashlight)
▼ Straight catheter kit: size 14–16 French for adult females and size 16–18 French for adult males

NOTE: A catheter kit contains a urine receptacle, catheter, specimen container, drape, label, lubricant, sterile gloves, antimicrobial swabs or solution with cotton balls and forceps and a receptacle for waste.

▼ Examination gloves
▼ Basin with soap and warm water, washcloth, and towel
▼ Biohazard bag
▼ Waterproof pad
▼ Sheet to be used as drape

▼ ACTION

1. Assess whether the client has had the procedure done previously.

2. Check the chart for a physician's order and the reason for the specimen collection.

3. Assess the client's ability to follow directions and cooperate.

4. Close the door and the curtains around the bed.

5. Raise the bed to a comfortable working height.

6. Position the client.

   a. A female client should be placed in the dorsal recumbent position with her feet spread apart.
   b. The male client should be placed in the supine position with his legs together. Raise the client's penis and scrotal sac to rest on top of his legs.

▼ RATIONALE

1. Teaching can be individualized based on prior experience. It also gives the client a chance to tell you what problems may have been encountered.

2. A physician's order is required. The reason for the catheterization should be explained to the client.

3. It may be necessary for another nurse to assist you if the client is uncooperative or unable to assist.

4. Provides privacy for the client.

5. Reduces the strain placed on your back.

6. These positions facilitate visualization of the urinary meatus.

▼ *ACTION*

▼ *RATIONALE*

7. a. For the female client: Place a drape over the client in a diamond configuration with one corner at the client's sternum, one corner over each of her knees, and one corner over her perineum.
   b. For the male client: Cover the client's chest and lower extremities with a sheet, leaving only his genital area exposed.

7. a. Allows you to expose the client's perineal area while covering the rest of her body.

8. Place a waterproof pad under the client's buttocks.

8. Prevents the bed linens from becoming soiled.

9. Put on examination gloves.

9. Decreases the transmission of microorganisms.

10. Wash the client's genital area with warm water and soap. Rinse and dry the area.

10. Removes secretions and feces.

11. Remove the examination gloves and wash your hands.

11. Decreases the transmission of microorganisms.

12. Using sterile technique, open the sterile prepackaged catheter insertion kit.
    a. For the female client: Open the kit on the bed between the client's feet.
    b. For the male client: Place the overbed table over the client's knees and open the kit on the overbed table (see Skill 1–9).

12. The inside of the wrapper will become your sterile working field.

13. Remove the sterile pad. Open it at the corners so as not to contaminate the pad and place it between the female client's legs to the perineal area. Place the pad on the male client's thighs.

13. The pad becomes an extension of the sterile work area.

14. Remove the catheter tray with its contents and place it within the sterile field.

14. Facilitates easy access to your equipment.

15. Remove the sterile gloves and put them on using sterile technique (see Skill 1–8).

15. Prevents the introduction of microorganisms into the urinary tract, which is normally sterile.

16. Remove the fenestrated drape and place it over the client's genital area so that only the genitalia are exposed. Do not move the drape once it has touched the client's skin. Do not allow your gloved hands to touch the client's skin.

16. The drape provides minimal exposure of the client's body. The client's skin is contaminated and if your gloved hands touch the skin, they will become contaminated. If moved, the drape also will become contaminated.

17. Open the disinfectant solution and pour the solution over the cotton balls. If disinfectant swabs are used, open this package.

17. Cotton balls or swabs are used to cleanse the urinary meatus.

18. Open the container of water-soluble lubricant and lubricate the tip of the catheter approximately 2 inches for a female client and approximately 6 inches for a male client.

18. The lubricant will decrease friction between the catheter and the urinary meatus during catheter insertion. The female urethra is approximately 2 inches long and the male urethra is approximately 6 inches long.

19. Place the open end of the catheter into the sterile specimen container.

19. When the client is catheterized, the urine flow will start. If the end of the catheter is not in a container, the urine will wet the sterile field and cause it to become contaminated.

▼ *ACTION* _ _ _ _ _ _ _ _ _ _ _ _ _ _ _ _

▼ *RATIONALE* _ _ _ _ _ _ _ _ _ _

20. a. For the female client: Using the thumb and middle finger of your nondominant hand, spread the client's labia. The labia should not be allowed to close during the entire procedure. If the labia do close, you should stop the procedure and start over at this step.

   b. For the male client: Use your nondominant hand to position the client's penis perpendicular to his body. Do not release the penis until the procedure is completed.

20. a. When the labia close, the area becomes contaminated.

21. Grasp the forceps in your dominant hand and pick up a cotton ball containing disinfectant solution

   a. For the female client: Using a separate cotton ball for each stroke, cleanse each side of the meatus with one downward stroke. Then clean from the client's meatus to the rectum with one stroke. Do not let the labia close (see Fig. 5–11).

   b. For the male client: The client's penis should be cleansed using a circular motion from the meatus to the base of the penis. Retract the foreskin on the uncircumcised male. The meatus and penis should be cleansed several more times using a new sterile disinfectant-soaked cotton ball each time (see Fig. 5–12).

21. The area around the meatus is cleansed to prevent contamination of the catheter by microorganisms and introduction of organisms into the client's urethra and bladder.

22. Visualize the client's urinary meatus. The female meatus may be near or in the anterior vaginal orifice in elderly or multiparous clients. A flashlight or lamp may be necessary to locate the female client's meatus.

22. The meatus may be difficult to locate on some female clients and extra light may be necessary.

23. Lift the lubricated tip of the catheter and gently insert it into the client's meatus. Ask the client to take a deep breath while you insert the catheter. The labia should still be spread with your nondominant hand. The foreskin of the male client should still be retracted and the penis should be held firmly and perpendicular to the client's body.

23. The client's deep breath will help to relax the urinary meatus. Since gentle pressure may cause an erection, the penis should be held firmly but not tightly. If held tightly, pressure will collapse the urethra and prevent advancement of the catheter. If the male client has an erection, stop the procedure until there is a nonerectile state. You should start insertion of the catheter again.

24. Insert the catheter 2 to 3 inches for adult females and 6 to 8 inches for adult males, or until urine begins to flow. Do not touch the client's perineal hair or skin as the catheter is advanced. If obstruction is encountered, do not force the catheter.

24. Hair or skin will contaminate the catheter. Forcing the catheter can cause trauma, bleeding, and possible scar formation, which can lead to strictures and obstruction of the urethra.

25. Let 15 to 20 ml of urine drain into a sterile specimen container. Allow the remaining urine to drain into the urine receptacle.

25. By draining the urine directly into the specimen container, the possibility of contaminating the specimen is decreased.

26. Remove the catheter.

26. Once the specimen is obtained, the catheter is no longer needed.

▼ *ACTION*	▼ *RATIONALE*
27. Put the lid on the container, label the specimen, and place it in a biohazard bag. Send the specimen to the laboratory immediately.	**27.** The results may be altered if urine is allowed to sit. Urine also will become alkaline.
28. Wash the client's perineal area and return the foreskin on the uncircumcised male.	**28.** Cleansing will promote the client's comfort and sense of well-being. The foreskin is returned to its normal position to prevent impairment of circulation to the penis. Failure to return the foreskin can lead to swelling of the penis and complications.
29. Return the client's bed to the lowest position.	**29.** Reduces potential injury from falls.
30. Remove your gloves and wash your hands.	**30.** Prevents the possible transmission of microorganisms.
31. Properly dispose of the equipment.	**31.** Prevents the transmission of microorganisms.
32. Record the procedure. Note the color, appearance, and odor of the urine.	**32.** Communicates the findings to the other members of the health care team and contributes to the legal record by documenting the care given to the client.

Example of Documentation

DATE	TIME	NOTES
10/25/93	0930	Number 16 French catheter inserted and 20 ml urine for culture was obtained. Urine was cloudy yellow. Specimen sent to lab.
		S. Williams, RN

Teaching Tips

Explain the purpose of the specimen to the client or the client's family, or both. This is a good time for a discussion related to perineal hygiene.

Home Care Variations

Transport the specimen in a cooler from the client's home to the laboratory. Dispose of all used equipment in a sealed plastic bag.

SKILL 5–13   COLLECTING A URINE SPECIMEN FROM A MINICATHETER

Clinical Situations in Which You May Encounter This Skill

A urine specimen is collected when a urinary tract infection is suspected and urine is needed for a urine culture and sensitivity test. A minicatheter is usually used in outpatient clinics and physicians' offices. This procedure is performed for female clients since the tubing in the kit is not of sufficient length for male clients.

Anticipated Responses

▼ You use sterile technique and the catheter is inserted and the specimen is obtained without contamination or trauma.

Adverse Responses

▼ No urine drainage occurs.

Materials List

Gather these materials before beginning the skill:

▼ Sterile gloves
▼ Sheet for drape
▼ Biohazard bag

▼ *ACTION*	▼ *RATIONALE*
1. Assess whether the client has had the procedure done previously.	1. Teaching can be individualized based on prior experience. It also gives the client a chance to tell you what problems may have been countered previously.
2. Check the chart for a physician's order and the reason for the catheterization.	2. A physician's order is required. The reason for the catheterization should be explained to the client.
3. Assess the client's ability to follow directions and cooperate.	3. It may be necessary for another nurse to assist you if the client is uncooperative or unable to assist.
4. Close the door and the curtains around the bed.	4. Protects the client's privacy.
5. a. If performing the procedure for a client in a hospital bed: Raise the bed to a comfortable working height and position the client in dorsal recumbent position with feet spread apart.	5. a. Reduces the strain placed on your back and aids in visualizing the client's urinary meatus.
b. If performing the procedure for a client on an examination table: Place the client's feet in stirrups and have the client move down on the table until his or her perineal area is even with the end of the table.	b. Aids in visualizing the client's urinary meatus.
6. Place the drape over the client in a diamond configuration with one corner at the client's sternum, one corner over each of his or her knees, and one corner over his or her perineum.	6. Allows you to expose the client's perineal area while covering the rest of his or her body.
7. Open the outer wrapper of the minicatheter kit. Keep the inside sterile.	7. Allows you to use the inner wrapper as a small sterile field.
8. Put on gloves using sterile technique.	8. Gloves should be worn whenever there is a chance of coming into contact with body fluids to prevent the transmission of microorganisms.
9. Tear open the top of the povidone-iodine (Betadine) swabs and place the container within easy reach.	9. Used to clean the client's perineal area.

▼ *ACTION* ▼ *RATIONALE*

10. Pull 3 to 4 inches of the length of the catheter out of the test tube (see Fig. 5–14).

10. Prepares the minicatheter for use.

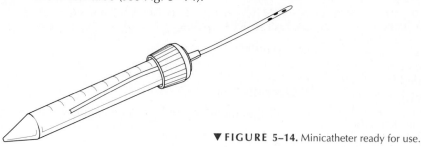

▼ **FIGURE 5–14.** Minicatheter ready for use.

11. Loosen and leave the cap on the test-tube portion of the minicatheter loose.

11. Urine will not flow into the test tube if the cap is too tight.

12. Place the minicatheter within easy reach on your sterile field.

12. Once the labia are spread, you may not release them to reach for the catheter.

13. Spread the client's labia with your nondominant hand.

13. Provides access to the client's urinary meatus for cleansing.

14. Clean the urinary meatus and the surrounding area by wiping from front to back once with each of the three povidone-iodine swabs.

14. Removes secretions and microorganisms that will contaminate the catheter and cause a urinary tract infection. Wiping from front to back prevents the introduction of fecal bacteria into the client's urinary meatus, and thus reduces the chance of introducing these bacteria into the bladder.

15. Grasp the test-tube portion of the minicatheter in your dominant hand and gently insert the tip of the minicatheter into the urinary meatus and advance it until urine begins to flow into the tube. (This requires insertion of 2–3 inches of the catheter.) Continue to hold the client's labia open during this process. If the labia close, the urinary meatus will be contaminated with microorganisms and you must clean the area again.

15. Promotes catheter insertion without contaminating the catheter tip, which will be inserted into the client's bladder.

16. Allow the test tube to fill with urine.

16. Collect 10 ml of urine for the culture and sensitivity test.

17. Withdraw the catheter from the client's urinary meatus.

17. A minicatheter is a single-use catheter only.

18. Pull the catheter out of the test tube and discard the catheter.

18. The specimen has been obtained and the catheter is no longer needed.

19. Tighten the lid on the test tube and close the stopper.

19. Seals the tube and prevents leakage of urine.

20. Return the client's bed to the lowest position.

20. Reduces potential injury from falls.

21. Fill out the identifying data on the adhesive label and place it on the tube. Place the tube in a biohazard bag.

21. Identifies the client to whom the specimen belongs.

22. Refrigerate the specimen or send it to the laboratory immediately.

22. Allowing the urine to sit will alter the results of the test.

23. Remove the gloves and wash your hands.

23. Prevents the possible transmission of microorganisms.

24. Record the procedure in the client's chart.

24. Communicates the findings to the other members of the health care team and contributes to the legal record by documenting the care given to the client.

Example of Documentation

DATE	TIME	NOTES
11/8/93	0900	Minicatheter inserted and 10 ml urine obtained for culture. Urine was cloudy yellow. Specimen sent to lab.

S. Williams, RN

Teaching Tips

Explain the purpose of the specimen collection to the client.

Home Care Variations

Transport the specimen from the client's home to the laboratory in a cooler. Dispose of all used equipment in a sealed plastic bag.

SKILL 5–14   COLLECTING A 24-HOUR URINE SPECIMEN

Clinical Situations in Which You May Encounter This Skill

Urine is collected over a 24-hour period to determine the excretion rate of certain hormones, proteins, and electrolytes. The laboratory will supply the container and add any necessary preservatives.

If urine is discarded accidentally after urine collection has begun, the physician should be notified and the test should be started again. Any loss of urine will invalidate the results of the test.

Anticipated Responses

▼ The urine is collected and put in the collection bottle without any loss of urine.

Adverse Responses

▼ Urine is discarded accidentally.

Materials List

Gather these materials before beginning the skill:

▼ Large capped collection bottle (containing preservative if necessary)
▼ Bedpan, toilet specimen container, or urinal if an indwelling catheter is not in place
▼ Large basin with ice
▼ Adhesive label or marker
▼ Signs: 24-Hour Urine in Progress
▼ Examination gloves

▼ ACTION

1. Determine the reason for the test and explain the reason and the procedure to the client.

2. Obtain a collection bottle from the laboratory. Determine if a preservative is needed by checking the laboratory manual.

3. Post signs on the door to the room, above the client's bed, and in the bathroom that a 24-hour urine test is in progress.

4. Have the client void to empty his or her bladder and discard the urine.

5. Note the time.

▼ RATIONALE

1. Explanation increases client's ability to participate in his care.

2. Allows you to check the bottle obtained from the laboratory for accuracy.

3. Reminds all nursing personnel and family members to save the client's urine.

4. Since the 24-hour urine is a timed quantitative determination, it is essential to start the test with an empty bladder.

5. This time will be the beginning of the 24-hour collection period.

▼ **ACTION** | ▼ **RATIONALE**

6. Instruct the client to save all urine for the next 24 hours and to notify you or another nurse of each voiding. If the urine is discarded, test results will be invalid. Also, instruct the client not to defecate with the urine or to place toilet tissue in the urine.

6. The total volume of urine collected during the 24-hour period is a factor used to calculate the excretion rate of the substance. The results will be altered if the urine is allowed to sit. Feces and toilet paper may alter the test results.

7. Pour urine from each voiding into the collection bottle and keep the collection bottle on ice or in the refrigerator unless the laboratory instructs you otherwise (see Fig. 5–15). Measure the amount of each voiding. Wear examination gloves when handling urine.

7. The results may be altered by urine that is not properly stored. Ice is used for preservation and to control bacterial growth. Gloves protect you from contact with blood or body fluids.

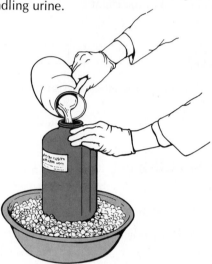

▼ **FIGURE 5–15.** The 24-hour urine specimen collection bottle must be kept on ice or refrigerated.

8. Fifteen minutes prior to the end of the 24-hour collection period, have the client void. Pour this final specimen into the collection bottle.

8. This is necessary for all urine excreted during the 24-hour time period to be collected.

9. Label the collection bottle and send it to the laboratory immediately.

9. The results may be altered since the urine is no longer on ice or refrigerated.

10. Wash your hands.

10. Decreases the transmission of microorganisms.

11. Assess the color and clarity of the urine and the presence of any sediment each time the client voids.

11. These data will be necessary for charting.

12. Record the time you began the collection. Note any preservatives added to the collection bottle and where the bottle is located. At the completion of the specimen collection, record the time completed and the color, appearance, and odor of the urine.

12. Communicates the findings to the other members of the health care team and contributes to the legal record by documenting the care given to the client.

Example of Documentation

DATE	TIME	NOTES
10/25/93	0900	24-hour urine for potassium begun. No preservative added to the bottle. Specimen container in bathroom on ice.
		S. Williams, RN

Teaching Tips

Explain the purpose of the sample and the procedure to the client or the client's family member.

Home Care Variations

Write instructions to leave for the client or his or her family member. Take a collection bottle with an appropriate preservative. If the specimen is to be kept cool, make sure that the family has ice or refrigeration. Make specific arrangements to return for the specimen and transport the specimen in a cooler.

SKILL 5–15 COLLECTING A CAPILLARY BLOOD SPECIMEN USING A LANCET OR AN AUTOMATIC PUNCTURE DEVICE

Clinical Situations in Which You May Encounter This Skill

A finger stick, earlobe stick, or heel stick is used to collect a small amount of blood for tests such as a hematocrit or blood glucose. The procedure may be done by a health care worker or by the client monitoring blood glucose at home. Capillary blood specimens also are performed to collect blood samples from neonates, infants, and young children, since venipuncture may be difficult or painful for these young clients.

Anticipated Responses

▼ The finger, earlobe, or heel bleeds when stuck and the specimen is collected.

Adverse Responses

▼ The finger, earlobe, or heel does not bleed sufficiently.

Materials List

Gather these materials before beginning the skill:

▼ Blood lancet or automatic puncture device
▼ 70% alcohol swab
▼ Dry gauze or cotton ball
▼ Small adhesive bandage
▼ Examination gloves
▼ Appropriate collection container for the test you are performing (filter paper, capillary tubes, sealing clay, etc.)

▼ ACTION	▼ RATIONALE
1. Check the physician's order for the blood to be drawn.	1. Allows you to gather the correct materials for the test. The reason for the test should be explained to the client or the client's parents.
2. Put on gloves.	2. When there is a chance of coming into contact with blood, gloves should be worn to prevent the possible transmission of microorganisms.

▼ *A C T I O N*

▼ *R A T I O N A L E*

3. Select a puncture site on the client's second or third finger. Avoid calluses, scars, or lesions. The heel is commonly used in infants and children up to 18 months of age. The earlobe is a puncture site that is less commonly used (Fig. 5–16).

3. Calluses and scars will make it more difficult to stick. Lesions are avoided to prevent the transfer of microorganisms.

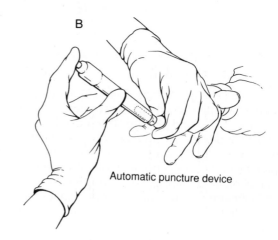

Lancet

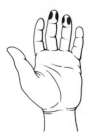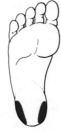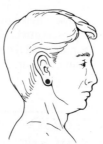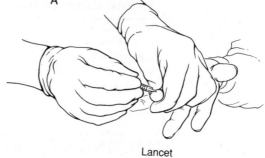

Finger stick   Heel stick   Earlobe stick

▼ **FIGURE 5–16.** Puncture sites for capillary blood specimen.

▼ **FIGURE 5–17.** Obtaining a capillary blood specimen using a lancet or an automatic puncture device.

Automatic puncture device

4. Place the client's extremity in a dependent position when using the finger or heel site. If you are using the heel, you should dorsiflex the client's foot.

4. A dependent position facilitates blood flow to the area.

5. Gently "milk" the client's extremity by alternately squeezing and releasing.

5. "Milking" will facilitate blood flow to the area.

6. Cleanse the site with a 70% alcohol swab and allow the area to dry.

6. Decreases the transfer of microorganisms.

7. a. If using a lancet: Puncture the site with a sterile lancet using a sharp quick flexion motion.
   b. If using an automatic puncture device: Load the automatic puncture device with a needle, place the autolet against the intended site, and pull the trigger (see Fig. 5–17).

7. a. This motion will help pierce the client's skin with the lancet.

8. Wipe off the first two drops of blood with a piece of dry gauze or a cotton ball.

8. An alcohol wipe would cause the site to burn.

9. Collect the specimen in the container appropriate for the test you are performing.

9. Filter paper may be used for a blood glucose test and a capillary tube may be used for a hematocrit test.

▼ *ACTION*   ▼ *RATIONALE*

a. If collecting a specimen on filter paper, thoroughly saturate the area indicated on the paper by placing the paper directly on the puncture site and milking the blood onto the paper (Fig. 5–18)

a. Thorough saturation of filter paper ensures adequate blood sample for the test to be performed.

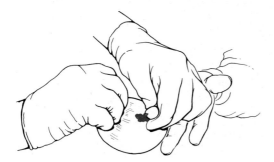

▼ **FIGURE 5–18.** Collecting a blood specimen on filter paper.

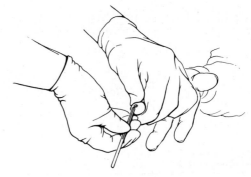

▼ **FIGURE 5–19.** Collecting a blood specimen in a capillary tube.

b. If using a capillary tube hold it horizontally and fill the tube two-thirds to three-fourths full (Fig. 5–19). Cover the end of the tube with your finger when transferring the specimen to sealing clay or other testing materials (Fig. 5–20).

b. Blood should flow to the marked end of the tube. The tube is held horizontally to facilitate blood flow into the tube. Covering the tube with your finger prevents blood from spilling.

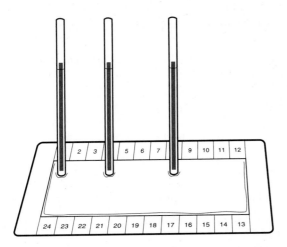

▼ **FIGURE 5–20.** Transferring filled capillary tube to sealing clay.

10. Apply pressure to the puncture site using a cotton ball or gauze pad.

10. Stops the bleeding.

11. Apply a small adhesive bandage over the puncture site.

11. Protects the site and prevents any further bleeding from soiling clothes or linen.

12. Properly dispose of the lancet.

12. Decreases the transmission of microorganisms.

13. Remove the gloves and wash your hands.

13. Decreases the transmission of microorganisms.

14. Check to make sure that bleeding has stopped. If it hasn't, apply pressure and then a small adhesive bandage.

14. Clients with hematologic disorders or who are taking Coumadin or heparin may continue to bleed.

▼ ACTION	▼ RATIONALE
15. Record the procedure.	15. Communicates the findings to the other members of the health care team and contributes to the legal record by documenting the care given to the client.

Example of Documentation

DATE	TIME	NOTES
11/15/93	1100	Finger stick on right middle finger for blood glucose. Blood glucose 124.
		T. White, RN

Teaching Tips

If the client is to perform finger sticks for home glucose monitoring, teach the procedure to the client or his or her family. Explain the purpose of a finger stick.

Home Care Variations

Periodically verify the client's ability to monitor his or her own blood glucose if home monitoring is being done. Talk to the client about the proper disposal of used equipment.

SKILL 5–16   COLLECTING A VENOUS BLOOD SPECIMEN BY VENIPUNCTURE USING A SYRINGE

Clinical Situations in Which You May Encounter This Skill

A syringe is used when a single tube of blood is needed. Principles of surgical asepsis should be followed when collecting the blood.

Anticipated Responses

▼ The blood is collected without contamination.

Adverse Responses

▼ Bleeding continues after the specimen has been collected.
▼ You are unable to obtain a blood sample.

Materials List

Gather these materials before beginning the skill:

▼ Five- to 10-cc syringe with a 19- to 21-gauge 1-inch needle
▼ 70% alcohol wipe
▼ Dry gauze or cotton ball
▼ Appropriate test tube for the test
▼ Labels for test tubes
▼ Small adhesive bandage
▼ Examination gloves
▼ Tourniquet
▼ Biohazard bag

▼ ACTION	▼ RATIONALE
1. Check the physician's order for the blood to be drawn.	1. Allows you to gather the correct materials for the test. The reason for the test should be explained to the client or the client's parent.

▼ *A C T I O N*

▼ *R A T I O N A L E*

2. Put on gloves.

2. When there is a chance of coming into contact with blood, gloves should be worn to prevent the possible transmission of microorganisms.

3. Select a puncture site (Fig. 5–21). Use distal aspects of the vein first. Avoid scars and lesions, or a vein with an intravenous (IV) infusion in place.

3. Scars will make sticking more difficult. Lesions are avoided to prevent the transfer of microorganisms. IV fluids will alter test results.

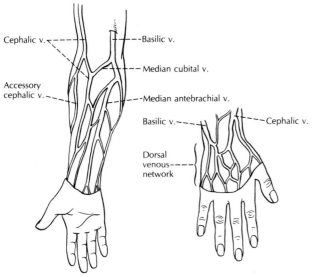

▼ **FIGURE 5–21.** Venipuncture sites.

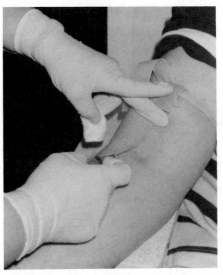

▼ **FIGURE 5–22.** Filling the syringe.

4. Place the site in a dependent position.

4. A dependent position facilitates blood flow to the area.

5. Ask the client to make a fist.

5. Helps to distend the vein.

6. Apply a tourniquet around the client's extremity above the site.

6. The tourniquet obstructs venous blood flow and causes the vein to distend. Distended veins are easier to see and palpate.

7. Cleanse the site with a 70% alcohol swab and allow the area to dry.

7. Decreases the transfer of microorganisms.

8. Anchor the vein with the thumb on your nondominant hand.

8. Stabilizes the vein.

9. Hold the syringe with the needle bevel up and the needle positioned at a 45-degree angle over the client's vein.

9. Allows the needle to be placed parallel to the vein.

10. Puncture the site (Fig. 5–22) and pull back on the plunger. Fill the syringe with the required amount of blood.

10. If the needle is in the vein, the syringe should begin to fill with blood.

11. Immediately loosen the tourniquet.

11. Prevents blood from entering the surrounding tissue.

12. Withdraw the syringe and apply pressure to the puncture site with a cotton ball or gauze pad.

12. Pressure is applied to stop the bleeding.

13. Apply a small adhesive bandage over the puncture site.

13. Helps to prevent further bleeding.

14. Carefully remove the needle from the syringe and the stopper from the test tube. Gently inject the blood into the correct collection tube. Take care to avoid needle stick.

14. Gentle transfer is necessary to prevent damage to the erythrocytes.

▼ A C T I O N	▼ R A T I O N A L E
15. Properly dispose of the syringe and needle.	**15.** Decreases the transmission of microorganisms.
16. If the tube contains an additive, gently rotate or invert the tube.	**16.** Facilitates mixing the blood with the contents of the collection tube.
17. Place the tube of blood in a biohazard bag for transport to the laboratory.	**17.** Bag protects you from blood contact.
18. Remove the gloves and wash your hands.	**18.** Decreases the transmission of microorganisms.
19. Record the procedure.	**19.** Communicates the findings to the other members of the health care team and contributes to the legal record by documenting the care given to the client.

Example of Documentation

DATE	TIME	NOTES
11/15/93	1000	Blood collected for a potassium level and sent to lab.
		T. White, RN

Teaching Tips

Explain the procedure and the purpose of the procedure to the client or the client's family, or both.

Home Care Variations

Take a sealed needle collection bottle to the client's home. After the procedure, dispose of the needle in the bottle, and remove the sealed needle collection bottle and used syringe from the client's home.

SKILL 5–17   COLLECTING A VENOUS BLOOD SPECIMEN BY VENIPUNCTURE USING A VACUUM CONTAINER

Clinical Situations in Which You May Encounter This Skill

A vacuum container may be used to collect a single tube or multiple tubes of blood. Principles of surgical asepsis should be followed when collecting blood.

Anticipated Responses

▼ Blood is collected without contamination.

Adverse Responses

▼ Bleeding continues after the specimen has been collected.
▼ You are unable to collect a blood specimen.

Materials List

Gather these materials before beginning the skill:

▼ Vacuum container
▼ Vacuum container needle
▼ 70% alcohol wipe
▼ Dry gauze or cotton ball
▼ Small adhesive bandage
▼ Appropriate stoppered tubes for the test
▼ Labels for test tubes
▼ Tourniquet
▼ Examination gloves
▼ Biohazard bag

▼ *ACTION*   ▼ *RATIONALE*

1. Check the physician's order for the blood to be drawn.

    1. Allows you to gather the correct materials for the test. The reason for the test should be explained to the client or the client's parent.

2. Put on gloves.

    2. When there is a chance of coming into contact with blood, gloves should be worn to prevent the possible transmission of microorganisms.

3. Insert the vacuum container needle into the vacuum container with the short end on the inside and screw the needle into place.

    3. The vacuum container is reusable and does not come with a needle attached.

4. Insert the stoppered tube into the vacuum container but do not puncture the stopper (Fig. 5–23).

    4. If the stopper is punctured, the tube will lose its vacuum and blood will not enter the tube.

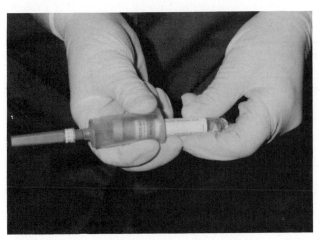

▼ FIGURE 5–23. Assembling the vacuum container collection device.

5. Select a puncture site (see Fig. 5–21). Use the distal aspect of the vein first. Avoid scars and lesions, or a vein with an IV infusion in place.

    5. Scars will make sticking more difficult. Lesions are avoided to prevent the transfer of microorganisms. IV fluids will alter test results.

6. Place the site in a dependent position.

    6. A dependent position facilitates blood flow to the area.

7. Ask the client to make a fist.

    7. Helps to distend the vein.

8. Apply a tourniquet around the client's extremity above the site.

    8. The tourniquet obstructs venous blood flow and causes the vein to distend. Distended veins are easier to see and palpate.

9. Cleanse the site with a 70% alcohol swab and allow the area to dry.

    9. Decreases the transfer of microorganisms.

10. Anchor the client's vein with the thumb on your nondominant hand.

    10. Stabilizes the vein.

11. Hold the vacuum container with the needle bevel up and the needle positioned at a 45-degree angle over the vein.

    11. Allows the needle to be placed parallel to the vein.

12. Puncture the site and push in on the tube to puncture the stopper.

    12. If the needle is in the vein, the tube should begin to fill with blood.

13. Immediately loosen the tourniquet.

    13. Prevents blood from entering the surrounding tissue.

14. Withdraw the vacuum container and apply pressure to the puncture site with a cotton ball or gauze pad.

    14. Pressure is applied to stop the bleeding.

▼ *ACTION*	▼ *RATIONALE*
15. Apply a small adhesive bandage over the puncture site.	**15.** Helps to prevent further bleeding.
16. Remove and properly dispose of the needle.	**16.** Decreases the transmission of microorganisms.
17. Remove the tube of blood from the vacuum container, label it, place in biohazard bag, and send it to the laboratory.	**17.** The label helps to ensure that the correct test is performed for the correct patient. The bag protects you from blood contact.
18. Remove the gloves and wash your hands.	**18.** Decreases the transmission of microorganisms.
19. Chart the procedure.	**19.** Communicates to the other members of the health care team and contributes to the legal record by documenting the care given to the client.

Example of Documentation

DATE	TIME	NOTES
11/15/93	1000	Blood collected for electrolytes and sent to the lab.
		T. White, RN

Teaching Tips

Explain the procedure and the purpose of the procedure to the client or the client's family, or both.

Home Care Variations

Take a sealed needle collection bottle to the client's home. After the procedure, dispose of the used needle in the bottle, and remove the bottle from the client's home.

SKILL 5–18   COLLECTING A SPUTUM SPECIMEN

Clinical Situations in Which You May Encounter This Skill

Sputum specimens are collected when the client is suspected of having a respiratory infection or malignancy; this suspicion is raised if the client has had a cough for more than 2 weeks, or the mucus that is expectorated has a color or an odor.

In certain circumstances, an induced sputum specimen may be ordered. This is usually accomplished by requiring the client to receive an ultrasonic nebulizing treatment (usually 15–30 ml of distilled water) for 20 minutes prior to the collection of the specimen. The following procedure then is used to obtain the specimen. The induced sputum specimen is useful when the microorganism in question has been difficult to identify. If a client is unable to cough productively, a sputum specimen may be obtained through nasotracheal suctioning using a sputum trap device.

Anticipated Responses

▼ The sputum specimen that is collected consists of mucus from the lungs and bronchi, but not saliva.
▼ The specimen is free of contamination from unrelated sources.
▼ The amount of sputum collected is adequate for the tests required.
▼ After the procedure, the client has no adverse change in respiratory status.

Adverse Responses

▼ Saliva is collected.
▼ The specimen is contaminated from external sources.
▼ No specimen or an inadequate amount of sputum is collected.
▼ After the procedure, the client's respiratory status is further impaired.

Materials List

Gather these materials before beginning the skill:

- ▼ Drinking cup with fresh drinking water
- ▼ Emesis basin
- ▼ Appropriate sterile specimen cup

- ▼ Biohazard bag
- ▼ Label
- ▼ Pen
- ▼ Tissues
- ▼ Trash can
- ▼ Examination gloves

▼ ACTION	▼ RATIONALE
1. Assess the client's ability to learn.	1. If the client is able to learn, he or she can be taught to collect his or her own sputum specimen correctly.
2. Provide the client with a drinking cup and water, an emesis basin, a collection cup, tissues, and a waste can.	2. Facilitates execution of the procedure.
3. Tell the client that: a. Sputum and saliva are not alike. b. Sputum, not saliva, should be analyzed. c. Sputum should be brought up from the lower respiratory tract.	3. a. and b. Saliva moistens food and helps with digestion, and sputum is secreted from the trachea, bronchi, and lungs. c. Sputum must be coughed up from the lower respiratory tract for adequate detection of pathogens.

NOTE: One to 2 tablespoons of sputum are needed for an accurate analysis.

4. Instruct the client to: a. Rinse his or her mouth with fresh water before obtaining a specimen. b. Wait until the client has the urge to cough and have him or her expectorate the sputum (mucus) into the cup without touching the insides of the cup or c. Take three deep breaths and as he or she exhales on the third breath, expectorate into the cup as above. (If this does not produce sputum, encourage the client to try again.) d. The optimal time to obtain the specimen is upon arising in the morning. e. After obtaining the specimen, put the top onto the cup without touching the inside of the top or the cup. f. Call you as soon as the specimen is collected.	a. Decreases contamination of the specimen by clearing the oral cavity of potentially unrelated organisms. b. The cough reflex may be initiated by mucus that then can be expectorated. c. Deep breathing encourages the movement and expectoration of secretions from the respiratory tract. d. Pooling of respiratory secretions occur during periods of rest with infrequent position changes. This facilitates the expectoration of sputum. e. Decreases contamination of the specimen with other organisms. f. The specimen should be taken to the laboratory immediately after collection.
5. Put on gloves.	5. Gloves should be worn when there is a chance of coming in contact with any body fluid to prevent the possible transmission of microorganisms.

▼ *ACTION*   ▼ *RATIONALE*

6. With gloved hands, take the sputum cup from the client (Fig. 5–24).

6. Decreases the transmission of microorganisms.

7. Label the specimen with appropriate information.

7. Helps ensure that results obtained are for the correct client so that treatment can be specified appropriately.

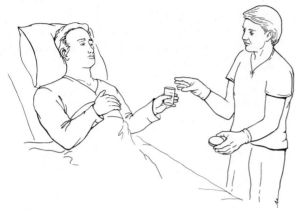

▼ FIGURE 5–24. Use gloves when handling sputum specimen.

8. Place the labeled container into a biohazard bag and close it securely.

8. Decreases the transmission of microorganisms.

9. Remove the gloves and discard them in a proper container.

9. Decreases the transmission of microorganisms.

10. Wash your hands.

10. Decreases the transmission of microorganisms.

11. Observe the sputum for color, odor, amount, and consistency.

11. Assists in the diagnosis of respiratory illnesses.

12. Send the specimen to the laboratory immediately.

12. The results may be altered if the specimen is allowed to sit.

13. Record the procedure and note the color, odor, amount, and consistency of the sputum.

13. Communicates the findings to the other members of the health care team and contributes to the legal record by documenting the care given to the client.

Example of Documentation

DATE	TIME	NOTES
10/23/93	0800	Approximately 2 tablespoons thick, white, odorless sputum collected and sent to lab for analysis. Client's respiratory status unchanged from 0700 assessment.
		S. Williams, RN

Teaching Tips

Remind the client that for an accurate analysis of the specimen, he or she should cough and produce sputum from as deep in the chest as possible. The client should be well hydrated to be able to produce sputum that may be expectorated readily. This skill lends itself to the teaching of basic hygiene principles including: proper and frequent handwashing, covering the mouth and nose when coughing, and proper disposal of contaminated tissues.

SKILL 5–19   COLLECTING A STOOL SPECIMEN

Clinical Situations in Which You May Encounter This Skill

Stool specimens may be obtained to examine for bile, bilirubin, blood, microorganisms, ova, and parasites. The presence of bacteria is noted through cultures, whereas microscopic examination reveals meat fibers and fat that indicate malabsorption. Stool specimens are often collected from clients who are experiencing diarrhea, constipation, bleeding, or other symptoms of a gastrointestinal disorder.

Anticipated Responses

▼ The stool specimen is collected.

Adverse Responses

▼ The stool specimen is discarded accidentally.
▼ The stool specimen is contaminated with urine or toilet tissue.

Materials List

Gather these materials before beginning the skill:

▼ Cardboard specimen cup or, if for a culture, sterile prepackaged swab with culture medium in the tube
▼ Adhesive label or marker
▼ Tongue blade
▼ Clean or sterile toilet specimen container or bedpan
▼ Label
▼ Examination gloves
▼ Air freshener
▼ Biohazard bag

▼ *A C T I O N*	▼ *R A T I O N A L E*
1. Ask the client if he or she has taken barium, bismuth, mineral oil, iron, or antibiotics.	1. These substances may interfere with the results of the test. The laboratory sheet should note that the client has taken these substances. If the stool is collected for ova and parasites, you should wait 7 days after the client has taken barium to collect the specimen. Antibiotic use should be noted on the laboratory sheet if the specimen is for a culture.
2. Check the physician's order for the test to be performed.	2. Facilitates proper collection of the specimen. If the stool is collected for both ova and parasites and culture and sensitivity, specimens should be sent in separate cups. If the test is for pinworms, the specimen should be collected early in the morning.
3. If you are collecting the specimen from a bedpan, close the door and the curtains around the client's bed.	3. Provides privacy for the client.
4. Instruct the client to void prior to collecting the stool specimen. If the client is menstruating, provide perineal care and place a tampon or a 4- × 4-inch gauze pad in her vaginal orifice. Caution the client not to put toilet paper in the specimen.	4. Urine can alter the results of the test. Menstrual blood can alter the test results. Toilet paper will alter the results.
5. When the client needs to defecate, either place the client on a clean bedpan or place a clean toilet specimen container in the toilet.	5. Urine and toilet paper can alter the test results.

▼ *ACTION*	▼ *RATIONALE*
6. Put on gloves.	**6.** When there is a chance of coming into contact with feces, gloves should be worn to prevent the possible transmission of microorganisms.
7. Obtain the specimen. 　a. If the specimen is for a culture, use the sterile prepackaged swab and collect a piece of stool on the end of the swab. Then return the swab to the tube, put the top on, and crush the end with the culture medium. 　b. If the stool is for ova and parasites, collect all of the stool. 　c. If the stool is for other tests, use the tongue blade and put approximately 15 ml of stool in the specimen container.	**7.** a. A sterile swab and culture tube are used to prevent the introduction of other bacteria into the sample. 　b. Since the ova and parasites are not distributed evenly in the feces, the entire amount is needed. Several specimens often are needed to find the parasites.
8. Label the specimen, place it in a biohazard bag, and send it to the laboratory immediately.	**8.** The specimen should either be kept warm or refrigerated depending on the test. If the test is for a culture, an overgrowth of organisms can occur when the specimen is allowed to sit. If the specimen for ova and parasites is not kept warm, the ova and parasites may die, which would prevent accurate diagnosis.
9. Cleanse the client, position him or her, and leave him or her comfortable. An air freshener may be used.	**9.** Cleansing the client will help to prevent the spread of microorganisms and will promote the client's comfort.
10. Properly dispose of equipment.	**10.** Prevents the transmission of microorganisms.
11. Remove the gloves and wash your hands.	**11.** Prevents the possible transmission of microorganisms.
12. Record the procedure. Note the color, consistency, odor, amount of stool, and time and disposition of the specimen.	**12.** Communicates the findings to the other members of the health care team and contributes to the legal record by documenting the care given to the client.

Example of Documentation

DATE	TIME	NOTES
10/19/93	0730	Moderate amount of formed brown stool. Specimen for ova and parasites collected. Sent immediately to the laboratory. *S. Williams, RN*

Teaching Tips

Explain the purpose of the stool specimen sample to the client or the client's family, or both. Explain the collection procedure.

Home Care Variations

The client can place a piece of plastic wrap under the seat over the opening of the toilet to collect the specimen and may use a tongue depressor to transfer the specimen to the container. Dispose of used equipment in a sealed plastic bag. Immediately transport the specimen to the laboratory.

SKILL 5–20   COLLECTING A URETHRAL SPECIMEN

Clinical Situations in Which You May Encounter This Skill

A urethral specimen is usually collected when signs of infection are present. Culture and sensitivity tests are performed to identify pathogenic organisms such as *Neisseria gonorrhoeae, Treponema pallidum,* and *Trichomonas vaginalis* and to identify the drug that will best eradicate the organisms. The specimen is collected using sterile technique.

Anticipated Responses

▼ The specimen is collected without contamination.

Adverse Responses

▼ The specimen is contaminated in the process of collection.

Materials List

Gather these materials before beginning the skill:

▼ Sheet
▼ Sterile prepackaged swab with culture medium in the tube
▼ Biohazard bag
▼ Lamp or flashlight
▼ Label
▼ Examination gloves
▼ Towel and washcloth
▼ Soap
▼ Basin of warm water

▼ *ACTION*

1. Determine the reason for the test.

2. Assess the client's ability to follow directions and cooperate.

3. Place the female client in the dorsal recumbent position and drape her. Position the male client in the supine position and drape him.
   a. For the female client: Place a drape over the client in a diamond configuration, with one corner at the client's sternum, one corner over each of her knees, and one corner over her perineum.
   b. For the male client: Expose only the client's penis while covering the remainder of his body with a sheet.

4. Position a light.

5. Put on gloves.

6. Open the culture tube. Hold the swab with your dominant hand.

▼ *RATIONALE*

1. The reason should be explained to the client.

2. It may be necessary for another nurse to assist you if the client is uncooperative or unable to assist.

3. These positions facilitate visualization of the urinary meatus. Draping provides privacy for the client.

4. Aids in visualization of the urinary meatus.

5. Gloves should be worn when there is a chance of coming in contact with bodily secretions to prevent the possible transmission of microorganisms.

6. Your nondominant hand will be used to spread the client's labia or hold the client's penis.

▼ ACTION	▼ RATIONALE

7. a. For the female client: Spread the client's labia with your nondominant hand. Observe the meatus.

    b. For the male client: Hold the client's penis vertically with your nondominant hand and retract the foreskin on an uncircumcised male to expose the urinary meatus. Observe the meatus.

8. Insert the swab gently through the meatus into the anterior portion of the urethra and obtain the drainage on the end of the swab (Fig. 5–25). (Return the foreskin on the uncircumcised male to the original position.)

7. a. The labia are spread to visualize the meatus for any drainage. Note the amount and characteristics of the drainage.

8. Drainage accumulates in the anterior portion of the urethra.

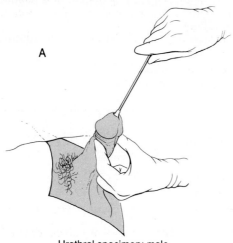
Urethral specimen: male

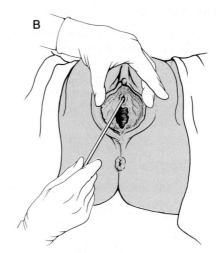
Urethral specimen: female

▼ **FIGURE 5–25.** Using a swab to obtain a urethral specimen from a male and a female client.

9. Put the swab into the tube with the culture medium, squeeze the end, push the swab into the medium, and put the top on the culturette (Fig. 5–26).

9. Squeezing the end of the tube activates the culture medium.

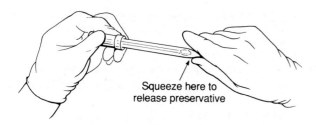
Squeeze here to release preservative

▼ **FIGURE 5–26.** Putting the swab into the culture medium tube.

10. Wash the client's perineal area with warm water and soap. Rinse and dry the area.

11. Remove the gloves and wash your hands.

12. Label the specimen and place it in a biohazard bag, and send it to the laboratory immediately.

10. Helps the client to feel better and removes the discharge that is irritating to the client's skin.

11. Prevents the possible transmission of microorganisms.

12. The results may be altered if the specimen is allowed to sit. An overgrowth of organisms could occur.

▼ _ACTION_	▼ _RATIONALE_
13. Note the color, amount, and odor of the drainage.	**13.** Presence of these data may be indicative of an infection.
14. Chart the procedure.	**14.** Communicates the findings to the other members of the health care team and contributes to the legal record by documenting the care given to the client.

Example of Documentation

DATE	_TIME_	_NOTES_
10/25/93	1000	Complained of itching. A small amount of yellowish discharge noted around urethra. Culture obtained and sent to the lab.
		S. Williams, RN

Teaching Tips

Explain the purpose of the specimen to the client or the client's family, or both. Explain the collection procedure. Discuss perineal hygiene.

Home Care Variations

Dispose of all used equipment in a sealed plastic bag according to your agency policy.

SKILL 5–21 COLLECTING A THROAT SPECIMEN

Clinical Situations in Which You May Encounter This Skill

A culture may be needed for clients who present with signs or symptoms of an upper respiratory, throat, or sinus infection.

Anticipated Responses

▼ The specimen is collected without contamination.

Adverse Responses

▼ The specimen is contaminated in the process of collection.

Materials List

Gather these materials before beginning the skill:

▼ Tongue blade
▼ Penlight or flashlight
▼ Sterile cotton-tipped swabs and blood agar plate or sterile prepackaged swab with culture medium in the tube
▼ Examination gloves
▼ Biohazard bag

▼ _ACTION_	▼ _RATIONALE_
1. Assess the client's ability to follow directions and cooperate.	**1.** It may be necessary for another nurse to assist you if the client is uncooperative or unable to assist.

▼ _A C T I O N_ _____ ▼ _R A T I O N A L E_ _____

2. Assess whether the client has had the procedure done previously.

2. Teaching can be individualized based on prior experience.

3. Put on gloves.

3. When there is a chance of coming into contact with bodily secretions, gloves should be worn to prevent the possible transmission of microorganisms.

4. Ask the client to sit facing you and to tilt his or her head back.

4. Facilitates collection of the specimen.

5. Ask the client to open his or her mouth and say "ah."

5. Allows you to visualize the pharynx. If the pharynx is not visualized, depress the anterior one-third of the tongue with a tongue blade.

6. Illuminate the pharyngeal area with a penlight.

6. Illumination is needed for good visualization.

7. Note any redness or white exudate.

7. The appearance of the pharynx should be charted.

8. Holding the tongue blade in your nondominant hand, depress the client's tongue.

8. The tongue is depressed so the swab can reach the client's pharyngeal area.

9. With your dominant hand, insert the swab and quickly swab the tonsillar area (Fig. 5–27).

9. The area is swabbed quickly to avoid stimulating the gag reflex.

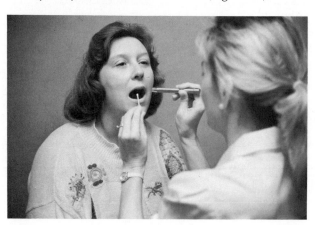

▼ **FIGURE 5–27.** Using a swab to obtain a throat specimen.

10. Avoid touching any oral structures.

10. If the oral structures are touched, the specimen is contaminated.

11. a. Agar plate: Swab the agar plate using a back-and-forth Z-shaped motion.
  b. Culturette: Put the swab into the tube with the culture medium, squeeze the end, push the swab into the medium, and put the top on the culturette (see Fig. 5–26).

11. a. Distributes any organisms.

  b. Squeezing the end of the tube activates the culture medium.

12. Label the specimen, place it in a biohazard bag, and send it to the laboratory immediately.

12. Allowing the specimen to sit may alter the results.

13. Remove the gloves and wash your hands.

13. Decreases the transmission of microorganisms.

14. Record the procedure.

14. Communicates the findings to the other members of the health care team and contributes to the legal record by documenting the care given to the client.

Example of Documentation

DATE	TIME	NOTES
11/17/93	1000	Complaining of a sore throat. Culture obtained and sent to lab.
		S. Williams, RN

Teaching Tips

Explain the procedure for and the purpose of the test to the client or the client's family, or both.

Home Care Variations

Dispose of all used equipment in a sealed plastic bag to decrease the transmission of microorganisms according to your agency policy.

SKILL 5–22 COLLECTING A NASAL SPECIMEN

Clinical Situations in Which You May Encounter This Skill

A culture may be needed for clients with signs and symptoms of sinus infections or upper respiratory infections.

Anticipated Responses

▼ The specimen is collected without contamination.

Adverse Responses

▼ The specimen is contaminated in the process of collection.

Materials List

Gather these materials before beginning the skill:

▼ Examination gloves
▼ Sterile prepackaged swab with culture medium in the tube
▼ Nasal speculum (optional)
▼ Label
▼ Biohazard bag

▼ *ACTION*	▼ *RATIONALE*
1. Assess whether the client has had the procedure done before.	1. Teaching can be individualized based on prior experience.
2. Assess the client's ability to follow directions and cooperate.	2. It may be necessary for another nurse to assist you if the client is uncooperative or unable to assist.
3. Put on gloves.	3. When there is a chance of coming into contact with bodily secretions, gloves should be worn to prevent the possible transmission of microorganisms.
4. Ask the client to sit facing you and to tilt his or her head back.	4. Facilitates collection of the specimen.

▼ *ACTION*   ▼ *RATIONALE*

5. Insert the nasal speculum (optional) or use your finger to push the tip of the client's nose upward.

5. Pushing up tip of client's nose or use of the nasal speculum exposes nasal cavity.

6. Insert the swab through the client's nasal cavity and gently swab the posterior part of the nasal canal as shown in Figure 5–28.

6. This is necessary in order to culture any organisms that may be present.

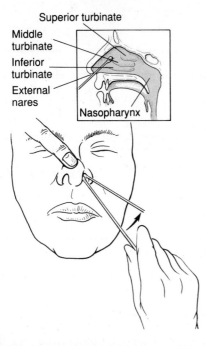

▼ **FIGURE 5–28.** Using a swab to obtain a nasal specimen.

7. Put the swab into the tube with the culture medium, squeeze the end, push the swab into the medium, and put the top on (see Fig. 5–26).

7. Squeezing the end of the tube activates the medium. The swab is pushed into the medium to ensure that any organisms come into contact with the medium.

8. Label the specimen, place it in a biohazard bag, and send it to the laboratory immediately.

8. Allowing the specimen to sit may alter the results.

9. Remove the gloves and wash your hands.

9. Decreases the transmission of microorganisms.

10. Record the procedure.

10. Communicates the findings to the other members of the health care team and contributes to the legal record by documenting the care given to the client.

Example of Documentation

DATE	TIME	NOTES
11/17/93	0900	Draining greenish fluid from nose. Culture obtained and sent to the lab.
		T. White, RN

Teaching Tips

Explain the procedure and the purpose of the test to the client or the client's family, or both.

Home Care Variations

Dispose of all used equipment in a sealed plastic bag to decrease the transmission of microorganisms.

SKILL 5–23   COLLECTING A WOUND OR LESION CULTURE

Clinical Situations in Which You May Encounter This Skill

A culture may be needed for clients with wounds or lesions that are draining.

Anticipated Responses

▼ The specimen is collected without contamination.

Adverse Responses

▼ The specimen is contaminated in the process of collection.

Materials List

Gather these materials before beginning the skill:

▼ Examination gloves
▼ Sterile prepackaged swab with culture medium in the tube
▼ Anaerobic culture tube
▼ Label
▼ Biohazard bag

▼ ACTION

1. Determine the reason for the test.

2. Assess whether the client has had the procedure done before.

3. Put on gloves.

4. Position the area containing the wound or lesion within easy reach.

5. Gently swab the wound or lesion, making sure to swab any drainage.

6. a. For an aerobic culture: Put the swab into the tube with the culture medium, squeeze the end, push the swab into the medium, and put the top on the culturette (see Figure 5–26).
   b. For an anaerobic culture: Be sure to follow the manufacturer's directions for use of anaerobic culture tubes. Collect the specimen on a swab. Quickly transfer the specimen to the anaerobic culture tube and close the tube.

7. Label the specimen, place it in a biohazard bag, and send it to the laboratory immediately.

8. Remove the gloves and wash your hands.

▼ RATIONALE

1. The reason should be explained to the client.

2. Teaching can be individualized based on prior experience.

3. When there is a chance of coming into contact with bodily secretions, gloves should be worn to prevent the possible transmission of microorganisms.

4. Facilitates collection of the specimen.

5. This is necessary in order to culture any organisms that may be present.

6. a. Squeezing the end of the tube activates the culture medium.

   b. Anaerobic culture tubes contain a carbon dioxide–rich environment that allows the anaerobic bacteria to thrive. You must avoid exposing the specimen to oxygen, since anaerobic bacteria cannot live in the presence of oxygen.

7. Allowing the specimen to sit may alter the results.

8. Decreases the transmission of microorganisms.

▼ ACTION	▼ RATIONALE
9. Record the procedure.	9. Communicates the findings to the other members of the health care team and contributes to the legal record by documenting the care given to the client.

Example of Documentation

DATE	TIME	NOTES
11/17/93	1000	Abdominal incision draining yellowish fluid. Culture obtained and sent to the lab.
		T. White, RN

Teaching Tips

Explain the procedure for and the purpose of obtaining the culture to the client.

Home Care Variations

Dispose of all used equipment and dressings in a sealed plastic bag to decrease the transmission of microorganisms.

References

Daly, J. (1993). Meeting bowel elimination needs. In V. Bolander (Ed.), *Basic nursing* (3rd ed.). Philadelphia: W. B. Saunders.

Dodaro-Surrusco, D., and Zweig, N. (1993). Meeting urinary elimination needs. In V. Bolander (Ed.), *Basic nursing* (3rd ed.). Philadelphia: W. B. Saunders.

Fischbach, F. (1988). *A manual of laboratory diagnostic tests* (3rd ed.). Philadelphia: J. B. Lippincott.

Kersten, L., and Cronin, S. N. (1993). Meeting respiration needs. In V. Bolander (Ed.), *Basic nursing* (3rd ed.). Philadelphia: W. B. Saunders.

Yannelli, B., et al. (1988). Yield of stool cultures, ova and parasite tests, and *Clostridium difficile* determinations in nosocomial diarrheas. *American Journal of Infection Control*, 16, 246–249.

CHAPTER 6

Assisting with Diagnostic Procedures and Screening Tests

Medical diagnostic procedures are used to identify the source of a disorder, assess structural pathologic changes, assess physiologic responses to a disorder, and assess functional impairments related to a disorder. Diagnostic procedures involve assessing a client's body systems through analysis of his or her organs, tissues, body fluids, excretions, and cells.

You will assist the client before, during, and after diagnostic procedures. General nursing responsibilities before a diagnostic test include:

▼ Preparing the person and his or her significant others for the procedure.
▼ Verifying that informed consent has been obtained for the procedure.
▼ Scheduling the diagnostic procedure.
▼ Carrying out preprocedure orders.
▼ Preparing the equipment for the procedure.
▼ Transporting the client to the examination room and his or her significant others to the waiting area.

General nursing responsibilities during a diagnostic test include:

▼ Supporting the client.
▼ Collecting baseline data such as vital signs and continuing to assess the client throughout the procedure.
▼ Assisting with the procedure.

General nursing responsibilities after a diagnostic test include:

▼ Providing postprocedure care and comfort measures.
▼ Notifying the client's significant others of procedure completion.
▼ Processing specimens.
▼ Cleaning or disposing of used equipment, or both.
▼ Documenting the procedure.

- -

SKILL 6–1 ASSISTING WITH ABDOMINAL PARACENTESIS

Clinical Situations in Which You May Encounter This Skill

Paracentesis, a sterile procedure to aspirate fluid from the peritoneal cavity, is used primarily to relieve dyspnea associated with ascites; for diagnostic analysis of the fluid (specific gravity, cell count, protein, culture, and sensitivity); and as a preliminary to other procedures, including surgery, radiography, or ascites reinfusion. Usually only 2 to 3 liters of fluid are removed at one time. Ascites tends to recur rapidly and protein depletion may follow the procedure.

Anticipated Responses

▼ The client does not experience any cardiovascular or respiratory distress or infection as a result of the procedure.
▼ If the paracentesis was done for massive ascites, the client experiences relief of the dyspnea.

Adverse Responses

▼ The client experiences respiratory and cardiovascular distress that results in shock.
▼ During or after the procedure, the client experiences increased pulse, decreased blood pressure, pallor, fainting, or sweating.

Materials List

Gather these materials before beginning the skill:

▼ Disposable paracentesis tray OR 16-gauge 3.5-inch aspiration needle
▼ 5-ml ampule of 1% lidocaine
▼ 21-gauge 1.5-inch needle
▼ 25-gauge 5/8-inch skin needle
▼ 5-ml syringe
▼ 50-ml syringe
▼ Two-way valve
▼ Three specimen tubes
▼ Drainage bag
▼ Sterile drape
▼ Adhesive bandage
▼ Prep applicators
▼ Sponges
▼ Prep tray
▼ Sterile gloves
▼ Masks (optional)
▼ Biohazard bag

▼ *A C T I O N*

▼ *R A T I O N A L E*

1. Ask the client if he or she has ever had the procedure before. Tell the client that the procedure is usually not painful. It may take 15 minutes to obtain a specimen and 1 hour to remove ascitic fluid.

2. Check the physician's order for the reason for the test.

3. Verify that a consent form has been signed by the client.

4. Ask the client if he or she is allergic to local anesthetics or antiseptic solutions.

5. Ask the client to void as completely as possible.

6. Measure the client's abdominal girth and weight.

7. Wash your hands.

8. Open the sterile abdominal paracentesis tray using sterile technique (see Skill 1–9).

9. Help the client to assume a fully supported upright position in the bed or chair. If the client can sit in a chair, support his or her feet on a stool.

10. Place a blood pressure cuff on one of the client's arms.

11. As the physician performs the procedure, help the client to maintain an upright position (Fig. 6–1). Assist the physician as needed.

1. Gives you the opportunity to clarify any questions and to explain exactly what the client should expect.

2. Allows you to provide the correct collection container. If the procedure is for a cell count, you will need a test tube for a small amount of fluid to be sent to the laboratory.

3. This is a surgical procedure that requires that the client understands the potential associated risks.

4. Protects the client from an avoidable allergic reaction.

5. Lessens the danger of inadvertently piercing the client's bladder. If urination is not possible, catheterization will be necessary.

6. Gives an indication of the amount of fluid removed and serves as a comparison if fluid reaccumulates.

7. Decreases the transmission of microorganisms.

8. This is a sterile procedure and sterility must be maintained.

9. In a sitting position, the client's intestines will float away from the paracentesis site and the danger of punctured intestines will be lessened.

10. Allows you to assess the client's blood pressure continuously.

11. Lessens the danger of punctured intestines.

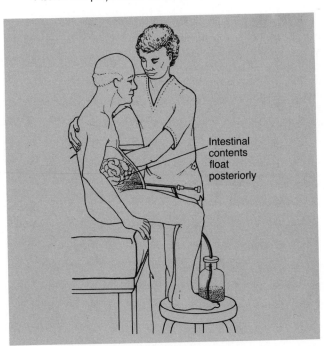

Intestinal contents float posteriorly

▼ **FIGURE 6–1.** Client position for paracentesis.

▼ ACTION	▼ RATIONALE
12. Reassure the client during the procedure.	12. Helps the client cope with the situation and reduces his or her anxiety.
13. Record the client's blood pressure readings and pulse rate at 15-minute intervals and observe the client for signs of pallor or sweating.	13. Indicates if the client is experiencing vascular collapse.
14. When the procedure is completed, assist the client to assume a comfortable position.	14. Fosters the client's relaxation after the procedure.
15. Obtain a measurement of the client's abdominal girth and weight.	15. Serves as a comparison with the preparacentesis assessment.
16. Monitor the client's vital signs, urine output, and dressing for drainage or bleeding every 15 minutes ×4, then every hour ×4, or as ordered by the physician.	16. Monitors the client for complications of shock or hemorrhage.
17. Label the fluid specimen, place in biohazard bag, and send it to the laboratory.	17. If the fluid is for culture and sensitivity, an overgrowth of microorganisms will occur if the fluid is allowed to sit. Label identifies specimen. Bag protects you from contact with body fluids.
18. Record and describe the amount of fluid drained.	18. Communicates the findings to the other members of the health care team and contributes to the legal record by documenting the care given to the client.
19. Dispose of equipment according to your agency guidelines.	19. Proper disposal decreases the transmission of microorganisms.
20. Assess the laboratory results.	20. Based on the results, further medical intervention may be necessary.

Example of Documentation

DATE	TIME	NOTES
11/2/93	0900	Abdominal paracentesis performed by Dr. Jones. BP = 140/86, wt. = 182 lb, abd. girth = 140 cm at beginning of procedure; BP = 138/88, wt. = 179 lb, abdominal girth = 130 cm at end of procedure. 1,500 ml cloudy fluid removed. Pulse remained 88–92 throughout the procedure. 15-ml specimen sent immediately to lab for culture and sensitivity. Resting in low Fowler's position with no complaints of dyspnea or discomfort. S. Williams, RN

SKILL 6–2 ASSISTING WITH BONE MARROW ASPIRATION AND BIOPSY

Clinical Situations in Which You May Encounter This Skill

A bone marrow biopsy is performed when marrow cells (the cells within the bone) need to be aspirated for study. The marrow is usually aspirated from the client's sternum or the upper iliac crest (Fig. 6–2).

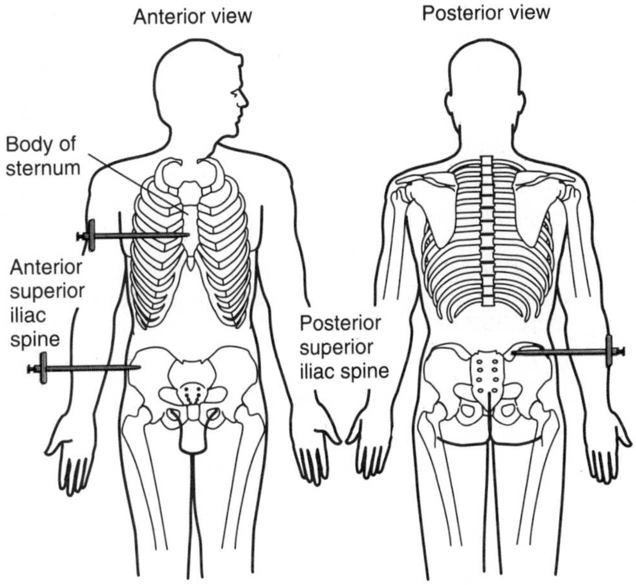

Anticipated Responses

▼ The client experiences some discomfort as the marrow is aspirated. The site may ache for 1 to 2 days after the procedure.

Adverse Responses

▼ The client hemorrhages from the site of aspiration.

Materials List

Gather these materials before beginning the skill:

▼ Bone marrow tray
▼ Antiseptic (such as povidone-iodine), if not supplied on the tray
▼ Lidocaine, if not supplied on the tray
▼ Masks (optional)
▼ Biohazard bag
▼ Sterile gloves

▼ **FIGURE 6–2.** Common sites for bone marrow biopsy.

▼ *ACTION*	▼ *RATIONALE*
1. Check the order to determine the site for the bone marrow aspiration.	1. Allows you to adequately prepare the client for what to expect.
2. Ask the client if he or she has ever had bone marrow aspiration. Tell the client that the procedure may be uncomfortable. The person may hear the needle as it is pushed through the bone and feel pain as marrow is aspirated.	2. Simple explanations of what to anticipate alleviate the client's apprehension and reduce his or her fear.
3. Verify that a consent form has been signed by the client.	3. This is a surgical procedure and the client must be informed about potential complications.
4. Ask the client if he or she has any bleeding disorders.	4. Bleeding disorders may predispose the client to bleeding after the biopsy.
5. Check the client's medications for any that may interfere with clotting.	5. Drugs such as heparin, warfarin, and aspirin can interfere with clotting.
6. Ask the client if he or she is allergic to local anesthetics or antiseptic solutions.	6. Protects the client from an avoidable allergic reaction.
7. Take the client's vital signs.	7. Provides a basis for comparison with postbiopsy vital signs.
8. If ordered, give the client preoperative medication.	8. If the client is very anxious, a preoperative medication may be ordered to allay apprehension and anxiety.

▼ _ACTION_	▼ _RATIONALE_
9. Position the client supine when the sternum or anterior iliac crest is to be used and prone when the posterior iliac crest is to be used.	9. The supine position allows the physician access to the client's sternum and anterior iliac crest and the prone position facilitates access to the posterior iliac crest.
10. Wash your hands.	10. Decreases the transmission of microorganisms.
11. Open the tray on the overbed table using sterile technique (see Skill 1–9).	11. This is a sterile procedure and sterility must be maintained.
12. As the biopsy is performed, reassure the client and assist the physician as necessary.	12. Decreases the client's anxiety.
13. After the biopsy, carefully label the specimens, place in biohazard bag, and send them to the laboratory.	13. Identifies the tests to be performed on the specimens. Bag protects you from contact with body fluids.
14. After bone marrow aspiration: a. Apply direct pressure to the site for 5 to 15 minutes. b. Apply a small dressing, such as a small adhesive bandage or a 4- × 4-inch piece of gauze. c. If a bone marrow biopsy is performed, apply direct pressure and a pressure dressing for 60 minutes.	14. The site may bleed because of the large-bore needle used.
15. Assist the client to assume a recumbent position with pressure on the site.	15. There is minimal discomfort after the procedure, so a position of comfort that will minimize bleeding is indicated.
16. Explain to the client that discomfort will be felt at the site for 1 to 2 days.	16. Reduces the client's apprehension.
17. Dispose of equipment according to your agency guidelines.	17. Decreases the transmission of microorganisms.
18. Ask the client if he or she is experiencing any pain.	18. Pain medication may need to be administered if the client is still experiencing pain after the procedure.
19. Take the client's vital signs and assess for bleeding at the puncture site.	19. An increase in pulse rate or a decrease in blood pressure from the measurements before the bone marrow aspiration and biopsy could indicate bleeding or shock, or both.
20. Chart the procedure. Note how the client tolerated the procedure.	20. Communicates to the other members of the health care team and contributes to the legal record by documenting the care given to the client.

Example of Documentation

DATE	TIME	NOTES
10/18/93	0900	Bone marrow aspiration, posterior iliac crest per Dr. Jones. 5-ml specimen sent to lab. VS = 120/68, 76, 20. No signs of bleeding on dressing. S. Williams, RN

SKILL 6–3   ASSISTING WITH BRONCHOSCOPY

Clinical Situations in Which You May Encounter This Skill

A physician may perform a bronchoscopy for diagnostic or therapeutic purposes. A rigid or a fiberoptic flexible bronchoscope is passed into the bronchi via the client's mouth while he or she is under local or general anesthesia (Fig. 6–3). The larynx, trachea, and bronchial tree then may be visualized to examine tissue, collect secretions, determine the location of pathology, determine if surgery is possible to resect a tumor, or diagnose the site of bleeding. Bronchoscopy also may be performed to remove a foreign body or to remove obstructing secretions.

Anticipated Responses

▼ The client coughs and experiences some hoarseness after the procedure.

Adverse Responses

▼ The client experiences hypoxia.
▼ The client has hemoptysis (bloody sputum) or hemorrhages, or both.
▼ The client experiences laryngospasm or bronchospasm.

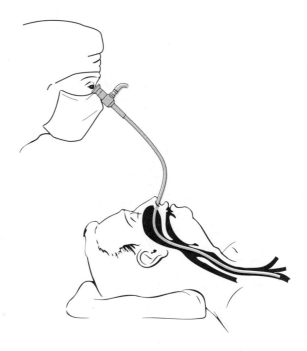

▼ **FIGURE 6–3.** Insertion of a fiberoptic flexible bronchoscope.

Materials List

Gather these materials before beginning the skill:

▼ Bronchoscopy tray
▼ Sterile gloves
▼ Laboratory requisition
▼ Specimen label
▼ Mask(s)

▼ *ACTION*

1. Verify that a consent form has been signed by the client.

2. Explain to the client what to expect before and after the procedure.

3. Ensure that the client has eaten nothing by mouth (NPO) since midnight before the procedure.

4. Ask the client if he or she is allergic to the local anesthetic spray to be used on his or her throat.

5. Have the client void.

▼ *RATIONALE*

1. This is a surgical procedure. The client must know what the procedure entails and the potential complications.

2. Reduces the client's apprehension and fear.

3. Reduces the risk of aspiration when gag reflexes are impaired.

4. Protects the client from an avoidable allergic reaction.

5. The client should not get out of bed after the preoperative medication is given.

▼ *ACTION*	▼ *RATIONALE*
6. Administer the preoperative medication (usually a sedative or narcotic and atropine).	**6.** Inhibits vagal stimulation, and guards against bradycardia, dysrhythmias, and hypotension. Suppresses the cough and gag reflex, sedates the client, and reduces the client's anxiety.
7. Have the client remove any dentures, contact lenses, or prostheses.	**7.** Dentures could break. Glasses or prostheses could be lost or broken.
8. Position the client in a supine, lateral (sidelying), or semi-Fowler's position with his or her neck hyperextended.	**8.** Promotes easy insertion of the bronchoscope.
9. Monitor the client's heart rate and respiratory status during the procedure.	**9.** The client may experience hypoxia.
10. Support the client during the procedure.	**10.** Reduces the client's anxiety.
11. After the procedure, check the gag reflex by gently touching the posterior portion of client's tongue with a tongue blade.	**11.** Preoperative medication and local anesthesia impair the laryngeal reflex and swallowing for several hours after the procedure.
12. Do not allow the client to eat until the gag reflex returns.	**12.** The client may choke or aspirate, or both, because of an impaired ability to swallow.
13. Once the client's cough and gag reflex return, administer ice chips and eventually fluids by mouth.	**13.** The client may experience nausea after the procedure. It is best to see if the client can tolerate ice chips without nausea.
14. Observe the client for dizziness, lethargy, cyanosis, bradycardia, hemoptysis, dyspnea, respiratory distress, hypotension, and dysrhythmias.	**14.** Lidocaine used during the procedure may cause respiratory depression, dizziness, hypotension, apnea, and bradycardia. Hemoptysis may occur.
15. Chart the procedure and the client's response to it.	**15.** Communicates to the other members of the health care team and contributes to the legal record by documenting the care given to the client.

Example of Documentation

DATE	TIME	NOTES
11/11/93	0800	Demerol 25, atropine 0.1 mg given IM right gluteal area. Dentures removed. VS = 144/80, 80, 18. To OR for bronchoscopy. S. Williams, RN
	0900	Returned to room. No cough or gag reflex present. VS = 140/78, 76, 20. NPO at present.
		S. Williams, RN

SKILL 6–4 ASSISTING WITH AN ELECTROCARDIOGRAM

Clinical Situations in Which You May Encounter This Skill

An electrocardiogram (EKG or ECG) records the electrical activity generated in the heart during the cardiac cycle. A 12-lead EKG may be ordered for a client who has a cardiac dysrhythmia, an enlarged heart, a rate or rhythm disturbance, a conduction disorder, a myocardial infarction, or an electrolyte disturbance. If a recording of cardiac electrical activity for several hours or several days is needed, a device called a Holter monitor may be used to record the EKG on a continuous basis. The Holter monitor is portable and can be worn by the client as he or she goes about normal daily activities.

Anticipated Responses

▼ A visual representation of the electrical conduction pattern of the client's heart is reflected by changes in electrical potential at the skin surface.

Adverse Responses

▼ The client is unable to remain still for a good tracing.

Materials List

Gather these materials before beginning the skill:

▼ EKG machine
▼ Electrodes
▼ Electrode paste or alcohol swabs

▼ ACTION	▼ RATIONALE
1. Elicit and record the client's age, sex, height, weight, blood pressure, symptoms, and medications; unusual position of the client during the examination; and the presence of thoracic deformities, amputation, respiratory distress, or muscle tremors.	1. Facilitates interpretation of the EKG.
2. Ask the client if he or she has ever had an EKG before. Explain that the procedure will take only 10 to 15 minutes and is painless.	2. Simple explanation reduces the client's anxiety. If the client has had an EKG, the old EKG should be obtained for comparison.
3. Assist the client to assume a supine position.	3. Facilitates a good recording.
4. Close the door and bedside curtains.	4. Provides privacy for the client.
5. Secure electrodes on the flat inner aspects of the client's wrists and ankles with extremity straps adjusted to hold the electrodes firmly in place. (Use electrode paste or alcohol swabs between the electrodes and the client's skin.)	5. If the straps are placed too tightly, circulation to the extremity could be compromised. Electrode paste or alcohol swabs ensure good contact between the client's skin and the electrode.

▼ *ACTION*

   ▼ *RATIONALE*

6. Attach the chest leads (Fig. 6–4):
   a. V_1—at the fourth intercostal space, at the right sternal border.
   b. V_2—at the fourth intercostal space, at the left sternal border.
   c. V_3—at the midpoint between V_1 and V_4.
   d. V_4—at the fifth intercostal space, at the midclavicular line.
   e. V_5—at the level of V_4, at the left anterior axillary line.
   f. V_6—at the level of V_4, at the left midaxillary line.

6. The recording will vary according to the placement of the leads.

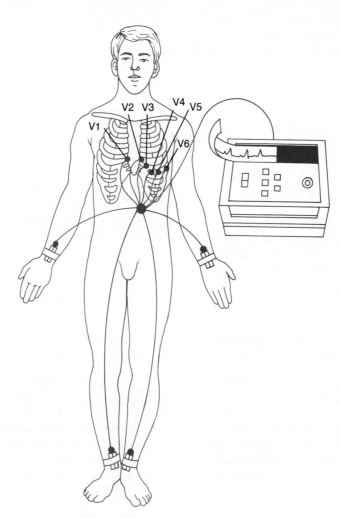

▼ **FIGURE 6–4.** Placement of chest leads for an EKG.

▼ *A C T I O N*   ▼ *R A T I O N A L E*

7. Turn on the lead selection switch to record all 12 leads.

8. Remove the leads and any paste that may be remaining.

8. Promotes the client's comfort.

9. Place the EKG results on the chart and note the time and condition of the client.

9. Communicates to the other members of the health care team and contributes to the legal record by documenting the care given to the client.

Example of Documentation

DATE	TIME	NOTES
10/12/93	0100	EKG recorded. C/O dull aching chest pains. V/S = 170/90, 120, 28. Skin cold and clammy. Dr. Jones notified.
		S. Williams, RN

SKILL 6–5   ASSISTING WITH ENDOSCOPY

Clinical Situations in Which You May Encounter This Skill

Upper and lower gastrointestinal (GI) endoscopic examinations (esophagogastroduodenoscopy and colonoscopy) are performed on individuals with GI complaints or symptoms. In an upper GI endoscopy, the physician directly visualizes the client's esophagus, stomach, and duodenum with a flexible endoscope (Fig. 6–5). Therapeutic procedures that may be completed include foreign-body removal, coagulation of bleeding lesions, laser photocoagulation, dilatations, and percutaneous endoscopic gastrostomy or jejunostomy.

A colonoscopy is an examination of the lower GI tract. The physician can visualize the client's anus, colon, cecum, and adjacent terminal ileum. Indications for a colonscopy include abnormal or questionable barium enema findings, stool that is positive for occult blood, lower GI bleeding, and unexplained symptoms

(such as diarrhea or abdominal pain). Colonoscopies also are done for preoperative and postoperative evaluation of patients with colon cancer; cancer surveillance; or therapeutic reasons such as polypectomy, hemostasis, or volvulus decompression.

Anticipated Responses

▼ The client's upper or lower GI tract is examined without adverse effects

Adverse Responses

▼ As a result of the medication used as a sedative, the client experiences respiratory depression and cardiac arrhythmias. The client experiences vasovagal reactions (slowed pulse, decreased blood pressure, cold clammy skin) or signs and symptoms of perforation, and hemorrhage.

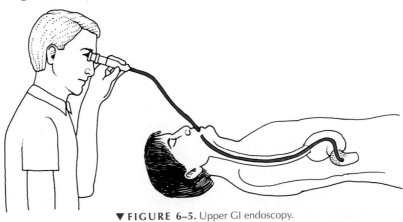

▼ **FIGURE 6–5.** Upper GI endoscopy.

Materials List

Gather these materials before beginning the skill:

▼ Endoscope
▼ Light source with cable and air or water pump
▼ Light source adaptors
▼ Portable instrument table with lower tray
▼ Examination gloves

▼ Gauze pads
▼ Cotton-tipped applicators
▼ Sheet
▼ Towels
▼ Washcloths
▼ Water-soluble lubricant jelly
▼ Viscous lidocaine or other local anesthetic jelly
▼ Masks (optional)

▼ ACTION

1. Verify that a consent form has been signed by the client.

2. Ask the client if he or she has ever had this procedure before.

3. Ask the client if he or she is allergic to any medications.

4. Verify that all preprocedure requirements have been carried out (NPO, bowel prep, preoperative medication).

5. Make sure that the client is wearing a hospital gown with no underwear underneath.

Prior to the Procedure

6. Take and record the client's blood pressure, pulse, and respirations.

7. Insert an intravenous line, if requested by the physician.

8. Assist the client to assume the position indicated by the type of endoscopy:
   a. Left sidelying position with his or her head on a small pillow, for upper GI endoscopy.
   b. Left sidelying position with his or her knees flexed at 90 degrees, for colonoscopy.

During the Procedure

9. Monitor the client's vital signs (especially rate and depth of respirations).

10. Reassure the client by talking in a calm and soothing voice.

11. Assist the physician as indicated during the procedure.

After the Procedure

12. Help the client to assume a position of comfort.

13. Assess the client's level of consciousness and vital signs every 15 minutes for 1 hour, then every hour for 4 hours. If upper GI endoscopy, assess for presence of gag reflex.

14. Assess the client for pain, abdominal distention, rectal bleeding, and hematemesis.

▼ RATIONALE

1. The client must be informed about the procedure, including any potential complications that may result from the procedure.

2. Simple explanations of what to anticipate alleviate the client's apprehension and reduce fear.

3. Medications will be administered before or during the examination. All allergies must be known.

4. Preparation varies depending on the reason for the examination and preferences of the physician.

5. Nylon is a fire hazard.

6. Serves as a baseline for comparison throughout the procedure.

7. Analgesics are often administered during the procedure.

8. Facilitates entry of the flexible endoscope into the client's GI tract.

9. Analgesics given to the client may depress respirations.

10. Allays the client's apprehension and reduces fear.

12. Promotes the client's relaxation.

13. Provides a means of monitoring the client's recovery from the analgesia.

14. May indicate that a perforation has occurred.

▼ *A C T I O N*	▼ *R A T I O N A L E*
15. Notify the physician of any change in the client's baseline status from the preoperative status.	**15.** Bleeding, perforation, respiratory depression, and arrhythmias may occur as a result of the procedure.
16. Chart the procedure, analgesia given, and client's reaction to the endoscopy.	**16.** Communicates to the other members of the health care team and contributes to the legal record by documenting the care given to the client.

Example of Documentation

DATE	TIME	NOTES
10/12/93	0800	To endoscopy per stretcher. V/S = 118/76, 78, 20. Colonscopy per Dr. Jones. 10 mg Valium IV slow push. V/S = 120/76, 78, 18. 2-mm biopsy specimen sent to lab. No abdominal distention, bleeding, or pain. *S. Williams, RN*

SKILL 6–6   ASSISTING WITH A LIVER BIOPSY

Clinical Situations in Which You May Encounter This Skill

A liver biopsy is a sterile procedure performed to aspirate liver tissue when a hepatic disorder is suspected. The procedure is usually accomplished at the client's bedside.

If the client complains of pain or manifests apprehension, an increase in respiratory rate, or a decrease in blood pressure, notify the physician immediately

Anticipated Responses

▼ The client does not experience any bleeding, pain, or infection after the procedure.

Adverse Responses

▼ The client experiences hepatic bleeding, severe hemorrhage, or bile peritonitis after the liver biopsy.

Materials List

Gather these materials before beginning the skill:

▼ Liver biopsy tray or sterile sponges
▼ Antiseptic, such as povidone-iodine
▼ Lidocaine 1%
▼ 2-ml syringe
▼ 22-gauge 6-inch needle
▼ 25-gauge 6-inch needle
▼ Sterile drapes or towels
▼ Sterile normal saline
▼ Specimen container with formalin
▼ Laboratory requisition
▼ Specimen label
▼ Face masks (for physician and optional for you)
▼ Sterile gloves (for physician)
▼ Examination gloves (for you)
▼ Biohazard bag

▼ *A C T I O N*	▼ *R A T I O N A L E*
1. Verify that a consent form has been signed by the client.	**1.** The client must be informed about the procedure, including any complications that may result from the procedure.
2. Check the physician's order for preprocedural medications to be given, such as vitamin K or a sedative.	**2.** Vitamin K may be administered for several days before the biopsy to reduce the risk of hemorrhage. Sedative reduces anxiety.
3. Check the physician's order for food or fluid restrictions for 2 hours before the procedure.	**3.** Many physicians require that the client have nothing by mouth before the procedure.

▼ *ACTION*   ▼ *RATIONALE*

4. Ask the client if he or she has any disorders that affect clotting.	**4.** Alerts you to problems that may interfere with clotting and cause bleeding after the procedure.
5. Check the client's medication record for any drugs that may interfere with clotting.	**5.** Drugs such as heparin, warfarin, and aspirin may prolong clotting.
6. Measure and record the client's pulse, respirations, and blood pressure immediately before the procedure.	**6.** Provides a basis from which to compare measurements after the procedure.
7. Describe the procedure to the client including: a. The steps in the biopsy. b. The position to be assumed. c. What to expect during the procedure. d. What to expect after the procedure, such as activity restriction.	**7.** Reduces the client's apprehension.
8. Open the sterile biopsy tray on the client's bedside table using sterile technique (see Skill 1–9).	**8.** This is a sterile procedure and sterility must be maintained.
9. Put on examination gloves.	**9.** You will be applying pressure to the biopsy site after the procedure is complete. Any time you may come in contact with bodily secretions, wear gloves to prevent the transmission of microorganisms.
10. Position the client supine with the right side of his or her upper abdomen exposed. The client's right arm is raised and extended over the left shoulder behind the head and the rest of the client is draped.	**10.** The liver is located in the right hypochondriac area. This position provides for maximal exposure of the right intercostal space. The biopsy needle will be inserted through the transthoracic (intercostal) or transabdominal (subcostal) route.
11. Tell the client when the physician is to inject the lidocaine.	**11.** Reduces the client's apprehension and anxiety.
12. Ask the client to lie still.	**12.** Prevents accidental lung puncture.
13. Instruct the client to take a deep breath and hold it for up to 10 seconds while the physician inserts the biopsy needle (Fig. 6–6).	**13.** Holding the breath after exhalation immobilizes the chest wall and liver. The diaphragm is in its highest position, injury is avoided to the diaphragm, and the liver is not lacerated.

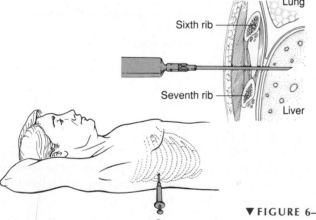

▼ **FIGURE 6–6.** Insertion site for a liver biopsy needle.

14. After the needle is withdrawn, instruct the client to resume breathing normally.	**14.** Lightheadedness may occur if the breath is held for a prolonged period.
15. Apply pressure to the puncture site with a sterile gauze pad.	**15.** Helps to stop any bleeding.

▼ *ACTION*	▼ *RATIONALE*
16. Apply a 4- × 4-inch gauze dressing to the puncture site.	**16.** Helps to prevent infection by occluding the site for potential entry of microorganisms.
17. After the procedure, assist the client to assume a right sidelying position with a small pillow or folded towel under the puncture site for at least 3 hours (Fig. 6–7).	**17.** Compresses the liver biopsy site against the chest wall and minimizes the escape of blood or bile through the puncture site.

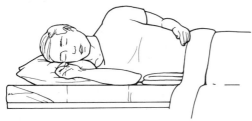

▼ **FIGURE 6–7.** Client position after liver biopsy.

▼ *ACTION*	▼ *RATIONALE*
18. Label specimen and place in a biohazard bag. Send the biopsy specimen to the laboratory immediately.	**18.** Labeling ensures that the correct tests will be performed on the specimen. Bag protects you from contact with body fluids.
19. Remove gloves and wash hands.	**19.** Decreases transmission of microorganisms.
20. Assess the client's vital signs and dressing every 10 to 20 minutes until they have been stable for 2 hours and no bleeding is evident.	**20.** Hemorrhage is a potential adverse response that should be reported immediately to the physician.
21. Chart the procedure and how the client tolerated the procedure.	**21.** Communicates the findings to the other members of the health care team and contributes to the legal record by documenting the care given to the client.

Example of Documentation

DATE	*TIME*	*NOTES*
11/11/93	1030	Liver biopsy per Dr. Jones. Specimen sent immediately to lab. V/S = 128/74, 88, 12. Right sidelying position with folded towel under puncture site. 2-cm area of bleeding noted and circled
		S. Williams, RN

SKILL 6–7   ASSISTING WITH A LUMBAR PUNCTURE

Clinical Situations in Which You May Encounter This Skill

A lumbar puncture (LP), or spinal tap, is a sterile procedure done to obtain a specimen of cerebrospinal fluid (CSF) for therapeutic or diagnostic purposes. The specimen may be used to determine the presence of microorganisms, red blood cells, white blood cells, sugar, or protein. An LP also may be done to remove CSF for the symptomatic relief of increased intracranial pressure, to administer pharmacologic agents or spinal anesthetic, or to inject dye or air for further diagnostic tests.

Anticipated Responses

▼ A clear specimen of CSF is removed.
▼ The client experiences no discomfort or infection.

Adverse Responses

▼ Swelling or bleeding occurs at the LP site.
▼ Numbness, tingling, or pain occurs in the client's legs.
▼ The client experiences a headache after the procedure.

▼ The most serious adverse response occurs when the brain stem herniates down through the tentorium when an LP is performed to relieve pressure associated with an intracranial mass.

▼ Lidocaine injection materials (if not on the tray)
▼ Antiseptic solution (if not on the tray)
▼ Mask (optional)
▼ Biohazard bag

Materials List

Gather these materials before beginning the skill:

▼ Diagnostic LP tray
▼ Sterile gloves (if not on the tray)

▼ ACTION	▼ RATIONALE
1. Verify that a consent form has been signed by the client.	1. Informed consent is essential. The client must know the potential complications of the procedure.
2. Explain the procedure to the client.	2. Anxiety is reduced if the client knows what to expect. If the client is very anxious and becomes tense, the pressure reading may be increased.
3. Ask the client if he or she is allergic to local anesthetics or antiseptic solutions.	3. Protects the client from an avoidable allergic reaction.
4. Have the client empty his or her bladder.	4. The procedure will take approximately 30 minutes and the client will not be able to get up during the procedure to void.
5. Wash your hands.	5. Reduces the transmission of microorganisms.
6. Open the sterile tray, pour the antiseptic solution into the sterile medicine cup using sterile technique, and if not included on the tray, add sterile gloves and lidocaine injection materials (see Skill 1–9).	6. This is a sterile procedure and sterility must be maintained.
7. Assist the client to assume the lateral recumbent position with his or her back bowed at the edge of the examining table, knees flexed up to the abdomen, and head bent so that his or her chin is resting on the chest (Fig. 6–8).	7. Separates the spinal processes and facilitates needle insertion into the subarachnoid space.

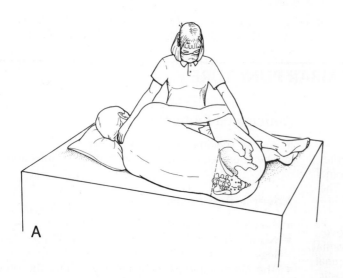

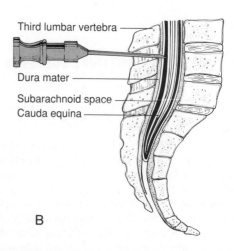

Third lumbar vertebra

Dura mater

Subarachnoid space
Cauda equina

A   B

▼ **FIGURE 6–8.** Client position for lumbar puncture.

▼ *A C T I O N*	▼ *R A T I O N A L E*
8. Place a pillow between the client's legs and under his or her head.	**8.** Keeps the client's upper leg from rolling forward and keeps the spine in a horizontal position.
9. Ask the client to take slow, deep breaths while the physician is inserting the needle.	**9.** Helps the client to relax and maintain the position.
10. Assist the physician with Queckenstedt's test, if asked.	**10.** When pressure is applied to the client's jugular veins, the CSF pressure normally increases. The Queckenstedt's test is used to identify a blockage of CSF.
11. Carefully number the CSF specimens sequentially.	**11.** The physician will order specific tests on each of the tubes.
12. After the procedure is complete, help the client to lie in the prone position for 4 to 12 hours. If 20 ml or more of CSF is removed, the client should be positioned prone for 2 hours, flat sidelying for 2 hours, then supine or prone for 6 hours.	**12.** Allows the tissue surfaces along the needle track to come together and prevent CSF leakage. A prone position helps to decrease the possibility of a spinal headache.
13. Immediately label the specimen and place in a biohazard bag. Send the CSF specimens to the laboratory.	**13.** Label identifies specimen. Bag protects you from contact with body fluids. Changes in the CSF will take place and bacteria may grow if the specimens are allowed to stand.
14. Dispose of the equipment according to your agency procedure.	**14.** Decreases the transmission of microorganisms.
15. Encourage the client to drink plenty of fluids.	**15.** Replaces the CSF removed and may help decrease the possibility of a spinal headache.
16. Assess the puncture site for bleeding or local swelling and apply a small bandage-type dressing to the needle insertion site.	**16.** The site may bleed if the blood vessels are punctured during the needle insertion.
17. Chart the procedure, the character of the CSF, and how the client tolerated the procedure.	**17.** Communicates the findings to the other members of the health care team and contributes to the legal record by documenting the care given to the client.

Example of Documentation

DATE	**TIME**	**NOTES**
10/19/93	1800	Lumbar puncture per Dr. Jones. 10 ml clear CSF removed, labeled, and immediately sent to lab. Client placed in prone position.

S. Williams, RN

SKILL 6–8 ASSISTING WITH PROCTOSIGMOIDOSCOPY

Clinical Situations in Which You May Encounter This Skill

A proctosigmoidoscopy is performed by the physician to examine the client's anus, rectum, and sigmoid colon by using a rigid instrument called a sigmoidoscope. A biopsy may be taken as part of the examination. The procedure is performed to screen clients at risk of developing colon cancer; clients with abnormal or questionable barium enema findings; clients with stool that is positive for occult blood; and clients with lower GI bleeding or unexplained symptoms such as diarrhea or abdominal pain. The procedure also is used for preoperative and postoperative evaluation of clients with colon cancer, cancer surveillance, or for therapeutic reasons such as polypectomy or control of bleeding.

Anticipated Responses

▼ The diagnostic or therapeutic procedure is completed with no adverse effects on the client.

Adverse Responses

▼ The client has cardiopulmonary complications related to the sedative medication, vasovagal reaction (slow pulse, drop in blood pressure, cold clammy skin), perforation of the colon, or bleeding after a biopsy.

Materials List

Gather these materials before beginning the skill:

▼ Rigid proctoscopic and sigmoidoscopic instrument
▼ Biopsy forceps long enough to extend the entire length of the sigmoidoscope
▼ Air insufflation bulb (suction apparatus with flexible tubing and suction head long enough to extend the length of the sigmoidoscope)

▼ Rectal swabs long enough to extend the length of the sigmoidoscope
▼ Examination gloves
▼ Gauze pads
▼ Water-soluble lubricant
▼ Glass microscope slides
▼ Cover slips
▼ Test reagent (for determination of occult blood)
▼ Filter paper
▼ Biopsy bottle and fixative
▼ Dropper bottle of normal saline and dropper bottle of Lugol's iodine solution
▼ Applicator sticks
▼ Small basin of water
▼ Silver nitrate sticks and holder
▼ Additional equipment may be used, such as syringes, tourniquets, IV medication, antiseptics, and sterile culture equipment
▼ Biohazard bag

▼ ACTION

1. Verify that a consent form has been signed by the client.

2. Ask the client if he or she has ever had a sigmoidoscopic examination before and explain that he or she will have to maintain a certain position for about 30 minutes.

3. Check the physician's order for an enema or a suppository to be administered to the client prior to the examination.

4. Help the client to assume one of the following positions:
   a. Knee-chest (Fig. 6–9).
   b. Left lateral (the hips should be fully flexed and the knees should be drawn up to a 90-degree angle with the trunk). The buttocks should be positioned slightly over the edge of the bed. The client lies on his or her left shoulder with the right arm extended out of the way. His or her head may rest on a small pillow.
   c. Jackknifed position on the examining table.

5. Drape the client so that only his or her anal area is exposed.

6. Open the proctoscopy tray on the overbed table.

7. Put on examination gloves.

8. Assess the client for pallor, diaphoresis, and change in pulse, respiration, or blood pressure during the examination.

▼ RATIONALE

1. The client must be informed about what will be done during the procedure and any complications that may result.

2. Alleviates the client's apprehension and reduces fear.

3. A suppository or enema will evacuate the colon contents and allow for adequate visualization of the rectum and lower colon.

4. These positions facilitate adequate visualization of the anus, rectum, and sigmoid colon.

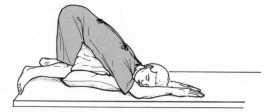

▼ **FIGURE 6–9.** Client's knee-chest position for proctosigmoidoscopy.

5. Provides for privacy and makes the client feel unexposed.

6. The tray should be ready for the examination and within easy reach.

7. Reduces the chance of transmission of microorganisms.

8. Provides an objective means of assessing how the client is tolerating the procedure and if any adverse responses are occurring.

▼ *A C T I O N* ▼ *R A T I O N A L E*

After the Procedure

9. Wipe the client's anus with gauze.

10. Assist the client from the position assumed during the examination to a position of comfort.

11. Label any specimens that were collected, place in biohazard bag, and transport to laboratory.

12. Assess the client's vital signs every 15 minutes × 4, then every hour × 4, noting any discomfort in or drainage from the anal area.

13. Document the procedure in your notes and include the objective and subjective data.

9. Provides for the client's comfort and removes any fecal material that can cause irritation of the anal area.

10. The position assumed during the examination is uncomfortable and the client may need assistance to change to a comfortable position.

11. Label identifies specimen. Bag protects from exposure to body fluids.

12. A decreased blood pressure or an increased pulse rate is indicative of bleeding. Drainage may be a sign of inadvertent tissue damage.

13. Communicates the findings to the other members of the health care team and contributes to the legal record by documenting the care given to the client.

Example of Documentation

DATE	TIME	NOTES
11/11/89	1300	Proctocopic exam per Dr. Jones. Biopsy sent immediately to lab. VS = 120/76, 76, 18. No complaints of pain or discomfort.

S. Williams, RN

SKILL 6–9   ASSISTING WITH THORACENTESIS

Clinical Situations in Which You May Encounter This Skill

Thoracentesis, the aspiration of pleural fluid or air, is performed to relieve pressure, pain, or dyspnea. Fluid may be removed to get specimens of the client's pleural fluid for analysis (Gram-stain culture and sensitivity, acid-fast staining and culture, differential cell count, cytology, pH, specific gravity, total protein, or lactic dehydrogenase). A pleural biopsy also may be done or medications may be instilled into the pleural space.

Anticipated Responses

▼ The client is comfortable during the procedure and experiences no dyspnea, coughing, or respiratory distress.

Adverse Responses

▼ The client has respiratory distress and exhibits symptoms such as increasing respiratory rate; uncontrollable cough; blood-tinged, frothy mucus; rapid heart rate; or signs of hypoxia.

Materials List

Gather these materials before beginning the skill:

▼ Thoracentesis tray OR
▼ 16-gauge 3.5-inch aspiration needle
▼ 5-ml ampule of 1% lidocaine
▼ 21-gauge 1.5-inch needle
▼ 25-gauge 5/8-inch needle
▼ 5-ml syringe
▼ 50-ml syringe
▼ Two-way valve
▼ Three specimen tubes
▼ Drainage bag
▼ Drape
▼ Adhesive bandage
▼ Prep applicators
▼ Sponges
▼ Prep tray
▼ Sterile gloves

▼ *ACTION*

▼ *RATIONALE*

1. Check the physician's order for a chest x-ray or an ultrasound examination to be completed before the procedure.

2. Verify that a consent form has been signed by the client.

3. Ask the client if he or she is allergic to the local anesthetic or antiseptic to be used.

4. Explain to the client what to expect during and after the procedure:
   a. He or she must remain immobile.
   b. Lidocaine may sting when injected.
   c. A pressure sensation will be felt during the procedure.
   d. No pain is expected after the procedure.

5. Assist the client to assume one of the three following positions:
   a. Sitting on the side of the bed with his or her feet supported on a stool, and his or her arms and head on the overbed table (Fig. 6–10A).
   b. Straddling a chair with his or her head and arms resting on the back of the chair (Fig. 6–10B).
   c. Lying in bed on the unaffected side with the head of the bed elevated 45 degrees (Fig. 6–10C).

1. X-rays are used to locate fluid or air in the client's pleural cavity to determine the puncture site. Ultrasound may be used to locate the area of fluid.

2. This is a surgical procedure that requires informed consent as to the nature and potential complications of the procedure.

3. The physician should be notified and another anesthetic should be made available.

4. Reduces the client's apprehension and prevents complications that may occur due to the client moving during the procedure.

5. Facilitates the removal of fluid from the chest wall.

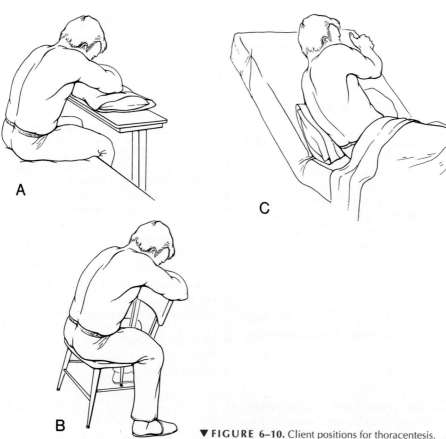

A

C

B

▼ FIGURE 6–10. Client positions for thoracentesis.

▼ *ACTION* _ _ _ _ _ _ _ _ _ _ _ _ _ _ _ ▼ *RATIONALE* _ _ _ _ _ _ _ _ _ _

6. Wash your hands.

7. Open the sterile thoracentesis tray using sterile technique (see Skill 1–9).

8. Expose the client's entire chest.

9. Adjust the lights for brightness.

10. During the procedure, provide emotional and physical support to the client and prepare the client for what to expect:
    a. The client will feel a cold sensation from the antiseptic.
    b. Encourage the client to be very still and not to cough.
    c. Tell the client when the lidocaine is to be injected.

11. After the procedure, apply pressure to the needle insertion site and apply a sterile dressing.

12. Assist the client to a position of comfort.

13. Verify with the physician if a chest x-ray is needed.

14. Dispose of equipment according to your agency procedure.

15. Assess the client for any adverse responses, such as increasing respiratory rate, faintness, vertigo, tightness in the chest, cough, blood-tinged sputum, rapid pulse, or cyanosis.

16. Chart the procedure. Note how the client tolerated the procedure and the character and amount of drainage.

6. Decreases the transmission of microorganisms.

7. This is a sterile procedure and sterility must be maintained.

8. After reviewing the client's x-ray films or ultrasound, the physician may percuss the client's chest to further delineate the area for dullness to determine the exact site for needle insertion.

9. Provides for visualization of the area for the thoracentesis.

10. a–b. Any sudden movements may cause trauma to the pleura or accidental puncture of the lungs.

    c. Lidocaine often stings when injected. If the client is unprepared for the anesthetic, he or she may move suddenly.

11. Reduces any bleeding. Protects the insertion site from the entry of microorganisms.

12. Promotes the client's relaxation.

13. X-ray films may be taken to verify that a pneumothorax has not occurred.

14. Proper disposal decreases the transmission of microorganisms.

15. Assesses for signs of pneumothorax.

16. Communicates the findings to the other members of the health care team and contributes to the legal record by documenting the care given to the client.

Example of Documentation

DATE	TIME	NOTES
10/18/93	1000	Thoracentesis completed by Dr. Jones. 100 ml of cloudy fluid drained from left posterior chest area. Specimen sent to lab. No respiratory distress noted.
		S. Williams, RN

SKILL 6–10   MEASURING BLOOD GLUCOSE

Clinical Situations in Which You May Encounter this Skill

Blood glucose may be measured using a blood sample from a finger stick whenever an immediate measurement is needed. Clients with diabetes mellitus often require frequent measurements of blood glucose to determine the status of their carbohydrate metabolism.

The fasting blood glucose value is 70 to 100 mg/dl. One to 2 hours after a meal, the fasting value may increase 40 to 80 mg/dl.

Hyperglycemia occurs when the values are consistently above 300 mg/dl. If blood glucose is consistently greater than 300 mg/dl, a check for ketones in the urine should be performed. Hyperglycemia requires a physician's attention to regulate the client's blood sugar.

Hypoglycemia occurs when the value is less than 50 mg/dl for an adult or child or the value is less than 30 mg/dl for a neonate. Hypoglycemia can pose a serious threat and usually calls for immediate treatment such as the ingestion of 10 g of a simple carbohydrate.

Anticipated Responses

▼ The value is within normal limits.

Adverse Responses

▼ The values indicate hyperglycemia or hypoglycemia.

Materials List

Gather these materials before beginning the skill:

▼ Appropriate reagent strip
▼ Cotton balls
▼ Lancet or automatic puncture device
▼ Alcohol swab
▼ Dry gauze
▼ Bandage
▼ Watch with second hand
▼ Examination gloves
▼ Wash bottle (used in some types of glucose tests)

▼ ACTION

1. Check the client's chart for a history of diabetes or any other factor or condition that may alter his or her blood sugar.

2. Put on examination gloves.

3. Obtain a blood specimen from the client's finger. Refer to Skill 5–15 for obtaining a blood specimen with a lancet if necessary.

4. Check the expiration date on the reagent strip bottle.

5. Remove one test strip and recap the bottle. Observe the strip for discoloration.

▼ RATIONALE

1. Alerts you to factors that may alter the client's blood sugar such as diabetes, receipt of corticosteroid drugs, or receipt of insulin.

2. Decreases the transmission of microorganisms.

3. A large droplet of blood will be required to cover both test pads.

4. Expired test strips may yield inaccurate results.

5. Prolonged exposure to humidity or temperature extremes may inactivate test strips. Discoloration indicates strip deterioration.

▼ *A C T I O N* _____ ▼ *R A T I O N A L E* _____

6. Touch one large drop of blood to the reagent test pad or pads (Fig. 6–11). Ensure that the pads are completely covered. *Do not* smear the blood.

6. The test pads must be well saturated with blood.

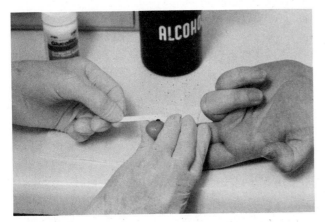

▼ **FIGURE 6–11.** Taking a blood sample from the client's finger.

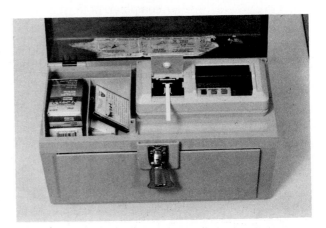

▼ **FIGURE 6–12.** Using a blood glucose meter.

7. Cover the puncture site with dry gauze and apply pressure. Apply a bandage if needed.

7. Aids in stopping the flow of blood.

8. Follow the manufacturer's directions regarding the developing time and method for removing blood from the test pad. It should be wiped off of some strips and rinsed with a wash bottle off of others.

8. Proper developing time and proper use of test strips are critical for accurate results.

For Visual Reading

9. Under a good light source, compare the test pad colors to the color scale on the bottle label from which the test strip came.

9. Each bottle has a color chart that corresponds to the specific reaction characteristics of the test strips within that vial.

For Instrument Reading

10. Follow the directions in the operations manual for the blood glucose meter that corresponds to the test strip you are using (Fig. 6–12).

10. Correct use of a glucose meter is necessary to ensure accurate test results. Use only the glucose meter recommended by the test strip manufacturer.

11. Dispose of soiled equipment in the proper container.

11. Decreases the transmission of microorganisms.

12. Remove the gloves and wash your hands.

12. Decreases the transmission of microorganisms.

13. Explain the results to the client if appropriate.

13. Keeps the client informed of his or her health status and allows the client to actively participate in his or her care.

14. Record the results on the client's record.

14. Communicates the findings to the other members of the health care team and contributes to the legal record by documenting the care given to the client.

Example of Documentation

DATE	TIME	NOTES
1/5/93	1100	Blood glucose is 360. Urine ketones moderate. Client complains of thirst and abdominal pain. Dr. Smith notified.
		C. Lammon, RN
1/5/93	1115	10 units regular insulin subcutaneously to right lower quadrant of abdomen.
		C. Lammon, RN

Teaching Tips

The procedure for and the purpose of measuring blood glucose should be explained to the client. Allow adequate time for the client to practice the procedure. If the client has been measuring blood glucose at home, check his or her technique.

Home Care Variations

The same procedure is used to check the client's blood sugar in his or her home.

SKILL 6–11   PERFORMING AN AUDIOMETRIC EXAMINATION

Clinical Situations in Which You May Encounter This Skill

Hearing screening is performed to assess for hearing deficiencies. Chronic otitis media or excessive cerumen often contributes to conductive hearing loss in children. Sensory neural damage may contribute to hearing loss in the elderly. There are three basic types of hearing loss:

1. Conductive hearing loss occurs because of decreased function in all or a part of the mechanical conducting parts of the auditory system. Common causes of conductive hearing loss include anatomic malformations, excessive cerumen, and otitis media. Clients with conductive hearing loss experience impaired hearing in the lower frequencies.
2. Sensorineural hearing loss occurs because of decreased function of the inner ear or neural pathways of the auditory system. Common causes of sensorineural hearing loss include severe viral infections, loud noise or music, and toxic effects of some drugs. Clients with sensorineural hearing loss experience impaired hearing in the higher frequencies and, therefore, their speech perception is poorer than it would be with conductive hearing loss.

3. Mixed hearing loss occurs in clients with significant conductive loss and sensorineural loss.

Anticipated Responses

▼ The client is able to hear all frequencies tested at 25 decibels (dB).

Adverse Responses

▼ The client is unable to hear all frequencies at 25 dB.

Materials List

Gather these materials before beginning the skill:

▼ Audiometer
▼ Two chairs
▼ Table
▼ Otoscope
▼ Notepad
▼ Pencil
▼ Audiogram
▼ Bucket and 5 blocks (optional use for young child)

▼ *ACTION*

▼ *RATIONALE*

1. Select a quiet room.

2. Place the audiometer on a table facing you. Place the client's chair so that he or she will be facing away from the audiometer.

3. Plug in the audiometer and turn the power switch on.

4. Instruct the client to raise his or her hand whenever a tone is heard and lower his or her hand when the tone stops. Give young children five blocks and a bucket. Instruct the child to throw a block into the bucket whenever a tone is heard.

5. Ask the client to remove earrings and pull his or her hair back behind the ears.

6. Place the earphones snugly over the client's ears and adjust them for comfort.

7. Administer a test tone in the client's right and left ear with a frequency of 1,000 Hertz (Hz) and an intensity of 40 dB (Fig. 6–13). Observe the client for the correct response.

1. A quiet environment is necessary for an accurate hearing test.

2. Allows you to adjust the audiometer settings without the client's knowledge.

3. The audiometer requires power to generate tones.

4. Notifies you that the client heard the tone. Young children may be shy about raising their hands. The blocks and bucket make the test seem like a game and elicits cooperation.

5. Facilitates a snug fit of the earphones.

6. Maximizes sound.

7. The loud test tone allows the client to become familiar with the sound. It also allows you to evaluate the client's understanding of your instructions.

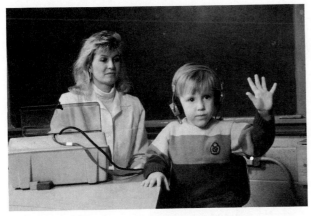

▼ **FIGURE 6–13.** Using an audiometer.

8. Turn the intensity to 25 dB and test each of the client's ears at 1,000 Hz, 2,000 Hz, 4,000 Hz, 8,000 Hz, and 500 Hz. Complete the testing of the right ear before testing the left ear.

9. Observe the client's response after each tone is given and keep a record of missed frequencies.

10. Explain the results to the client or send a letter home to the child's parents describing the test findings.

11. If the client's hearing was not satisfactory, examine his or her internal ear with an otoscope to determine the presence of excessive cerumen, otitis media, etc. Make any referrals that are needed based on your findings.

8. The normal ear should be able to hear these frequencies at 25 dB of intensity.

9. An audiogram communicates to a hearing specialist which frequencies were tested and at which decibel level each frequency was heard. Failure to hear tested frequencies at 25 dB indicates the need for a referral to a hearing specialist.

10. Keeps the client informed of his or her health status and allows the client to actively participate in his or her care.

11. Excessive cerumen, a foreign body, or otitis media may result in a hearing deficit.

▼ ACTION	▼ RATIONALE
12. Record your findings in the client's record.	**12.** Communicates the findings to the other members of the health care team and contributes to the legal record by documenting the care given to the client.
13. If the client's hearing was not satisfactory on the first test, make an appointment to rescreen the client's hearing.	**13.** A second screening decreases the chance of making an unnecessary referral.
14. After the second unsatisfactory screening test, refer the client to an appropriate hearing specialist.	**14.** Further evaluation and treatment are indicated if the client fails two successive hearing tests.

Example of Documentation

See Figure 6–14.

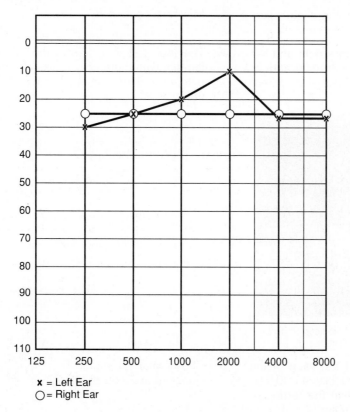

x = Left Ear
◯ = Right Ear

▼ **FIGURE 6–14.** An audiogram.

Teaching Tips

Explain the procedure, the purpose of the test, and the results to the client or the client's family, or both.

Home Care Variations

This test is not usually performed in the client's home.

SKILL 6–12   MEASURING HEMATOCRIT (CAPILLARY METHOD)

Clinical Situations in Which You May Encounter This Skill

The hematocrit is measured to determine the percent of erythrocytes in a given volume of blood. Decreased values indicate the presence of anemia, bleeding, leukemia, hyperthyroidism, cirrhosis, or hemolytic reaction (due to transfusion of incompatible blood, reaction to chemicals, reaction to infectious agents, or physical agents such as burns and prosthetic heart valves). Increased values are found in erythrocytosis, polycythemia, severe dehydration, and shock (when hemoconcentration rises considerably).

The normal values for hematocrit are: men, 40–54%; women, 37–47%; and newborns, 50–62%.

The normal values for the microhematocrit (done by finger stick) are: men, 45–47%; women, 42–44%; and newborns, 44–62% (Fischbach, 1988).

Anticipated Responses

▼ The value is within normal limits.

Adverse Responses

▼ The client's hematocrit is decreased or increased.

Materials List

Gather these materials before beginning the skill:

▼ Centrifuge
▼ Lancet or automatic puncture device
▼ Alcohol wipe
▼ Capillary tubes
▼ Sealing clay
▼ Dry gauze
▼ Small adhesive bandage
▼ Examination gloves

▼ ACTION	▼ RATIONALE
1. Check the client's chart for conditions that may alter the hematocrit.	1. Alerts you to reason hematocrit may be altered.
2. Examine the client's chart to determine the previous hematocrit level.	2. Needed for determining any change in the client's hematocrit.
3. Put on examination gloves.	3. Decreases the transmission of microorganisms.
4. Collect a blood sample from a finger or heel stick. Refer to the procedure for collecting capillary blood specimen with a lancet if necessary (Skill 5–15).	4. The hematocrit test may be performed on a capillary sample.
5. Fill two capillary tubes three-quarters full.	5. A sufficient sample is needed to obtain accurate results. Second sample will be used if 1st sample is accidentally damaged in centrifuge.
6. Seal one end of each capillary tube with sealing clay.	6. Prevents loss of the blood sample during centrifugation.
7. Place one of the sealed capillary tubes into the slot in the high-speed microhematocrit (HSM) centrifuge head. The sealed end should lie in contact with the peripheral rim of the HSM centrifuge head that contains a rubber gasket.	7. Prevents loss of the blood sample during centrifugation.
8. Place an empty capillary tube in the slot opposite the blood sample.	8. Balances the centrifuge head.
9. Replace the head cover and tighten the nut on the head cover with your fingers.	9. The head cover prevents blood and glass from flying out of the machine during processing.
10. Close and latch the HSM centrifuge cover.	10. The cover must be closed before starting the machine.

▼ *ACTION*   ▼ *RATIONALE*

11. Turn the time switch on the dial and set it for at least 5 minutes at 1,000–1,300 revolutions per minute or as the manufacturer recommends.

11. Adequate time must be allowed to completely separate the red blood cells from the plasma.

12. After the centrifuge head has spontaneously ceased to rotate, lift the outside cover and unscrew the head cover.

12. *Do not* touch the centrifuge until the head has ceased to rotate.

13. Remove the capillary tubes. Note the color of the plasma and use a Spiracrit (hematocrit reader) (Fig. 6–15) to read the percent volume of packed red blood cells.

13. A Spiracrit graph allows you to accurately measure the volume percent of erythrocytes present in the plasma.

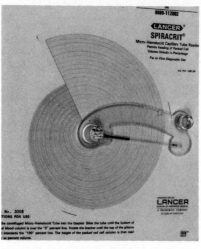

▼ **FIGURE 6–15.** Reading hematocrit on a Spiracrit graph.

14. Dispose of contaminated equipment in an appropriate container.

14. Decreases the transmission of microorganisms.

15. Remove the gloves and wash your hands.

15. Decreases the transmission of microorganisms.

16. Discuss the findings with the client if appropriate.

16. Keeps the client informed of his or her health status and allows the client to actively participate in his or her care.

17. Record the results in the client's record.

17. Communicates the findings to the other members of the health care team, and contributes to the legal record by documenting the care given to the client.

Example of Documentation

DATE	TIME	NOTES
1/5/93	1100	150 ml coffee ground emesis. Positive guaiac test. HCT = 34%. BP = 110/60. Dr. Smith notified.
		C. Lammon, RN

Teaching Tips

Explain the procedure, the purpose of the test, and the results to the client or the client's family, or both.

Home Care Variations

This procedure is usually not performed in the home.

SKILL 6–13   TESTING STOOL FOR OCCULT BLOOD

Clinical Situations in Which You May Encounter This Skill

The guaiac (Hemoccult) test is performed to evaluate the client's stool for the presence of hidden (occult) blood.

Anticipated Responses

▼ The stool specimen is collected without contamination with urine or toilet paper.

Adverse Responses

▼ The stool specimen is discarded.
▼ The stool specimen contains blood.

Materials List

Gather these materials before beginning the skill:

▼ Stool specimen cup
▼ Wooden spatula
▼ Toilet specimen container or bedpan
▼ Adhesive label or marker
▼ Examination gloves
▼ Guaiac test kit and developer

▼ *ACTION*

1. Assess the client's diet and medication for the last 48 to 72 hours.

2. Help the client to implement any dietary or medication changes that are ordered.

3. If the specimen is to be collected from a bedpan, screen the client while he or she is using the bedpan by closing the door and closing the curtains around the bed.

4. Put on gloves.

5. Collect the stool specimen. Refer to Skill 5–19 regarding the collection of a stool specimen.

▼ *RATIONALE*

1. Medicines such as bromides, colchicine, iodides, iodine, iron, oxidizing agents excreted in the urine, and phenazopyridine hydrochloride may cause increased values or false positives. Ascorbic acid may cause decreased values or false negatives. A meat-free diet may be prescribed for 72 hours before the test to prevent a false-positive result.

2. Helps to obtain accurate test results.

3. Provides privacy for the client.

4. Decreases the transmission of microorganisms.

▼ _ACTION_   ▼ _RATIONALE_

6. Open the flap of the guaiac test kit and using the wooden spatula (Fig. 6–16), make a thin smear of stool in the first box.

6. The guaiac developer may not penetrate thick stool smears.

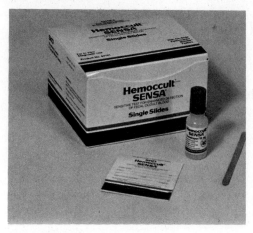

▼ **FIGURE 6–16.** Hemoccult slide, developer, and wooden spatula.

7. Take another stool sample from a different part of the stool specimen and make a thin smear in the second box.

7. Use of a second part of the stool sample increases the chance of detecting blood if it is present in the stool specimen. One sample can be taken from the interior and one from the exterior of the stool.

8. Close the flap on the guaiac test kit, turn the kit over, and open the flap on the reverse side of the test kit.

8. Exposes the area where the guaiac developer is to be applied.

9. Apply two drops of guaiac developer to each box and one drop between the positive and negative controls located below the test boxes.

9. The developer will react with the stool sample if blood is present.

10. Wait 60 seconds and compare the test to the controls.

10. A blue color indicates a positive test.

11. Discard the soiled supplies in an appropriate container.

11. Decreases the transmission of microorganisms.

12. Cleanse the client, position him or her, and make him or her comfortable.

12. Cleansing the client will help to prevent the spread of microorganisms and will promote the client's comfort.

13. Remove the gloves and wash your hands.

13. Decreases the transmission of microorganisms.

14. Explain the results of the test to the client if appropriate.

14. Keeps the client informed of his or her health status and allows the client to actively participate in his or her care.

15. Record the results in the client's chart.

15. Communicates the findings to the other members of the health care team and contributes to the legal record by documenting the care given to the client.

Example of Documentation

DATE	TIME	NOTES
11/8/93	1030	Stool specimen obtained and tested for occult blood. Results were positive. Physician notified.
		S. Williams, RN

Teaching Tips

The procedure and the purpose of the test should be explained to the client or the client's family, or both. Encourage the client to avoid any medications (such as vitamin C, aspirin, or nonsteroidal antiinflammatory drugs) that may alter the results and to eat a diet free of red meat and raw fruits and vegetables for 3 days prior to the test.

Home Care Variations

The client may be given a guaiac test kit to take home, collect the specimen, and mail to the physician's office or clinical laboratory. Often this is a serial test kit. The stool sample should consist of three consecutive bowel movements. The slides should be protected from heat and light. A developer usually is not used with these kits.

SKILL 6–14   SCREENING FOR LICE

Clinical Situations in Which You May Encounter This Skill

You may screen clients for lice in a school or camp. Head lice (*Pediculus capitis*) and body lice (*Pediculus corporis*) are small and grayish white in color. Pubic lice or crab lice (*Pediculus pubis*) are small with gray bodies and red legs.

Anticipated Responses

▼ The client is free of nits or lice.

Adverse Responses

▼ The client has nits or lice.

Materials List

Gather these materials before beginning the skill:

▼ Examination gloves

▼ ACTION

1. Determine if the client has been exposed to others with known lice infection.

2. Put on gloves.

3. Standing away from the client, separate his or her hair shafts and inspect the scalp and hair follicles to determine the presence of lice or nits.

4. Inspect for bites or pustules behind the client's ears, along the hairline at the base of skull, and in the groin.

5. Remove your gloves and dispose of them in an appropriate container.

6. Wash your hands.

7. Explain the results to the client or send a letter home to the child's parents or caretakers.

8. Make an appropriate referral for treatment.

9. Schedule a follow-up appointment to recheck for lice after the treatment is completed.

▼ RATIONALE

1. Lice are spread to others through close contact such as sharing a comb or hairbrush.

2. Protects you from potential contact with lice.

3. Position yourself to prevent your clothes from coming in contact with lice.

4. Bites are seen most frequently where skin surfaces are in contact with each other.

5. If lice were found, the gloves should be sealed in an airtight container or bag and burned.

6. Decreases the transmission of microorganisms.

7. Keeps the client informed of his or her health status and allows the client to actively participate in his or her care.

8. Medication must be prescribed to rid the client of lice.

9. Evaluates the success of the treatment.

Example of Documentation

DATE	TIME	NOTES
1/4/93	0900	Client referred to school nurse by teacher for lice detection. Inspection of child's head reveals *Pediculus capitis*. Letter sent home to parents stating findings and instructions for using shampoo containing benzene hexachloride (or lindane). Repeat shampoo application 12–24 hours later. I will reevaluate child upon return to school.
		C. Lammon, RN

Teaching Tips

Emphasize to the parents that the shampoo treatment should be repeated to kill the lice that hatch after the first shampoo.

Home Care Variations

This procedure is primarily done in the client's home according to the steps described above.

SKILL 6–15   TESTING URINE

Clinical Situations in Which You May Encounter This Skill

Urine testing may be performed using urine dipsticks to measure specific gravity, pH, protein, glucose, ketones, bilirubin, blood, nitrates, and urobilinogen. Normal results are:

SPECIFIC GRAVITY: 1.003–1.030

PH: 4.6–8 (average 6)

PROTEIN: Negative to trace

GLUCOSE: Negative

KETONES: Negative

BILIRUBIN: Negative

BLOOD: Negative

NITRATES: Negative

UROBILINOGEN: 0.1–1.0 Ehrlich units

Many different disturbances can alter one or more of the above values:

PH: Normally the urine is acid. If urine is allowed to stand at room temperature, it will become alkaline from bacterial growth. Urine also may become alkaline in renal acidosis syndrome.

PROTEIN: The presence of protein indicates that the kidneys are allowing protein, usually albumin, to be excreted into the urine.

GLUCOSE: Glucose in the urine usually indicates an elevated blood glucose. The normal renal threshold for glucose is a 180 mg/dl blood glucose level. However, the renal threshold can vary with the individual.

KETONES: Ketones are classically found in clients with diabetic acidosis. However, they also may be found in cases of starvation and dehydration. The presence of ketones indicates that the body is burning fats for energy. Ketones are acidic; therefore, expect acidic pH if ketones are present in the urine.

BILIRUBIN: Bilirubin usually appears in the urine as a result of a liver dysfunction such as a hepatic obstruction. The urine will be dark in color because of the presence of bile pigments.

BLOOD: Blood in the urine indicates bleeding in the renal system or rapid destruction of blood cells elsewhere in the body because of trauma or burns. Assess menstruation as a possible source of bleeding in female clients.

NITRATES: The presence of nitrates may indicate bacteria.

UROBILINOGEN: Bilirubin is converted to urobilinogen in the intestinal tract. It may be increased by hemolytic processes or impaired liver function.

Anticipated Responses

▼ Results are within normal limits.

Adverse Responses

▼ One or more of the results are not within normal limits.

Materials List

Gather these materials before beginning the skill:

▼ Appropriate urine test strip (dipstick)
▼ Urine cup
▼ Examination gloves

▼ ACTION	▼ RATIONALE
1. Check the client's chart for any present and past medical diagnoses.	1. Alerts you to conditions that may cause altered results.
2. Collect a routine voided urine specimen (see Skill 5–9).	2. Urine screening should be performed with fresh uncentrifuged urine. If the test cannot be performed within 1 hour after collection, refrigerate the specimen immediately and allow it to return to room temperature prior to testing.
3. Check the expiration date on the bottle of urine dipsticks.	3. Expired strips may give inaccurate data because of deterioration of the reagent pads.
4. Check the test strip for discoloration or darkening of the reagent areas.	4. Discoloration or darkening may indicate deterioration of the reagent pads.
5. Recap the bottle after removing the test strip.	5. Maintains freshness of the test strips.
6. Put on gloves.	6. Gloves are needed when there is a chance of coming into contact with body secretions to prevent the possible transmission of microorganisms.
7. Observe the urine for color, clarity, sediment, and odor.	7. The color may range from yellow to amber. Urine should be clear and without sediment. Fresh urine normally has a slight odor of ammonia.

For Visual Inspection

8. a. Completely immerse the reagent areas of the test strip in fresh (less than 1 hour old), well-mixed, uncentrifuged urine and remove it immediately.	8. a. Saturates the reagent strip with urine.
b. While removing the strip from the urine, tap the edge of the strip against the rim of the urine container to remove excess urine.	b. Excess urine may flow from one reagent pad to another and may cause the chemicals to mix and distort the tests.
c. Hold the strip in a horizontal position.	c. See Step 8.b.

▼ ACTION   ▼ RATIONALE

d. Compare the test areas to the corresponding color chart on the bottle label at the time specified (Fig. 6–17).

d. Proper reading time is critical for optimal results. Colors may continue to change after the specified reading time.

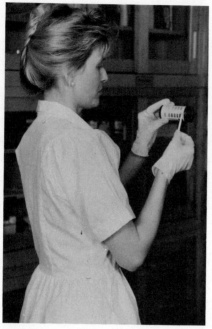

▼ **FIGURE 6–17.** Comparing a urine dipstick to the bottle color chart.

For Instrument Reading

9. Use the urine chemistry analyzer recommended by the test strip manufacturer and follow the directions given in the operations manual.

9. Provides more accurate analysis of specimen.

10. Discard the soiled equipment in an appropriate container.

10. Proper disposal decreases the transmission of microorganisms.

11. Remove the gloves and wash your hands.

11. Decreases the transmission of microorganisms.

12. Explain the results to the client if appropriate.

12. Keeps the client informed of his or her health status and allows the client to actively participate in his or her care.

13. Record the results in the client's record.

13. Communicates the findings to the other members of the health care team, and contributes to the legal record by documenting the care given to the client.

Example of Documentation

DATE	TIME	NOTES
1/1/93	0800	Urine specimen negative for glucose and protein.
		C. Lammon, RN

SKILL 6–16 SCREENING FOR PHENYLKETONURIA

Clinical Situations in Which You May Encounter This Skill

Phenylketonuria (PKU) is an inherited disease characterized by deficiency of the enzyme phenylalanine hydroxylase, which converts phenylalanine to tyrosine. Phenylalanine is an essential amino acid and is necessary for growth; however, any excess must be degraded by conversion to tyrosine. An infant with PKU lacks the ability to make this necessary conversion.

Routine screening of the newborn infant's blood for PKU is mandatory in the United States and usually is done 2 to 3 days after birth. A urine test to detect phenylalanine is also done when the infant is 6 weeks old (Pagana and Pagana, 1986).

The normal blood level is less than 4 mg/100 ml and the urine should be negative (no color change) on a dipstick. An elevated PKU blood level or positive urine can indicate a defective gene, liver disease, or galactosemia. If the PKU test is abnormal, it should be followed up with further diagnostic testing to determine the specific origin of the problem. Treatment usually consists of a low-phenylalanine diet. However, if the elevation is not due to a deficiency of the enzyme, harm can be done by a prolonged low-phenylalanine diet.

Anticipated Responses

▼ The child is found to have normal serum PKU and negative urine.

Adverse Responses

▼ The child is found to have positive urine or an elevated serum PKU, or both.

Materials List

Gather these materials before beginning the skill:

▼ PKU test paper
▼ Lancet or automatic puncture device
▼ Alcohol swab
▼ Small adhesive bandage
▼ Dry gauze
▼ Examination gloves
▼ Biohazard bag

▼ ACTION

1. Determine the age of the child and the type of PKU test to be done (urine or blood).

To collect a blood sample for PKU testing:

2. Put on examination gloves.

3. Collect a blood specimen from the child's heel. Refer to Skill 5–15 for collecting a blood specimen from the heel with a lancet if necessary.

4. Thoroughly saturate all the designated areas on the PKU test paper with blood from the heel stick (Fig. 6–18).

▼ RATIONALE

1. Allows you to gather the proper supplies to collect the specimen.

2. Decreases the transmission of microorganisms.

3. A sufficient amount of blood will be needed to saturate four circles the size of a dime on the test paper.

4. An adequate sample is needed to yield accurate results.

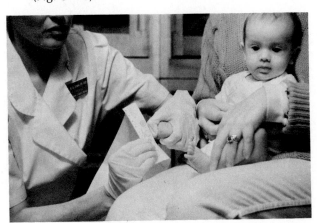

▼ **FIGURE 6–18.** Heel stick for PKU test.

▼ ACTION	▼ RATIONALE
5. Label the specimen and place in biohazard bag.	**5.** Identifies the test to be done, the date the specimen was obtained, and the identity of the client. Bag protects your from blood contact.
6. Send the specimen to the laboratory.	**6.** Results may be altered if specimen is allowed to sit.
7. Discard soiled equipment in the appropriate container.	**7.** Decreases the transmission of microorganisms.
8. Remove the gloves and wash your hands.	**8.** Decreases the transmission of microorganisms.
9. Record the procedure in the client's record.	**9.** Communicates to the other members of the health care team and contributes to the legal record by documenting the care given to the client.

Example of Documentation

DATE	TIME	NOTES
1/5/93	0800	PKU 3 mg/dl at 3 days of age.
		C. Lammon, RN
2/15/93	0900	Urine negative for PKU at 6-week checkup.
		C. Lammon, RN

Teaching Tips

Explain the purpose of the test and the results to the child's family.

Home Care Variations

This procedure usually is not performed in the child's home.

SKILL 6–17   SCREENING FOR SICKLE HEMOGLOBIN

Clinical Situations in Which You May Encounter This Skill

Sickle cell testing is done to detect the presence of an abnormal type of hemoglobin gene called sickle hemoglobin (HbS). In heterozygous form this gene causes sickle cell trait and in homozygous form it causes a hereditary chronic form of anemia with characteristic sickle-shaped erythrocytes. The gene that causes this disease occurs most frequently in Mediterranean and African populations.

Positive tests are 99% accurate. Differential diagnosis of the hemoglobin pattern is done by hemoglobin electrophoresis. Electrophoresis is necessary to differentiate between sickle cell trait and sickle cell disease.

Anticipated Responses

▼ The client's blood does not contain HbS.

Adverse Responses

▼ The blood test shows the presence of HbS.

Materials List

Gather these materials before beginning the skill:

▼ Sickle cell test paper
▼ Lancet or automatic puncture device
▼ Alcohol swab
▼ Small adhesive bandage
▼ Dry gauze
▼ Examination gloves
▼ Biohazard bag

▼ A C T I O N	▼ R A T I O N A L E
1. Determine if there is a history of sickle cell disease in the client's family.	1. This information will be helpful in counseling the client or the client's family, or both, about a hereditary disorder.
2. Put on examination gloves.	2. Decreases the transmission of microorganisms.
3. Collect a blood sample from a finger stick. Refer to Skill 5–15 for collecting a blood sample with a lancet if necessary.	3. An adequate sample will be needed to yield accurate results.
4. Thoroughly soak an area the size of a quarter or larger on the sickle cell test paper.	4. Sufficient blood must be provided to perform the test.
5. Label the specimen and place in biohazard bag.	5. Identifies the test to be done, the date the specimen was obtained, and the client's identity. Bag protects your from blood contact.
6. Send the specimen to the laboratory.	6. Test results may be altered if allowed to sit.
7. Discard soiled equipment in the appropriate container.	7. Decreases the transmission of microorganisms.
8. Remove the gloves and wash your hands.	8. Decreases the transmission of microorganisms.
9. Record the procedure in the client's chart.	9. Communicates the findings to the other members of the health care team, and contributes to the legal record by documenting the care given to the client.

Example of Documentation

DATE	TIME	NOTES
1/5/93	1000	Positive result on sickle cell test. Client's mother counseled regarding the results and referred to physician for examination and hemoglobin electrophoresis.
		C. Lammon, RN

Teaching Tips

Explain the purpose of the test and the results to the child's parents.

Home Care Variations

The same procedure can be used in the child's home and the specimen should be transported immediately to the lab.

SKILL 6–18   MEASURING THE SPECIFIC GRAVITY OF URINE

Clinical Situations in Which You May Encounter This Skill

Specific gravity reflects the ability of the kidney to concentrate urine. Concentrated urine has a high specific gravity and dilute urine has a low specific gravity. Diabetes mellitus, dehydration, and an increased secretion of antidiuretic hormone (ADH) cause elevated specific gravity. Diabetes insipidus, a decreased secretion of ADH, renal disease, and overhydration cause low specific gravity.

If the specific gravity is increased, nursing care may involve increasing intravenous (IV) or oral (PO) fluids. If the specific gravity is decreased, nursing care may involve decreasing the IV rate or amount of PO fluids. Drugs such as vasopressin may be used to decrease fluid loss.

Anticipated Responses

▼ The specific gravity is between 1.003 and 1.030.

Adverse Responses

▼ The specific gravity is increased or decreased.

Materials List

Gather these materials before beginning the skill:

▼ Cylinder
▼ Urinometer (Fig. 6–19)
▼ Urine specimen
▼ Clean specimen cup
▼ Washcloth
▼ Soap
▼ Towel
▼ Bath basin
▼ Examination gloves

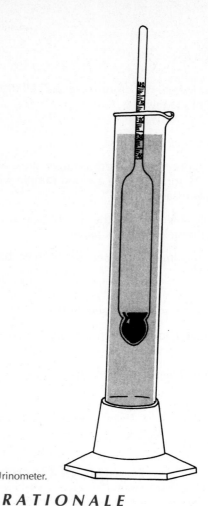

▼ **FIGURE 6–19.** Urinometer.

▼ ACTION	▼ RATIONALE
1. Assess the client for history of renal disease, diabetes insipidus, diabetes mellitus, and use of diuretics.	1. These conditions will alter the specific gravity of urine.
2. Assess the hydration of the client by checking skin turgor, intake and output, and the moistness of his or her mucous membranes.	2. The client's hydration will affect the concentration of his or her urine.
3. Put on gloves.	3. When there is a chance of coming into contact with urine, gloves should be worn to prevent the possible transmission of microorganisms.
4. Collect a fresh, nonsterile urine specimen without contaminants such as toilet paper or stool. You need to collect 20 ml of urine. If necessary, refer to Skill 5–9 on collection of urine specimens.	4. Contaminants will alter the results of the test. Urine must fill the cylinder at least two-thirds full.
5. Assist the client with perineal hygiene.	5. Provides for the client's comfort.
6. Check the accuracy of the urinometer by placing it in a cylinder filled two-thirds full with water. The reading should be 1.000.	6. The specific gravity measurement compares the weight of urine to that of water. If the water reading is greater than 1.000, distilled water should be used. Check the calibration of the urinometer.
7. Fill the cylinder two-thirds full of urine.	7. The urinometer must float in the cylinder.
8. Place the urinometer in the cylinder and wait until all movement ceases.	8. Allows for accurate measurement.
9. At eye-level, read the highest point on the urinometer scale where the urine touches the scale (Fig. 6–19).	9. The point where the urine level touches the scale is the specific gravity.
10. Discard the urine and clean the cylinder with soap and water. Rinse well.	10. Prepares the equipment for further use.

▼ *A C T I O N* _ _ _ _ _ _ _ _ _ _   ▼ *R A T I O N A L E* _ _ _ _ _ _ _ _

11. Remove the gloves and wash your hands.

12. Record the results.

11. Decreases the transmission of microorganisms.

12. Communicates the findings to the other members of the health care team and contributes to the legal record by documenting the care given to the client.

Example of Documentation

DATE	TIME	NOTES
1/7/93	0900	Specific gravity 1.001. Ten units vasopressin SC to right dorsolateral aspect of upper arm. IV 0.9 NaCl infusing to replace 200 ml urine lost in previous hour.

C. Lammon, RN

Teaching Tips

Explain the procedure, the purpose of the test, and the results to the client.

Home Care Variations

The procedure can be performed in the client's home using the same steps.

SKILL 6–19   PERFORMING TUBERCULIN SKIN TESTS

Clinical Situations in Which You May Encounter This Skill

Tuberculin skin tests are used for detecting exposure to *Mycobacterium tuberculosis* (tubercle bacillus). The tine test is a sterile multipuncture, single-use device and is used for mass screening for the presence of *M. tuberculosis*. If the results of a tine test are positive or doubtful, the client should be given a Mantoux test.

The Mantoux text is a diagnostic test in which purified protein derivative (PPD) is administered intradermally. A positive Mantoux test indicates past or present infection with the tubercle bacillus and indicates the need for further evaluative procedures before a diagnosis of tuberculosis (TB) can be made.

Reactions can be interpreted as positive, doubtful, or negative. A positive reaction occurs when there is an induration of 10 mm or more. If the induration measures 5 to 9 mm, a reaction is doubtful. A negative reaction occurs when the induration is less than 5 mm. Recent viral infections, the receipt of a live virus vaccine, or HIV infection can depress the reactivity to the tuberculin skin test.

Anticipated Responses

▼ The client has a negative reaction that indicates no exposure to the tubercle bacillus.

Adverse Responses

▼ The client has a positive reaction that indicates exposure to the tubercle bacillus.
▼ The client has a doubtful reaction.
▼ The client has a false negative reaction.

Materials List

Gather these materials before beginning the skill:

For a Tine Test

▼ Alcohol wipe
▼ Tine test

For a Mantoux Test

▼ Alcohol wipe
▼ Tuberculin syringe with 25-gauge 5/8-inch needle or smaller
▼ Purified protein derivative (PPD)
▼ Examination gloves

▼ *ACTION*

▼ *RATIONALE*

1. Ask the client if he or she has ever had a positive tuberculin skin test or a bacille Calmette-Guérin (BCG) vaccination.

2. Ask the client if he or she has had a vaccination or viral illness in the last 4 weeks.

3. Put on examination gloves.

4. Select a test site on the anterior ventral surface of the client's forearm.

5. Using a circular motion, cleanse the site with an alcohol wipe.

6 a. For a tine test:
   Open the tine test and press the prongs firmly on the client's forearm.

   b. For a Mantoux test:
   Administer the intradermal skin test using 0.1 ml of PPD (Fig. 6–20). Refer to the procedure for administering an intradermal injection (Skill 18–12) if necessary.

1. TB screening will always be positive in these individuals and therefore cannot be used as a screening test.

2. A viral illness and vaccination can suppress a reaction to the tuberculin skin test.

3. Decreases the transmission of microorganisms.

4. The site should be free of blood vessels, moles, hairs, or other marks.

5. Reduces the number of microorganisms on the skin surface.

6 a. Delivers a premeasured amount of PPD intradermally.

   b. A wheal at the injection site indicates the skin test was administered correctly.

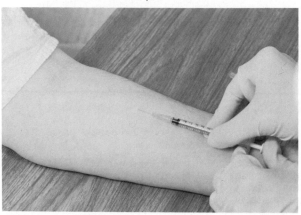

▼ **FIGURE 6–20.** Mantoux test.

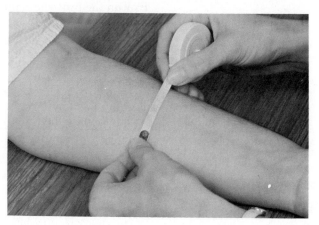

▼ **FIGURE 6–21.** Measuring an induration after a TB skin test.

7. Discard soiled supplies in an appropriate container.

8. Remove the gloves and wash your hands.

9. Tell the client to return for evaluation of the TB skin test in 48 to 72 hours.

10. After 48 to 72 hours, measure any induration present at the site of one puncture mark (Fig. 6–21).

11. Explain the results to the client.

12. If the test is positive, make a referral for further screening or treatment with the appropriate health care professional.

13. Record the TB skin test and results in the client's record.

7. Proper disposal decreases the transmission of microorganisms.

8. Decreases the transmission of microorganisms.

9. The maximum result will be observed during this interval of time.

10. An induration with a diameter greater than 10 mm is considered a positive test.

11. Keeps the client informed of his or her health status and allows the client to actively participate in his or her care.

12. A positive test indicates that the client has been exposed to tuberculosis and further evaluation is indicated.

13. Communicates the findings to the other members of the health care team and contributes to the legal record by documenting the care given to the client.

Example of Documentation

DATE	TIME	NOTES
1/4/93	0800	0.1 ml PPD given ID to Rt. forearm. No history of previous positive TB test or BCG vaccine.
		C. Lammon, RN
1/6/93	0900	15-mm induration noted at site of TB skin test. Client referred to chest clinic at public health department for further evaluation.
		C. Lammon, RN

SKILL 6-20   SCREENING VISION

Clinical Situations in Which You May Encounter This Skill

Visual acuity may be assessed in clinics, physician's offices, health fairs, or schools to detect myopia, hyperopia, or amblyopia. The client with myopia (nearsightedness) is able to see well at close distances but will exhibit poor distant vision. The person with myopia is unable to reach the referral line on the eye chart. Myopia results from light rays focusing in front of the retina rather than on the retina as in normal vision.

With hyperopia (farsightedness), the client is able to see well at far distances but exhibits poor near vision. The person with hyperopia is able to read an eye chart without difficulty. Further testing with a +2 diopter lens is needed to confirm the presence of hyperopia. Hyperopia results from light rays focusing behind the retina rather than on the retina as in normal vision.

Amblyopia is a condition of reduced vision with no apparent pathologic condition. It is usually seen unilaterally on eye screening and is indicated when the client is able to read two or more lines on the eye chart better with one eye than with the other.

Anticipated Responses

▼ The adult has 20/20 vision.
▼ The child of 3 to 4 years has 20/40 vision.
▼ The child 5 years or older has 20/30 vision.

Adverse Responses

▼ The client has myopia, hyperopia, or amblyopia.

Materials List

Gather these materials before beginning the skill:

▼ Snellen chart
▼ Tape measure
▼ Masking tape
▼ Butcher paper
▼ Index card
▼ +2 diopter lens

▼ ACTION

1. Select a well-lighted area with 20 feet of distance from the wall.

2. Cover any distractions that cannot be removed from the wall with butcher paper.

3. Hang charts on the wall with the referral line at eye-level.

4. Measure 20 feet from the wall and place a tape line on the floor.

5. Ask the client to wear corrective lenses if he or she has them.

▼ RATIONALE

1. Most eye charts require that the client stand 20 feet away.

2. Prevents the client from becoming distracted by extraneous visual stimuli.

3. Facilitates an accurate test of visual acuity at the referral line on the eye chart.

4. The client should stand with his or her heels on the tape line and face the eye chart.

5. Vision screening should determine the client's best visual acuity with correction.

▼ *A C T I O N*   ▼ *R A T I O N A L E*

6. Cover the client's right eye with an index card or cupped hand and instruct the client to keep both of his or her eyes open (Fig. 6–22).

6. Squinting or winking can alter the client's ability to read the eye chart.

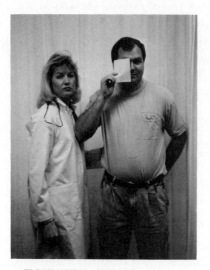

▼ **FIGURE 6–22.** Vision screening.

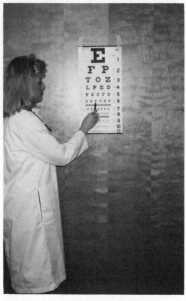

▼ **FIGURE 6–23.** Snellen chart for vision screening.

7. Beginning at the first line that the client can see clearly on the Snellen's chart, hold a pointer vertically below each symbol and ask the client to read each line (Fig. 6–23).

7. Holding the pointer vertically below each symbol prevents obstruction of the client's view.

8. Observe the client for squinting, tearing of his or her eyes, tilting of the head, or leaning forward.

8. Behavioral cues suggest problems with visual acuity.

9. Continue to have the client read progressively smaller lines on the eye chart until he or she can no longer read a *majority* of the symbols correctly on any given line. The client must be able to read a line correctly with no more than two errors. *Do not* ask the client to read lines below the referral line that is appropriate for his or her age.

9. A majority of the symbols must be correctly identified for each line in order to progress to the next line. Asking a client, especially a child, to read symbols beyond the referral line may cause feelings of inadequacy and failure.

10. Determine the client's visual acuity.

10. Visual acuity is recorded as a fraction. The numerator is the distance from the chart in feet. The denominator is the smallest line for which the client reads a majority of symbols correctly. This is actually the distance to which a person with normal vision can read a particular line.

11. Cover the client's left eye and repeat the test.

11. Both eyes should be assessed individually.

12. **NOTE:** If the client is unable to read the 20/200 line, walk toward the chart with him or her until he or she can identify the symbol on the 20/200 line. Measure the distance from the client to the chart and record this number over 200 as the client's vision (e.g., 13/200).

12. Determines the numerator of the client's visual acuity.

▼ *ACTION*	▼ *RATIONALE*
13. If the client is able to read the 20/200 line and does not wear corrective lenses, ask him or her to read the 20/200 line with the +2 diopter lens on.	**13.** Assesses for hyperopia.
14. If the client's vision was not satisfactory, schedule an appointment for a second screening test.	**14.** A second screening confirms initial findings prior to making a referral.
15. If the client's vision is not satisfactory on the second vision screening, make a referral to an appropriate eye care specialist.	**15.** Assists the client in receiving further eye evaluation and treatment.
16. Record the results of the vision testing in the client's record.	**16.** Communicates the findings to the other members of the health care team and contributes to the legal record by documenting the care given to the client.

Example of Documentation

DATE	*TIME*	*NOTES*
1/4/93	1000	Teacher reports client squinting in class and doing poorly in schoolwork when blackboard is used. Vision is 20/50 right eye and 20/60 left eye on second screening. Letter sent home describing screening results and need for further evaluation by an eye specialist.
		C. Lammon, RN

Teaching Tips

The purpose of the test and the procedure should be explained to the client.

Home Care Variations

Vision screening is not usually performed in the client's home.

SKILL 6–21   ASSISTING WITH A VAGINAL EXAMINATION

Clinical Situations in Which You May Encounter This Skill

A Pap smear involves removing a cell sample from the client's vaginal vault and cervical area to assess for abnormal or malignant cells. A normal Pap smear (Class I) indicates that no abnormal or atypical cells are present. If the smear is abnormal, the results may be reported as Class II to V. Classes II to V require further testing. A repeat Pap smear or a biopsy, or both, may be performed. The cytologic findings for Classes II to V are:

CLASS II: Atypical cytology—dysplastic, borderline but not neoplastic cells.

CLASS III: Cytology suggestive of but not inclusive of malignancy—"suspect."

CLASS IV: Cytology suggestive of malignancy—"strongly suspect."

CLASS V: Cytology conclusive of malignancy—cancerous cells present.

A wet prep is done to determine the presence and identity of any microorganisms that may be infecting the vagina. A gonorrhea culture is done to detect the presence of a *Neisseria gonorrhoeae* infection. Since vaginal infections and gonorrhea are sexually transmissible diseases, a sexual history is required to trace contacts and provide appropriate treatment. Finally, a bimanual examination is performed to detect the presence of abnormal masses in the client's ovaries, fallopian tubes, or uterus.

Anticipated Responses

▼ The client is able to tolerate the lithotomy position and pelvic examination with no more than a minimum amount of discomfort.

▼ The results of the Pap smear are Class I.
▼ There is no infection.

Adverse Responses

▼ The client has difficulty assuming the lithotomy position.
▼ The client experiences discomfort during insertion of the speculum.
▼ The findings are abnormal.

Materials List

Gather these materials before beginning the skill:

▼ Speculum
▼ Slide
▼ Cytology fixative or hair spray
▼ Wooden spatula (Ayre spatula)
▼ Sterile cotton-tipped applicators
▼ Examination gloves
▼ Water-soluble lubricant
▼ Drape
▼ Gown
▼ Light source
▼ Mayo stand
▼ Disposable towelette
▼ Basin with disinfectant solution
▼ Test tubes
▼ NaCl solution
▼ Chocolate agar plate (Thayer-Martin medium), air-tight plastic bag, and carbon dioxide tablet; or culture bottle with Thayer-Martin medium

▼ ACTION

1. Ask the client if she has had the procedure performed before. Explain the procedure if necessary.

2. Determine if the client has had an abnormal Pap smear in the past and previous medical management.

3. Ask the client to empty her bladder.

4. Ask the client to undress and provide a gown for her to put on.

5. Assist the client onto the examining table and ask her to lie down.

6. Place the drape over the client in a diamond configuration with one corner at her sternum, one corner over each of her knees, and one corner over her perineum.

7. Adjust the stirrups to a comfortable position.

8. Assist the client into the lithotomy position with her feet positioned in the stirrups (Fig. 6–24).

▼ RATIONALE

1. This information will assist you in individualizing the client teaching.

2. If the results are abnormal from this testing, the client's history will be important in determining future treatment. Also, repeat Pap smears are often needed to confirm results.

3. Facilitates bimanual examination and prevents accidental voiding during the examination.

4. Protects the client's dignity. All clothing is removed since the examiner will likely perform a breast examination at this time also.

5. Provides for the client's safety. The lithotomy position is used for a pelvic examination.

6. Allows you to expose the client's perineal area while covering the rest of her body.

7. Provides for the client's comfort and prevents leg cramps.

8. Facilitates examination of the pelvic area.

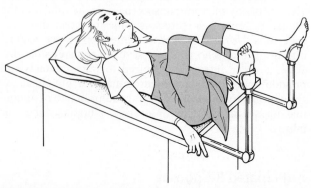

▼ **FIGURE 6–24.** Client's lithotomy position for vaginal examination.

▼ *ACTION* _ _ _ _ _ _ _ _ _ _ _ _ _ _ _ _   ▼ *RATIONALE* _ _ _ _ _ _ _ _ _ _ _ _ _ _ _

9. Direct the light source toward the client's perineum.

10. Place a waste disposal receptacle near the foot of the examining table.

11. Arrange the necessary equipment on a Mayo stand between you and the examiner.

12. Put on gloves.

13. Provide gloves for the examiner.

14. Hand the examiner a speculum moistened with warm water.

For a Pap Smear

15. a. Hand the wooden spatula and the cotton-tipped applicator to the examiner. An endocervical sample and a vaginal smear from the vaginal pool can be obtained with the cotton-tipped applicator. A cervical sample can be obtained by scraping the client's outer cervix with the wooden spatula (Fig. 6–25).

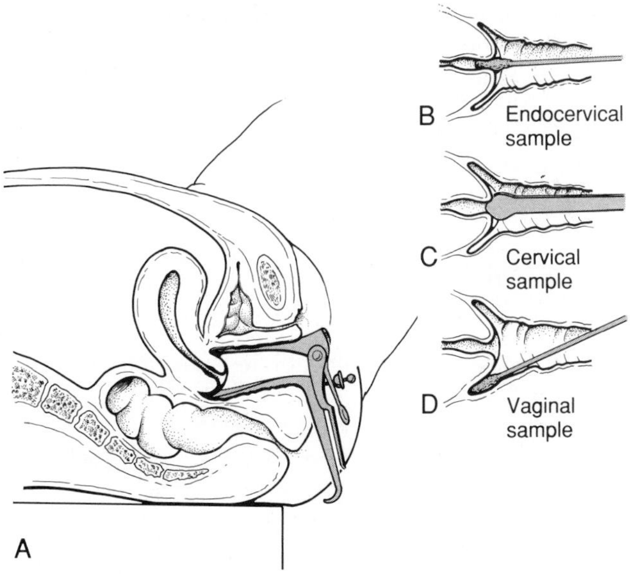

▼ FIGURE 6–25. Pap smear.

b. Hold the slide on the frosted end to allow the examiner to smear the vaginal specimen on the slide.

c. Hold cytology fixative 1 foot from the slide and lightly spray the slide

d. Label the specimen and set it aside for processing when the examination is completed.

9. Adequate light is needed for good visualization of the perineal and pelvic area.

10. Facilitates disposal of used supplies.

11. Facilitates passing supplies to the examiner.

12. Gloves should be worn whenever there is a chance of coming into contact with bodily secretions to prevent the transmission of microorganisms.

13. Decreases the transmission of microorganisms.

14. Aids in insertion of the speculum. Lubricating gels are not used as they may alter the results of the tests to be performed.

15. a. Used to obtain a sample of the client's endocervical, cervical, and vaginal cells.

b. The cells will be examined to determine the presence of abnormal or malignant cells.

c. Preserves the specimen.

d. Identifies to whom the specimen belongs.

▼ ACTION	▼ RATIONALE

For a Wet Prep

15. a. Hand the examiner a cotton-tipped applicator.

b. Place 2 to 3 drops of saline in a test tube.

c. Place the cotton-tipped applicator with the specimen into the tube with the saline solution.
d. Label the specimen and immediately take it to the laboratory for processing.

15. a. Used to collect a sample of the client's vaginal secretions.
b. A wet mount slide is made to examine the vaginal secretions for any organisms that may be present.
c. Disperses organisms into saline solution.

d. Identifies the client to whom the specimen belongs. The wet prep slide should be examined immediately after collecting the specimen.

For a Gonorrhea Culture

15. a. Hand the examiner a cotton-tipped applicator.

b. If using an agar plate: Streak the agar with the specimen-laden cotton-tipped applicator, cover the plate, and seal it in an airtight bag with a carbon dioxide tablet.

If using a culture bottle: Hold the bottle neck in an elevated position. Do not open the bottle until you are ready to inoculate the medium. Open the bottle and soak up the excess moisture in the bottle with a specimen swab. Roll the swab from side to side across the medium, beginning at the bottom of the bottle.
c. Discard the swab properly.
d. Label the specimen and send it to the laboratory for incubation.

e. Soak the soiled speculum in the disinfectant solution.

15. a. Used to collect a specimen from the client's endocervical canal.
b. *Neisseria gonorrhoeae* is an anaerobic organism. The carbon dioxide creates an environment that allows the organism (if present) to thrive until the culture medium can be examined.

Prevents loss of carbon dioxide from the bottle.

c. Decreases the transmission of microorganisms.
d. Identifies the client to whom the specimen belongs. Incubation helps the organisms to grow and multiply.
e. This is the first step in cleansing the instrument.

For a Bimanual Examination

15. a. Place a small amount of water-soluble lubricant on the examiner's fingers for the bimanual examination.
b. Instruct the client to breath deeply and relax her pelvic muscles as the examiner performs the internal examination.
c. Dispose of soiled equipment in an appropriate container.

16. Help the client to get off the examination table.

17. Offer the client a towelette for personal hygiene.

18. Wash your hands.

19. Record the procedure in the client's record.

15. a. Aids in insertion.

b. Makes the examination less uncomfortable.

c. Decreases the transmission of microorganisms.

16. Provides for the client's safety.

17. Removes any vaginal secretions or excess lubricant jelly.

18. Decreases the transmission of microorganisms.

19. Communicates the findings to the other members of the health care team and contributes to the legal record by documenting the care given to the client.

Example of Documentation

DATE	TIME	NOTES
1/2/93	1300	Pap smear and gonorrhea culture performed and specimen sent to laboratory. Large amount white cheesy vaginal discharge noted.
		C. Lammon, RN
1/4/93	1000	Wet prep reveals *Candida* infection. Prescription for miconazole nitrate given per physician. Client instructed in use of medication and measures to take to avoid infections in future such as use of cotton underwear and avoiding tight restrictive clothing.
		C. Lammon, RN

Teaching Tips

Explain the procedure and the purpose of the procedure to the client or her family, or both.

Home Care Variations

These tests are not usually performed in the client's home.

References

Fischbach, F. T. (1988). *A manual of laboratory diagnostic tests.* Philadelphia: J. B. Lippincott.

Lammon, C. A., and Adams, M. H. (1994). Assisting with diagnostic procedures. In V. Bolander (Ed.), *Basic nursing* (3rd ed.). Philadelphia: W. B. Saunders.

Pagana, K. D., and Pagana, T. J. (1986). *Diagnostic testing and nursing implications.* St. Louis: The C. V. Mosby Company.

UNIT III

THERAPEUTIC SKILLS

CHAPTER 7

Meeting Mobility Needs

- -

When a client is unable to move about independently or change positions in bed, he or she is at risk for complications due to immobility. These complications include development of pneumonia caused by stasis of pulmonary secretions; urinary retention; pressure ulcers; and contractures. The client is also at risk for psychologic complications such as anger or depression attributable to dependence on others for help. Helping the client to meet his or her mobility needs can aid in preventing these complications.

You can help increase the client's mobility by assisting with ambulation. Devices such as ambulation belts, canes, crutches, and walkers can provide the support necessary for the client to achieve more independent mobility.

You should help the immobilized client to change positions in bed at least every 2 hours. More frequent position changes may be required if the client is susceptible to skin breakdown or has a condition such as hemiparesis.

- -

- -

SKILL 7–1   HELPING THE CLIENT TO MOVE UP IN BED

Clinical Situations in Which You May Encounter This Skill

You may need to help the client who has had an operation or is weak or debilitated to move up in bed. Another nurse may need to assist you, depending on how much assistance the client can provide. If the client's bed is equipped with an overhead frame and trapeze, the client can use this to move up in the bed. A drawsheet also can be used to move the client up in bed. The drawsheet reduces the amount of effort expended by the nurses. It should extend from the client's shoulder to his or her knees. When you use a drawsheet, two other nurses should assist you.

Anticipated Responses

▼ You help the client to move up in bed without injury to you or to the client.

Adverse Responses

▼ The client or nurses receive an injury.

Materials List

Gather these materials before beginning the skill:

▼ Bed with side rails, overhead frame, and/or trapeze attached
▼ Drawsheet
▼ Bed linens and gown if needed
▼ Examination gloves if needed

▼ ACTION

1. Check the physician's order to see how much movement the client is allowed.

2. Assess the client's level of consciousness and ability to follow directions.

3. Lock the wheels of the bed and lower the side rails.

4. Lower the head of the bed. If body fluids are present in bed linens, put on examination gloves.

5. Adjust the bed to a comfortable working height.

6. Remove all of the pillows except one. Place the remaining pillow at the head of the bed.

7. Position urinary drainage, nasogastric (NG), and intravenous (IV) tubing so that there is slack in the tubing.

8. Stand facing the head of the bed diagonally and place your foot that is closest to the bed behind your other foot while flexing your knees.

9. Place one of your hands under the client's shoulders and one of your hands under the client's hips.

▼ RATIONALE

1. The client's condition may not allow him or her to assist.

2. It may be necessary to ask another nurse to help.

3. The wheels should be locked to prevent the bed from rolling when the client is moved.

4. If the head of the bed is not lowered, you will be trying to move the client against the pull of gravity. Gloves reduce transmission of microorganisms.

5. Reduces the strain placed on your body.

6. Protects the client's head as he or she is moved toward the top of the bed.

7. Prevents the tubing from being dislodged when the client is moved.

8. A principle of body mechanics is to face the direction in which you are working to reduce or prevent back strain. Your feet should be positioned as described to provide a wide base of support. Flexing your knees lets your legs do the work.

9. Your arms will be used for power and for guiding the client.

▼ *A C T I O N* _____   ▼ *R A T I O N A L E* _____

10 a. Ask the client to grasp the headboard of the bed, flex his or her knees, and place his or her feet flat on the mattress. On the count of three, ask the client to push with his or her feet and pull with his or her arms to assist you in moving him or her toward the head of the bed. Shift your weight to your forward foot as you help the client to move (Fig. 7–1).

10 a. If possible, the client should assist in moving to reduce the strain on you. By shifting your weight, you keep your weight over your base of support.

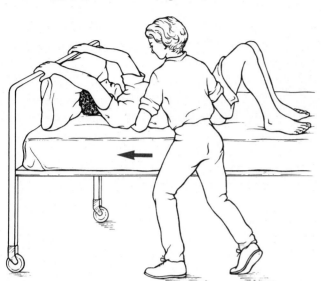

▼ **FIGURE 7–1.** Assisting client to move up in bed.

b. If you are using a trapeze: Ask the client to hold the trapeze and pull up to lift his or her upper body, flex his or her knees, and push on the count of three.

b. When the client pulls up, you can easily guide the client toward the head of the bed. The client should flex his or her knees in order to use his or her legs as levers.

c. If you are using a drawsheet:
   i. Two nurses should stand on one side of the bed and one nurse should stand on the other side. Place the client's arms on his or her abdomen and ask the client to flex his or her knees if permitted.

   i. Prevents any additional force against the client as he or she is moved.

   ii. Loosen the drawsheet on both sides of the bed and roll it toward the client.

   ii. Grip the rolled drawsheet to move the client.

   iii. On the side of the bed with two nurses, the nurse closest to the head of the bed should support the client's head with one hand and grasp the uppermost third of the drawsheet with the other hand. The other nurse on that side should grasp the middle and bottom one-third of the drawsheet. The nurse on the opposite side of the bed should grasp the top and bottom of the drawsheet.

   iii. The client's head should be supported to prevent injury. By grasping the drawsheet in the manner described, the client's entire body can be lifted and moved at one time and the client's head is supported.

   iv. On the count of three, all three nurses should shift their weight back and away from the client and toward the most forward foot in order to move the client to the head of the bed.

   iv. When the nurses shift their weight back and away from the client, it will lift the client from the bed. As the weight is shifted forward, the client can be moved toward the head of the bed.

▼ ACTION	▼ RATIONALE
11. Help the client to assume good body alignment, and reconnect the tubing and make sure it is functioning properly.	11. Reduces the strain on the client's muscles and joints. When the tubing is properly positioned, optimal functioning is promoted.
12. Replace the call signal, raise the side rails, lower the bed, and discard any soiled laundry.	12. Promotes client safety and comfort.
13. Remove gloves and discard them. Wash your hands.	13. Decreases the transmission of microorganisms.
14. Assess the client for skin breakdown, pain caused or relieved by the move, and proper body alignment.	14. Gives you the opportunity to make sure the client is comfortable and cared for before you leave the room.
15. Record the procedure.	15. Communicates the findings to the other members of the health care team and contributes to the legal record by documenting the care given to the client.

Example of Documentation

DATE	TIME	NOTES
10/26/93	1000	Mr. B. moved up in bed and repositioned. Body in good alignment.
		L. White, RN

Teaching Tips

The procedure for moving the client up in bed should be explained to the client and the client's family. The family should be taught how to help the client to assume good body alignment.

Home Care Variations

The same techniques can be used to assist the client to move up in bed at home.

SKILL 7–2   HELPING THE CLIENT TO SIT ON THE SIDE OF THE BED

Clinical Situations in Which You May Encounter This Skill

The client should sit on the side of the bed in preparation for getting out of bed to sit in a chair or to walk. Sitting on the side of the bed also can help the client to cough, deep breathe, overcome orthostatic hypotension, and increase muscle activity.

The client who has been confined to the bed will be weak and may experience orthostatic hypotension. The client who has just had an operation or who has been in the bed for a prolonged period of time may complain of dizziness or faintness. If so, do not keep the client in the sitting position, but help him or her to lie down. A client with impaired balance should be supported while sitting to prevent injury.

Anticipated Responses

▼ The client sits on the side of the bed without injury to the client or to you.

Adverse Responses

▼ You receive a back injury.
▼ The client complains of dizziness or faintness.

Materials List

Gather these materials before beginning the skill:

▼ Footstool
▼ Client's footwear

▼ *A C T I O N*	▼ *R A T I O N A L E*
1. Check the physician's order to determine the length of time the client may sit.	1. The physician may want the client to sit only for a specified length of time or for as long as possible.
2. Check the client's medical diagnosis.	2. Assists you in determining any problems that sitting may cause or any restrictions that are needed.
3. Prepare the client:	
a. Ask the client how long ago he or she last sat.	a. If the client has been in the bed for several days, he or she may experience dizziness or lightheadedness.
b. Take the client's vital signs.	b. Baseline vital signs are needed in order to evaluate changes such as orthostatic hypotension.
c. Place the footwear on the client.	c. Footwear protects the client's feet and prevents slipping.
4. Lock the wheels of the bed.	4. Prevents the bed from rolling when the client is moved.
5. Adjust the bed to a comfortable working height.	5. This will reduce the strain placed on your body.
6. Lower the side rails and move the client to the side of the bed closest to you.	6. By moving the client to the side of the bed, you can avoid reaching over and placing added strain on your body.
7. Raise the head of the bed to the maximum height that the client can tolerate.	7. Minimizes the distance required for the client to reach a sitting position.
8. Face the opposite side of the bed. If you are working from the left side of the bed, place your right foot closest to the bed.	8. Prevents twisting of your spine.
9. Place your right hand under the client's shoulders and your left hand under the client's thighs, with your palms up (Fig. 7–2*A*).	9. Your hands and arms will be used to pivot the client to a sitting position.
10. Shift your weight from your right foot to your left foot (Fig. 7–2*B*) and pivot the client to a sitting position (Fig. 7–2*C*).	10. By shifting your weight, you are keeping your weight over your base of support.
11. Stand in front of the client and support him or her until he or she is stable.	11. The client may experience some dizziness after assuming a sitting position.
12. Lower the bed to the lowest position.	12. The bed should be lowered for the client's safety.
13. If the client's feet do not touch the floor, place the client's feet on a footstool. Stay with the client while he or she is sitting.	13. The client may experience weakness or dizziness and you should be available to help him or her to lie down.
14. After the prescribed period, or if the client cannot tolerate sitting up any longer, help the client to lie back down by reversing the procedure.	14. The client probably will be tired and will need your assistance.

▼ *ACTION*   ▼ *RATIONALE*

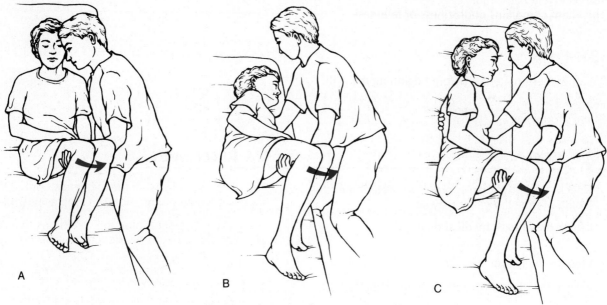

▼ **FIGURE 7–2.** Pivoting client to a sitting position.

15. Help the client to assume good body alignment and reposition any tubing. Lower the bed to lowest position.

15. The client's body should be in good alignment to promote optimal body functioning. Bed in low position promotes client safety.

16. Wash your hands.

16. Decreases the transmission of microorganisms.

17. Assess how well the client tolerated the procedure and whether any dizziness was experienced.

17. These data are necessary for charting the client's response

18. Record the procedure. Note the length of time the client sat and whether he or she experienced any dizziness.

18. Communicates the findings to the other members of the health care team and contributes to the legal record by documenting the care given to the client.

Example of Documentation

DATE	TIME	NOTES
10/26/93	1000	Helped Mrs. T. to sit on the side of the bed. She sat for 10 minutes without complaints of dizziness. Helped back to bed.
		L. White, RN

Teaching Tips

Encourage the client to assist you in moving him or her as much as possible. Explain that it is less painful for the client to move on his or her own and that it helps to increase muscle strength.

Home Care Variations

The client can be helped to sit on the side of the bed at home using the same technique.

SKILL 7–3 TRANSFERRING THE CLIENT FROM A BED TO A STRETCHER

Clinical Situations in Which You May Encounter This Skill

If the client is weak or has had an operation, you may need to help him or her to move from a bed to a stretcher or from a stretcher to a bed. If the client is able to assist, have him or her assist as much as possible. If the client is obese, a mechanical lift can be used. If the client is confused, sedated, immobile, or unresponsive, you probably will need to have another nurse assist. Alignment of the spine should be maintained for clients with a spinal cord injury or who have had spinal surgery.

Anticipated Responses

▼ You help the client to move from a bed to a stretcher without injury to the client or to you.

Adverse Responses

▼ Client's alignment is compromised during transfer.
▼ You receive a back injury.

Materials List

Gather these materials before beginning the skill:

▼ Stretcher
▼ Sheets
▼ Drawsheet

▼ *ACTION*	▼ *RATIONALE*
1. Determine the client's activity orders.	1. Alerts you to how much the client may be able to assist.
2. Determine the client's diagnosis and any other health problems.	2. If the client has an unstable spine, you will need to ensure alignment of the spine.
3. Assess the client's level of consciousness and ability to follow directions.	3. It may be necessary to ask another nurse to help. If the client is unresponsive or unable to follow directions, you will need assistance.
4. Determine whether the client has an IV, NG, or urinary drainage tube in place.	4. The tubing should be repositioned on the side of the bed toward which the client will be moved.
5. Position urine drainage, NG, and IV tubing, with slack in the tubing, on the side of the bed where the stretcher will be placed.	5. Prevents the tubing from being dislodged when the client is moved.
6. Clamp and disconnect any tubing if permitted.	6. NG suction tubing and tube-feeding tubing are often allowed to be clamped. This will make moving the client easier.
7. Lock the wheels of the bed.	7. Prevents the bed from rolling.

Assisting the Client Who Is Mobile (Steps 8 through 12)

8. Position the stretcher next to the bed and raise the bed to the level of the stretcher.	8. Promotes the client's safety.
9. Lock the wheels of the stretcher.	9. Prevents the stretcher from rolling.
10. Lower the head of the bed and loosen the top sheet.	10. The head of the bed is lowered so that the entire bed is the same height as the stretcher.
11. Stand on the side of the stretcher opposite the bed.	11. By standing on the side of the stretcher opposite the bed, you are in a position to assist the client if needed.

▼ _A C T I O N_	▼ _R A T I O N A L E_
12. Ask the client to move to the edge of the bed by flexing his or her knees and pushing with his or her feet to move his or her hips, trunk, and head to the edge of the bed. The client then should move his or her feet to the edge and then to the stretcher. Have the client flex his or her knees and use this same procedure to move to the center of the stretcher.	**12.** The client moves his or her body in segments using this technique.

Assisting the Client Who Is Immobile, Confused, Sedated, or Unresponsive (Steps 13 through 22)

13. Two additional persons will be needed to help. Three nurses should stand on the side of the bed to which the client is to be moved.	**13.** Positioning the nurses on the side to which the client will be moved allows you to pull instead of push.
14. Place the client's arms on his or her abdomen.	**14.** Prevents injury to the client and facilitates moving.
15. Lower head of bed. Loosen the drawsheet and roll it toward the client.	**15.** It is easier to move client if bed is flat. The nurses will grip the rolled drawsheet to move the client.
16. The nurse closest to the head of the bed should support the client's head with one hand and grasp the uppermost third of the drawsheet with the other hand. The second nurse should grasp the middle one-third of the drawsheet. The third nurse should grasp the bottom of the drawsheet and the client's legs.	**16.** The client's head should be supported to prevent injury. By grasping the drawsheet in the manner described, the client's entire body can be lifted and moved at one time.
17. On the count of three, lift and move the client to the side of the bed closest to the stretcher.	**17.** Makes it easier to move the client to the stretcher. Transfer the client across the shortest possible distance.
18. The first nurse should go to the opposite side of the bed and reach across the bed to hold the client in place. The remaining nurses should position the stretcher next to the bed and lock the wheels.	**18.** The wheels should be locked for the client's safety.
19. Raise the bed to the level of the stretcher.	**19.** The bed and stretcher should be at the same level for the client's safety.
20. The two nurses should move to the side of the stretcher opposite the bed and grasp the drawsheet as previously described.	**20.** The two nurses will pull the client toward the stretcher.
21. The first nurse on the opposite side of the bed should kneel in the bed at the level of the client's waist and grasp the drawsheet at the client's shoulder and hip.	**21.** The nurse kneels in the bed to avoid reaching over the bed and straining the back.
22. On the count of three, all nurses should lift and move the client to the stretcher.	**22.** Remember to use the your biceps since they are stronger than your triceps.

After Transfer of Both the Mobile and Immobile Client (Steps 23 through 26)

23. Help the client to assume good body alignment and reposition any tubing.	**23.** The client's body should be in good alignment to promote optimal body functioning.
24. Raise the side rails on the stretcher.	**24.** Protects the client from injury.
25. Wash your hands.	**25.** Decreases the transmission of microorganisms.

▼ ACTION	▼ RATIONALE
26. Record the procedure.	**26.** Communicates the findings to the other members of the health care team and contributes to the legal record by documenting the care given to the client.

Example of Documentation

DATE	TIME	NOTES
11/7/93	0700	Client to O.R. per stretcher.
		S. Smith, RN

Teaching Tips

The reason and the procedure for transfer should be explained to the client's family. If the client is to be moved in the home, the family should do a return demonstration.

Home Care Variations

The client can be moved in the home using the same technique.

SKILL 7–4 TRANSFERRING THE CLIENT FROM A BED TO A CHAIR OR WHEELCHAIR

Clinical Situations in Which You May Encounter This Skill

You may need to help the client who is weak or who has had an operation to move from a bed to a chair. The client who has just had an operation or who has been in bed for a long time may complain of dizziness or faintness. If this happens, assist the client in getting back into bed.

Anticipated Responses

▼ You help the client to sit in a chair without injury to the client or to you.

Adverse Responses

▼ You receive a back injury.
▼ The client complains of dizziness or faintness

Materials List

Gather these materials before beginning the skill:

▼ Chair
▼ Wheelchair
▼ Ambulation (gait) belt (optional)

▼ ACTION	▼ RATIONALE
1. Determine the client's activity orders.	**1.** Alerts you to how much the client may be able to assist.
2. Assess the client's level of consciousness and ability to follow directions.	**2.** It may be necessary to ask another nurse to help. If the client is unresponsive or unable to follow directions, you will need assistance.
3. Ask the client how long ago he or she last sat.	**3.** If the client has been in the bed for several days, he or she may complain of dizziness.

▼ *ACTION*   ▼ *RATIONALE*

4. Determine the client's diagnosis and any other health problems

4. If the client has an unstable spine, you will need to ensure alignment of his or her spine.

5. Determine whether the client has an IV, NG, or urinary drainage tube in place

5. The tubing should be repositioned on the side of the bed toward which the client will be moved.

6. Lock the bed wheels.

6. Prevents the bed from rolling when the client is moved.

7. Position the chair or wheelchair parallel to the bed or at a 40-degree angle facing the bed. If the client has more strength on one side than the other, place the chair so that the client gets out of the bed toward the stronger side and moves toward the chair with the stronger side leading. If a wheelchair is used, lock the wheels.

7. The parallel chair placement allows more room for you to assist the client. The angled chair placement puts the chair handle closer to the client and makes it easier for him or her to grasp the handle and swivel into the chair. Locking wheels of wheelchair prevents accidental movement of chair during the transfer.

8. Position urine drainage, NG, and IV tubing on the side of the bed where the chair or wheelchair was placed. Ensure slack in the tubing.

8. Prevents the tubing from being dislodged when the client is moved.

9. Clamp and disconnect any tubing if permitted.

9. NG suction tubing and tube-feeding tubing are often allowed to be clamped. This will make moving the client easier.

10. Lower the bed to its lowest position.

10. Promotes the client's safety.

11. Help the client to a sitting position on the side of the bed (see Skill 7–2).

11. Helps the client to overcome any dizziness before he or she stands.

12. Apply an ambulation (gait) belt if needed.

12. Aids in transferring the client safely.

13. Help the client to stand and move to the chair (Fig. 7–3):

13. The client may be weak upon first standing.

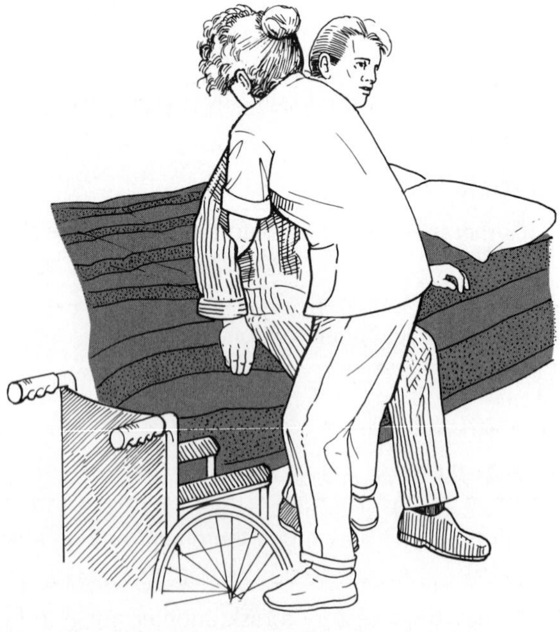

▼ FIGURE 7–3. Helping client move from bed to wheelchair.

a. Face the client as he or she sits on the side of the bed.

a. Provides for use of your body to move client.

▼ *A C T I O N*   ▼ *R A T I O N A L E*

b. Ask the client to move his or her buttocks to the edge of the bed.

    b. Allows client's weight to assist in moving.

c. Ask the client to place his or her feet in a wide stance on the floor with the strongest foot slightly back.

    c. Provides stability.

d. Grasp an ambulation belt or encircle the client with your arms under his or her arms and clasp your hands under the client's scapula.

    d. Provides safety.

e. Ask the client to lean forward and stand as you shift your weight backward while pulling the client forward and upward. Using a rocking motion forward and backward to gain momentum may help in lifting the client to a standing position. The client can assist by pushing off the mattress with his or her fists. If you are concerned that the client's arms may interfere with the transfer, have the client put his arms around your neck.

    e. Allows use of client's weight and good body mechanics to help client stand. Rocking uses both client's and nurse's weight to gain momentum and move client.

f. Ask the client to stand up straight and balance in an upright position. Place your knee against the client's weaker forward knee to prevent sliding.

    f. Provides stability.

g. Ask the person to grasp the arm of the chair. Then pivot with the client so that his or her back faces the chair.

    g. Pivoting allows for greatest movement with least expenditure of energy.

h. Lower the client into the chair.

14. Reposition and reconnect any tubing. The client's legs may need to be elevated. Also extra covering may be provided.

14. Tubing should not be left disconnected. The client may want to sit for a while and will need all the equipment to function properly. Elevating legs decreases edema. Covers provide comfort.

15. Wash your hands.

15. Decreases the transmission of microorganisms

16. Assess how well the client tolerated the move and whether any dizziness was experienced.

16. These data are necessary for charting whether the client experienced any problems.

17. Record the procedure. Note the length of time the client sat in the chair and whether he or she experienced any dizziness.

17. Communicates to the other members of the health care team and contributes to the legal record by documenting the care given to the client.

18. Reverse the procedure to return the client to bed.

Example of Documentation

DATE	TIME	NOTES
11/8/93	1000	Mrs. T. sat in chair at side of bed for 15 minutes. No complaints of dizziness. Assisted back to bed.
		L. White, RN

Teaching Tips

Encourage the client to assist you in moving him or her. Activity will help to increase the client's muscle strength. The client should wear street shoes to provide support while standing.

Home Care Variations

The same technique can be used to move the client to a chair or wheelchair in the home.

SKILL 7–5 TRANSFERRING THE CLIENT WITH A HYDRAULIC LIFT

Clinical Situations in Which You May Encounter This Skill

You may need to use a hydraulic lift (Fig. 7–4A) to transfer a client who is immobile or obese. The client can be transferred to a chair, stretcher, bedside commode, or scale using a hydraulic lift. Follow the specific manufacturer's directions. Do not use a hydraulic lift on any client who exceeds the weight limits. The hydraulic lift should not be used for a client with a spinal cord injury. Another nurse should assist you. The client who has just had an operation or who has been in bed for a long time may complain of dizziness or faintness. If this happens, help the client get back to bed.

Anticipated Responses

▼ You move the client without injury to the client or to you.

Adverse Responses

▼ You receive a back injury.
▼ The client complains of dizziness or faintness.

Materials List

Gather these materials before beginning the skill:

▼ Hydraulic lift
▼ Chair
▼ Blanket

▼ *A C T I O N* ▼ *R A T I O N A L E*

1. Check the weight capacity of the lift.

2. Check the physician's order to determine the length of time the client may sit.

3. Check the client's medical diagnosis and any other medical problems.

4. Ask the client how long ago he or she last sat.

5. Lock the wheels of the bed.

6. Position the chair close to the bed.

7. Position urine drainage, NG, and IV tubing on the side of the bed where the chair will be placed. Ensure slack in the tubing.

8. Clamp and disconnect any tubing if permitted.

9. Roll the client on his or her side and position the sling on the bed behind the client.

1. The weight capacities of lifts vary.

2. The physician may want the client to sit only for a specified length of time or for as long as possible.

3. Assists you in determining any problems that sitting may cause or any restrictions needed.

4. If the client has been in the bed several days, he or she may complain of dizziness or faintness.

5. Prevents the bed from rolling when the client is moved.

6. Always transfer the client the shortest possible distance.

7. Prevents the tubing from being dislodged when the client is moved.

8. NG suction tubing and tube-feeding tubing are often allowed to be clamped. This will make moving the client easier.

9. The sling is positioned behind the client so that he or she can be turned in the opposite direction and the sling can be pulled through.

▼ _ACTION_ _____ ▼ _RATIONALE_ _____

10. Roll the client to his or her opposite side, pull the sling through, and position the sling smoothly on the bed.

10. Prevents skin breakdown.

11. Roll the client back onto the sling and fold his or her arms over his or her chest.

11. Prevents injury to the client's arms during the transfer.

12. Make sure that the sling is centered.

12. Evenly distributes the client's weight.

13. Lower the side rail and position the lift on the side of the bed with the chair. Protect the client from falls while the side rail is down.

13. The side rail must be down to use the lift. Always transfer the client the shortest possible distance.

14. Lift the frame and pass it over the client. Carefully lower the frame and attach the hooks to the sling. Raise the client from the bed by pumping the handle (Fig. 7–4B).

14. Read the manufacturer's directions to determine the mechanism for raising the particular lift you are using. The various models do not operate in the same manner.

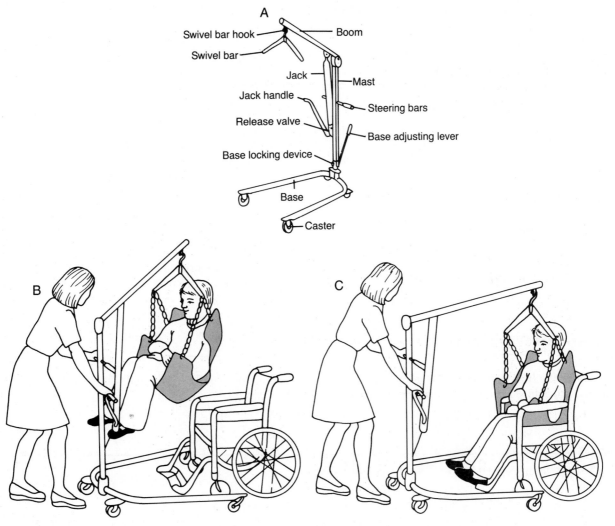

▼ FIGURE 7–4. Moving client with a hydraulic lift.

15. Secure the client with a safety belt and cover the client with a blanket.

15. Provides safety and comfort.

16. Steer the client away from the bed and slide a chair through the base of the lift.

16. It is safer to slide the chair through the base than to slide the base around the chair.

▼ ACTION	▼ RATIONALE
17. Lower the client into the chair and disconnect the sling from the lift (Fig. 7–4C).	17. The sling can be disconnected and the lift can be moved out of the way while the client is sitting in the chair.
18. Reposition and reconnect any tubing if necessary.	18. Tubing should not be left disconnected. The client may sit for a while and will need all the equipment to function properly.
19. Wash your hands.	19. Decreases the transmission of microorganisms.
20. Assess how well the client tolerated the move and whether any dizziness or faintness was experienced.	20. These data are necessary for charting whether the client experienced any problems.
21. Record the procedure. Note the length of time the client sat in the chair and whether he or she experienced any dizziness or faintness.	21. Communicates to the other members of the health care team and contributes to the legal record by documenting the care given to the client.
22. Repeat the procedure to return the client to the bed.	

Example of Documentation

DATE	TIME	NOTES
11/8/93	0900	Hydraulic lift used to help Mrs. T. to move to chair. Sat in chair for 15 minutes. No complaints of dizziness. Lift used to return Mrs. T. to bed.
		S. Shaw, RN

Teaching Tips

Explain to the client and the client's family why the lift is used and the procedure for using the lift. If the family will be using a lift at home, demonstrate the procedure and allow the family to do a return demonstration.

Home Care Variations

Hydraulic lifts usually are not used in the home. However, if the family has rented one, the procedure for transfer would be the same.

SKILL 7–6 LOGROLLING THE CLIENT

Clinical Situations in Which You May Encounter This Skill

Logrolling is used to turn a client who has a spinal cord injury or a spinal disorder, or who has had a spinal cord operation or a hip operation (with a prosthesis or pinning). Another nurse should assist you with this procedure.

Anticipated Responses

▼ You help the client to turn without injury to the client or to you.

Adverse Responses

▼ You receive a back injury.

Materials List

Gather these materials before beginning the skill:

▼ Pillow
▼ Drawsheet
▼ Wedge
▼ Pillows and extra linens as needed

▼ *A C T I O N*	▼ *R A T I O N A L E*
1. Determine the reason for logrolling the client and the client's diagnosis.	1. The reason for the procedure should be explained to the client.
2. Raise the bed to a comfortable working level.	2. A principle of body mechanics is to always position work at a comfortable height to prevent back strain.
3. Lock the wheels of the bed. Gently remove supportive devices around client.	3. Prevents the bed from rolling. Prepares client for position change.
4. The two nurses should position themselves on opposite sides of the bed and roll the edges of the drawsheet toward the client.	4. The nurses will grip the rolled drawsheet to roll the client.
5. With the drawsheet, slide the client to the edge of the bed opposite the direction to which the client is to be turned.	5. Allows ample room for positioning the client once he or she is rolled to the opposite side.
6. Place a pillow lengthwise between the client's legs.	6. Helps to maintain the correct alignment of the client's lower extremities as he or she is turned.
7. Position the client's arms. To turn the client to the right, place his or her left arm to the side and his or her right arm either flexed above the head or at the side. Raise the bedrails. Both nurses should move to the side of the bed that the client will turn toward.	7. The client's arms are positioned as described to prevent injury to them and to make their final positioning easier.

> **NOTE:** If the client has a cervical spinal cord injury, a third person should assist and support the client's neck.

8. One nurse should grasp the client at the client's shoulders and waist, supporting the neck. The other nurse should grasp the client at the client's buttocks and knees, supporting the legs. Roll the client all in one motion to a side-lying position.	8. Allows the client's spine to remain straight and not rotate. The client is turned as a unit to prevent further spinal cord damage. Grasping the client rather than the drawsheet gives you better control of the client's body.
9. Place the client in correct body alignment and put the wedge against his or her back.	9. The client is aligned correctly to prevent any contractures and damage to the spinal cord.
10. Flex the client's top leg at the knee and place a pillow under the knee and lower leg. A small pillow or folded linen may be placed under the head and shoulders.	10. Maximizes the client's comfort and provides good body alignment.
11. Wash your hands.	11. Decreases the transmission of microorganisms.
12. Assess the client's comfort and body alignment.	12. Proper body alignment aids in the client's comfort and assists in preventing complications.
13. Record the procedure.	13. Communicates to the other members of the health care team and contributes to the legal record by documenting the care given to the client.

Example of Documentation

DATE	TIME	NOTES
11/8/93	0800	Mr. W. turned on his side and positioned. Stated he was comfortable.
		T. Anderson, RN

Teaching Tips

The purpose of logrolling should be explained to the client and the client's family. Emphasize that logrolling will help to protect the client's spinal cord. Demonstrate to the family the logrolling procedure and how to correctly position the client.

Home Care Variations

The same technique can be used to logroll the person in the home.

SKILL 7–7   MOVING THE CLIENT TO THE SUPINE POSITION

Clinical Situations in Which You May Encounter This Skill

In the supine position (Fig. 7–5), the client lies down on his or her back. The client's head, neck, and upper shoulders rest on a pillow, and the arms and legs are extended. The legs should be abducted slightly to prevent skin breakdown as a result of the skin of the inner thighs touching. The ankles should be supported at 90 degrees to prevent plantar flexion.

The supine position is one of the common positions for rest. It also allows for physical assessment of the anterior portion of the client's body. Some clients with back and cervical problems are required to lie in this position.

Clients who must lie in this position for a long time may develop a respiratory impairment such as atelectasis. The client's back may become tired. A pillow that is too thick can cause cervical flexion contractures. Other problems that may arise if a client is left too long in this position are footdrop, external rotation of the hips, and pressure sores, especially on the heels and sacrum.

Anticipated Responses

▼ The client is comfortable and his or her respiratory effort is not compromised.
▼ The client's body is in proper alignment and the skin is free from pressure sores.

Adverse Responses

▼ The client is uncomfortable.
▼ The client's respiratory effort is compromised.

Materials List

Gather these materials before beginning the skill:

▼ Bed that can be positioned either manually or electrically
▼ Several pillows
▼ Sheet and other covers as needed

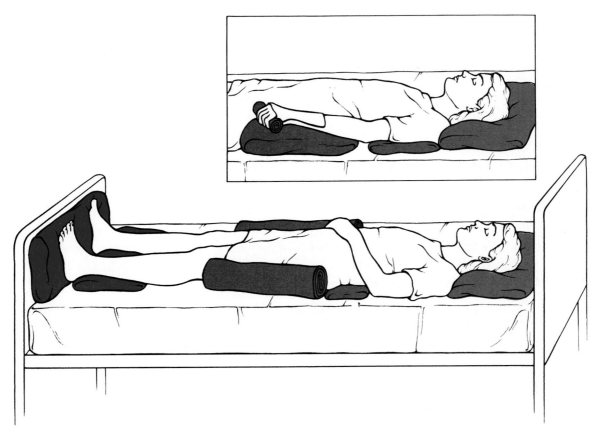

▼ **FIGURE 7–5.** Supine position.

▼ *A C T I O N*

▼ *R A T I O N A L E*

1. Review the chart for the client's condition.

1. Provides information for the plan of care.

2. Help the client to lie down on his or her back in the middle of the bed. Raise the bed to working height.

2. Promotes proper body alignment. Raising the bed provides for proper body mechanics.

3. Assist the client to the head of the bed. Use proper body mechanics and obtain help if needed.

3. Prevents the client from assuming an abnormal position when his or her head is raised. Provides comfort. Obtaining help prevents you from receiving muscle strain and related injuries.

4. Align the client's body with a straight spine in the center of the bed.

4. Promotes proper body alignment.

5. Place a trochanter roll on either side of the client's hips and thighs.

5. Prevents external rotation of the hips.

▼ *ACTION* _____ ▼ *RATIONALE* _____

6. Place a small pillow behind the client's head, under each arm, and under the lower legs.

6. The pillow for the client's head prevents pulling his or her shoulders into poor alignment and hyperextension of the neck. The pillow under the client's arms helps to prevent dependent edema. The pillow under the client's lower legs helps to prevent skin breakdown on the heels and hyperextension of the knees.

7. If not contraindicated, the bed frame may be raised slightly at the client's knees. If you are unable to gatch the bed frame, a thin pillow may be placed under the client's thighs. It should not extend into the back of the knees.

7. Raising the knee gatch of the bed frame relieves the pressure on the client's lower back. Pillows under the knees can compromise the client's circulation.

8. If the client is to be in this position long, his or her feet should be supported with a footboard.

8. Protects the client's feet from developing plantar flexion.

9. Place covers over the client. Lower the bed to the lowest position.

9. Provides comfort and safety.

10. Wash your hands.

10. Decreases the transmission of microorganisms.

11. Record the procedure and other relevant information.

11. Communicates the information to other members of the health care team and contributes to the legal record by documenting the care given to the client.

12. a. Check the client's body alignment and his or her comfort.
    b. Observe the client's heels, sacrum, and other areas of the skin for pressure sores. Check for cervical flexion.
    c. Assess the client's feet for footdrop.
    d. Assess the client's respiratory status frequently.

12. a. Provides you with information that is useful for the client's optimal wellness.
    b. The pillow may be too thick.

    c. Without support, footdrop will occur.
    d. This position will cause pooling of respiratory secretions.

Example of Documentation

DATE	TIME	NOTES
6/24/93	1030	Client in supine position. States he is comfortable and breathing easily. RR = 18. Skin color pink. Skin clear, no pressure areas noted. No accessory muscle use noted. Lungs auscultated. Breath sounds bilaterally clear and equal. Feet against footboard. No plantar flexion noted.
		H. White, RN

Teaching Tips

The purpose of the supine position and the procedure for assuming it should be explained to the client or to the client's caregiver, or both. Emphasize that the client's position should be changed frequently to prevent complications and that pressure sores can develop on any area of the body that has experienced prolonged pressure, including the back of the head and ears.

Home Care Variations

For clients who are homebound with family members caring for them, the purchase or rental of a hospital bed might be worthwhile to help change the client's position more readily. If circumstances are not conducive to such a purchase, families must be made aware of the need for frequent position changes in bedridden clients.

SKILL 7–8 MOVING THE CLIENT TO THE PRONE POSITION

Clinical Situations in Which You May Encounter This Skill

In the prone position, the client lies facedown with his or her head turned to one side. The client's shoulders are both abducted and rotated 90 degrees. The arms are flexed at the elbow with palms facing downward along the side of the head. The legs are extended and slightly separated. The feet should extend over the bottom of the mattress with the ankles at a 90-degree angle (Fig. 7–6A) or supported at a 90-degree angle with sandbags (Fig. 7–6B).

Clients who require a change of position or who require a procedure or treatment involving the back may be placed in this position. The prone position facilitates respiratory secretion drainage. The prone position also helps to prevent footdrop. Modifications may need to be made in the position according to the client's condition.

Limitations of the prone position include poor body alignment if the ankles are in prolonged plantar flexion and the lumbar spine has continuous hyperextension. It is also difficult to assess respiratory status in this position. Because of decreased visual cues in this position, some clients become disoriented. Thus, the client should not be left in the prone position for prolonged periods of time.

Anticipated Responses

▼ The client is fairly comfortable and without respiratory compromise.
▼ The client's body is in correct alignment.

Adverse Responses

▼ The client is uncomfortable.
▼ The client's respiratory effort is compromised.

Materials List

Gather these materials before beginning the skill:

▼ Bed that can be positioned either manually or electrically
▼ Pillows
▼ Bed linens and gown if needed
▼ Lift sheet

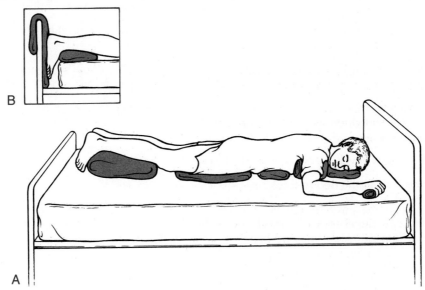

▼ FIGURE 7–6. Prone position.

▼ *ACTION* _____ ▼ *RATIONALE* _____

1. Review the chart to assess the client's condition.

   1. Allows for an adequate plan of care.

2. Plan activities for the client that will help with the client's orientation.

   2. Decreases the likelihood of the client becoming disoriented.

3. Raise bed to working height.

   3. Provides for proper body mechanics.

4. Help the client to lie chestdown on the bed. If the client is unable to assume this position, place him or her in the supine position.

   4. This is the beginning position for the prone position.

5. Remove all pillows and positioning devices. A nurse should stand at each side of the bed and a third nurse should support the client's head. Using a lift sheet, move the client to the side of the bed opposite that of the planned turn.

   5. The lift sheet prevents the client from being dragged across the sheets and reduces skin damage.

6. Place pillows in the bed next to the client to protect the following pressure points when the turn is completed: the lower chest and abdomen for females and the waist to groin for males; the thighs; and the lower leg between the knee and the ankle.

   6. Protects the client's breast and scrotum from pressure. Decreases pressure on the client's knees and prevents stress on the client's knee joints and lumbar spine.

7. Be sure the client's gown is not wrinkled or constricting at the neckline.

   7. Protects the client's skin from injury and promotes comfort.

8. Place the client's arms against his or her body. Stand on the side of bed toward which the client will turn.

   8. Prevents injury to the client's limbs. It is easier to pull than to push.

9. Roll the client over his or her arm into a facedown position. The nurses should control the person's head and leg movement so that the client's body rolls as a unit.

   9. Moving the person as a unit maintains his or her spinal alignment.

10. Assess the client's respiratory status. Turn his or her head to the side. A small pillow may be used to relieve pressure from the person's facial bones.

    10. Ensures that the client's airway is not obstructed by the mattress.

11. Position the client's arms flexed at the elbows with the palms facing downward, along the side of the person's head.

    11. Maintains the client's spinal alignment.

12. Adjust pillow supports if needed.

    12. Promotes the client's comfort.

13. Use small pillows or linen rolls in the space between the client's axilla and clavicle.

    13. Reduces pressure on the client's shoulders.

14. Observe the client from the foot of the bed and the side of the bed for proper body alignment.

    14. Promotes the client's comfort and reduces stress on his or her joints.

15. Be sure the client's feet are hanging over the end of the mattress or are supported with the person's ankles at a 90-degree angle.

    15. Prevents plantar flexion of the client's feet.

16. Provide the client with a cover.

    16. Provides comfort.

17. Raise the side rails. Lower the bed to lowest position.

    17. Provides safety.

18. Ascertain that the call signal is within reach. (A clock where the client can see it may be beneficial.)

    18. Provides safety. A clock will help orient the client to time spent in prone position.

▼ _A C T I O N_	▼ _R A T I O N A L E_
19. Periodically change the client's arm positions and encourage deep breathing and coughing.	19. Provides comfort and respiratory hygiene.
20. Wash your hands.	20. Decreases the transmission of microorganisms.
21. Observe male clients for scrotal edema when they are in this position.	21. Dependent edema due to obstructed circulation may cause scrotal edema when the client is in the prone position.
22. Record the procedure.	22. Communicates to the other members of the health care team and contributes to the legal record by documenting the care given to the client.
23. Assess the client's comfort and physical condition while he or she is in this position.	23. Provides updated information for planning client care. Respirations may be compromised in this position.

Example of Documentation

DATE	TIME	NOTES
4/4/93	1000	Client placed in prone position for 1 hour. No respiratory distress noted. Client states she has no discomfort.
		H. White, RN

Teaching Tips

The purpose of the prone position and the procedure for assuming it should be explained to the client or to caregiver, or both. Emphasize that the client should not remain in this position for an extended period of time and that any difficulty in breathing should be reported.

Home Care Variations

If the prone position will be used at home, make sure the people responsible for putting the client in this position are aware of the problems associated with it and know how to assess for respiratory distress. Reinforce the fact that clients should not be left in this position for a long period of time.

SKILL 7–9   MOVING THE CLIENT TO THE SIDE-LYING POSITION

Clinical Situations in Which You May Encounter This Skill

In the side-lying position (Fig. 7–7), the client lies on his or her right or left side with the head and shoulders aligned with the hips and the spine parallel to the edge of the mattress. A pillow supports the client's head and neck. The upper arm is supported with a pillow. A small pillow or folded linen can support the waist if needed. The lower shoulder is pulled forward (protracted) slightly and the lower shoulder and elbow are flexed 90 degrees. The client's legs may be flexed or extended. The ankles are supported at 90 degrees to prevent footdrop.

The side-lying position places pressure on the body prominences of the greater trochanter and iliac crest and therefore should not be used for persons at risk for developing pressure ulcers. A modified position that limits the degree of turn to no more than 30 degrees to either side with the head of the bed elevated no more than 30 degrees is recommended by the National Pressure Ulcer Advisory Panel.

Clients who require position changes are placed in the side-lying position, alternating the right and left side if possible. Clients who have lobar pneumonia or acute pleurisy also may be positioned on one side or the other. The left side-lying position is used for certain gynecologic and obstetric procedures and treatments and for large pericardial effusions. The right side-lying position is used after a liver biopsy.

Anticipated Responses

▼ The client is fairly comfortable.
▼ The client's respiratory effort is not compromised.
▼ The client's proper body alignment is maintained.

Adverse Responses

▼ The client is uncomfortable.
▼ The client's respiratory effort is compromised.
▼ The client's proper body alignment is not maintained.
▼ The client's neck is laterally flexed.
▼ There is internal rotation of the client's hip or shoulder joints.
▼ Footdrop occurs.
▼ Pressure sores develop on the dependent areas of the client's skin.

Materials List

Gather these materials before beginning the skill:

▼ Bed or examination table
▼ Pillows and folded linens
▼ Sheet or other cover

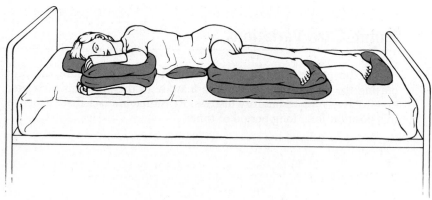

▼ FIGURE 7–7. Side-lying position.

▼ *A C T I O N*

▼ *R A T I O N A L E*

1. Review the chart for the client's condition and any contraindications to the client assuming this position.

2. Raise the bed to working height. Using proper body mechanics, position the client on his or her back and remove all pillows and positioning devices.

3. Ask the client to turn onto his or her right or left side. If the client is unable to turn, assist the client using proper body mechanics.

4. Move the client to the side of the bed opposite the one the client will face when turned.

5. Place a small pillow or folded linen at the client's waist level on the side to which he or she will turn. Position a head pillow to support the client's head and neck during and after the turn.

6. Go to the opposite side of the bed. Position the client's arm closest to you by abducting the shoulder 90 degrees and flexing the elbow 90 degrees.

7. Cross the client's other arm over his or her abdomen and place the client's far leg across his or her leg closest to you.

8. Place your fingers around the client's body at the shoulder and hip and roll the person toward you. A drawsheet also could be used to roll the client toward you.

9. Position the client's lower shoulder by gently pulling it slightly toward you.

10. Elevate the client's upper arm and hand on the pillow. Maintain client's hand higher than the upper arm.

11. Position the client's upper leg with the hip and knee at 45 to 90 degrees of flexion and the ankle at 90 degrees. Place pillows between the client's legs to support the upper leg and foot.

12. Use a sandbag to hold the client's lower foot in place with the ankle at 90 degrees of flexion.

13. Cover the client with adequate blankets for comfort.

14. Assess the client's comfort, including body alignment and respiratory status. Place a call light within the client's reach. Lower the bed to the low position. Raise the side rails.

15. Wash your hands.

16. Record the procedure.

1. Provides information for the plan of care.

2. Use of body mechanics prevents injury to your back. The supine position is the starting point for the side-lying position.

3. Use of proper body mechanics prevents injury to you.

4. Allows space for the client to turn toward the center of the bed.

5. The support helps to maintain the client's spinal alignment.

6. Prevents the client from rolling over on his or her arm during the turn.

7. Uses the client's body weight to facilitate turning.

8. Whenever possible, pull rather than push to move a person.

9. Prevents the weight of the client's body from compressing the circulation to his or her arm.

10. Supports the client's arm in proper alignment and promotes venous return. The most distal part of the extremity should be highest to prevent edema.

11. Maintains the client's leg alignment and prevents pressure on the bony knee prominences.

12. Prevents footdrop.

13. Provides comfort.

14. Provides information important for the client's care and comfort. Provides for safety.

15. Decreases the transmission of microorganisms.

16. Communicates to the other members of the health care team and contributes to the legal record by documenting the care given to the client.

Example of Documentation

DATE	TIME	NOTES
6/5/93	1000	Client placed on left side for 1 hour. Respiratory status unchanged.
		H. White, RN

Teaching Tips

The purpose of the side-lying position and the procedure for assuming it should be explained to the client or to caregiver, or both. The client should be encouraged to change positions frequently.

Home Care Variation

The same procedure can be used to help the client to assume the side-lying position at home.

SKILL 7–10   MOVING THE CLIENT TO THE SIMS POSITION

Clinical Situations in Which You May Encounter This Skill

The Sims position (Fig. 7–8) is midway between the prone and side-lying positions. In the Sims position, the client lies on his or her left side with his or her body turned approximately 45 degrees. The spine is parallel with the mattress and the shoulders and hips are aligned. The person's face is supported by a small pillow. The lower arm is behind the body and the shoulder is retracted and hyperextended. The elbow is flexed slightly. The upper arm and upper right chest are supported by a pillow. The lower leg is extended and the upper leg is flexed at the hip and knee approximately 45 to 90 degrees. The ankles are supported at 90 degrees to prevent footdrop. The client also may assume this position on his or her right side. This is called a right Sims position.

The Sims position may be used for clients who require a curettement of the uterus, irrigation of the uterus after delivery, or rectal or cervical procedures. It also may be used for unconscious or paralyzed clients. The Sims position also facilitates drainage of oral secretions.

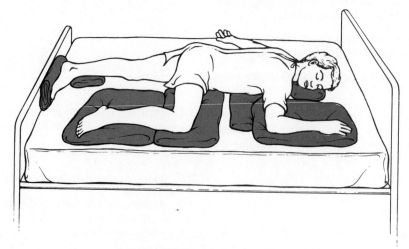

▼ **FIGURE 7–8.** Sims' position.

Anticipated Responses

▼ The client is fairly comfortable without respiratory compromise.
▼ There is adequate visualization of the required area.

Adverse Responses

▼ The client is uncomfortable.
▼ The client's respiratory effort is compromised.
▼ There is inadequate visualization of the required area.

Materials List

Gather these materials before beginning the skill:

▼ Bed that can be positioned either manually or electrically (sometimes an examination table is used)
▼ Pillows and folded linens
▼ Sheet

▼ ACTION	▼ RATIONALE
1. Review the chart to assess the client's condition and the reason for the position.	1. Allows for an adequate plan of care.
2. Raise the bed to working height. Position the client on his or her back and assist the client if needed. Use proper body mechanics. Remove all pillows and positioning devices.	2. Promotes the client's body alignment. Provides for safety. Use of proper body mechanics helps to prevent injury to you.
3. Move the client to the right side of the bed.	3. Allows adequate room for the client to turn to the left side.
4. Place a pillow or folded linen in line with the client's body near the shoulder and upper chest, between the waist and knees, and between the knee and lower leg.	4. Provides support for the client's upper torso, arms, and legs when the turn is completed.
5. Extend the client's arms next to his or her body with the client's palms touching his or her thighs.	5. Prevents injury to the client's arms during the turn.
6. If not contraindicated by spine or hip injuries, place the client's right leg over the left leg.	6. Uses the client's weight to facilitate the turn.
7. Standing on the left side of the bed, cup your fingers around the client's shoulder and hip and roll him or her 45 degrees toward you. Control the client's head, neck, and legs during the turn, moving the client's entire body as a unit.	7. Pulling requires less work than pushing. Moving the client's body as a unit maintains spinal alignment.
8. Position the client's head and neck, making certain that the client's airway is not obstructed. A small pillow may be used to support the head.	8. Ensures that the client's airway is open and he or she is comfortable.
9. Make sure the client's hips and shoulders are aligned and his or her spine is parallel with the mattress.	9. Maintains the client's good body alignment and prevents strain on his or her body structures.
10. Place the client's lower arm behind him or her, with the shoulder retracted and hyperextended.	10. Prevents a pressure injury to the soft tissues of the arm and alteration in circulation or innervation.
11. Cover the client as needed.	11. Provides comfort and privacy.
12. Wash your hands.	12. Decreases the transmission of microorganisms.
13. Record the procedure.	13. Communicates to the other members of the health care team and contributes to the legal record by documenting the care given to the client.
14. Assess the client's comfort and physical condition while he or she is in this position.	14. Provides updated information for planning client care. Respirations may be compromised in this position.
15. If the client is to be left alone, lower the bed and raise the side rails.	15. Provides client safety.

Example of Documentation

DATE	TIME	NOTES
4/8/93	1000	Client placed in Sims' position for rectal examination. No respiratory distress noted.
		H. White, RN

Teaching Tips

The purpose of the Sims position and the procedure for assuming it should be explained to the client or the caregiver, or both. Frequent position changes and the necessity for the client's body to be positioned in good alignment should be emphasized so complications can be avoided.

Home Care Variations

The client can be placed in this position in the home setting using the same technique.

SKILL 7–11 MOVING THE CLIENT TO THE TRENDELENBURG POSITION

Clinical Situations in Which You May Encounter This Skill

In the Trendelenburg position (Fig. 7–9), the client lies supine in bed with his or her head lowered and the legs raised on an incline plane. This position is used for postural drainage, to assist venous return from lower extremities, especially those with decreased peripheral perfusion, or in abdominal operations in which upward displacement of the abdominal organs is needed.

The Trendelenburg position is contraindicated in shock because it (1) allows abdominal organs to place pressure against the diaphragm, resulting in decreased respiratory excursion; (2) may increase intracranial pressure if a head injury is present; (3) may result in myocardial ischemia due to decreased filling of coronary arteries; and (4) may impair cerebral blood flow by stimulating aortic and carotid sinus reflexes.

The preferred position for shock is supine with legs elevated 20 degrees.

Anticipated Responses

▼ The client's clinical condition is improved when he or she is placed in this position.
▼ The person's abdominal organs are displaced in the direction needed.
▼ If the position is used for pulmonary toilet, the client produces sputum.

Adverse Responses

▼ The client's clinical condition does not improve or it deteriorates.
▼ The person's abdominal organs are not displaced in the direction needed.
▼ The client does not produce sputum and respiratory efforts become impaired.

Materials List

Gather these materials before beginning the skill:

▼ Bed that can be positioned either manually or electrically, or shock blocks
▼ Sheet

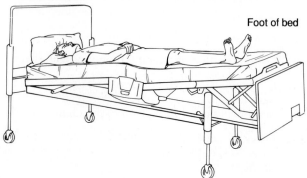

Head of bed

Foot of bed

▼ **FIGURE 7–9.** Trendelenburg's position.

▼ *ACTION*	▼ *RATIONALE*
1. Review the client's record to determine the basis for the position.	1. Helps you to plan care.
2. Ask the client to lie down on his or her back. If the client is unable to cooperate, you should position the client on his or her back. Use proper body mechanics.	2. Promotes the client's proper body alignment. Proper body mechanics help to prevent injury to you.
3. Elevate the lower portion of the bed 45 degrees and raise the head of the bed while maintaining the client's spine and the bed frame in a straight line. This may be done by using the controls on the bed, or by placing shock blocks under the foot of the bed. Make sure the bed is secure on the blocks. A small pillow may be placed between the client's head and the head of the bed, if a headboard is present.	3. Increases the blood flow to the client's brain and other vital, central organs. Allows for displacement of the person's abdominal organs toward the head. Provides for client safety. Provides comfort.

> **NOTE:** This position is usually contraindicated for clients with head injuries, some chest injuries, and some respiratory conditions. Each case should be assessed individually.
> The Trendelenburg position increases intracranial pressure and may cause more bleeding from above-waist injuries. Since abdominal organs move up against the diaphragm, respiratory difficulties may occur.

4. Cover the client with a sheet.	4. Provides comfort and protects the client's modesty.
5. Wash your hands.	5. Decreases the transmission of microorganisms.
6. Record the procedure.	6. Communicates to the other members of the health care team and contributes to the legal record by documenting the care given to the client.
7. Assess the client's condition frequently. The client may need to be repositioned occasionally.	7. Provides updated information on which to base care. Because of the client's position and gravity, the client may slip upward toward the head of the bed.
8. If the client is to be left alone, raise the side rails and place the call light within his or her reach.	8. Provides safety.

Example of Documentation

DATE	TIME	NOTES
6/16/93	1450	Client states "I feel like I have stuff down there I need to cough up." RR = 20, color pink, no respiratory distress. Ronchi auscultated over right anterior lung fields. Patient placed in Trendelenburg position for 10 minutes. Tolerated well. Client coughing up small amounts of yellow mucus. States "feels like it's moving up now."
		H. White, RN

Teaching Tips

The purpose of the Trendelenburg position and the procedure for placing the client in this position should be explained to the client or the client's family, or both. Explain that the client will be assessed frequently while he or she is in this position.

Home Care Variations

This position usually is not used in the home setting.

SKILL 7–12   MOVING THE CLIENT TO THE REVERSE TRENDELENBURG POSITION

Clinical Situations in Which You May Encounter This Skill

In the reverse Trendelenburg position (Fig. 7–10), the client lies in a supine position in a bed with the head of the bed elevated and the foot of the bed lowered and on an incline plane. The client who must have his or her spine remain straight and unbent, yet needs the upper body elevated, may be placed in the reverse Trendelenburg position. An example is a client who has been placed in cervical traction and needs to have arterial circulation promoted to the lower extremities.

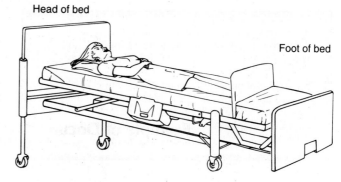

Head of bed

Foot of bed

▼ **FIGURE 7–10.** Reverse Trendelenburg's position.

Anticipated Responses

▼ The client's body is in correct alignment and the upper body is elevated appropriately.
▼ The client is comfortable.

Adverse Responses

▼ The client's body is out of correct alignment and the upper body is not elevated.
▼ The client has slipped to the lower portion of the bed.
▼ The client is uncomfortable.

Materials List

Gather these materials before beginning the skill:

▼ Bed that can be positioned either manually or electrically, or shock blocks
▼ Footboard
▼ Pillow(s)
▼ Sheet

▼ *ACTION*

1. Review the client's record to determine the basis for the position or any contraindications for this position.

2. Ask the client to lie down on his or her back. If the client is unable to cooperate, you should position the client on his or her back. Use proper body mechanics. The person should be rolled as a unit, especially if cervical injuries are suspected.

▼ *RATIONALE*

1. Helps you to plan the client's care.

2. Promotes proper body alignment. Proper body mechanics prevent injury to you. Protects the client's spine from injury.

▼ *A C T I O N*

▼ *R A T I O N A L E*

3. Raise the upper portion of the bed 30 degrees and lower the foot of the bed while maintaining the client's spine and the bed's frame in a straight line. At times the two upper legs of the bed may be raised by placing them on "shock" blocks. Be sure the legs of the bed are secure.

3. Puts the client in the correct position. Provides safety.

4. Place a footboard at the end of the bed and, if appropriate, position the client's feet against it.

4. Keeps the client at the head of the bed. Helps to prevent footdrop.

5. If not contraindicated, place a small pillow under the client's head.

5. Provides comfort.

6. Cover the client with a sheet.

6. Provides comfort. Protects the person's modesty.

7. Wash your hands.

7. Decreases the transmission of microorganisms.

8. Record the procedure.

8. Communicates to the other members of the health care team and contributes to the legal record by documenting the care given to the client.

9. Assess the client's condition frequently and provide appropriate support as needed. The client may need to be repositioned occasionally.

9. Provides updated information on which to base care. Because of the client's position and gravity, the client may slip downward toward the foot of the bed.

Example of Documentation

DATE	TIME	NOTES
5/24/93	1400	Client placed in reverse Trendelenburg's position. Body in correct alignment. Resting comfortably.
		H. White, RN

Teaching Tips

The purpose of the reverse Trendelenburg position and the procedure for assuming this position should be explained to the client or caregiver, or both. The client should be told to notify you if he or she slips too far down in the bed.

Home Care Variations

This position can be used in the home using the same procedure.

SKILL 7–13   MOVING THE CLIENT TO THE FOWLER POSITION

Clinical Situations in Which You May Encounter This Skill

There are actually three Fowler's, or sitting positions. In the low Fowler position (Fig. 7–11*A*), the client is supine in the bed with the head of the bed raised 30 degrees. This position is frequently used for clients with cardiac or respiratory conditions. The low Fowler position also is used during bed rest for relaxing and socializing. In the Fowler (Fig. 7–11*B*), or sitting position, the client is supine in the bed with the head of the bed raised 45 degrees. During bed rest, this position may be used to facilitate breathing and drainage and to promote client comfort. The Fowler position also is used for eating, drinking, and socializing while the client is on restricted bed rest. In the high Fowler position (Fig. 7–11*C*), the client is supine in the bed with the head of the bed raised 90 degrees. This position is used for clients who have had thoracic operations or have severe respiratory conditions. The high Fowler position also may be used in general position changes for comfort.

Problems that may arise if a client is left too long in the Fowler position are: footdrop; external rotation of the hips; and pressure sores, especially on the heels and sacrum. Clients with back problems may find this position uncomfortable even for a short period of time. Use of pillows that are too thick may cause cervical flexion contractures.

Anticipated Responses

▼ The client is comfortable and respiratory effort is not compromised.

Adverse Responses

▼ The client is uncomfortable.
▼ The client's respiratory effort is compromised.

Materials List

Gather these materials before beginning the skill:

▼ Bed that can be positioned either manually or electrically
▼ Several pillows
▼ Sheet and other covers as needed
▼ Footboard

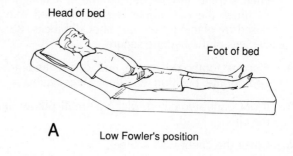

A   Low Fowler's position

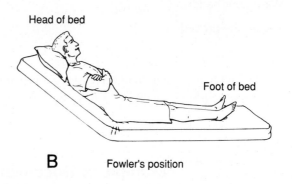

B   Fowler's position

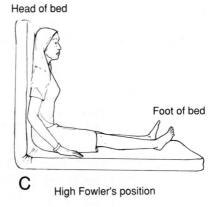

C   High Fowler's position

▼ **FIGURE 7–11.** The three Fowler's positions.

▼ *ACTION*	▼ *RATIONALE*
1. Review the client's chart to ascertain any medical reason that the client might not be allowed to assume the Fowler position.	**1.** Some medical conditions (e.g., if the client has had a back operation or spinal cord injury) may contraindicate this position.
2. Ask the client to lie down on his or her back in the middle of the bed. Provide assistance as needed.	**2.** Promotes the client's proper body alignment.
3. Raise bed to working height. Assist the client to the head of the bed. Use proper body mechanics. Obtain help if needed.	**3.** Raising bed provides proper body mechanics. Prevents the client from assuming an abnormal position when the head of the bed is raised. Promotes comfort. Assistance with the procedure prevents muscle strain and related injuries to you.
4. Use the bed control to raise the head of the bed to the proper angle (30–90 degrees).	**4.** Facilitates breathing and drainage and allows the client more interaction with the environment.
5. Place a small pillow behind the client's head and under each of his or her arms. The client's fingertips should extend over the edge of the pillow.	**5.** Provides comfort and prevents the client from pulling his or her shoulders into poor alignment. Maintains normal arching of the client's hand.
6. Use a footboard to keep the client's ankles flexed at 90 degrees.	**6.** Prevents plantar flexion.
7. Place covers over the client, as appropriate. Lower bed to lowest position.	**7.** Provides comfort and safety.
8. Wash your hands.	**8.** Decreases the transmission of microorganisms.
9. Record the procedure.	**9.** Communicates to the other members of the health care team and contributes to the legal record by documenting the care given to the client.
10. Check the body alignment and comfort of the client. Alternate the client's position so that his or her hips are not always in a flexed position. Observe the client's heels, sacrum, and other areas of the skin for pressure sores, and check for cervical flexion.	**10.** Provides you with useful information for the client's optimal wellness. In the Fowler position, the client's hips are flexed, and alternate positions should be used to prevent flexion contractures.

Example of Documentation

DATE	*TIME*	*NOTES*
6/24/93	1030	Client in Fowler's position. States he is comfortable and breathing easily. RR = 18. Skin color pink. No accessory muscle use noted.
		H. White, RN

Teaching Tips

The purpose of the Fowler position should be explained to the client or caregiver, or both. Emphasize that positions need to be alternated to prevent complications.

Home Care Variations

For clients who are homebound with family members caring for them, the purchase or rental of a hospital bed might be worthwhile to ease the client's position changes. If circumstances are not conducive to such a purchase, pillows may be used or a back wedge may be constructed with plywood and foam padding. Also, a straight-back or recliner chair may be useful. Clients with respiratory problems frequently sleep in recliner chairs in order to facilitate their nocturnal breathing.

SKILL 7–14   ASSISTING THE CLIENT WITH AMBULATION

Clinical Situations in Which You May Encounter This Skill

The client who has been confined to bed or who is weak may need assistance with ambulation. If the client is unsteady, a second nurse should assist. The client may complain of dizziness or faintness. If this happens, help the client to sit down or return to bed.

Anticipated Responses

▼ The client is able to ambulate without injury.
▼ The client does not complain of dizziness or faintness.

Adverse Responses

▼ The client complains of dizziness or faintness.

Materials List

Gather these materials before beginning the skill:

▼ Slippers
▼ Housecoat
▼ Ambulation (gait) belt (optional)

▼ ACTION

1. Check the client's medical diagnosis and any other medical problems.

2. Ask the client how long ago he or she last walked and how far.

3. Clear the path of any obstacles.

4. Lock the wheels of the bed.

5. Help the client to sit on the side of the bed (see Skill 7–2).

6. Lower the client's bed to the lowest position.

7. Help the client to put on slippers and a housecoat.

8. Apply an ambulation (gait) belt if needed.

▼ RATIONALE

1. May assist you in determining any problems that may be encountered.

2. Helps you to determine how far the client may be able to walk.

3. Obstacles present a safety hazard to the client.

4. Prevents the bed from rolling when the client is moved.

5. Helps the client to overcome any dizziness before standing.

6. Ensures the client's safety.

7. Slippers protect the client's feet. The shoes should have nonslip soles.

8. Helps you support the client.

▼ *ACTION* | ▼ *RATIONALE*

9. Help the client to stand. Walk slightly behind and to the side of the client. Support the client with one of your hands under the client's axilla and the other hand around his or her waist (Fig. 7–12), or grasping ambulation belt. If the client has weakness on one side, you should support that side.

9. Helps you control the client's lateral, backward, and forward movements. Provides support and safety for weakened side.

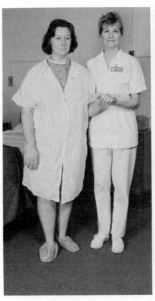
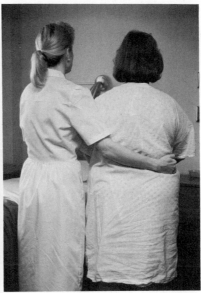

▼ **FIGURE 7–12.** Assisting client to walk.

10. After the walk is completed, help the client to return to bed.

10. The client may be tired and may need your assistance.

11. Wash your hands.

11. Decreases the transmission of microorganisms.

12. Assess how well the client tolerated the walk and whether any dizziness was experienced.

12. These data are necessary for charting whether the client experienced any problems.

13. Record the procedure.

13. Communicates to the other members of the health care team and contributes to the legal record by documenting the care given to the client.

Example of Documentation

DATE	TIME	NOTES
11/8/93	0900	Mrs. M. walked the length of the hall one time. No complaints of dizziness.
		T. Smith, RN

Teaching Tips

The procedure should be explained and demonstrated to the client's family. The family should inspect the home for any obstacles such as throw rugs or small articles that may cause the person to trip. The client should be encouraged to wear street shoes with nonslip soles for support.

Home Care Variations

The same procedure can be used at home to assist the client in walking.

SKILL 7-15   ASSISTING THE CLIENT WITH THE USE OF A CANE

Clinical Situations in Which You May Encounter This Skill

Clients who have sustained an injury to one side of the body, hemiparesis, or hemiplegia may need the assistance of a cane. Canes are used for balance and support. They are made of either aluminum or wood. Aluminum canes can be adjusted. Wood canes are made in various sizes. Canes have a rubber tip on all points that touch the floor. The cane handle should be even with the client's greater trochanter. There should be 25 to 30 degrees of flexion at the client's elbow.

There are three types of canes (Fig. 7-13): the standard cane, the quad cane, and the T-handle cane. The standard cane has a straight shaft with a hooked handle. The quad cane has four points and is broad-based. The T-handle has a bent shaft and a straight handle.

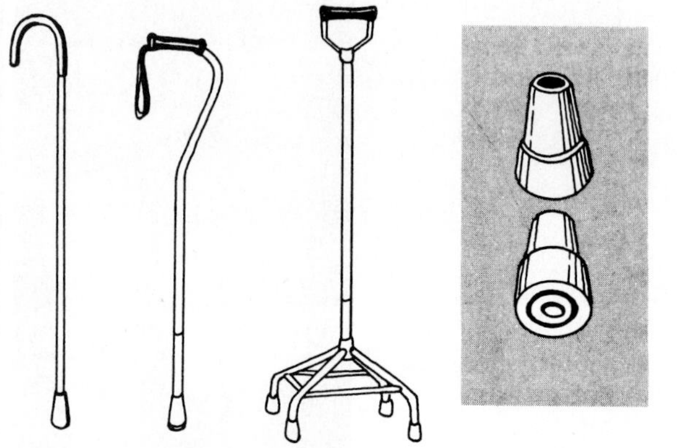

| A | B | C | D |
| Standard cane | T-handle cane | Quad cane | Rubber cane tips |

▼ FIGURE 7–13. (A) Standard cane. (B) T-handle cane. (C) Quad cane. (D) Rubber tips provide traction.

Anticipated Responses

▼ The client learns to use the cane to ambulate.

Adverse Responses

▼ The client has difficulty or is unable to learn to ambulate with the cane correctly.
▼ The client experiences instability and/or falls.

Materials List

Gather these materials before beginning the skill:

▼ Cane
▼ Walking shoes with nonslip soles

▼ ACTION	▼ RATIONALE
1. Assess the client's readiness to learn to use the cane.	1. The client's ability to learn is affected by the readiness to learn.
2. Assess the client's knowledge of how to use a cane.	2. You should individualize your teaching based on the client's knowledge.
3. Explain to the client the following points about walking with a cane: a. The cane should be used on the unaffected side. b. The cane should be held close to the body. c. The rubber tip should be inspected daily for worn places. d. The cane and the affected side should work together.	3. a. Shifts the client's weight away from the affected side. b. Prevents the client from leaning. c. Worn places could cause the client to slip and fall. d. The cane helps to support the affected side as it moves forward. It also helps the client to maintain balance.

▼ ACTION	▼ RATIONALE
4. Help the client to put on his or her shoes and stand to measure the cane for correct height.	**4.** A cane of the incorrect height will not allow the client's center of gravity to go through his or her base of support.
5. Explain and demonstrate the correct cane-walking gait. Move the cane forward, then move the affected side forward parallel to the cane. Next, the unaffected leg should move forward.	**5.** A demonstration helps to reinforce the explanation.
6. Help the client to practice.	**6.** Reinforces teaching.
7. Help the client to return to bed.	**7.** The client may be tired and may need your assistance.
8. Wash your hands.	**8.** Decreases the transmission of microorganisms.
9. Assess the client's ability to use the cane.	**9.** These data are necessary for charting and for further client education.
10. Record the procedure. Note the client's balance, ability to walk with a cane, and the distance walked.	**10.** Communicates to the other members of the health care team and contributes to the legal record by documenting the care given to the client.

Example of Documentation

DATE	TIME	NOTES
11/8/93	1000	Taught the proper use of a cane. The proper technique was demonstrated. Mr. R. walked 10 feet with his standard cane. No problems with balance.
		E. Shaw, RN

Teaching Tips

The procedure should be explained to the client and the client's family. The client should be encouraged to wear street shoes at all times for support. The family should assess the house for any objects that may be a hazard for the client.

Home Care Variations

The same technique can be used for walking with a cane in the home.

SKILL 7–16   ASSISTING THE CLIENT WITH THE USE OF CRUTCHES

Clinical Situations in Which You May Encounter This Skill

Crutch walking may be indicated for clients with arthritis, a lack of coordination, muscle weakness, orthopedic problems, or paraplegia. It also may be indicated for clients who have not recieved a prosthesis after amputation. There are three types of crutches (Fig. 7–14): the axillary crutch, the Lofstrand crutch, and the elbow extension (Canadian) crutch. Selection of the specific type is based on the client's needs, physical condition, arm strength, and balance. The crutches are measured to fit the client by measuring the client in the supine position from the anterior axillary fold and adding 2 inches. When the client is standing, there should be 2 to 3 finger breadths between his or her axilla and the top of the crutch. The handgrip is positioned to allow 25 to 30 degrees of flexion at the elbow.

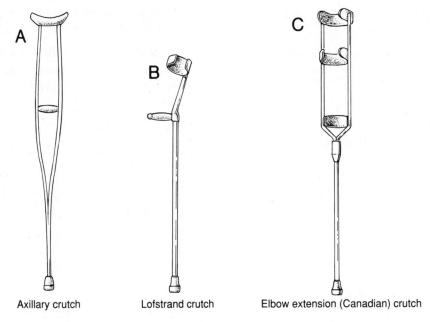

Axillary crutch   Lofstrand crutch   Elbow extension (Canadian) crutch

▼ FIGURE 7–14.

Several gait patterns exist for crutch walking. The four-point gait (Fig. 7–15) is used for clients with muscle weakness or poor balance who can bear weight on both legs. The gait is safe but slow. The client always has three points in contact with the floor. Instruct the client to move the crutches and his or her feet in the following manner:

1. Move the right crutch forward.
2. Move the left foot forward.
3. Move the left crutch forward.
4. Move the right foot forward.

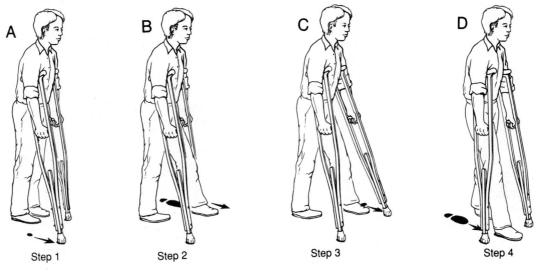

Step 1 Step 2 Step 3 Step 4

▼ **FIGURE 7–15.** Four-point gait.

The two-point gait (Fig. 7–16) is faster than the four-point gait and requires more balance. It is used when weight bearing is allowed on both feet. Only two points are in contact with the floor. The two-point gait closely resembles normal walking. Instruct the client to move the crutches and his or her feet in the following sequence:

1. Advance the right crutch and the left foot forward, and
2. Advance the right foot and left crutch forward.

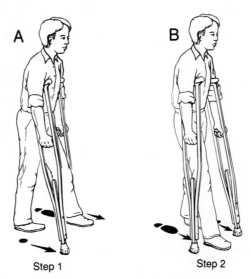

Step 1 Step 2

▼ **FIGURE 7–16.** Two-point gait.

A three-point gait (Fig. 7–17), or orthopedic gait, is used for amputees and orthopedic clients. It requires that the client have normal use of one leg and both arms. Instruct the client to simultaneously move both crutches and the affected leg forward. Then the unaffected leg should move forward.

A swing-to gait (Fig. 7–18) is used for paraplegic client or clients with other central nervous system (CNS) disorders. The client must have good upper arm strength and his or her legs must be able to bear some weight in order to use this gait. Instruct the client to move both crutches forward and then swing both feet forward to the crutches.

The swing-through gait (Fig. 7–19) also may be used for paraplegic clients or clients with other CNS disorders. It offers less stability than the swing-to gait. Instruct the client to move both crutches forward and then swing both feet through and slightly forward of the crutches.

Anticipated Responses

▼ The client learns to use the crutches correctly with the proper gait.

Adverse Responses

▼ The client is unwilling or unable to learn to use the crutches.
▼ The client experiences instability and/or falls.

Materials List

Gather these materials before beginning the skill:

▼ Crutches
▼ Walking shoes with nonslip soles

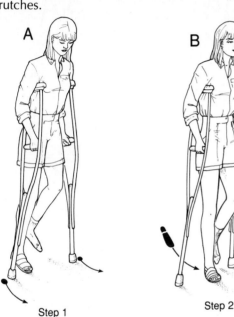

Step 1   Step 2

▼ **FIGURE 7–17.** Three-point gait.

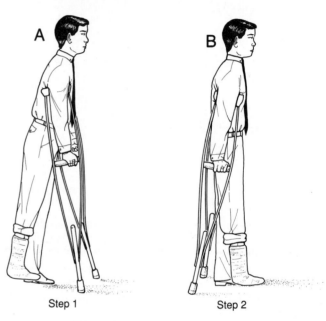

Step 1   Step 2

▼ **FIGURE 7–19.** Swing-through gait.

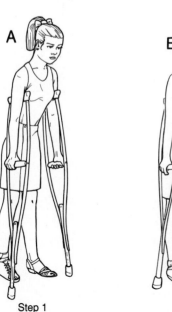

Step 1   Step 2

▼ **FIGURE 7–18.** Swing-to gait.

▼ _ACTION_

1. Assess the client's readiness to learn to use crutches.

2. Assess the client's knowledge of walking with crutches and the gait to be used.

3. If necessary, explain crutch walking to the client. The explanation should include the following:
   a. Bear the body weight on the hands and not on the axilla.
   b. Rubber tips should be inspected daily for worn places.
   c. The selected gait pattern.

   d. The method for going up and down stairs. To go up the stairs (Fig. 7–20), the client should move the unaffected leg up first. Then he or she should move the affected leg and crutches up. To go down the stairs (Fig. 7–21), the client should move the crutches and the affected leg down. Then he or she should move the unaffected leg down.

▼ _RATIONALE_

1. The client's ability to learn is affected by the readiness to learn.

2. You will need to individualize the teaching based on the client's knowledge.

3. The client will be more likely to be compliant if he or she understands the proper technique.
   a. If the axilla bears body weight, it can cause crutch paralysis.
   b. Worn places could cause the client to slip and fall.
   c. The client should understand that there are several different patterns and the client should understand the reason why he or she should use the particular pattern selected.
   d. The client should understand the correct technique for his or her own safety. Even a task as simple as stepping out of a door requires this knowledge.

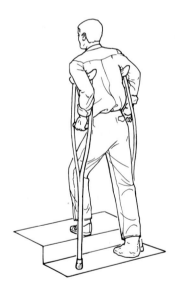

▼ **FIGURE 7–20.** Going up stairs.

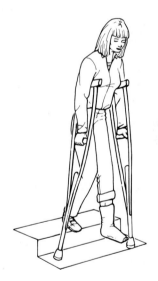

▼ **FIGURE 7–21.** Going down stairs.

▼ *ACTION*   ▼ *RATIONALE*

e. To stand from a sitting position (Fig. 7–22): Place the crutches together on the affected side and hold them on the inside by the handgrips. Use the other hand to push down on the chair while straightening the strong leg.

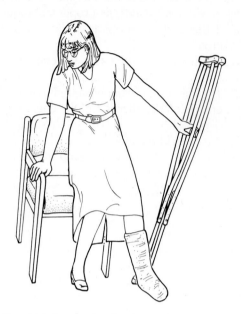

▼ **FIGURE 7–22.** Standing from a sitting position.

f. To sit: Reverse the above procedure.

4. Measure the crutches for the correct length.

5. Help the client to put on his or her shoes and stand.

6. Demonstrate the selected gait.

7. Help the client to practice.

8. Help the client to return to bed.

9. Wash your hands.

10. Assess the client's ability to use the crutches and to use the selected gait.

11. Record the procedure. Note the client's balance, ability to walk with crutches, and the distance walked.

4. Incorrectly fitted crutches will not allow the client's line of gravity to go through his or her base of support.

5. The client should have a wide base of support.

6. Helps to reinforce the explanations.

7. Reinforces the teaching.

8. The client may be tired and may need your assistance.

9. Decreases the transmission of microorganisms.

10. These data are necessary for charting and for further client education.

11. Communicates to the other members of the health care team and contributes to the legal record by documenting the care given to the client.

Example of Documentation

DATE	TIME	NOTES
11/8/93	1000	Crutch walking was explained and a demonstration of the three-point gait was provided. Mrs. M. walked 10 feet with the crutches. Going up and down steps should be explained tomorrow. No problem with balance.
		E. Reed, RN

Teaching Tips

Crutch walking and care of the crutches should be explained to the client and the client's family. The gait should be demonstrated for the client and the client should be allowed to practice. The family should assess the home for any obstacles. The client should be encouraged to wear street shoes for support.

Home Care Variations

The same gait is used in the home setting.

SKILL 7–17   ASSISTING THE CLIENT WITH THE USE OF A WALKER

Clinical Situations in Which You May Encounter This Skill

A walker provides more support than a cane or crutches. It is used when maximum support is required. Mobility is limited more with a walker than with a cane or crutches.

Anticipated Responses

▼ The client learns to use the walker correctly.

Adverse Responses

▼ The client is unable or unwilling to learn to use the walker.
▼ The client experiences instability and/or falls.

Materials List

Gather these materials before beginning the skills:

▼ Walker
▼ Walking shoes with nonslip soles

▼ ACTION	▼ RATIONALE
1. Assess the client's readiness to learn.	1. The client's ability to learn is affected by his or her readiness to learn.
2. Assess the client's knowledge about the use of the walker.	2. Teaching can be individualized based on the client's knowledge.

▼ *ACTION* _ _ _ _ _ _ _ _ _ _ _ _ _ _ _ _ ▼ *RATIONALE* _ _ _ _ _ _ _ _ _ _

3. If necessary, explain to the client how to use a walker (Fig 7–23). The explanation should include the following:
   a. Rubber tips should be inspected daily for worn places.
   b. Pick up the walker and move it forward and then walk into the walker one step at a time.

3. a. Worn places could cause the client to slip and fall.
   b. Helps the client to maintain a wide base of support.

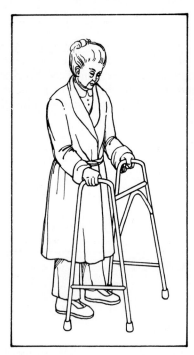

▼ **FIGURE 7–23.** Using a walker.

4. Help the client to put on his or her shoes and to stand to measure the walker for the correct length. In a standing position, there should be 25 to 30 degrees of flexion at the client's elbow.

4. A walker of an incorrect height will not allow the client's line of gravity to go through his or her base of support.

5. Demonstrate the correct walking technique.

5. Helps to reinforce the explanation.

6. Help the client to practice.

6. Reinforces the teaching.

7. Help the client to return to bed.

7. The client will be tired and will need your assistance.

8. Wash your hands.

8. Decreases the transmission of microorganisms.

9. Assess the client's ability to use the walker.

9. These data are necessary for charting and for further client education.

10. Record the procedure. Note the client's ability to walk with the walker and the distance walked.

10. Communicates to the other members of the health care team and contributes to the legal record by documenting the care given to the client.

Example of Documentation

DATE	TIME	NOTES
11/8/93	1030	Use of the walker was explained and a demonstration was provided. Mrs. T. walked 20 feet with the walker.
		S. Smith, RN

Teaching Tips

The purpose of a walker and care of a walker should be explained to the client and the client's family. The gait should be demonstrated for the client and the client should be allowed to practice. The family should assess the home for any obstacles. The client should be encouraged to wear street shoes for support.

Home Care Variations

The same technique is used for the walker at home.

References

Bolander, V. B. (1993). Meeting mobility needs. In V. Bolander (Ed.), *Basic nursing* (3rd ed.). Philadelphia: W. B. Saunders.

CHAPTER 8

Preventing Complications of Immobility

When a person loses mobility because of illness or injury, he or she is susceptible to many complications of immobility. Psychologic complications may include anger or depression because of the loss of independence. Physical complications may include pneumonia, urinary retention, pressure ulcers, and contractures.

You must be skillful in assessment techniques as well as nursing procedures to prevent these complications. Many devices can aid you in protecting the client from hazards such as skin breakdown and contractures. These devices include special beds, frames, mattresses, and other equipment.

OVERVIEW OF RELATED RESEARCH

Conine, T. A., et al. (1990) Costs and acceptability of two special overlays for the prevention of pressure sores. *Rehabilitation Nursing,* 15, 133–137.

One hundred and eighty-seven clients were assigned to use either an alternating air mattress or a silicone overlay for 3 months. Of these, 148 clients completed the trial. Costs were calculated for each overlay. The alternating air mattress was found to be 54% more costly per year than the silicone overlay. Factored into the annual costs were depreciation, maintenance, and operating and repair costs.

Forty-five primary nurses for the clients were interviewed and completed questionnaires regarding the acceptability of the two types of overlays. No significant differences were found in the nurses' views of the alternating air mattress and silicone overlay in relation to overall ease of client and overlay care, client complaints, or efficacy. Significantly more nurses recommended the silicone overlay for use at home. However, nurses reported significantly more problems with transfer positioning and linen displacement with the silicone overlay than with the alternating air mattress. Nurses were concerned about the necessity of frequent monitoring, cleaning, and repair of the alternating air mattress.

No differences were found between the two overlays in relation to client satisfaction. More clients found the silicone overlay to be more comfortable. However, more clients found odor buildup and instability to be a problem with the silicone overlay than with the alternating air mattress.

Counsell, C., et al. (1990). Interface skin pressures on four pressure-relieving devices. *Journal of Enterostomal Therapy,* 17, 150–153.

This study evaluated the effectiveness of four pressure-relieving devices (2-inch polyurethane foam, air mattress, and two air flotation low–air-loss beds) by measuring interface pressures in 15 healthy subjects who were selected according to their body builds. The two air flotation low–air-loss beds had the lowest mean interface pressures. Body build did not significantly influence the interface pressures. Of the pressure points measured (head, sacrum, heel, shoulder, and trochanter), the heel, head, and trochanter had the highest interface pressures.

Jacobs, M. S. (1989). Comparison of capillary blood flow using a regular hospital bed mattress, ROHO mattress, and Mediscus bed. *Rehabilitation Nursing,* 14, 270–272.

This was a pilot study that examined capillary blood flow in 9 clients with spinal cord injuries who did not have preexisting pressure sores. The subjects were positioned for 1 hour on a regular hospital bed mattress and for 4 hours each on a ROHO mattress and a Mediscus bed. Results indicated that pressure relief and improvement in capillary blood flow were comparable for the ROHO mattress and the Mediscus bed.

SKILL 8–1 ASSISTING WITH RANGE-OF-MOTION (ROM) EXERCISES

Clinical Situations in Which You May Encounter This Skill

Clients who have normal joints and are on bed rest need exercise to prevent musculoskeletal complications of inactivity such as contractures, ankylosis, osteoporosis, muscle atrophy, and weakness. In addition, range-of-motion (ROM) exercises stimulate circulation. These exercises are usually performed several times a day.

Clients may perform these exercises by themselves (active ROM exercises). If clients are unable to do this, you should assist with full ROM exercises at least once per day (passive ROM exercises). Often it is most time efficient to do this during the morning bath; however, other times are also acceptable. At times the client may assist you with the performance of some parts or all of the exercises (assisted ROM exercises).

As with any exercise, ascertain that the exercise is appropriate for the client's physical condition. Increased circulation and increased mobility of joints occur with both active and passive ROM; however, increases in respiratory and cardiac functioning and increased muscle mass, tone, and strength occur only with active exercise.

Anticipated Responses

▼ The client experiences full ROM in all joint and muscle groups. If the client did not have full ROM prior to starting the exercises, then no deterioration of motion should be seen and improvement of motion may occur. The client's pre–bed rest energy level should be maintained or improved.

Adverse Responses

▼ The client experiences pain or resistance.
▼ There is deterioration in motion.
▼ Energy level decreases.

Materials List

Gather these materials before beginning the skill:

▼ Bath blanket or sheet

Passive Range-of-Motion Exercises: General Guidelines

▼ _ACTION_	▼ _RATIONALE_
a. Unless contraindicated, most of the exercises are performed while the client is in a supine position. Some exercises are performed while the client is in the prone or Fowler's position.	a. Provides for proper body alignment.
b. Conduct the exercises in a cephalocaudal direction first on one side of the client's body and then on the other. Then turn the client to a prone position and conduct the exercises in a cephalocaudal direction. Finally, place the client in Fowler's position.	b. Allows for the most efficient use of energy.
c. Exercises should be performed with smooth, slow, even movements. Remember to support the client's body part above and below the involved joint.	c. Promotes efficiency of movement and safety.
d. The client should perform each exercise 5 to 10 times. Unless otherwise ordered, ROM exercises should be done twice a day.	d. Provides symmetry and proper exercise.
e. When the client feels discomfort or resistance to passive movement is experienced, stop that exercise.	e. If the joint is moved past the point of pain or resistance, injury can occur.
f. At the completion of each ROM exercise, return the client's body part to its proper anatomic position.	f. Promotes proper body alignment.
g. Minimize friction between the client's skin and the linens as much as possible.	g. Reduces skin shearing.
h. Observe the client for fatigue and respiratory and cardiac compromise.	h. If symptoms of these conditions occur, the exercises should be stopped and the client should be assessed.
i. Wear gloves if contamination with body fluids is possible.	i. Prevents transmission of microorganisms.
1. Review the client's chart and assess the client for contraindications to the procedure.	1. ROM exercises may be contraindicated in conditions such as arthritis, acute cardiac disease, dislocated joints, and fractures.
2. Raise the bed to a comfortable working level and lower the side rail on the working side.	2. Promotes proper body mechanics.
3. Assess vital signs.	3. Provides baseline data.
4. Place the client in a supine position.	4. Allows for exercises of the front of the client's body.
5. Remove the pillow from under the client's head.	5. Allows for full ROM for the neck and shoulders.
6. Cover the client with a bath blanket and fold the top covers to the end of the bed.	6. Protects the client's modesty and provides warmth.
7. Proceed in the following order.	

▼ *A C T I O N* _ ▼ *R A T I O N A L E* _ _ _ _ _ _ _ _ _ _ _ _

Supine Position Exercises
Neck

8. Begin with neck ROM exercises.

    a. *Flexion* (Fig. 8–1): Bring the client's head forward until the chin is as close to the chest as possible.

    b. *Extension* (Fig. 8–2): Bring the client's head back to an upright position.

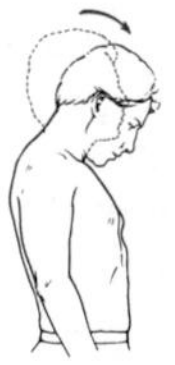

▼ **FIGURE 8–1.** Flexion. 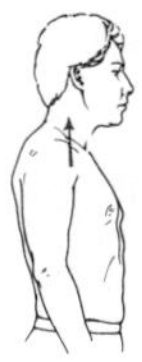   ▼ **FIGURE 8–2.** Extension.

    c. *Lateral flexion* (Fig. 8–3): Bring the person's right ear down to touch the right shoulder. Repeat on the left side.

    d. *Rotation* (Fig. 8–4): Turn the person's head to the right side. Attempt to have the person's chin end up over the shoulder. Repeat on the left side.

 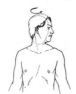

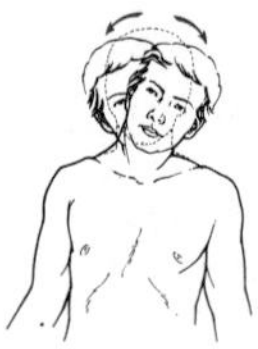

▼ **FIGURE 8–3.** Lateral flexion.   ▼ **FIGURE 8–4.** Rotation.

Shoulder

9. Continue with shoulder ROM exercises.

    a. *Flexion* (Fig. 8–5): While supporting the client's elbow, bring his or her arm straight up from the side to reach over the head (approximately 180 degrees).

    b. *Extension* (Fig. 8–6): Bring the client's arm back down to the side.

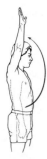 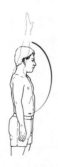

▼ **FIGURE 8–5.** Flexion.   ▼ **FIGURE 8–6.** Extension.

8. Neck ROM exercises prevent flexion contractures of the neck.

9. ROM exercises assist in keeping the shoulder mobile.

▼ *A C T I O N*   ▼ *R A T I O N A L E*

c. *Abduction* (Fig. 8–7): Bring the person's arm away from his or her body. Make an approximate 110-degree angle.

d. *Adduction* (Fig. 8–8): Bring the client's arm back to the side of his or her body.

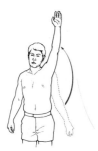 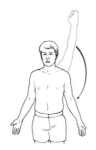

▼ **FIGURE 8–7.** Abduction.   ▼ **FIGURE 8–8.** Adduction.

e. *Horizontal adduction* (Fig. 8–9): Bring the client's arms straight out to the side. Then move them straight out in front of the client and across his or her chest to the opposite side.

f. *Horizontal abduction* (Fig. 8–10): Bring the person's arms back to the beginning position—straight out to the side.

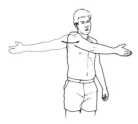 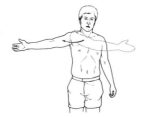

▼ **FIGURE 8–9.**
Horizontal adduction.   ▼ **FIGURE 8–10.**
Horizontal abduction.

g. *External rotation* (Fig. 8–11): Position the client's arm at the side of his or her body with the elbow bent to form a 45-degree angle between the upper and lower arm. Bring the arm forward and turn the palm upward as the arm is straightened.

h. *Internal rotation* (Fig. 8–12): Position the person's arm at the same starting position as above. Bring the arm back to the side of the body with the palm facing toward the bed.

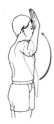 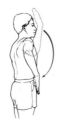

▼ **FIGURE 8–11.**
External rotation.   ▼ **FIGURE 8–12.**
Internal rotation.

▼ *ACTION*   ▼ *RATIONALE*

    i. *Circumduction* (Fig. 8–13): While supporting the client's elbow, move his or her shoulder in as wide a circle as possible.

    j. *Elevation* (Fig. 8–14): If possible, ask the client to shrug.

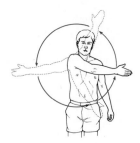 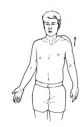

▼ **FIGURE 8–13.** Circumduction.   ▼ **FIGURE 8–14.** Elevation.

    k. *Depression* (Fig. 8–15): If possible, ask the client to stretch his or her neck upward while pushing the shoulders down.

    l. *Protraction* (Fig. 8–16): Position the client's arm straight out in front of him or her. Then stretch the arm farther forward from the shoulder.

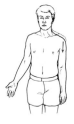 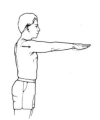

▼ **FIGURE 8–15.** Depression.   ▼ **FIGURE 8–16.** Protraction.

Elbow

10. Continue with elbow ROM exercises.

    a. *Flexion* (Fig. 8–17): While the client's upper arm remains at his or her side, bend the elbow so that the fingers touch the shoulder.

    b. *Extension* (Fig. 8–18): Straighten the person's elbow from a flexed position and return it to the original position.

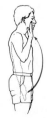 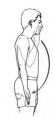

▼ **FIGURE 8–17.** Flexion.   ▼ **FIGURE 8–18.** Extension.

10. Prevents flexion or extension contractures of the elbow. Performance of activities of daily living is limited by flexion and extension contractures.

▼ *ACTION* — — — — — — — — ▼ *RATIONALE* — — — — — —

Wrist and Forearm

11. Continue with wrist and forearm ROM exercises.

    a. *Flexion* (Fig. 8–19): Bend the client's wrist so that the palm of his or her hand forms a 90-degree angle with the lower arm.

    b. *Extension* (Fig. 8–20): Straighten the person's wrist so that his or her arm and hand form a straight line.

11. Flexion and extension contractures can alter a client's grasp.

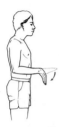

▼ **FIGURE 8–19.** Flexion.

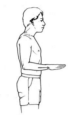

▼ **FIGURE 8–20.** Extension.

    c. *Hyperextension* (Fig. 8–21): Bend the person's wrist so that the back of the hand forms a 90-degree angle with the lower arm.

    d. *Abduction (ulnar deviation)* (Fig. 8–22): Bend the person's wrist sideways so that the little finger bends toward the ulnar side of the forearm. A deviation of a couple of inches is sufficient.

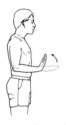

▼ **FIGURE 8–21.** Hyperextension.

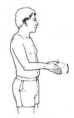

▼ **FIGURE 8–22.** Abduction (ulnar deviation).

    e. *Adduction (radial deviation)* (Fig. 8–23): Keeping the client's fingers and thumb together, bend the wrist sideways so that the thumb bends toward the radial side of the forearm. A deviation of approximately 1 inch is sufficient.

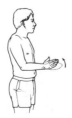

▼ **FIGURE 8–23.** Adduction (radial deviation).

▼ *ACTION* _ _ _ _ _ _ _ _ _ _ _ _ _ _ _ _ ▼ *RATIONALE* _ _ _ _ _ _ _ _ _ _ _ _ _

f. *Supination* (Fig. 8–24): While supporting the client's forearm, turn his or her wrist so that the palm faces upward.

g. *Pronation* (Fig. 8–25): While supporting the client's forearm, turn his or her wrist so that the palm faces downward.

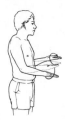 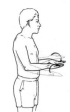

▼ **FIGURE 8–24.** Supination. ▼ **FIGURE 8–25.** Pronation.

Fingers and Thumb

12. Continue with ROM exercises of the fingers and thumb.

a. *Flexion* (Fig. 8–26): Bend all of the client's fingers inward so that a fist is made.

b. *Extension* (Fig. 8–27): Straighten all of the client's fingers so that a straight line is formed with the forearm, hand, and fingers.

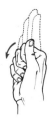 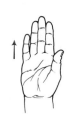

▼ **FIGURE 8–26.** Flexion. ▼ **FIGURE 8–27.** Extension.

c. *Hyperextension* (Fig. 8–28): Gently bend the person's fingers backward slightly.

d. *Abduction* (Fig. 8–29): After interlacing your fingers with the client's, gently spread the client's fingers apart.

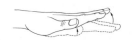

▼ **FIGURE 8–28.** Hyperextension.

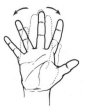

▼ **FIGURE 8–29.** Abduction.

12. Grasp and fine motor coordination can be altered by contractures of the fingers and thumb.

▼ *ACTION* _____   ▼ *RATIONALE* _____

e. *Adduction* (Fig. 8–30): While grasping the client's thumb and fingers in one hand, gently bring his or her fingers and thumb together.

f. *Thumb flexion* (Fig. 8–31): Have the person's thumb reach as far across the palm as possible.

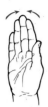 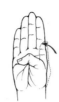

▼ **FIGURE 8–30.** Adduction.   ▼ **FIGURE 8–31.** Thumb flexion.

g. *Opposition* (Fig. 8–32): One finger at a time, have the tips of each finger touch the tip of the thumb.

h. *Circumduction* (Fig. 8–33): Move the person's thumb in as wide a circle as possible, first in one direction and then the other.

 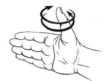

▼ **FIGURE 8–32.** Opposition.   ▼ **FIGURE 8–33.** Circumduction.

Hip and Knee

13. Continue with ROM exercises of the hip and knee.

   a. *Flexion* (Fig. 8–34): While supporting the client's heel and upper leg, flex his or her knee as the leg is lifted toward the body as much as possible.

   b. *Extension* (Fig. 8–35): Straighten the client's leg back to the original position.

13. Contractures of the hip and knee can alter the client's ability to ambulate and sit in a comfortable position.

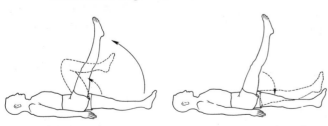

▼ **FIGURE 8–34.** Flexion.   ▼ **FIGURE 8–35.** Extension.

▼ *ACTION*   ▼ *RATIONALE*

c. *External rotation* (Fig. 8–36): Rotate the client's leg outward away from the center of his or her body.

d. *Internal rotation* (Fig. 8–37): Rotate the client's leg inward toward the center of his or her body.

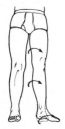   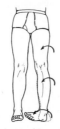

▼ **FIGURE 8–36.**   ▼ **FIGURE 8–37.**
External rotation.   Internal rotation.

e. *Abduction* (Fig. 8–38): Keeping the person's leg straight, move it away from the midline of his or her body.

f. *Adduction* (Fig. 8–39): Keeping the person's leg straight, move it toward the midline of his or her body.

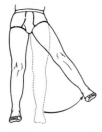   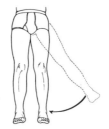

▼ **FIGURE 8–38.** Abduction.   ▼ **FIGURE 8–39.** Adduction.

g. *Circumduction* (Fig. 8–40): Keeping the person's leg straight, circle the leg in as big a semicircle as possible.

h. *Cross adduction* (Fig. 8–41): Move each of the client's legs across his or her body to the opposite side.

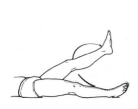   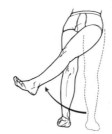

▼ **FIGURE 8–40.** Circumduction.   ▼ **FIGURE 8–41.** Cross adduction.

▼ _ACTION_ ▼ _RATIONALE_

Ankle and Foot

14. Continue with ROM exercises of the ankle and foot.

    a. *Dorsiflexion* (Fig. 8–42): Move the client's foot back toward his or her body.

    b. *Plantar flexion* (Fig. 8–43): Move the client's foot away from his or her body (point the toes).

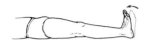   

▼ **FIGURE 8–42.** Dorsiflexion. 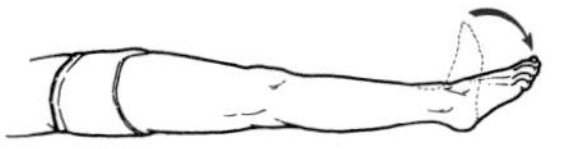   ▼ **FIGURE 8–43.** Plantar flexion.

    c. *Inversion* (Fig. 8–44): Move the sole of the person's foot toward the midline of his or her body.

    d. *Eversion* (Fig. 8–45): Move the sole of the person's foot away from the midline of his or her body.

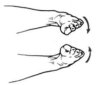   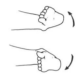

▼ **FIGURE 8–44.** Inversion.   ▼ **FIGURE 8–45.** Eversion.

Toes

15. Continue with ROM exercises of the toes.

    a. *Flexion* (Fig. 8–46): Bend the person's toes down toward the sole of his or her foot.

    b. *Hyperextension* (Fig. 8–47): Bend the person's toes back toward the top of his or her foot. Movement of 1 inch is sufficient.

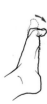   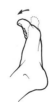

▼ **FIGURE 8–46.** Flexion.   ▼ **FIGURE 8–47.** Hyperextension.

14. Contractures of the ankle and foot can limit the client's ability to walk.

15. Contractures of the toes can interfere with walking.

▼ *A C T I O N*   ▼ *R A T I O N A L E*

c. *Abduction* (Fig. 8–48): After interlacing the client's toes with the fingers of one of your hands, spread the toes gently.

d. *Adduction* (Fig. 8–49): Grasping all of the client's toes in one hand, gently bring the toes together.

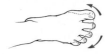   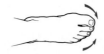

▼ **FIGURE 8–48.** Abduction.   ▼ **FIGURE 8–49.** Adduction.

Prone Position Exercises

Neck

16. Position the client in a prone position. Continue with ROM exercises of the neck.

   a. *Hyperextension* (Fig. 8–50): Gently bend the client's head backward so that the base of his or her skull almost touches the top of the back.

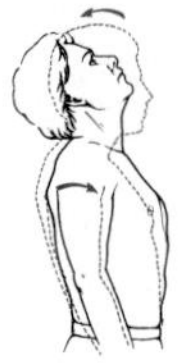

▼ **FIGURE 8–50.** Hyperextension.

16. ROM helps to prevent extension contractures of the neck.

Shoulder

17. Continue with ROM exercises of the shoulder.

   a. *Hyperextension* (Fig. 8–51): Keeping the client's arm straight, gently lift his or her arm upward from the side of his or her body.

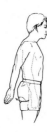

▼ **FIGURE 8–51.** Hyperextension.

17. ROM assists in maintaining the mobility of the shoulder.

▼ *A C T I O N* _____   ▼ *R A T I O N A L E* _____

Hip

18. Continue with ROM exercises of the hip.

   a. *Hyperextension* (Fig. 8–52): Keeping the client's leg straight, gently lift his or her leg upward.

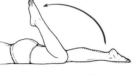

▼ **FIGURE 8–52.** Hyperextension.

Knees

19. *Flexion* (Fig. 8–53): Move the client's heels toward his or her buttocks; bend the leg at the knee.

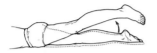

▼ **FIGURE 8–53.** Flexion.

Trunk

20. Position the client in a supine position and then raise the head of the bed so the client is in Fowler's position. With the client in the Fowler's position, continue with the following exercises.

   a. *Flexion* (Fig. 8–54): Support the client's head, neck, and torso. Gently bend the client forward.

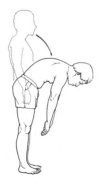

▼ **FIGURE 8–54.** Flexion.

18. Contractures of the hip interfere with sitting and walking.

▼ *ACTION*   ▼ *RATIONALE*

b. *Lateral flexion* (Fig. 8–55): While the client is upright, gently pull his or her waist toward you while pushing, his or her shoulders and neck away from you.

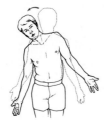

▼**FIGURE 8–55.** Lateral flexion.

c. *Rotation* (Fig. 8–56): Place the client's forearm that is farthest away from you across his or her waist. Place your hand that is closest to the client's head on the client's shoulder that is closest to you. Place your other hand behind the client's other shoulder and rotate the client toward your side of the bed. Return to the starting position.

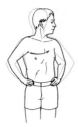

▼**FIGURE 8–56.** Rotation.

21. Position the client in a position of comfort. Raise the side rails.

21. Provides comfort.

22. Lower the bed to a low position.

22. Promotes safety.

23. Record the procedure and other relevant information.

23. Communicates the information to the other members of the health care team and contributes to the legal record by documenting the care given to the client.

24. Assess the client's comfort and physical condition, especially his or her respiratory and circulatory status, including vital signs.

24. Provides updated information for planning the client's care.

Example of Documentation

DATE	TIME	NOTES
10/31/93	1100	Full ROM exercises performed. Client tolerated procedure fairly well. States he is less tired than after the exercises yesterday. No decrease in function noted from previous times. BP = 132/78, HR = 88, RR = 22.
		S. Long, RN

Teaching Tips

The purpose of the exercises should be explained to the client or the client's family, or both. The client should be encouraged to participate as much as possible. If the exercises are to be performed in the client's home, they should be demonstrated to the family and time should be allowed for the family to do a return demonstration.

Home Care Variations

Clients who are bedridden at home need to have ROM exercises performed twice daily. These exercises should be taught to caretakers of homebound clients. Care must be taken not to overstress joints and muscles during exercise.

SKILL 8–2   ASSISTING WITH ANTIEMBOLIC HOSE

Clinical Situations in Which You May Encounter This Skill

Antiembolic hose are useful in the treatment of clients who have vascular disorders such as thrombophlebitis, varicose veins, or other conditions that may lead to impaired circulation in the legs. They also are used to prevent thrombophlebitis of the legs after surgery or in clients who are confined to bed.

The hose are available in different lengths (toes-to-knee or toes-to-thigh) and sizes (small, medium, and large). The stockings should be applied before the client's legs fill with blood, as they do when the client stands or dangles his or her legs over the side of the bed.

Each leg should be inspected for color, temperature, intact skin, infection, ulcers, or absence of (or unequal) peripheral pulses below the femoral artery before the hose are applied for the first time. If there are positive findings, the physician should be notified.

The hose should be removed and reapplied twice a day (usually at bathtime and once later in the day). If the stockings are needed for a prolonged period, it is helpful to have two pairs so they can be alternated.

The condition of the client's skin should be assessed and the skin should be cleansed before reapplying the hose. Heel ulcerations are a side effect of antiembolic stockings when they are used for some clients with vascular diseases such as diabetes mellitus, peripheral vascular disease, peripheral neuropathy, and severe arteriosclerosis.

Anticipated Responses

▼ The client's venous return is enhanced and the development of thrombophlebitis is suppressed.
▼ The client's legs have popliteal, posterior tibial, and dorsalis pedis pulses while the stockings are on.
▼ The color of the client's extremities indicates good circulation (specific color is race-dependent); the temperature is warm; and the skin is intact with no swelling or edema noted.

Adverse Responses

▼ The client's venous return is compromised and thrombophlebitis develops.
▼ The condition of the client's extremities deteriorates. For example, there is a decrease in the quality of the popliteal, posterior tibial, and dorsalis pedis pulses; the color of the extremities becomes lighter or more cyanotic; the skin temperature is cooler; the skin is not intact; or there is increased swelling or edema.

Materials List

Gather these materials before beginning the skill:

▼ Package of antiembolic stockings
▼ Talc or cornstarch (if client is not allergic)
▼ Tape measure

▼ *ACTION* ▼ *RATIONALE*

1. Ascertain the reason for the order for antiembolic hose.

2. Review the physician's order for the type of stocking needed (knee or thigh).

3. Check the diagnosis of the client's illness and complete an assessment of the client's extremities.

4. Ask the client to lie in a supine position on his or her bed.

5. Take the following measurements to ascertain the correct stocking size:
   a. Below-the-knee stockings (Fig. 8–57):
      i. From the Achilles tendon to the popliteal fold (Fig. 8–57A).
      ii. Circumference of the midcalf (Fig. 8–57B).
   b. Thigh-high stockings (Fig. 8–58):
      i. From the Achilles tendon to the gluteal fold (Fig. 8–58A).
      ii. Circumference of the midthigh (Fig. 8–58B).

1. Allows you to prepare for the procedure and to explain the reason for the hose to the client.

2. Allows for accurate completion of the order.

3. Provides baseline data for decision making and alerts you to potential problems.

4. Encourages venous return and decreases swelling, thereby allowing for accurate measurements for the stockings.

5. Correct stocking size is essential in order for the stockings to apply the pressure needed for adequate venous return without interfering with circulation.

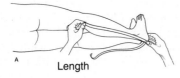

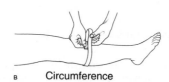

▼ **FIGURE 8–57.** Measurements for below-the-knee stockings.

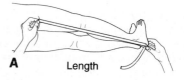

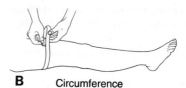

▼ **FIGURE 8–58.** Measurements for thigh-high stockings.

6. Compare the obtained measurements with the graph included in the stocking envelope and choose the appropriate-sized stockings.

7. Evenly spread approximately 1 tablespoon of talc or cornstarch on the client's legs and feet.

8. Although it is best to apply the stockings early in the day before the client gets out of bed, this is not always possible. Therefore, keep the client in a supine position with his or her legs elevated until the stockings can be applied.

9. Open the package and ascertain that the stockings are "inside out." Place your hand deep enough inside the stocking to grasp the stocking toe.

6. Allows for the selection of the correct stocking size. Stockings that are too tight will impair circulation and stockings that are too loose will not improve circulation.

7. Assists in a smooth, more comfortable application of the stockings by absorbing moisture and decreasing friction between the stockings and the client's skin.

8. Allows for the most venous return.

9. Steps 9 through 16 describe one method of applying stockings that allows for the least wrinkles, which increases client comfort and decreases areas of potential skin breakdown, and encourages venous return.

▼ *ACTION* ▼ *RATIONALE*

10. Then hold onto the client's left toes with the same hand. Invert the stocking with the other hand and pull it over your hand that is holding the client's toes. Then remove your hand from inside the stocking.

10. Arranges the stocking into the most convenient position from which to apply it efficiently.

11. Hold onto each side of the stocking and pull the left inverted stocking toe over the client's left toes.

11. See above.

12. Gently but firmly pull the stocking from the person's toes to the heel in one motion. Do not allow the stocking to fall back. Pull the stockings up by using the insides of your fingers and hands.

12. Allows for the most venous return without pooling. Fingernails can tear the material.

13. Grasp the stocking by the outside and pull it past the client's ankle.

13. Helps to keep the material tension evenly placed and prevents bunching of the material.

14. Continue to pull the stocking up the client's leg toward the buttocks in approximately 2-inch increments until you reach the appropriate length.

14. Allows you the most control of the stocking, thereby allowing for the most venous return and the least pooling.

15. Repeat Steps 9 to 14 on the client's right leg.

16. Remove the wrinkles in both stockings and smooth over the covered area.

16. Wrinkles in stockings are uncomfortable and can lead to skin irritation and pressure sores.

17. Remove both stockings for 30 minutes twice a day. At this time bathe and thoroughly dry the client's legs and reapply the talc (or cornstarch).

17. Helps to decrease the potential for undiscovered skin lesions and aids in client comfort and hygiene. Allows you to assess for changes in the client's peripheral vascular system.

> **NOTE:** Always reassess the client's peripheral pulses (posterior tibial, dorsalis pedis, and popliteal) before reapplying the stockings. Also reassess the rest of the client's peripheral circulatory system.

18. Wash and dry the stockings as needed. Be sure to follow the manufacturer's directions.

18. Assists in hygiene maintenance and promotion of the client's comfort.

19. Wash your hands.

19. Decreases the transmission of microorganisms.

20. Record the procedure.

20. Communicates to the other members of the health care team and contributes to the legal record by documenting the care given to the client.

21. Ascertain the proper fit of the stockings at frequent intervals by checking:
    a. That the stocking does not roll at the top.
    b. For swelling above the stocking top. (If swelling occurs, remove the stocking.)
    c. Circulation in client's legs.

21. Stockings that are too tight can compromise necessary circulation and lead to tissue damage. Stockings that are too loose will not assist in venous return.

Example of Documentation

DATE	TIME	NOTES
5/25/93	1010	Medium-sized thigh-high antiembolic stockings applied. Popliteal, posterior tibial, and dorsalis pedis pulses are 2+. Extremities are pink, warm, and dry and the skin is intact. No edema noted.
		S. Williams, RN

Teaching Tips

The client or the client's family, or both, should be taught how to assess the client's circulation, apply and remove the stockings, and wash the stockings. The client also should be encouraged to remove the stockings twice a day and cleanse the skin beneath the hose.

Home Care Variations

Family members should be taught how to assess the client's extremities for compromises in circulation. Since heat will break down the elastic, the stockings should not be dried in a clothes dryer, but should be allowed to drip-dry. It is very helpful to have two sets of stockings at home so that proper hygiene may be maintained.

SKILL 8–3   ASSISTING WITH POSTOPERATIVE EXERCISES

Clinical Situations in Which You May Encounter This Skill

Clients who have had an operation need a variety of exercises to assist them in recovering their optimum health. These exercises increase blood flow to the lower extremities, thereby decreasing venous stasis and the possibility of deep-vein thrombosis.

Other skills that should be considered for inclusion in a complete postoperative exercise regimen are: turning, range-of-motion exercises, deep breathing, and coughing. Antiemboli hose are also beneficial in preventing venous stasis, deep-vein thrombosis, and related complications.

Anticipated Responses

▼ The client has increased venous flow, decreased venous stasis, no decrease in joint mobility and muscle strength from the preoperative state, and a negative Homans' sign.

Adverse Responses

▼ The client's venous flow is impaired and venous stasis is present.
▼ The client's joint mobility decreases and his or her muscle strength is less than in the preoperative state.
▼ The client has a Homans' sign.

Materials List

Gather these materials before beginning the skill:

▼ None

▼ *ACTION* _ _ _ _ _ _ _ _ _ _ _ _ _ _ _ _ _ _ _ ▼ *RATIONALE* _ _ _ _ _ _ _ _ _ _

1. Before the operation, assess the client to determine:
   a. Any conditions that may contraindicate leg exercises.
   b. His or her muscle strength and mobility.

2. Assess the client's knowledge of the leg exercises to be done after surgery.

1. Provides information for optimum care. Leg deformities may affect the client's ROM and therefore contraindicate some leg exercises. Provides baseline data with which to compare the postoperative assessments.

2. Allows for clarification. Generally, the client has better retention when he or she is taught the exercises before the operation.

> **NOTE:** Teach the exercises to the client before the operation, if possible.

3. After the operation, ascertain whether Homans' sign is present.

4. Assess the client's ability to assist actively with leg exercises. (If the client is unable to actively assist, the exercises may be done passively—see Skill 8–1. If passive exercises are done, raise the bed to a comfortable working level.)

5. Perform appropriate postoperative assessment of the client. Include the vital signs.

6. Assess the client's comfort level and medicate him or her as needed.

7. Ask the client to lie in a supine position. (Assist him or her to get into this position if needed.)

8. Repeat each exercise five to seven times every 2 hours while the client is awake.

9. Starting with the client's feet, ask the client to:
   a. Rotate each ankle so that his or her toes draw an imaginary big circle in the air (Fig. 8–59).
   b. Alternate inversion and eversion of each ankle (see Figs. 8–44 and 8–45).
   c. Alternate dorsiflexion and plantar flexion of each foot (see Figs. 8–42 and 8–43).

3. A positive sign indicates deep-vein thrombosis.

4. The client may be unable to cooperate because of surgery, emotions, or medications. Raising the bed helps to protect your back.

5. Provides information for implementing and evaluating care.

6. Clients in pain are not able to participate well.

7. A supine position helps with performance of the exercises.

8. Decreases the client's venous stasis and increases joint mobility.

9. Promotes venous return. Increases ankle joint mobility and muscle movements of the foot, ankle, and calf.

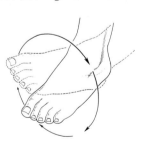

▼ **FIGURE 8–59.** Rotation.

▼ *ACTION*	▼ *RATIONALE*

10. Ask the client to:
  a. Slowly bend one leg until the heel is as close as is comfortable to his or her buttocks.
  b. Slowly straighten the leg until the knee is flat on the bed (Fig. 8–60).
  c. Repeat with the opposite leg.
	10. Maintains knee mobility and muscle movement in the upper legs.

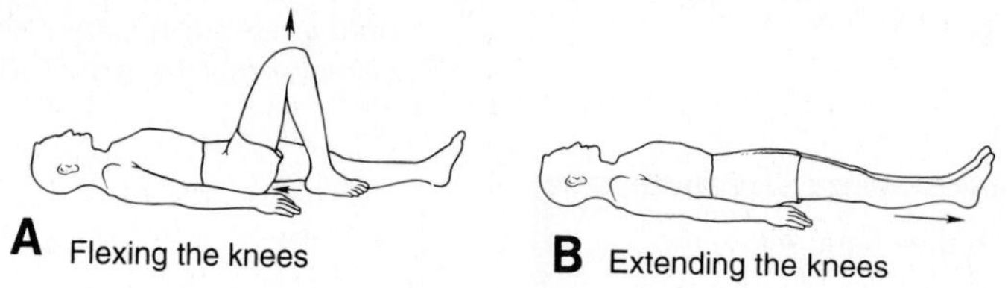

A Flexing the knees   **B** Extending the knees

▼ **FIGURE 8–60.** Straightening the leg.

11. If the bed is raised, lower it to the lowest level and raise the side rails, as appropriate.	**11.** Provides for the client's safety.
12. Obtain the client's vital signs and compare them to pre-exercise vital signs.	**12.** Helps determine if the exercises were too exhausting.
13. Determine the client's mobility and strength.	**13.** Indicates if the exercises are maintaining muscle strength and mobility.
14. Record your observations regarding the client's performance of the postoperative exercises.	**14.** Communicates the findings to the other members of the health care team and contributes to the legal record by documenting the care given to the client.

> **NOTE:** If the client will be immobile for more than a few days, other exercises should be added to those mentioned above. See Skill 8–1. Active exercises are better than passive exercises.

Example of Documentation

DATE	TIME	NOTES
12/28/93	1100	Postoperative Day 2. Active leg exercises performed by client. Tolerated well. RR = 24, AP = 86, BP = 132/78. Neg. Homans' sign. *K. Smith, RN*

Teaching Tips

Explain the purpose of the exercises and the procedure to the client or the client's family, or both. Allow the client to perform a return demonstration.

Home Care Variations

The client can be taught to perform these exercises at home and should be encouraged to do them after same-day or 1-day surgery.

SKILL 8–4 SPECIAL MATTRESSES, BEDS, AND POSITIONING DEVICES

Clinical Situations in Which You May Encounter this Skill

Several devices are available to assist in protecting the client from the hazards of immobility. These devices are usually used for clients who are confined to the bed for prolonged periods of time.

Devices to support pressure areas and reduce pressure include egg crate or foam mattresses, sheepskin heel protectors, gel cushions and pads (flotation pads), and alternating pressure air mattresses.

Special beds are also available to reduce development of pressure areas in immobilized clients.

Positioning devices to prevent contractures include pillows, bolsters, and trochanter rolls; foam abduction wedges; bed cradles; hand rolls; footboards; and sandbags.

Since use of this equipment varies with each manufacturer, and with the individual needs of the client, specific steps are not given in this text for use of these devices. However, the information discussed below will assist you in selecting the correct device for your client's needs.

Pressure-relieving Devices

Egg Crate or Foam Mattresses

The egg crate mattress consists of a thin foam mattress with peaks and valleys much like an egg carton. The egg crate mattress is placed over the client's regular mattress and helps to equalize and disperse pressure and promote air circulation to the skin. A single sheet is usually placed between the client and the egg crate mattress.

Sheepskins

Synthetic sheepskins are placed directly against the client's skin to disperse pressure over a wider body area, reduce friction and shearing forces, and absorb moisture away from the client's skin. Contoured sheepskin elbow and heel protectors (Fig. 8–61) are available to protect those pressure points from breakdown. Sheepskins should be laundered when soiled.

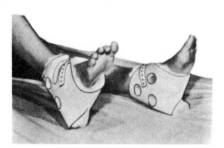

▼ FIGURE 8–61. Heel protector.

Flotation Pads

Flotation pads are filled with a pliable substance such as silicone, water, or foam that aids in spreading pressure over a larger area to protect bony prominences such as the sacral area. These pads are frequently used in wheelchairs.

Alternating Pressure Air Mattresses

An alternating pressure air mattress consists of a vinyl mattress with air cells and an electric pump that alternately inflates and deflates the various cells of the mattress. This air movement results in continually changing pressure points on the client's skin. Manufacturers recommend not using other devices such as sheepskins with air mattresses as they may decrease the effectiveness of the mattress.

Table 8–1 compares the benefits and disadvantages of each of these pressure-relieving devices.

TABLE 8–1. Pressure-Relieving Devices.

Category	Definition	Benefits	Disadvantages
Foam mattress	A mattress made of foam that is placed on top of the client's regular mattress	Maintenance-free Low cost Helps to relieve pressure	Not soilproof Can be damaged by cleaning solutions
Sheepskin	A pad made of sheepskin that is placed between the client and the sheet	Helps to relieve friction and to decrease moisture	Can cause the client to perspire
Gel cushion or pad	A vinyl pad filled with a gelatinous substance	Helps to relieve pressure Soilproof Fire-resistant	Expensive Cold to the touch Gel may harden when exposed to cold
Air mattress	A vinyl mattress that is either filled once with air (static) or is connected to a device that intermittently inflates and deflates the mattress (alternating)	Helps to relieve pressure Lightweight Durable Easily cleaned Fire-resistant	Easily punctured Difficult to transfer the client to and from the bed Alternating air mattress is expensive Must be monitored frequently Feels cold Relatively high maintenance costs

Special Beds

Many manufacturers make special beds that reduce the complications of immobility and make caring for the immobilized client easier. Table 8–2 describes these special beds and their individual benefits.

TABLE 8–2. Special Beds.

Category	Definition	Benefits
Spinal stabilization Roto Rest	A bed that continuously rotates the client from a right lateral to a left lateral position	Good for highly immobile clients
CircOlectric bed	An electric bed that allows you to turn the client vertically between a prone and a supine position on a circular frame	Good for highly immobile clients
Stryker wedge frame	A bed that has a thin, narrow anterior and posterior frame that permits the client to be turned to either the supine or prone position	Allows turning of the client who needs strict spinal immobilization
Air-fluidized bed Clinitron, FluidAir, Skytron	A bed that is air-fluidized	Reduces pressure by distributing the client's weight over the surface of the bed
Low–air loss beds Flexicare, KenAir, Mediscus	A bed with a mattress composed of a series of air sacs connected by a hose to an air-supply system	Good for clients with intractable pain Less chance of dehydration Waterproof
Oscillating low–air loss beds BioDyne	A bed that oscillates and has a series of air sacs that continuously inflate and deflate	Good for clients who are highly immobile but who have no spinal instability Beneficial for hemodynamically unstable clients
Orthopedic bed Nelson bed	An electric bed that can place the client in a chair, contour, standing, Trendelenburg's, or normal flat position	The client can walk off the bed in the standing position The chair position can be used for the client who is tube-fed

Positioning Devices

Pillows, Bolsters, and Trochanter Rolls

Pillows, bolsters, and trochanter rolls are used to maintain alignment of body parts, separate pressure points such as the knees, or to lift a pressure point such as the knees off the bed. Trochanter rolls also are used to prevent external rotation of the hips when the client is in the supine position.

Trochanter rolls (Fig. 8–62) are available commercially or can be made from folded and rolled bath towels. To make a trochanter roll, fold a bath towel in half lengthwise. Then, tightly roll the towel on one end, leaving approximately 1 foot at the other end unrolled. Turn the roll over and place the flat part of the towel under the client's hips. Be sure to smooth out any wrinkles. Position the roll so that the midpoint supports the client's greater trochanter to prevent external rotation.

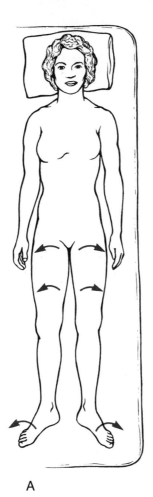
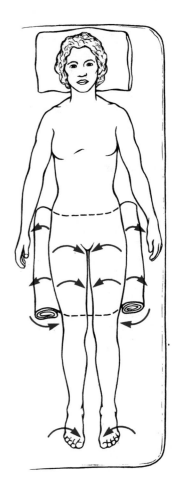

A

B

▼ FIGURE 8–62. Using a trochanter roll.

Hip Abduction Wedges

A hip abduction wedge (Fig. 8–63) is a wedge-shaped piece of dense foam that fits between the client's legs to maintain the hips in an abducted position. These devices are often used after surgical hip replacements to prevent dislocation of the new joint when the client is turned.

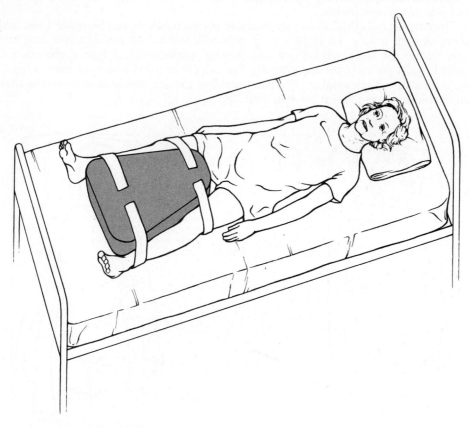

▼ FIGURE 8–63. Hip abduction wedge.

Bed Cradles

A bed cradle (Fig. 8–64) is a frame used to lift the top sheet off the client's skin and protect the skin from irritation. Bed cradles are often used to protect the skin and decrease pain in clients with burns. Cradles usually are made of a lightweight metal such as aluminum or heavy steel wire. For stability, they should be secured to the bed beneath the mattress. At home, a bed cradle can be made from a cardboard box that has been cut out on one side.

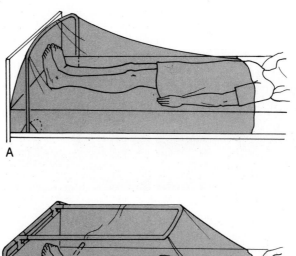

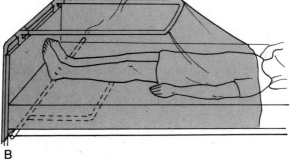

▼ **FIGURE 8–64.** Bed cradle.

Hand Rolls

Hand rolls (Fig. 8–65) are devices that when placed in the palms of the hands help to prevent contractures of the fingers. They can be purchased commercially or can be made from a washcloth or abdominal pad dressing by folding it in half, rolling it up, and securing the roll with tape or gauze.

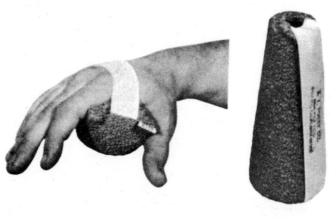

▼ **FIGURE 8–65.** Hand rolls.

Footboards

Footboards (Fig. 8–66) are rigid vertical devices that are placed at the foot of the bed to maintain the normal alignment of the client's ankle and foot at 90 degrees. Footboards also prevent the client from slipping down in the bed. The client's feet should firmly rest against the footboard. Footboards are not recommended for clients who have had a stroke since the stimulation of a footboard against the bottom of the foot may encourage plantar flexion.

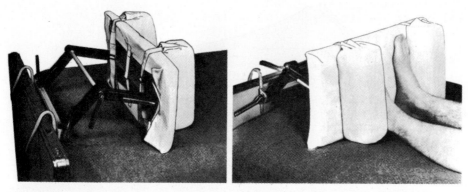

▼ **FIGURE 8–66.** Footboards.

Sandbags

Plastic bags filled with sand may be used to hold the person's body parts in proper alignment and prevent the client from slipping into a position that would promote development of contractures. Sandbags are often used to hold the feet in proper position when the client is turned.

SKILL 8–5 USING A STRYKER WEDGE TURNING FRAME

Clinical Situations in Which You May Encounter This Skill

Special frames such as the Stryker wedge turning frame (Fig. 8–67) may be used to assist in turning and positioning a client while maintaining his or her proper body alignment. These devices are especially useful for clients with spinal cord injuries.

Anticipated Responses

▼ The client's position is changed safely without undue stress to the client or damage to any tubes or devices attached to the client.
▼ There are no signs or symptoms of skin breakdown.
▼ The client's body is in good alignment.

Adverse Responses

▼ The client's skin shows areas of redness or edema.
▼ The client is excessively uncomfortable or anxious during the turning process or when left in the prone position.
▼ The client has difficulty breathing in the prone position.

Materials List

Gather these materials before beginning the skill:

▼ Anterior or posterior turning-frame restraining straps
▼ Clean linen (Custom-sized sheets with ties may be available for the Stryker frame.)
▼ Waterproof pads
▼ Pillows or other support devices
▼ Footboard
▼ Sheepskin or other skin protection device

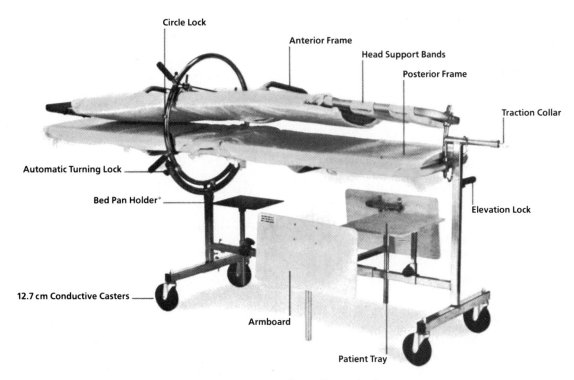

▼ FIGURE 8–67. Stryker wedge turning frame.

▼ ACTION	▼ RATIONALE
1. Before turning the client, assess his or her skin for pressure or breakdown (redness, irritation, or edema).	**1.** These areas should be protected from further pressure and skin breakdown.
2. Before turning the client, assess the neurologic status of his or her extremities for numbness, tingling, movement, sensation, and strength.	**2.** Provides baseline data with which to compare assessments made after turning the client.
3. Assess the client's level of knowledge and anxiety about being turned.	**3.** The client may need explanations regarding what to expect. Explanations provide reassurance and comfort.
4. Assess the client's tolerance for the new position.	**4.** Some clients cannot remain in the prone position for long periods of time. The supine position is usually better tolerated.

Preparing to Turn the Client

5. Find an assistant to help with monitoring the client's tubes, devices, and attachments as the client is turned.	**5.** Prevents accidental dislodgement or withdrawal of tubes.
6. Provide any appropriate nursing care before turning the client (e.g., skin care, back rub, dressing change).	**6.** Prevents unnecessary turning of the client.
7. Place all intravenous (IV) lines and feeding, drainage, and suction tubes at the head of the bed. If necessary, add extension tubing. Place a urinary drainage bag on the mattress beside the client.	**7.** Prevents accidental withdrawal or dislodgement of tubes. Extension tubing is long enough to accommodate the turn.
8. Lock the wheels of the frame.	**8.** Prevents the turning frame from rolling during the turn.

Turning the Client from a Supine to a Prone Position

9. Remove the top bed linen from the client and place a pillow lengthwise over the client's legs.	**9.** The pillow helps to prevent movement of the client's legs during the turn.
10. Place the client's arms at his or her sides. Make sure they do not extend beyond the turning frame and move the armboards out of the way.	**10.** Prevents injury to the client's arms during the turn.
11. Place a small pillow or folded towel beside the client's head.	**11.** Prevents lateral head movement during the turn.
12. Place clean linen on the anterior frame if needed.	**12.** Promotes the client's comfort and hygiene.
13. Place the anterior frame over the client and tighten the knurled nut at the head of the frame.	**13.** The anterior frame forms a wedge with the posterior frame. The tightened knurled nut holds the frame together during the turn.
14. Close and lock the turning ring over the anterior frame.	**14.** Helps to hold the client securely in place.
15. Fasten the foot with the nut and adjust the nuts on the anterior turning ring, if needed, to ensure a snug fit.	**15.** Holds the client in the frame.
16. Secure the restraining straps around the client and frame at the client's chest and legs.	**16.** The straps prevent the client's arms and legs from slipping during the turn.
17. Remove the lock pin at the head of the frame.	**17.** Allows the frame to turn.
18. Pull out the red turning lock knob located on the turning ring.	**18.** Allows the frame to turn.

▼ *ACTION*   ▼ *RATIONALE*

19. Stand by the narrow edge of the wedge, grasp the turning handle, and inform the client that you are going to turn him or her.	**19.** Makes the client aware that he or she is about to be turned.
20. Smoothly turn the frame toward the patient's right.	**20.** Turning the frame toward the patient's right makes use of the wedge and prevents the patient from slipping out of the frame.
21. Push in the silver lock knob on the turning ring.	**21.** Allows the turning ring to open.
22. Remove the restraining straps around the client and the frame.	**22.** The frame cannot be removed until the restraining straps are removed.
23. Loosen the knurled nut and remove the posterior frame.	**23.** Allows you to position and provide care to the client.
24. Replace the lock pin at the head of the frame.	**24.** Prevents the frame from turning and injuring an unrestrained client.
25. Replace the armboards and position the client.	**25.** Promotes the client's comfort and good body alignment.
26. Place a restraining strap around the client when he or she is sleeping or receiving sedatives or narcotics.	**26.** Prevents injury.
27. Cover the client with a sheet and, if needed, a blanket.	**27.** Provides warmth and promotes dignity.

Turning the Client from the Prone to the Supine Position

28. Follow Steps 1 to 8 when preparing to turn the client.	
29. If needed, position incontinence pads and sheepskin over the client's buttocks and back. A small pillow may be placed in his or her lumbar curve.	**29.** Reduces pressure and prevents soiling of the bed linens.
30. If needed, place clean linen on the posterior frame.	**30.** Promotes the client's comfort and hygiene.
31. Position the posterior frame over the client and secure it by tightening the knurled nut at the head of the frame.	**31.** The knurled nut holds the frame together during the turn.
32. Follow Steps 14 to 27 to complete the turn to the supine position.	
33. Assess the neurologic status of the client's extremities for numbness, tingling, movement, sensation, and strength.	**33.** The neurologic status of the extremities may have been compromised during the turn. If this occurs, the client should be repositioned and reassessed.
34. Record the procedure. Note the neurologic status assessments before and after turning and the client's response to turning.	**34.** Communicates the information to the other members of the health care team and contributes to the legal record by documenting the care given to the client.

Example of Documentation

DATE	TIME	NOTES
1/4/93	0900	Client turned from supine to prone position. No pressure areas noted on back or buttocks. Skin care and massage applied to back, sacrum, buttocks, heels, and elbows. Neurologic status of extremities unchanged after turn.

C. Smith, RN |

Teaching Tips

If the client's condition allows, teach the client arm and leg ROM exercises.

Home Care Variations

The Stryker wedge frame is not used in the home setting.

SKILL 8–6   CAST CARE

Clinical Situations in Which You May Encounter This Skill

The client who has any part of the body immobilized by a cast requires special care. The amount of area covered by the cast, the type of area covered by the cast, and the ability of the client to assume self-care all affect the type and amount of nursing care required.

Cast care is important in the prevention of decreased circulation and skin breakdown. After an injury, swelling often continues to increase for several days. Since swelling can increase the tightness of the cast, frequent assessment of the client's circulation is important.

Anticipated Responses

▼ The body part that is immobilized by the cast is in correct alignment.
▼ Circulation in the body part(s) distal to the cast area is not compromised.
▼ The client does not complain of numbness.
▼ There is no unanticipated increase in swelling.

Adverse Responses

▼ The body part immobilized by the cast is not in alignment.
▼ Circulation to the body part(s) distal to the cast area(s) is compromised.
▼ The client complains of numbness or increased pain.
▼ There is increased swelling beneath the cast.

Materials List

Gather these materials before beginning the skill:

▼ Examination gloves
▼ Adhesive tape
▼ Bandage scissors

▼ ACTION	▼ RATIONALE
1. Review the client's chart for the type of injury and the type of cast.	1. Alerts you to potential problems and allows for appropriate plans of care.
2. Wear gloves if there is any drainage.	2. Prevents the transmission of microorganisms.

▼ *A C T I O N* — — — — — — — — — — — — — — — ▼ *R A T I O N A L E* — — — — — — — — —

3. Elevate the person's entire extremity above the level of his or her heart by using pillows, a suspension device, or by electrically raising the bed (Fig. 8–68*A*).

3. Assists venous return and discourages dependent edema that can lead to compartment syndrome and impaired circulation.

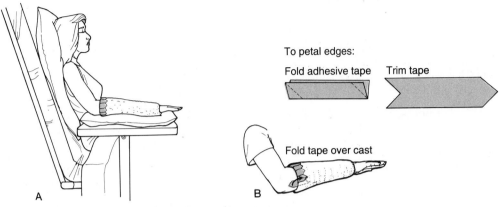

To petal edges:

Fold adhesive tape   Trim tape

Fold tape over cast

▼ **F I G U R E 8–68.** Petaling the edges of a cast.

4. Encourage drying of the newly applied cast by keeping the covers off and repositioning the client every 2 to 3 hours during the first 24 to 48 hours.

4. Casts must dry thoroughly and evenly to provide adequate support.

> **NOTE:** A plaster cast dries more slowly than a synthetic cast. After repositioning the client, check the cast for areas of flatness or impressions.

5. Assess the client's circulation and neurovascular functions in the affected area every 30 minutes for 4 hours, then every hour for 24 hours. After 24 hours, assessments can be performed every 4 hours as long as they are within acceptable limits for the client.

5. Impaired circulation can lead to necrotic areas and loss of body tissue. Impaired neurologic functioning can lead to irreversible loss of function.

6. Periodically, as the cast dries, check its edges for roughness, plaster crumbling, and pressure areas. When the cast is dry, petal the edges (Fig. 8–68*B*).

6. Petaling the edges of the cast creates a smooth edge that is less likely to crumble and injure the client's skin.

7. If areas of bleeding are seen through the cast, circle each area with a pen and write the date.

7. Provides for continued observation of the client's circulatory status. Monitors potential development of infection.

> **NOTE:** Check for drainage beneath the cast.

8. Assess for odors and swelling.

8. Swelling can impair circulation. An odor may indicate an infection.

▼ *ACTION* _____   ▼ *RATIONALE* _____

9. Assess for pressure areas under the cast as far as you can see.

9. Pressure areas can lead to pressure sores.

10. Assess the client for signs and symptoms of compartment syndrome (pain, numbness, tingling, loss of sensation, loss of movement, swelling, pallor).

10. Blood or drainage, or both, collect under damaged tissue and result in circulatory and neurovascular impairment. This is an emergency situation and the physician should be notified immediately.

11. Assess the client's circulation in the body parts distal to the cast, as well as the client's comfort.

11. Provides information about the client's well-being.

12. If the client has open wounds under the cast, observe for signs of infection.

12. Untreated infections can lead to loss of body parts and death.

13. Instruct the client not to insert any object into the cast.

13. Protects the client from injuries that might not be noticed or treated and could result in infection and further damage.

14. Assist the client in pain management.

14. Pain can inhibit recovery. Its correct assessment and alleviation is a major nursing role.

15. Perform range-of-motion exercises for the client unless they are contraindicated by his or her medical condition.

15. Prevents contractures and other complications of immobility.

16. Use a slightly damp cloth to clean soiled areas on the cast. Synthetic casts may be cleaned with mild soap and water and rinsed. They then can be blotted dry with towels and dried with a hand-held hair dryer on low settings. Do not get plaster casts wet, nor dry them with a hair dryer.

16. Provides for cleanliness. Plaster casts will lose their shape and support when wet.

NOTE: Do not immerse a cast. For clients who are able to bathe and request a bath or shower, wrap the cast in a waterproof covering. If a bath is taken, the client should keep the cast out of the water.

Allowing a cast to become too wet may weaken its necessary support.

17. Wash your hands.

17. Decreases the transmission of microorganisms.

18. Record the procedure.

18. Communicates to the other members of the health care team and contributes to the legal record by documenting the care given to the client.

19. Periodically evaluate whether or not the cast is providing immobilization as needed.

Example of Documentation

DATE	TIME	NOTES
5/23/93	1000	Left forearm cast dry and intact. Cast elevated on one pillow. Hand distal to cast is pink, warm, and dry. No swelling is noted, and skin is intact. The radial pulse is 2+. Capillary refill is <1 second. Client denies pain or numbness in the affected extremity.
		H. Morris, RN

Teaching Tips

The purpose of the cast and the need for frequent circulatory checks should be explained to the client or the client's family, or both. The client should be instructed not to put anything down the cast to scratch the skin.

Home Care Variations

Clients who are sent home after cast application must be taught the principles of cast care for both the newly applied and the older cast. It is especially important with a newly applied cast to observe for any compromise in circulation and to report it promptly.

SKILL 8–7   CARING FOR THE CLIENT IN TRACTION

Clinical Situations in Which You May Encounter This Skill

Traction is applied to fractures to assist in the alignment, reduction, support, and immobilization of broken bones in order for healing to take place. There are two methods of applying traction: skin traction and skeletal traction.

Skin traction (Fig. 8–69), the most common method of traction, is applied to the skin without pins or wires that break the skin's integrity. Skeletal traction (Fig. 8–70) is generally used for more complicated injuries. It is more dependable and successful than skin traction because pins or wires are inserted in the bone distal to the fracture and traction is applied.

Some types of traction such as cervical traction may be applied either as skin or skeletal traction. Halo cervical traction provides immobilization of the spine while allowing the client to ambulate.

Traction may be applied in three ways: straight, suspension, or fixed. With straight traction the pull or force is in a straight line on the affected part. Buck's traction is a straight type of skin traction.

Suspension traction provides support of the affected part in some type of device. This device is suspended by ropes, pulleys, and weights. Russell's traction is a type of suspension traction that may be either skin or skeletal. A balanced suspension traction is composed of two systems of ropes, pulleys, and weights. A common example of balanced suspension traction is the Thomas splint with Pearson attachment.

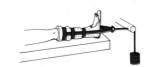

▼ **FIGURE 8–69.** Skin traction.

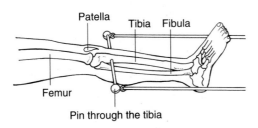

▼ **FIGURE 8–70.** Skeletal traction.

Fixed traction such as a cervical collar is used primarily for emergency treatment and during emergency medical service transportation, as it immobilizes the affected body part. Table 8–3 describes common types of traction and related nursing care.

There are general guidelines that apply to all clients in traction; this section will address these guidelines instead of providing steps.

Anticipated Responses

▼ Reduction, realignment, and proper immobilization of the fracture occurs.
▼ Circulation to the injured area and the area distal to it is maintained.
▼ Healing occurs within the expected time.
▼ Function of the unaffected body parts is maintained.

Adverse Responses

▼ Reduction, realignment, and proper immobilization of the fracture does not occur.
▼ Circulation to the injured area and the area distal to it is compromised.
▼ Healing does not occur or is delayed.

Materials List

Gather these materials before beginning the skill:

▼ Pillows
▼ Adhesive tape
▼ Other items determined by assessment

TABLE 8–3. Common Methods of Applying Traction.

Type	Use	Nursing Care
Skin traction: Buck's	Straight traction to immobilize fractures of the hip or femur; may be unilateral or bilateral	Assess for proper body alignment, nerve and circulatory impairment, skin breakdown, and allergic reaction to adhesive tape; make sure the weights hang freely
Bryant's	An adaptation of Buck's traction; used to stabilize fractured femurs or correct congenital hip dislocations in children who weigh less than 40 pounds; traction is applied to both legs with a spreader bar attached to maintain leg alignment	Assess for pressure at the bony prominences; the clients' buttocks should clear the mattress by 1 inch (see also nursing care for Buck's traction)
Russell's	Unilateral suspension traction used to immobilize fractures of the femur	Assess the sling for wrinkles and slippage (see also nursing care for Buck's traction)

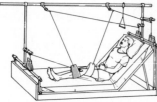

TABLE 8–3. Common Methods of Applying Traction *Continued*

Type	Use	Nursing Care
Cervical head halter	Intermittent or continuous skin traction to relieve muscle spasm and nerve compression in the neck	Assess for pressure at the chin, occipital area, and ears; maintain the client's good body alignment; be sure the weights hang freely
Pelvic belt or girdle	Provides traction to the client's hips to relieve back, hip, and leg pain	Keep the body in proper alignment; assess for pressure and skin irritation under the device; be sure the weights hang freely
Dunlop's	Horizontal traction to align fractures of the humerus; vertical traction maintains the forearm in proper alignment	(See Buck's traction)
Skeletal traction Thomas leg splint with Pearson attachment	Balanced suspension traction to stabilize fractures of the femur, acetabulum, hip, or lower leg	Assess for infection at the pin site; care for the pin site; maintain the person's body in good alignment to provide countertraction; the client may lift his or her buttocks for a bedpan or skin care without disturbing the traction; assess pressure areas for skin breakdown
Crutchfield tongs and other skull tongs	Provides immobilization of the cervical and upper thoracic vertebrae; halo traction is a variation that allows the client to move about freely while maintaining cervical traction	Maintain the client's body alignment; assess for infection at the pin site; care for the pin site

▼ *ACTION*

▼ *RATIONALE*

1. Assess the client for the neurovascular status of affected areas, vital signs, level of comfort, nutritional status, and skin condition.

1. Provides baseline data with which to compare future assessments.

2. Determine the type of traction being used.

2. Alerts you to the type of assessments you need to make to determine proper functioning of the traction device. For example, with skeletal traction, the pin sites should be examined for signs of infection.

3. Ascertain the type of position the client is allowed to assume.

3. Altering the client's position may change the direction of pull of the client's traction.

4. For all traction:
   a. Assess the neurovascular condition of the areas distal to the injury every hour immediately after application and every 2 to 4 hours as needed thereafter.
   b. Ascertain that the client is in the middle of the bed and has good body alignment with the traction lines correctly placed. The affected extremity should be in a neutral position unless otherwise ordered. Usually side-lying and semi-Fowler's positions are contraindicated.
   c. Do not allow the client's feet to rest against the foot of the bed.
   d. Keep all ropes in pulleys.

   e. Do not remove the traction weight except by a physician's order.
   f. Keep the weights hanging free. If the weights are removed and reapplied, they must be lowered smoothly and slowly.
   g. Every 3 to 4 hours, evaluate the affected and dependent skin areas. Look for signs of irritation and breakdown.
   h. Provide for special skin protection devices such as elbow and heel protectors as needed.
   i. Keep linens, Ace bandages, and other coverings as smooth as possible.
   j. When moving the client in bed, allow the client to use an overbed trapeze, if possible.
   k. Help the client to perform passive and active ROM exercises at least every shift.
   l. Affected extremities require isometric or isotonic exercises as ordered.
   m. Provide a fracture pan for the client's elimination needs.
   n. Make the bed from head to foot.

   o. Do not tuck in the top sheets or bedspreads.

   p. Provide for adequate hydration, nutrition, and respiratory hygiene every shift.

4. a. Provides data necessary to evaluate the client's progress. Possible compromise of circulation with loss of sensation, infection and necrosis may occur.
   b. Provides the correct alignment for healing to occur properly. Allows for the correct traction on the affected body part. The side-lying and semi-Fowler's positions alter the pull of the traction on the affected body parts.

   c. Alters the pull and counterpull of the traction.

   d. Allows for movement while maintaining proper traction.
   e. May allow the alignment to slip.

   f. Allows for correctly balanced traction. Prevents jerking of the client, which may cause spasms and pain.
   g. Determines skin integrity and helps to prevent skin breakdown.

   h. Decreases pressure at vital points and the potential for skin breakdown.
   i. Decreases skin irritation.

   j. Decreases skin shearing. The trapeze also facilitates self-movement by the client.
   k. Prevents loss of function of nonaffected body parts.
   l. Prevents further loss of function of the affected body parts. Strengthens the affected muscles.
   m. Decreases the negative effects of traction.

   n. Having the client roll from side to side can alter the pull of the traction.
   o. Tucking these in can interfere with the pull of the traction.
   p. Helps to prevent complications such as urinary stasis and infection, poor healing, and hypostatic pneumonia or atelectasis. Immobility can cause urinary stasis and pulmonary stasis.

▼ _A C T I O N_	▼ _R A T I O N A L E_
q. Assess the frequency and ease of the client's bowel movements.	q. Immobility decreases gastrointestinal peristalsis.
5. For skin traction: a. Cleanse, carefully dry, and massage the client's skin beneath the covered traction areas and dependent areas.	**5.** a. Removes debris and promotes circulation in these areas.
b. Assess the mobility of the joints affected by traction, if appropriate.	b. Allows for recognition and prevention of contracture development.
c. Maintain appropriate pressure with wraps and splints.	c. Inappropriate pressure can cause skin breakdown. Circumferential wraps can compromise the person's circulation.
6. For skeletal traction: a. Evaluate pin insertion sites for signs of infection and loosening.	**6.** a. The skin harbors bacteria and pin insertion may alter the integrity of the skin. The pin may become loose from client movement.
b. Use aseptic technique to cleanse the pin insertion sites and apply antimicrobial medication as ordered.	b. Decreases the possible transmission of microorganisms.
7. Record your observations and the care given to the client.	**7.** Communicates the findings to the other members of the health care team and contributes to the legal record by documenting the care given to the client.

Example of Documentation

DATE	TIME	NOTES
3/6/93	1000	Client in correct alignment with pelvic belt. 10-lb weights hanging freely. Skin areas under belt clear and intact. Client states he is without pain at this time. No tingling or loss of sensation noted in lower extremities. Pedal pulses strong, feet warm and dry, pink in color. *N. Francis, RN*

Teaching Tips

Explain the purpose of the traction and the observations to be made to the client or the client's family, or both. Encourage the client to eat a well-balanced diet to promote adequate healing and to prevent weight gain that may accompany activity.

Home Care Variations

If the client is instructed to set up skin traction at home, the related guidelines and safety measures should be explained to the client. Most clients who have skeletal traction will go home with some type of device and probably will require insertion-site care. Also, clients may require crutch-walking instructions. Prevention of further injuries is a very important aspect of home care.

References

Alterescu, V., and Alterescu, K. B. (1992). Pressure ulcers: Assessment and treatment. *Orthopaedic Nursing*, 11 (2), 37–49.

Bolander, V. B. (1994). Preventing complications of immobility. In V. Bolander (Ed.), *Basic nursing* (3rd ed.). Philadelphia: W. B. Saunders.

Ceccio, C. M. (1990). Understanding therapeutic beds. *Orthopaedic Nursing*, 9 (8), 57–70.

Conine, T. A., Choi, K. M., and Lim, R. (1989). The user-friendliness of protective support surfaces in prevention of pressure sores. *Rehabilitation Nursing*, 14 (5), 262–263.

Conine, T. A., et al. (1990). Costs and acceptability of two special overlays for the prevention of pressure sores. *Rehabilitation Nursing*, 15, 133–137.

Counsell, C., et al. (1990). Interface skin pressures on four pressure-relieving devices. *Journal of Enterostomal Therapy*, 17, 150–153.

Jacobs, M. S. (1989). Comparison of capillary blood flow using a regular hospital bed mattress, ROHO mattress, and Mediscus bed. *Rehabilitation Nursing*, 14, 270–272.

Lovell, H., and Anderson, C. (1990). Put your patient on the right bed. *RN*, 53, 66–72.

Martes, M. (1984). The Nelson bed on an orthopaedic unit. *Orthopaedic Nursing*, 3 (4), 51–54.

Willey, T. (1989). High-tech beds and mattress overlays: A decision guide. *American Journal of Nursing*, 89 (9), 1142–1145.

CHAPTER 9

Providing Physical Protection and Bodily Support

Restraints are devices used to restrict the client's movement. They are applied to keep the client from self-inflicted injury or from injuring others; from pulling out intravenous (IV) lines, catheters, or tubes; or from removing dressings. Restraints also may be used to keep children still and from injuring themselves during treatments and diagnostic procedures. Restraints should not be used as a form of punishment. Many institutions recommend using restraints only after all other measures have failed.

Restraints may be environmental, chemical, or physical. Environmental restraints involve manipulating the client's surroundings to make the client safer. They include side rails, "quiet" rooms, locked wards, and plastic domes on infant cribs. Side rails are particularly useful in a variety of settings. They are used for persons who are unconscious, disoriented, or receiving medications that depress the central nervous system; immobilized clients; clients on stretchers; and postoperative and postpartum clients.

Chemical restraints involve the use of sedative medications such as major and minor tranquilizers and hypnotics to assist the client in achieving control of his or her actions. Physical restraints are devices that limit a client's movement and prevent the client from harming himself or herself or others. Many types of physical restraints are available. Those more commonly used are the hand mitt restraint, wrist restraint, ankle restraint, chest (vest) restraint, waist (belt) restraint, elbow splint restraint, and total body (mummy) restraint.

Restraining a client has certain legal implications. Holding a person against his or her will is called false imprisonment. Therefore, you must give careful consideration to the decision to use restraints. Many institutions require a physician's order for the use of restraints. In other institutions, the nurse may make the decision to restrain a client. Be sure to document completely:

1. The client's behavior that led to the use of restraints
2. The time the restraint was applied
3. The type of restraining device used
4. The client's behavior after the restraint was applied
5. Nursing assessment and interventions to prevent physical complications from the use of restraints
6. The times of client assessment
7. The time the restraints were removed
8. The client's response to the removal of the restraints

The use of restraints can cause physical and psychologic harm to the client; therefore, you should implement nursing measures to avoid injury to the client. Table 9–1 lists possible complications that can occur in the restrained client.

When applying commercial restraining devices, always follow the manufacturer's directions. Use of restraints contrary to the company's instructions is potentially unsafe and may result in serious injury to or death of a client.

Restraints should not be used over skin areas that have abrasions, are irritated, or show signs of ischemia. Furthermore, they should not be applied over areas that have an IV line, arterial line, dialysis shunt, or other devices, and they should not be used for clients with tonic-clonic seizures.

SKILL 9–1 **APPLYING RESTRAINTS** 288

TABLE 9–1. Complications Resulting from the Use of Restraints

The restrained client may experience:

▼ Negative emotions such as frustration, stress, anxiety, fear, panic, combativeness, agitation, depression, despair, or hopelessness
▼ A sense of loss of personal control or loss of positive self-image, or both
▼ A sense of being viewed by others as disturbed, dangerous, or mentally incompetent
▼ Sensory deprivation
▼ Increased disorganized behavior
▼ Growing dependency
▼ Increased confusion from limited communication
▼ A heightened degree of disorientation
▼ Regressive behavior and withdrawal
▼ Diminished functional capacity resulting in decreased potential for rehabilitation
▼ Tissue or nerve damage from friction and pressure under the restraints
▼ Damage to other body parts, such as shoulder dislocation if a restrained client is combative or experiences a generalized tonic-clonic seizure
▼ Hypostatic pneumonia
▼ Pressure areas, skin abrasions, and edema
▼ Musculoskeletal damage such as contractures and bone loss due to immobility when restraints are used for a prolonged time
▼ Aspiration pneumonia
▼ Accidental or purposeful strangulation or entanglement
▼ Delays in resuscitation efforts due to time spent in releasing restraints
▼ Injury or death due to fires or other disasters

(Data from Morse, C., Harkveado, H.: Providing physical protection and body support. In Bolander, V. B. ed.: Basic Nursing, 3rd ed. Philadelphia, W.B. Saunders, 1994.)

SKILL 9–1 APPLYING RESTRAINTS

Clinical Situations in Which You May Encounter This Skill

Restraints are applied to prevent a combative person from self-inflicted harm or from harming others, to prevent a confused client from removing medical devices from his or her body, to protect a client from falls, and to aid a child in remaining still during medical procedures.

Anticipated Responses

▼ Restraints are safely applied without resulting complications (see Table 9–1).
▼ The client does not try to remove the restraints.

Adverse Responses

▼ The client suffers physical or psychologic harm, or both, from the use of restraints (see Table 9–1).

Materials List

Gather these materials before beginning the skill:

▼ Restraining device: wrist or ankle restraint, or both; waist (belt) restraint; chest (vest) restraint; hand mitt restraint; elbow restraint; mummy restraint
▼ Padding materials such as 4 × 4's or abdominal pads may be needed
▼ Gauze bandage for a homemade ankle or wrist restraint

▼ ACTION

1. Assess the client's behavior and the need for restraints.

2. Check to see if a physician's order has been written for restraints.

▼ RATIONALE

1. This information should be documented because you could be charged with false imprisonment.

2. Some states require a physician's order before restraints can be used.

▼ *A C T I O N* _ _ _ _ _ _ _ _ _ _ _ _ _ _ _ _

▼ *R A T I O N A L E* _ _ _ _ _ _ _ _ _ _ _

3. Decide what type of restraint is needed and obtain it. You also will need padding material for the client's bony prominences.

3. Avoid overrestraining or underrestraining the client. The restraint should limit the client's freedom only as much as is necessary. Padding protects the client's bony prominences from friction and prevents constriction of the client's circulation.

4. Obtain assistance.

4. Do not attempt to restrain a person without adequate assistance because of the possibility of injury to yourself and to the client.

5. Wash your hands.

5. Reduces the transmission of microorganisms.

6. If possible, explain the purpose of the restraint to the client and the client's family in a calm, reassuring manner. If the client is combative or incoherent, work with your assistants as a team to quickly and smoothly restrain the individual.

6. Attempts to elicit the client's cooperation.

7. Apply the restraint:
   a. Ankle and wrist restraints: Restraints may be made of leather (Fig. 9–1*A*), fabric (Fig. 9–1*B*), or a synthetic disposable material. If a commercial restraint is not available, one can be made using a strip of gauze bandage (Fig. 9–2).

   a. Prevents the client from self-inflicted injury or removal of tubes, etc.

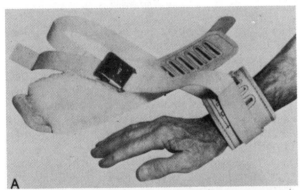

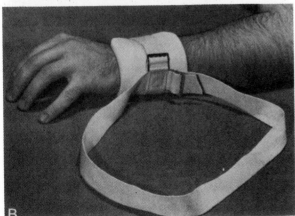

▼ **FIGURE 9–1.** Ankle and wrist restraints. *A,* leather; *B,* fabric. (Courtesy of J. T. Posey Co.)

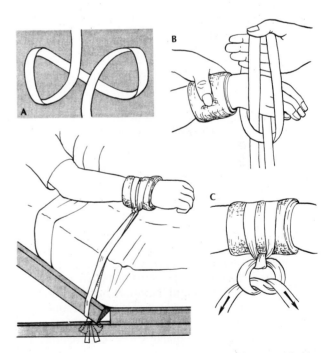

▼ **FIGURE 9–2.** Restraint made from gauze bandage. First fashion the bandage into a clove hitch (*A*). Slip the client's wrist through both loops of the clove hitch (*B*). Then tie a single knot on top of the clove hitch to prevent the restraint from becoming too tight if the client pulls hard against it (*C*).

▼ *ACTION*   ▼ *RATIONALE*

    i. Pad the skin under the restraint.

    ii. Place the restraint on the client's wrist or ankle and secure it according to the manufacturer's directions.

    iii. Fasten the straps of the wrist restraint below the level of the client's waist and the straps of the ankle restraint below the client's knees.

    iv. Use a bow knot to tie the ends of the restraint to the bed frame out of the client's reach (Fig. 9–2C).

    v. When using wrist and ankle restraints, avoid positioning the client in the supine position. A slightly turned position is safer.

  v. Avoids the risk of aspiration if the person vomits.

b. Chest (vest) and waist (belt) restraints: Chest restraints (Fig. 9–3) are usually made of muslin or mesh fabric and are washable. Belt restraints (Fig. 9–4) may be made of a woven fabric or leather.

b. Prevents falls when the client is in bed, on a stretcher, or sitting in a chair.

    i. Apply the chest or belt restraint, or both, following the manufacturer's directions.

    ii. Smooth out all wrinkles in the restraint.

  ii. Avoids pressure areas on the client's skin.

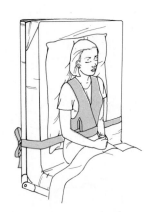

▼ **FIGURE 9–3.** Chest restraint.

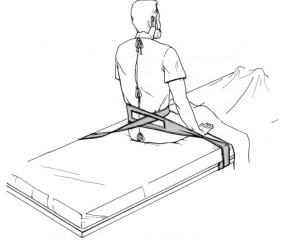

▼ **FIGURE 9–4.** Belt restraint.

c. Hand mitt: A hand mitt (Fig. 9–5) is a thumbless mitten that prevents effective use of the client's fingers and thumb. A hand roll may be used to keep the client's fingers in a functional position inside the hand mitt.

c. Prevents removal of medical devices and other restraining devices.

    i. Follow the manufacturer's directions for fastening the mitt around the client's wrist.

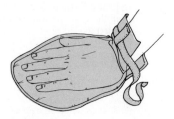

▼ **FIGURE 9–5.** Hand mitt.

▼ *ACTION*   ▼ *RATIONALE*

d. Elbow restraint: An elbow restraint (Fig. 9–6) is a cloth device that has a series of pockets that hold tongue blades around the client's elbow joint and render it immobile.

   i. Pad the client's elbow under the restraint and follow the manufacturer's directions for tying the restraint in place.

d. Prevents children from removing medical devices such as IV lines.

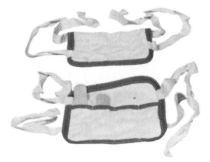
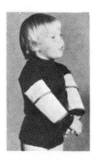

▼ **FIGURE 9–6.** Elbow restraint. (Courtesy of J. T. Posey Co.)

e. Body restraints (mummy restraints): Body restraints are used when the client's entire body must be immobilized. A mummy restraint for children can be made from a sheet folded to the appropriate size for the child (Fig. 9–7). Commercial body restraints such as the Olympic Papoose Board are also available (Fig. 9–8).

e. Commonly these restraints are used on children during medical procedures that require the child to remain perfectly still.

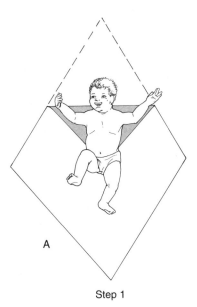

A

Step 1

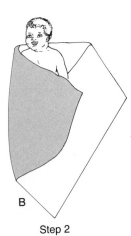

B

Step 2

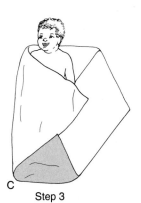

C

Step 3

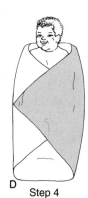

D

Step 4

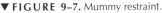
▼ **FIGURE 9–7.** Mummy restraint.

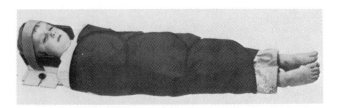

▼ **FIGURE 9–8.** Olympic Papoose Board with head immobilizer. (Courtesy of Olympic Medical, Seattle, WA.)

▼ *ACTION* _____ ▼ *RATIONALE* _____

8. Remove the restraint every 2 hours during the day and every 4 hours at night.

8. Allows you to assess the client's skin and to give care to prevent skin breakdown.

9. Do range-of-motion exercises, assess the condition of the client's skin, and provide skin care.

9. Range-of-motion exercises prevent ischemia and contractures. If all restraints are removed at one time, you will not be able to keep the client from injuring himself or herself or from removing equipment.

> **NOTE:** Only remove one restraint at a time.

10. Assess the client's circulatory status every 30 minutes (see Skill 4–11).

10. Ensures that the client's circulation is not altered.

> **NOTE:** Circulatory checks should be done distal to the restraint.

11. Change the client's position every 2 hours.

11. Prevents pneumonia and other complications.

12. Record the procedure. Note the client's behavior that necessitated the restraints; the type of restraint used; the time the restraint was applied; the client's behavior after the restraint was applied; and the client's skin condition and circulatory and respiratory status. When the restraints are removed, note the time and the client's response.

12. Communicates the findings to other members of the health care team and contributes to the legal record by documenting the care given to the client.

Example of Documentation

DATE	TIME	NOTES
11/18/93	0900	Mr. B. is confused and disoriented. Reorientation attempted s̄ success. Pulled out IV and attempted to pull out nasogastric tube. Wrist restraints applied. Importance of and need for restraint explained to client and his family. Fingers pink and warm with good capillary refill. No signs of skin breakdown noted over wrists. Client still attempting to remove devices, but stops when pull of restraint is felt.
		H. White, RN.

Teaching Tips

The purpose of the restraint and the proper procedure for applying the restraint should be explained to the client's family. Restraints can cause psychologic stress not only for the client but also for the client's family.

Home Care Variations

If restraints are used in the home, the client should be placed in a hospital bed. It is extremely difficult to tie the straps to a regular bed.

References

Morse, C., and Harkreader, H. (1993). Providing physical protection and bodily support. In V. Bolander (Ed.), *Basic nursing* (3rd ed.). Philadelphia: W.B. Saunders.

CHAPTER 10

Promoting Hygiene

- -

Assisting a client with grooming and hygiene practices is a basic function of nursing. Bathing and combing the hair are refreshing to the client and promote feelings of self-esteem.

Providing assistance with hygiene often involves invading the client's personal space. You should protect the client's dignity and modesty by using draping in an appropriate manner while providing care. Helping with hygiene also involves the use of therapeutic touch. Provide this care in an unrushed and gentle manner.

- -

OVERVIEW OF RELATED RESEARCH

MAKING THE OCCUPIED BED

Harrell, J., et al. (1992). Bedmaking in the coronary care unit. *Heart and Lung*, 21 (3), (abstract), 297.

To study the difference between making an occupied bed and allowing the client to sit in a chair while the bed was made, the effects on 20 stable persons recovering from myocardial infarction were examined. A noninvasive procedure, impedence cardiography, was used to measure cardiac performance as each client, on different days, either sat in a chair for 5 minutes or remained in bed during the bed linen change. The researchers found no clinically significant differences in heart performance whether the clients sat in the chair or remained in bed during bedmaking. Cardiac contractility did decrease slightly when clients sat in the chair but quickly returned to normal after the clients returned to bed. Based on information from this study, clients may actually conserve energy by getting out of bed for linen changes, rather than rolling from side to side while remaining in bed during bedmaking.

ORAL HYGIENE PRACTICES

Crosby, C. (1989). Method in mouth care. *Nursing Times*, 35 (85), 38–41.
Trenter, P., and Creason, N. (1986). Nurse administered oral hygiene: Is there a scientific basis? *Journal of Advanced Nursing Science*, 11 (3), 323–331.

There have been numerous research studies investigating nurse-administered oral hygiene. Various studies have compared one method of administering oral hygiene to another, one mouthwash to another, one dentifrice to another, or one product to another. The studies are too numerous to cite them all. The student is instead referred to these two articles, which do an excellent job of summarizing the body of research related to oral hygiene.

SKILL 10–1   ASSISTING WITH ORAL HYGIENE

Clinical Situation in Which You May Encounter This Skill

Clients who are able to take care of their own oral hygiene should be given the necessary supplies. Clients who are unable to take care of their own oral hygiene need your assistance. These clients include comatose individuals, postoperative clients, and clients who have intravenous fluids infusing into the dominant hand, as well as clients with mental impairment and other problems that affect the arms and hands.

Clients who are unresponsive are often mouth breathers and need oral care frequently. The complete procedure does not have to be done each time, but oral swabs moistened with normal saline or one-half strength hydrogen peroxide should be used to clean out the oral cavity and moisten the mucous membranes. This is also useful for clients who are not allowed to eat by mouth.

Oral hygiene decreases the microorganisms in the oral cavity and decreases the possibility of bad breath and oral infections. It also provides moisture and removes secretions that might interfere with the client's respiratory status.

Anticipated Responses

▼ The client's oral cavity is clean and free of infection.
▼ The client's gums are not irritated.
▼ The client does not have halitosis.

Adverse Responses

▼ The client's gums are irritated or have signs of infection or disease, or both.
▼ The client has halitosis.

Materials List

Gather these materials before beginning the skill:

▼ Soft nylon toothbrush or gauze swabs
▼ Toothpaste (preferably fluoridated) or other oral cleansing agent (at times, baking soda may be used)

▼ Drinking cup with water
▼ Straw, if needed
▼ 10-ml syringe (if the client is comatose)
▼ Suction equipment (for the comatose or dysphagic client)
▼ Mouthwash or hydrogen peroxide (one-half strength)
▼ Waxed dental floss
▼ Emesis basin or something to expectorate into
▼ Bite-block, if needed
▼ Towels
▼ Waterproof pads
▼ Examination gloves

▼ ACTION

1. Assess whether the client is able to take care of his or her own oral hygiene.

2. If you will be giving the oral care, position the bed at a comfortable working height.

3. Position the client in an upright position. If the client is unresponsive, position the client on his or her side and place a bite-block in between his or her teeth.

4. Protect the client's bed linens and garments with waterproof pads.

5. Fill the drinking cup with fresh cool water and place the emesis basin within the client's reach.

6. Put on gloves.

NOTE: If needed, a mask, goggles, and a protective gown should be worn.

7. Allow the client to rinse his or her mouth with water and expectorate the liquid into the basin. If the client is unresponsive:
   a. Place 2 to 5 ml of clear water in a syringe and rinse out the client's mouth. Allow the liquid to drain into the emesis basin.
   b. Watch for respiratory difficulties, choking, and strangling.
   c. Have suction equipment set up.

▼ RATIONALE

1. Allows for the client's independence if self-care is possible.

2. Decreases the strain to your back.

3. The client must be able to expectorate secretions. Turning the unresponsive client to the side allows for more complete drainage of secretions and helps prevent aspiration. The bite-block prevents the client from clenching his or her mouth and teeth shut.

4. Promotes comfort.

5. The client will need water to rinse his or her mouth. The client will need to expectorate into the emesis basin.

6. Decreases the transmission of microorganisms. Proper barrier precautions should be used to prevent exposure of your skin and mucous membranes when contact with blood or body fluids is anticipated.

7. Cleanses the mouth of large debris that can be removed easily. Allows for effective oral care.

   a. Rinsing removes debris.

   b. If water drains down the throat of an unconscious client, aspiration can occur.
   c. Provides for suctioning if needed to prevent aspiration.

▼ *ACTION*

▼ *RATIONALE*

8. Place a small amount of toothpaste or other cleansing agent on a toothbrush. If the client is unresponsive, gauze or oral hygiene "brushes" may be used (Fig. 10–1). Do not use foaming cleansing agents on unresponsive clients.

8. Aids in cleansing.

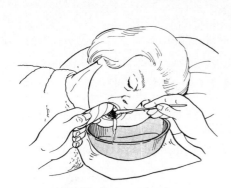

▼ **FIGURE 10–1.** Assisting the unresponsive person with oral hygiene.

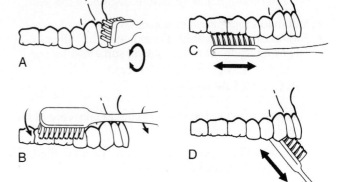

▼ **FIGURE 10–2.** Brushing the client's teeth.

9. Hold the toothbrush at a 45-degree angle. Point toward the client's gum line and use a gentle, circular motion to brush all exposed areas of the teeth (Fig. 10–2A). Then:
   a. Use short, angled strokes on the inner and outer surfaces of the client's back teeth (Fig. 10–2B).
   b. With the toothbrush held flat, brush the chewing surfaces of the back teeth (Fig. 10–2C).
   c. Tilt the toothbrush and use a circular motion to clean the inner surfaces of the front teeth (Fig. 10–2D).
   d. Gently brush the client's tongue. Be careful not to initiate the gag reflex.

9. Recommended American Dental Association (ADA) guidelines for proper hygiene.

   d. The gag reflex is uncomfortable for the client and may precipitate vomiting and potential aspiration.

10. Allow the client to expectorate and rinse his or her mouth as needed during the procedure. Irrigate, then drain the liquid into an emesis basin, or suction the liquid from the mouth of the unresponsive client, as needed.

10. Promotes comfort and allows for removal of debris.

11. Floss the client's teeth after brushing with approximately 1.5 ft of waxed floss.
    a. Wind most of the floss around the middle or index finger of one of your hands and the rest around the middle or index finger of your other hand. Leave an inch or two between the two fingers.

11. Recommended ADA guidelines for proper dental hygiene. Waxed floss should be used to discourage shredding of the floss on rough teeth.

▼ *ACTION*   ▼ *RATIONALE*

b. When flossing the client's bottom teeth, use your index fingers to press down on the unwound floss to pull it tight (Fig. 10–3*A*). When flossing the upper teeth, use your thumbs to press up on the unwound floss to pull it tight (Fig. 10–3*B*).

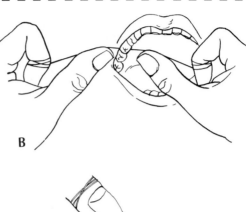

B

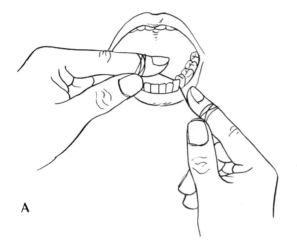

A

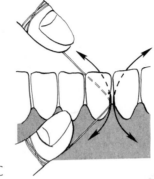

C

▼ **FIGURE 10–3.** Flossing the client's teeth.

c. Using a gentle sawing motion, slide the floss between the client's teeth, starting in the front.
d. Scrape the sides of the client's teeth with an up-and-down motion (Fig. 10–3*C*).

NOTE: Do not force floss into the gums.

e. Unwinding the floss as needed, work in a systematic pattern so that all of the client's teeth are flossed.

NOTE: If the client is not used to flossing, a small amount of bleeding or gum soreness may be present. If these conditions last longer than a few days, the client's physician should be notified. Be especially alert to this for the client taking anticoagulant medications.

Continued bleeding may indicate gum disease. Anticoagulants increase bleeding time.

▼ *A C T I O N*	▼ *R A T I O N A L E*
12. Give the client approximately an ounce of mouthwash or one-half strength hydrogen peroxide.	**12.** Provides fresh breath.

> **NOTE:** Depending on the client's level of orientation, remind the client not to drink mouthwash. The syringe may be used to rinse the mouth of an unresponsive client with one-half strength peroxide. Suction may be needed.

13. If the client's lips are dry, a protective ointment such as petroleum jelly should be applied sparingly.	**13.** Provides protection from dryness and cracking. Do not use petroleum jelly if client is receiving oxygen therapy since this poses a fire and burn safety risk.
14. Assess the client's comfort.	**14.** Provides information for planning further client care.
15. Lower the bed to a safe height.	**15.** Promotes the client's safety.
16. Clean the equipment and the area.	**16.** Decreases the transmission of microorganisms. Provides for a pleasing environment.
17. Remove the gloves and dispose of them properly.	**17.** Decreases the transmission of microorganisms.
18. Wash your hands.	**18.** Decreases the transmission of microorganisms.
19. Record the procedure and other relevant information.	**19.** Communicates information to the other members of the health care team and contributes to the legal record by documenting the care given to the client.

Example of Documentation

DATE	TIME	NOTES
6/14/93	1000	Oral care given. Oral mucosa pink, moist, and intact. RR = 16. Breath sounds bilaterally clear and equal.
		C. Lewis, RN
		(Note: Some agencies have a checklist for oral hygiene. Note any abnormalities in your notes.)

Teaching Tips

Families should be made aware of the importance of the client's oral hygiene. If the client is unresponsive, the person providing the care should be taught carefully how to prevent aspiration.

Home Care Variations

The same procedure can be used to provide oral hygiene in the client's home.

SKILL 10-2   ASSISTING WITH DENTURE CARE

Clinical Situations in Which You May Encounter This Skill

Clients who are unable to take care of their dentures because of a temporary or permanent condition need assistance with oral hygiene. Denture care decreases the number of microorganisms that can produce bad breath and oral infections. It also removes oral secretions that may interfere with respiratory status and promotes the client's comfort. The dentures should be handled carefully during cleaning to prevent breakage.

Anticipated Responses

▼ The client has clean and comfortable dentures.

Adverse Responses

▼ The client's dentures are broken.
▼ The client has halitosis.
▼ The client has oral irritation.

Materials List

Gather these materials before beginning the skill:

▼ Paper towel or washcloth
▼ Toothpaste or denture paste
▼ Toothbrush
▼ Two labeled denture cups
▼ Examination gloves
▼ Water
▼ Mouthwash or other oral rinse (if appropriate)
▼ Emesis basin
▼ Cup of water
▼ Gauze sponge

▼ *A C T I O N*	▼ *R A T I O N A L E*
1. Assess whether the client needs help with his or her oral hygiene.	**1.** Allows for the client's independence if self-care is possible.
2. Assemble supplies for the client if he or she is able to take care of oral hygiene.	**2.** Allows the client to remain as self-sufficient as possible.
3. If you will be performing denture care, put on gloves.	**3.** Decreases the transmission of microorganisms.
4. Grasp the dentures with a gauze sponge and gently remove them from the client's mouth (Fig. 10-4A and B). Place them in a denture cup that has water in it.	**4.** Allows the water to start the cleaning process by loosening any secretions and food particles.

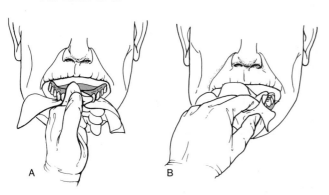

▼ **FIGURE 10-4.** Removing the client's dentures.

▼ *ACTION* ▼ *RATIONALE*

5. Place a washcloth or paper towel in the bottom of the sink with a small amount of water.

5. Cushions the dentures, if dropped. Helps to prevent breakage.

6. Place a small amount of toothpaste or denture paste on a toothbrush.

6. Assists in the proper cleaning of the dentures. The cleansing agent used should not be too abrasive in order to prevent damage to the denture surface.

7. Take one denture from the cup and hold it low over the sink. Grasping the denture firmly in the palm of one hand, use your other hand to thoroughly brush the denture (Fig. 10–5).

7. Allows for the most efficient and effective cleaning of the dentures with the least possibility of damage to them.

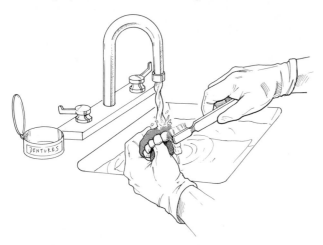

▼ **FIGURE 10–5.** Brushing the client's dentures.

8. Rinse the denture thoroughly and place it in a clean denture cup. A small amount of mouthwash may be used in the final soak.

8. Allows for removal of the cleansing agent. Provides for a pleasant taste when the dentures are replaced.

9. Using the same technique, brush the other denture.

10. If the client will not wear the dentures at this time due to sleep, surgery, procedures, or other reasons, soak the dentures in fresh water in the denture cup until they will be used. Mark outside of denture cup with client's name and room number.

10. Allows the dentures to remain moist. Provides a specific place for storage. Decreases the chance of lost dentures.

NOTE: Make sure the cup is labeled and placed where it will not accidentally be thrown away.

11. Provide the client with an emesis basin and a cup of warm water to rinse out his or her oral cavity. If appropriate, the client also may rinse with mouthwash.

11. Provides for the client's oral hygiene and comfort.

12. Using long, straight strokes with a soft nylon toothbrush, brush the client's oral mucosa (including the tongue) from the posterior to the anterior surfaces. If a toothbrush is not available, use gauze or a washcloth. Do not initiate the gag reflex.

12. Provides for the client's oral hygiene and comfort. The gag reflex is uncomfortable for the client and may precipitate vomiting.

▼ _ACTION_   ▼ _RATIONALE_

13. Massage the client's gums with the gloved fingers of your thumb and index finger. Use a press-and-release motion over the surfaces of the gum ridges and rub the hard palate with the end of your thumb, making sure your thumbnail does not cause trauma.

13. Promotes the increased circulation and toughening of the client's oral mucosa. This increases the health of the oral mucosa and denture-wearing comfort.

14. If the dentures are to be worn, carefully place them in their proper position in the client's mouth.

14. Provides for the client's comfort. Wearing dentures improves the client's eating technique, speech, mouth contour, and appearance.

15. Clean up the area.

15. Decreases the transmission of microorganisms and provides for a pleasing environment.

16. Remove the gloves and discard them in an appropriate container.

16. Decreases the transmission of microorganisms.

17. Wash your hands.

17. Decreases the transmission of microorganisms.

18. Record the procedure and other relevant information.

18. Communicates information to the other members of the health care team and contributes to the legal record by documenting the care given to the client.

Example of Documentation

DATE	TIME	NOTES
7/23/93	1000	Dentures cleaned. Oral mucosa pink, moist, and intact. No areas of irritation noted. Oral care given and dentures reinserted.

M. Moore, RN

(NOTE: Some agencies use a checklist for this procedure. Be sure to note any abnormal findings in your notes even if a checklist is used.)

Teaching Tips

Remind the client or the client's caregiver to be cautious when cleaning dentures to prevent breakage. Covering the bottom of the sink with a protective cover and keeping the hands low in the sink when cleaning are helpful.

Home Care Variations

The client's family should be taught the importance of the client's oral hygiene, including denture care. The importance of dentures for proper eating, facial structure, and appearance should be included in this discussion.

SKILL 10–3   PROVIDING EYE CARE FOR THE CLIENT WHO DOES NOT BLINK

Clinical Situations in Which You May Encounter This Skill

Clients who have lost the ability to blink due to various medical conditions such as coma, other neurologic disorders, and use of paralyzing medications need assistance to keep their eyes moist and prevent corneal abrasions, corneal ulcerations, and possible loss of vision. Eye care should be provided at least every 4 hours.

Anticipated Responses

▼ The client's eyes are moist and clear.
▼ No redness or corneal abrasions are noted.

Adverse Responses

▼ The client's eyes are dry, cloudy, or reddened.
▼ The client's eyes have corneal abrasions.

Materials List

Gather these materials before beginning the skill:

▼ Washcloth (one for each eye)
▼ Cotton balls (at least one for each eye)
▼ Bath towel
▼ Liquid tear solution or ointment (if ordered)
▼ Eye patch (if needed)
▼ Sterile gloves

▼ ACTION

1. Assess the client's eyes for abnormalities, including edema, inflammation, pain, secretions, lesions, and pupillary light response.

2. Review the client's chart for information concerning his or her eye care and condition.

3. Raise bed to working height.

4. Place a towel under the client's head.

5. Gently turn the client's head toward the side you will be treating.

6. Put on gloves using sterile technique.

7. Clean the client's eye by wiping with a wet, warm washcloth from the inner to the outer canthus. Do not use soap in the eye area. If crusting is present, place a warm, moist cotton ball over the eye until secretions are softened. This procedure may need to be repeated until the secretions are soft enough to remove without injury to the eye structures. Use separate washcloths and cotton balls for each eye.

8. Once the eye is clear of secretions, a liquid tear solution or an ointment may be instilled into the conjunctival sac or eye (see Skill 18–2).

9. Turn the client's head to the opposite side and repeat the procedure.

10. If the client's eyes remain open or appear dry and irritated even after the above procedure, the eyes may be closed gently and covered with a protective patch.

11. Remove your gloves and discard them in an appropriate container. Lower bed to lowest level.

▼ RATIONALE

1. Provides information for care.

2. Provides information for planning care.

3. Protects nurse from back injury.

4. Protects the linen from contamination.

5. Prevents cross-contamination of the eyes.

6. Decreases the transmission of microorganisms.

7. Follows the natural flow of tears for removal of debris from the eye. Warm water moistens dry secretions and facilitates easy removal. Prevents cross-contamination of the eyes.

9. Prevents contamination of the other eye.

10. Provides protection from corneal abrasions and ulcerations and possible loss of vision.

11. Decreases the transmission of microorganisms. Low position of bed promotes client safety.

▼ _ACTION_	▼ _RATIONALE_
12. Wash your hands.	**12.** Decreases the transmission of microorganisms.
13. Record the procedure.	**13.** Communicates to the other members of the health care team and contributes to the legal record by documenting the care given to the client.
14. Observe the client's eyes on a routine basis for anticipated and adverse responses.	**14.** Provides for optimal care.

Example of Documentation

DATE	TIME	NOTES
4/20/93	0930	Eye care completed with instillation of liquid tears in each eye. Both eyes clear and moist. No redness, swelling, or excessive tearing noted.
		L. Mead, RN

Teaching Tips

Explain the purpose of the eye care to the client or the client's family. If the family will be providing eye care at home, demonstrate the procedure for the family and allow an opportunity for a return demonstration.

Home Care Variations

Family members often care for clients who may need this procedure while at home. Proper understanding and teaching of this skill are important. Stress the importance of keeping eye medications sterile and the client's eyes moist, and observing for problems.

SKILL 10-4   TAKING CARE OF ARTIFICIAL EYES

Clinical Situations in Which You May Encounter This Skill

A client who has had an enucleation, or removal of the eyeball, will probably have an artificial eye. The prosthesis is made of either glass or plastic and is placed behind the eyelids. The artificial eye should be removed, cleaned, and replaced, or removed, cleaned, and stored. It can be stored in a sterile normal saline or distilled water solution.

Anticipated Responses

▼ The client's prosthesis is clean and intact.
▼ The client's eye socket and the area around it are clean and without redness, swelling, drainage, or irritation.

Adverse Responses

▼ The client's prosthesis is damaged.
▼ The client's eye socket and the area around it are reddened, swollen, draining, or irritated.

Materials List

Gather these materials before beginning the skill:

For cleansing of an artificial eye:

▼ Suction cup (optional) for eye removal
▼ Small clean basin
▼ Mild soap
▼ Clean tap water
▼ Towel
▼ Normal saline
▼ Gloves
▼ Case for eye (if appropriate)

For cleansing of an eye socket:

▼ Irrigating syringe with water or normal saline
▼ Gauze pad
▼ Washcloth
▼ Towel
▼ Gloves
▼ Any other materials that the client may use for this procedure

▼ ACTION

1. Determine the client's methods for cleansing the prosthesis and eye socket.

2. Assess the client's eyelids and socket for redness, swelling, drainage, and irritation.

3. Wash your hands and put on gloves. Raise the bed to working height.

4. Raise the client to a 45-degree angle.

5. Allow the client to remove the prosthesis or help the client to remove the prosthesis by:
   a. Lining a container with gauze and filling it with water.
   b. Pulling down and depressing the lower eyelid (Fig. 10–6).

▼ RATIONALE

1. Provides information for planning care.

2. Provides for early detection of an infection that could spread to surrounding tissue and structures.

3. Decreases the transmission of microorganisms. Raising the bed protects the nurse's back from injury.

4. Facilitates removal of the prosthesis.

5. The client should participate in his or her care as much as possible.
   a. Provides a protective cushion for the eye and prevents breakage.
   b. This is the least traumatic and most efficient way to remove the prosthesis.

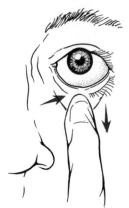

▼ **FIGURE 10–6.** Removing an artificial eye.

▼ *A C T I O N*   ▼ *R A T I O N A L E*

    c. Catching the prosthesis in your hand and placing it in the prepared container.

    d. If the prosthesis will not slide out, use a suction cup to remove it. Attach the suction cup to the prosthesis. Pull down the lower eyelid and use the handle of the suction cup to pull the prosthesis downward and out of the socket.

6. Allow the client to clean the prosthesis or place the prosthesis in a basin and wash it well with a washcloth, soap, and water.

7. Rinse the prosthesis well under running water.

8. Finally, rinse the prosthesis with normal saline.

9. If the prosthesis is to be stored, do so according to the client's or eye care specialist's directions (usually in sterile normal saline or distilled water solution).

10. Prior to reinserting the prosthesis, clean the client's eye socket area. Pull downward on the lower lid with your thumb and raise the upper lid with your index finger. Clean the socket by irrigating it with warm water or normal saline from the inner to the outer canthus or washing with a gauze pad soaked with saline or water (Fig. 10–7).

    c. Prevents accidental damage to prosthesis.

    d. Suction facilitates eye prosthesis removal.

6. Allows the client to participate in his or her care. Removes exudate and microorganisms.

7. Removes soap, which can be irritating to the eye socket.

8. Provides an isotonic solution around the prosthesis.

9. Helps to protect the prosthesis.

10. Decreases the microorganisms that can lead to infection and helps to provide for the client's comfort.

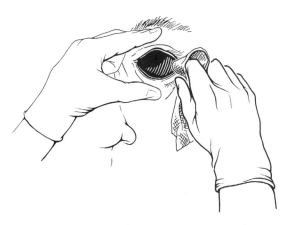

▼ **FIGURE 10–7.** Cleansing an empty eye socket.

11. Wash and dry the external eye well.

12. To reinsert the prosthesis, moisten it with water or normal saline.

13. Open the client's eye as described in Step 10.

14. The top portion of the prosthesis (usually marked) is placed under the upper eyelid.

11. Moisture can lead to the growth of microorganisms.

12. Lubricates the prosthesis and prevents traumatic insertion.

13. Exposes the client's eye socket.

14. Allows for proper placement.

▼ *ACTION*	▼ *RATIONALE*
15. Pull the lower eyelid down.	15. Allows the prosthesis to fall into the proper position under the lower eyelid.
16. Remove the gloves and dispose of them properly. Lower the bed to the lowest position.	16. Decreases the transmission of microorganisms. Lowering the bed promotes client safety.
17. Wash your hands.	17. Decreases the transmission of microorganisms.
18. Periodically, the prosthesis should be professionally cleaned and polished.	18. Removes dried protein secretions and provides for a more natural look.
19. Record the procedure and other relevant information.	19. Communicates information to the other members of the health care team and contributes to the legal record by documenting the care given to the client.

Example of Documentation

DATE	TIME	NOTES
9/24/93	1000	Eye prosthesis removed and cleaned with mild soap and water. Rinsed in normal saline prior to reinsertion. Eye socket clear, without redness, swelling, or drainage. No complaints of discomfort.
		S. White, RN

Teaching Tips

The client or the client's family may need to have the proper cleaning and storage techniques explained or reinforced. Emphasize to the family the necessity to report redness, swelling, drainage, or irritation.

Home Care Variations

The same procedure is used in the client's home to cleanse the socket and prosthesis.

SKILL 10–5 TAKING CARE OF CONTACT LENSES

Clinical Situations in Which You May Encounter This Skill

Contact lenses are small discs that are worn over the cornea of the eye to correct vision. There are two main types of contact lenses: hard lenses that are made of a nonpliable, nonabsorbent material, and soft lenses that are made of a plastic material that absorbs water, thereby becoming soft and pliable. There are three types of soft contact lenses: daily wear, which are removed daily for cleaning (as are hard contact lenses); extended wear, which are removed every 14 to 30 days for cleaning; and disposable lenses, which are discarded after use. Reusable soft lenses must be kept in a sterile saline solution when they are out of the eye or they will harden and crack.

Clients who are unable to remove their lenses because of an injury or other reasons need assistance in removing and cleaning their lenses. The lenses become dirty with wear. Cleaning is an important measure that assists in preventing infection and damage to the eyes. Insertion and cleaning procedures are similar for all types of lenses; however, it is important to use the cleaning and wetting solutions recommended by the lens manufacturer. The hands must be completely clean and free of oils, lotions, powder, and soaps when handling contact lenses in order to prevent contamination and damage to the lenses.

Anticipated Responses

▼ The client's lenses are removed intact, without obvious tears, chips, or cracks.
▼ The lenses are not dropped or lost.
▼ The lenses are cleaned, if proper solutions are available. If not, the lenses are stored in sterile normal saline.
▼ The outside of the case correctly identifies which contact is left and which is right.
▼ The case is marked correctly with identifying information.

Materials List

Gather these materials before beginning the skill:

▼ Cleaning kit specific for the type of contact lenses (if available)
▼ Sterile normal saline (usually unpreserved and specially developed for contact lenses)
▼ Storage case
▼ Examination gloves
▼ Tissues

Adverse Responses

▼ The client's lenses are torn, chipped, cracked, dropped, or lost during removal and storage.

▼ **ACTION**	▼ **RATIONALE**
1. If possible, discuss usual lens care with the client and gather necessary materials, if available.	1. Allows the client to participate in his or her care and assists in determining the required materials.
2. Assess the condition of the client's eyes prior to removal of the lenses. If there is an eye injury, do not remove the lenses, and document that the lenses are in place.	2. Removal can further damage an already injured eye. The eye specialist should be aware that the lenses are there and may be called on to remove them as part of the procedure.
3. Assess the ability of the client to clean his or her contacts.	3. The client may have physical or mental alterations that will prevent him or her from properly cleaning the contacts

Removing and cleaning lenses

4. Raise the bed to a comfortable working level.	4. Assists in preventing an injury to your back.
5. Open the storage case. Note which side is marked right and which is marked left. Place the case on a flat surface next to the client's bed.	5. Allows for the efficiency of the procedure. Assists in preventing a mix-up of lenses.
6. Do not touch the inside of the case.	6. Touching the inside of the case will lead to contamination.
7. Put on gloves.	7. Decreases the transmission of microorganisms.
8. Remove the lens from the client's right eye first.	8. Allows for the logical progression of the procedure.

Removing hard lenses

9. a. Observe the client's eye and determine if the lens is centered over the cornea. b. If not, center the lens by gently applying pressure on the lower eyelid and use it to nudge the lens into place.	9. a. Allows for the efficient removal of the lens. b. Centers the lens without discomfort.

▼ *ACTION* _ _ _ _ _ _ _ _ _ _ _ _ _ _ _ _ _ _   ▼ *RATIONALE* _ _ _ _ _ _ _ _ _

c. When the lens is centered, gently spread the eyelids apart so that they are above and below the rims of the lens (Fig. 10–8A).

c. Provides for efficient removal of the lens.

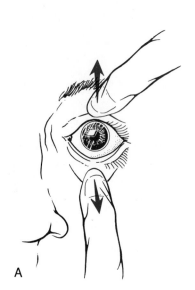
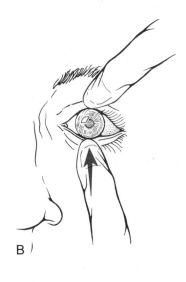
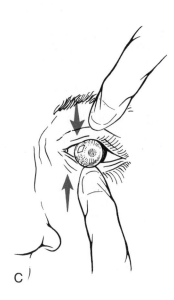

A   B   C

▼ **FIGURE 10–8.** Removing hard contact lenses.

d. Holding the upper eyelid in place, press the lower eyelid up under the bottom rim of the lens (Fig. 10–8B).

e. Once the lens loses its hold on the cornea and begins to tilt, move both eyelids toward each other (Fig. 10–8C).

f. Watch for the lens to drop out and intercept it with your lower hand.

g. Place the right lens in the storage container marked *R*.

h. Repeat steps 9a through 9g to remove the left lens.

d. Provides for the efficient removal of the lens with the least trauma to the eye.

f. Removes the lens without allowing it to become lost or contaminated.

g. Helps to prevent a mix-up of lenses on reinsertion.

Removing soft lenses

9. a. Pull down the client's lower eyelid with one hand (Fig. 10–9A).

9. a. Provides for efficient removal of the lens.

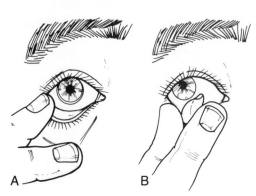

A   B

▼ **FIGURE 10–9.** Removing soft contact lenses.

▼ *ACTION*   ▼ *RATIONALE*

    b. Use gentle pressure on the top eyelid to move the lens partly onto the sclera.

    c. Using the pads of your thumb and the index finger of your lower hand, gently grasp the lens and remove it (Fig. 10–9*B*).

    d. Place the right lens in the storage container marked *R*.

    e. Repeat steps 9a through 9d to remove the left lens.

10. If materials for cleaning are available, clean the lens with cleaning solution and rinse well.

    b. Same as in 9a.

    c. Removes the lens without allowing it to become lost or contaminated.

    d. Helps to prevent a mix-up of lenses on reinsertion.

10. Provides for removal of microorganisms and debris from the lens.

NOTE: Clean only one lens at a time. Place the lenses in their respective sides of the storage case.   Prevents a mix-up of lenses when putting the lenses into the eyes.

---

11. If cleaning materials are unavailable, rinse the lens well with saline solution for soft lenses and water for hard lenses.

12. a. If the lenses are not reinserted into the client's eyes and are placed in a storage case, cover each lens completely with saline solution. Make sure the lenses stay centered in the case.

    b. Tightly close the lid on the case. Make sure the lid is not closed on the lens.

    c. Place the storage case on the client's bedside table or with the client's personal items. Make sure the client or a responsible family member knows where they are and chart the location of the lenses.

13. Remove gloves, if worn, and dispose of them properly.

14. Lower the bed to its lowest level and raise the side rails.

15. Assess the client's eyes for any damage or irritation.

11. Rinses off some debris.

12. a. Provides an isotonic medium for the lenses. Prevents them from drying out.

    b. Prevents spilling and evaporation of liquid.

    c. Provides for safe storage of lenses and helps prevent their loss.

13. Decreases the transmission of microorganisms.

14. Provides for the client's safety.

15. Provides information for planning care.

Inserting lenses

16. Remove each lens from its container and moisten with the appropriate wetting solution recommended by the manufacturer.

16. Dry lenses are uncomfortable and can damage the eye.

▼ *ACTION*   ▼ *RATIONALE*

17. Observe the lenses for damage and correct appearance (Fig. 10–10*A* and *B*).

17. Damaged lenses will damage the eye.

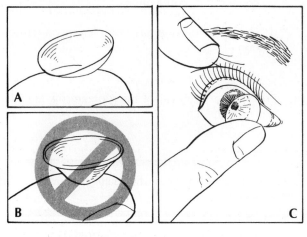

▼ FIGURE 10–10. Inserting soft contact lenses.

18. Place the lens on the index finger of your dominant hand.

19. Use your other hand to hold open the client's upper and lower eyelids. Ask the person to look straight ahead.

19. Stabilizes the eye structures for lens insertion.

20. Place the lens directly over the client's iris and pupil (Fig. 10–10*C*).

20. This is the proper lens position for use.

21. Release the client's eyelids and gently rub the upper lid with your finger to remove any air bubbles under the lens.

21. Facilitates proper lens placement.

22. Assess the patient's level of comfort. If the lens is uncomfortable, remove the lens, clean it, and reinsert it.

22. Discomfort may indicate that the lens is not clean.

23. Record the procedure and other relevant information.

23. Communicates information to the other members of the health care team and contributes to the legal record by documenting the care given to the client.

Example of Documentation

DATE	TIME	NOTES
6/10/93	1600	Contact lenses removed from both eyes. Placed in storage case with normal saline and then in the client's bedside drawer. Client's mother informed (by phone) of where contact lenses are. Eye assessment shows eyes to be clear, nonirritated, and without exudate. Client denies discomfort. Requests glasses be brought from home as "I'm blind as a bat without them."
		T. Reed, RN

Teaching Tips

Proper care and cleaning of contact lenses need to be stressed with clients who wear contact lenses. The continued health of the eye depends on this. The client should be told to stop wearing the contacts and notify his or her eye care specialist immediately if redness, excessive tearing, unusual or excessive exudate, vision changes, or eye discomfort is noticed. Corneal ulcers and other eye problems can develop rapidly.

Home Care Variations

The same technique can be used to care for contact lenses in the client's home.

SKILL 10–6   IRRIGATING THE EARS

Clinical Situations in Which You May Encounter This Skill

An ear irrigation provides for cleansing of the ear canal by flushing it with water or other solutions. The ear canal commonly has hardened cerumen (earwax) that inhibits visualization of the tympanic membrane or restricts hearing. A physician's order is usually required to irrigate the ear canal.

Anticipated Responses

▼ Secretions are removed from the client's ears.
▼ The client's hearing improves.
▼ The client's tympanic membrane remains intact and can be visualized.

Adverse Responses

▼ Secretions are not removed from the client's ears.
▼ The client's hearing does not improve or worsens.
▼ The client's tympanic membrane is perforated and the irrigating solution enters his or her middle ear.

Materials List

Gather these materials before beginning the skill:

▼ Emesis basin
▼ Appropriate solution
▼ Bath thermometer
▼ Bulb syringe
▼ 4- × 4-inch gauze dressing
▼ Towel
▼ Examination gloves
▼ Washcloth

▼ ACTION	▼ RATIONALE
1. Assess the client's pinna and meatus for redness, lesions, discharge, and pain. Use an otoscope to assess the client's ear canal and the integrity of the tympanic membrane.	1. Provides information on which to base care. Irrigation is contraindicated if the client's tympanic membrane is perforated.
2. Prepare approximately 500 ml of the solution.	2. This amount of solution is usually sufficient.
3. Warm the solution to 100° Fahrenheit.	3. Solutions that are not close to the client's body temperature can be uncomfortable and may cause injury, nausea, and vertigo.
4. Put on gloves. Raise the bed to working height.	4. Decreases the transmission of microorganisms. Raising the bed protects the nurse's back from injury.
5. Clean the client's outer ear and ear canal if necessary.	5. Prevents washing discharge into the ear canal.

▼ *ACTION*

▼ *RATIONALE*

6. Place a towel over the client and under the ear to be irrigated.

6. Protects the client's garments from getting wet.

7. Ask the client to turn his or her head so that the ear to be irrigated is facing downward.

7. Allows gravity to assist in removal of the earwax and solution.

8. Place an emesis basin below the client's ear and fill a bulb syringe with solution. The client may assist by holding the basin in position.

8. Prepares the area for the procedure. Allows for collection of the solution. Allows the client to participate in the procedure.

9. Straighten the adult client's ear canal by pulling the ear auricle up and back (or down and back for a child) (Fig. 10–11*A* and *B*).

9. Straightens the ear canal and allows access of the solution to the entire ear canal. The curves of the ear change with age.

10. Place just the tip of the bulb syringe inside the client's ear canal and gently squeeze the syringe. Direct a slow, steady stream of solution toward the upper wall of the ear canal (Fig. 10–11*C*). Use only enough force to remove secretions. (Do not close off the ear canal with the irrigating tip.)

10. Decreases injury to the client's ear canal and tympanic membrane. Decreases the possibility of pushing material farther into the ear. Too much force could cause the tympanic membrane to rupture. The in-and-out flow of solution prevents undue pressure in the ear.

11. After the irrigation, dry off the client's outer ear. Ask the client to lie on the affected side for a period of time. Place a gauze square under the client's ear.

11. Provides for the client's comfort. Allows the ear to finish draining. The gauze will collect any discharge from the ear.

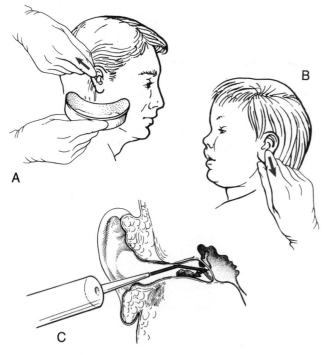

▼ **FIGURE 10–11.** Irrigating the ears.

12. Note any discharge obtained from the ear before discarding the solution.

12. Assists in diagnosis and treatment.

13. Clean up the area. Thoroughly clean and rinse the bulb syringe, and allow it to air-dry. Lower the bed to the lowest level.

13. Decreases the transmission of microorganisms and provides a pleasing environment. Lowering the bed promotes client safety.

14. Remove the gloves and discard them.

14. Decreases the transmission of microorganisms.

15. Wash your hands.

15. Decreases the transmission of microorganisms.

▼ *ACTION*	▼ *RATIONALE*
16. Assess the client's comfort.	**16.** Provides information on which to plan future client care.
17. Reexamine the client's ear with an otoscope.	**17.** Provides data for assessing the successfulness of the irrigation.
18. Record the procedure and other relevant information.	**18.** Communicates information to the other members of the health care team and contributes to the legal record by documenting the care given to the client.

Example of Documentation

DATE	TIME	NOTES
5/26/93	1100	Left ear irrigated with clear warm water. Approximately 1 cm yellow-brown wax obtained. Client states he can hear more clearly. Reexam shows ear canal to be clear and the eardrum intact. Light reflex seen, no redness or swelling of the tympanic membrane noted.

D. Lewis, RN |

Teaching Tips

If clients plan to irrigate their ears at home, be sure they understand that warm water must be used, the syringe should not be put far inside the ear canal, excessive force should not be used to irrigate, and any bleeding or pain should be reported immediately. Clients also need to be reminded not to put small objects into their ears.

Home Care Variations

An ear irrigation can be done in the client's home using the same procedure.

SKILL 10–7   TAKING CARE OF A HEARING AID

Clinical Situations in Which You May Encounter This Skill

Clients who wear hearing aids may need assistance in the care of their appliance while they are in the hospital. The hearing aid is delicate and requires special care to function properly. The following is general information about hearing aids:

▼ Keep a few extra batteries in a cool, dry place.
▼ Do not store a hearing aid in high temperatures.
▼ If a client lives in a humid climate, moisture is more likely to collect in the aid and cause problems.
▼ Keep the aid and its batteries out of the reach of young children and pets.

There are four basic types of hearing aids (Fig. 10–12): the body-worn aid, the eyeglasses aid, the behind-the-ear aid, and the in-the-ear aid.

Anticipated Responses

▼ The hearing aid is turned off when not in use.
▼ The aid is properly stored when not in use.
▼ The client wears the aid when appropriate.
▼ The aid is kept clean and in working order.

Adverse Responses

▼ The battery wears down because the hearing aid was left on when not in use.
▼ The aid is lost due to improper storage.
▼ The client misses interactions because the aid is not worn.
▼ The aid is dirty with earwax, which can plug up the earmold and interfere with hearing.

Materials List

Gather these materials before beginning the skill:

▼ Tissues
▼ Storage case for the hearing aid
▼ Washcloth
▼ Towel
▼ Soap
▼ Basin
▼ Otoscope

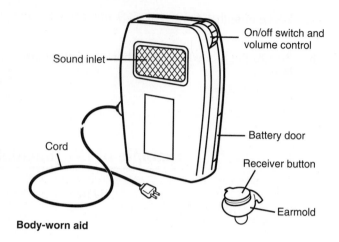

Body-worn aid

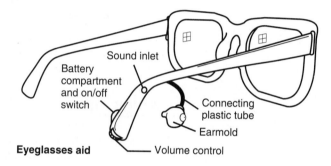

Eyeglasses aid

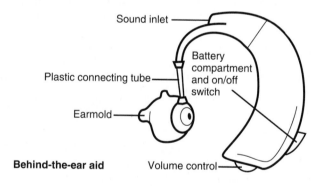

Behind-the-ear aid

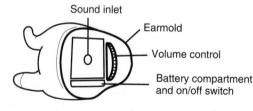

In-the-ear aid

▼ FIGURE 10–12. Hearing aids.

▼ *ACTION*   ▼ *RATIONALE*

1. Ascertain the number of hearing aids the client wears.	1. Provides information for the plan of care.
2. Ask the client how he or she usually cares for the aid or aids.	2. Helps to determine if the client is caring for the hearing aid properly.
3. Gently remove the hearing aid from the client's ear.	3. Prevents discomfort and damage to the client's outer ear.
4. Turn the aid off.	4. Saves the battery.
5. Wipe the aid with a dry tissue.	5. Aids must have earwax and moisture removed to prevent earwax plugs and the growth of bacteria in the aid.
6. Examine the aid for wax plugs, cracks, and twisting of the plastic tubing. Wax plugs that cannot be removed with the dry tissue and cracks need to be noted and the client's hearing specialist should be notified. Plastic tubing should be untwisted.	6. These will cause interference in the working ability of the aid. The hearing aid cannot conduct sound if the tubing is twisted.

NOTE: Never use water, alcohol, or cleaning fluids on a hearing aid. Do not use pipe cleaners or sharp objects to clean the aid.	Aids are not waterproof and can be permanently damaged. Sharp objects can make holes in the plastic aid.

7. Open the battery compartment of the hearing aid and remove the battery.	7. Removing the battery prevents damage to the hearing aid due to battery leaks.
8. Place the aid in its storage case and set it in the drawer of the client's bedside table.	8. Prevents accidental loss or damage of the aid.
9. With an otoscope, assess the client's ear canal for earwax, swelling, irritation, and discharge.	9. Provides information for the plan of care. Improperly cleaned aids may cause ear infections.

NOTE: If excessive earwax is noted, it should be recorded on the client's medical record and reported to the client's hearing specialist.	Earwax can interfere with hearing aid function. The specialist may have recommendations for treatment.

10. Ask the client if he or she has any ear discomfort and report pain promptly.	10. May indicate infection.
11. The client's ear should be gently washed with a clean washcloth and mild soap and warm water. Rinse and dry the ear well.	11. Removes microorganisms and earwax.

NOTE: Do not use cotton-tipped applicators to clean ears.	Packs earwax into the ear and creates a plug.

▼ *ACTION*	▼ *RATIONALE*
12. Prior to inserting the hearing aid: a. Close the battery compartment tightly.	a. Provides electrical power for the aid to function.
b. Cup the aid in one hand, turn the aid on, and adjust the volume to high. If it is working properly, the aid should whistle.	b. Provides feedback to determine proper functioning.
c. If the aid does not whistle, put in a new battery and test again.	c. Whistling may not occur because of an inadequate power source.
d. Check the tubing and untwist it if needed.	d. If the tubing is twisted, it interferes with sound transmission.
e. If the aid whistles, turn the aid off and gently insert it into the client's ear.	e. Prevents discomfort in the client's ear because of high volume.
f. Turn the aid on and adjust the volume for the client's hearing comfort.	f. Provides for the client's comfort and optimal hearing.
13. Record the procedure and other relevant information.	**13.** Communicates information to the other members of the health care team and contributes to the legal record by documenting the care given to the client.

Example of Documentation

DATE	TIME	NOTES
7/23/93	2100	Hearing aid removed, wiped with dry tissue, and placed in bedside table in storage case with aid off. Client's ear canal clear, tympanic membrane visualized with light reflex. *M. Allen, RN*

Teaching Tips

The client or a family member needs to understand the correct technique for cleaning and storing the hearing aid. Explain the necessity of keeping a few extra batteries on hand in a cool dry place. Since moisture can cause problems with the functioning of a hearing aid, advise the client not to go out in the rain without covering his or her head, and not to swim or shower with the hearing aid in place.

Home Care Variations

The same technique can be used to care for the hearing aid in the client's home.

SKILL 10–8   GIVING A COMPLETE BED BATH

Clinical Situations in Which You May Encounter This Skill

Clients who are unable to bathe themselves because of temporary or long-term physical or psychologic conditions need assistance with bathing. The bed bath provides an excellent opportunity for you to assess the client's physical condition and for the client to perform range-of-motion exercises. It also provides an opportunity for you to teach methods of self-care such as self–breast examination or self-testicular examination. Bathing usually is done at the same time the bed linens are changed. The client needs to be closely observed for fatigue, changes in vital signs, changes in the clinical condition, or a combination of these. Intermittent rest periods may be needed during the bathing procedure.

Anticipated Responses

▼ The client is clean and comfortable.

Adverse Responses

▼ The client may become chilled or overtired if appropriate care is not taken.

Materials List

Gather these materials before beginning the skill:

▼ Towels (at least three)
▼ Washcloths (at least two)
▼ Bath blanket or sheet
▼ Gown or other bed apparel
▼ Soap or other cleansing agent, soap dish
▼ Linen bag
▼ Bath basin
▼ Bath talc
▼ Other personal hygiene items such as deodorant and lotion
▼ Examination gloves

▼ _A C T I O N_

1. Review the client's chart to ascertain whether alterations in the procedure need to be implemented.

2. Position the client's bed at a comfortable working level.

3. Keep the side rail on the opposite side of the bed elevated. Put both side rails up when you are away from the bed.

4. Wash your hands and put on gloves.

5. Place a bath blanket over the client, and remove the top linens and discard them or fold them for reuse. Usually linens are changed during bathtime (Skill 10–16).

6. Position the client on the side of the bed closest to you and remove his or her gown. Keep the client covered with the bath blanket.

7. Fill the water basin one-half full of warm water (approximately 109–114° Fahrenheit [F]).

8. Remove the pillow from under the client's head and place a dry towel under his or her head.

9. Most of the bath is given with the washcloth folded into a mitt on your hand (Fig. 10–13).

▼ _R A T I O N A L E_

1. Some clinical conditions require rest periods or that certain positions be maintained.

2. Protects your back from strain.

3. Promotes the client's safety. The raised rail on the opposite side of the bed can be used by the client to assist in turning.

4. Decreases the transmission of microorganisms.

5. Protects the client's modesty. Decreases the transmission of microorganisms.

6. Enables you to reach the client more easily. Protects your back and promotes safety for you and the client.

7. Provides for the client's comfort and safety.

8. Prevents the pillow from getting wet. Protects the bottom linens from getting wet and the client from becoming chilled.

9. Prevents the wet cloth from dragging across the person's skin in an uncomfortable manner.

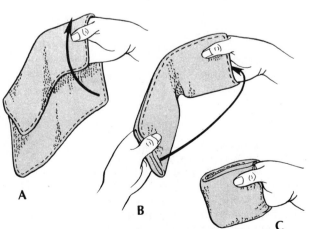

A   B   C

▼ **FIGURE 10–13.** Bath cloth mitt.

▼ *ACTION*

▼ *RATIONALE*

10. Throughout the bath, remember to obtain fresh water as needed.

10. Excessively cool or soapy water should be discarded.

11. Cleanse the client's face and neck:

a. Wet the washcloth. Using the wrung out washcloth, cleanse the client's eyes by wiping from the inner canthus toward the outer canthus of each eye (Fig. 10–14). Use opposite corners of the washcloth to cleanse each eye. Do not use soap to cleanse the eye area.

11. Working in a systematic manner allows for the most efficient and effective use of resources.
a. Follows the client's natural tear flow. Prevents the spread of microorganisms. Soap irritates and can burn the eyes.

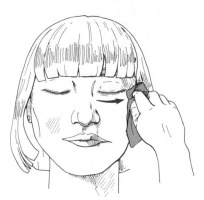

▼ **FIGURE 10–14.** Cleansing the eyes.

b. Rinse the washcloth and wash the client's forehead, cheeks, nose, and around his or her mouth.

b. Cleanses the skin.

c. Rinse the client well and dry him or her.

c. Removes the soap residue. Drying the client prevents chilling.

d. Rinse the washcloth and wash the client's outer ear.

d. Cleanses the ear. The ears should not be cleansed deeply, as the eardrum may be damaged.

e. Rinse the washcloth and wash the front and back of the client's neck.

e. Cleanses the client's neck.

12. Remove the bath towel from under the client's head and replace the pillow.

12. Prevents chilling. Provides for the client's comfort.

13. Place the bath towel under the client's entire arm. To cleanse the client's arms:
a. Wring out the washcloth and prepare the cloth with a cleansing agent.
b. With your nondominant hand, hold one of the client's arms up. Place a cloth mitt on your dominant hand, and cleanse up and down the client's arm with firm strokes, working from the anterior to the posterior arm. Make sure the total circumference of the client's arm is cleansed. Cleanse the axilla. Rinse these areas well and dry them. Cleanse the other arm and axilla.
c. After drying, remove the bath towel from under the client's arm. If it does not interfere with care, a small amount of deodorant may be used.

b. Cleanses the client's complete arm in a systematic way. Firm strokes create friction that removes debris and stimulates the client's circulation.

c. Provides for the client's comfort. Decreases chilling. Helps decrease body odor.

14. Cleanse the client's hands:

a. Place a bath towel under the basin and another towel beside the basin.

14. Decreases the transmission of microorganisms. Hands transmit many microorganisms.

▼ *ACTION* _____   ▼ *RATIONALE* _____

b. Place the client's hands in the basin and wash all of his or her hand surfaces well.

c. Place the client's hands on the towel to dry. If the person's fingernails need to be trimmed, do this now (see Skill 10–11).

    c. Soaking the nails before cutting them softens the nail and facilitates cutting.

d. Rinse the client's hands well and dry them with a bath towel.

15. Place the bath towel over the client's chest underneath the bath blanket and fold the bath blanket down to the client's lower abdomen for cleansing of his or her chest.

    15. Decreases chilling. Protects the client's modesty.

a. With your nondominant hand, hold one towel away from one side of the client's chest and wash the chest with firm strokes from top to bottom. Be sure to wash well under the client's breast.

    a. This area can become irritated easily and is a potential area for infection.

b. Rinse the client's chest well and dry it. Be sure the area under the client's breast is rinsed and dried well.

c. Cleanse the other side of the client's chest. Replace the towel over his or her chest between each step.

    b–c. You may wish to teach breast self-examination at this time.

d. If it does not interfere with care, a slight dusting of talc may be used under the breast area.

    d. Absorbs moisture.

NOTE: Clients with cardiac monitoring should not have talc or lotion applied to the chest area. | Decreases contact between electrodes and skin. May cause arcing of electrical current during cardioversion or defibrillation.

---

16. Leave the towel over the client's chest area and place another towel over his or her abdomen. Lower the bath blanket to the client's pubic area for cleansing of the abdomen.

    16. Decreases chilling. Protects the client's modesty. Allows for comfort. Decreases the transmission of microorganisms.

a. With your nondominant hand, lift the towel and with your dominant hand wash the client's abdomen with horizontal firm strokes. Be sure the area in and around the client's umbilicus is cleansed.

    a. Firm strokes decrease tickling. Decreases the potential for growth of microorganisms.

b. Rinse the client well and dry him or her.

c. Replace the bath blanket to the top of the client's shoulder and remove both towels from the client's torso.

    c. Decreases chilling and protects the client's modesty. Provides comfort. Decreases the transmission of microorganisms.

17. Cleanse the client's legs:

a. Place a towel lengthwise under the client's leg that is farthest from you. Raise the bath blanket covering that leg to the height of the inguinal fold.

    a. Protects the bed. Protects the client's modesty and decreases chilling.

b. Place the bath basin on a towel near the client's foot.

    b. Facilitates soaking the client's feet. The towel protects the bed from excessive wetting.

c. Using the appropriate arm, position your arm under the client's leg so that his or her heel will rest in your hand.

    c. Allows for movement of the client's leg with the least amount of strain on you and the client.

▼ *A C T I O N* ‾ ‾ ‾ ‾ ‾ ‾ ‾ ‾ ‾ ‾ ‾ ‾ ‾ ‾ ‾ ▼ *R A T I O N A L E* ‾ ‾ ‾ ‾ ‾ ‾ ‾

d. Slightly raise the client's leg and slide the basin into the proper position to place his or her foot into the basin of water (Fig. 10–15).

d. Allows for the most thorough cleansing of the client's feet. Provides for the client's comfort.

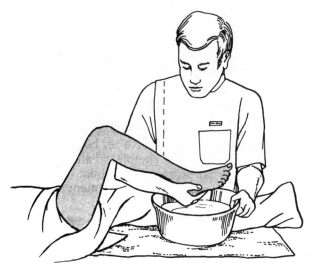

▼**FIGURE 10–15.** Cleansing the foot.

e. While continuing to support the client's leg, use your other hand with a washcloth to cleanse the client's leg. Use firm, lengthwise strokes to wash the circumference of the total leg. Also, wash the client's foot and toes.

f. Rinse the area well and dry it.

g. Remove the client's leg from the basin and place the leg on the bed. Repeat the procedure for the opposite leg. The client's toenails may be trimmed at this time if needed (see Skill 10–12).

e. Cleanses the client's leg. Firm strokes lessen tickling.

18. Remove the towel and reposition the bath blanket to cover the client's legs.

18. Protects the client's modesty. Decreases chilling. Provides for the client's comfort.

19. Help the client to assume a prone or side-lying position for cleansing of his or her back.

a. Position the bath blanket at the client's thighs. Place two towels horizontally across the client's back: one across the shoulders and one across the buttocks.

b. Use your nondominant hand to hold the towel away from the client's upper back as your dominant hand washes his or her back with a washcloth. Use firm, lengthwise strokes from the bottom of the client's neck to the top of his or her buttocks.

c. Rinse the client's back well, and dry him or her. Cover the client's back with a towel between steps.

d. A back rub may be given at this time (see Skill 11–1).

19. Enables you to cleanse the client's back.

a. Protects the client's modesty and prevents chilling.

d. Provides for the client's comfort.

▼ *ACTION* — — — — — — — — — — — — — — ▼ *RATIONALE* — — — — — — — — —

e. Cover the client's upper back with a towel. Using the same steps as above, cleanse his or her outer buttocks.

f. Wash, rinse, and dry the client's anal area. Discard this washcloth and towel.

g. Cover the client's back with the bath blanket up to his or her neck and remove the towels.

20. Help the client to assume a supine position.

21. Obtain a fresh washcloth and towel. Obtain fresh, warm water for cleansing of the client's perineal area. Allow the client to clean these areas, if possible. (If you need to cleanse these areas, see Skills 10–9 and 10–10).

22. Put a clean gown on the client. If combining a linen change with the bed bath, turn the client to a side-lying position facing away from you. Apply the clean gown to the upper side of his or her body. Change the linen on the side of the bed closest to you (see Skill 10–16). Next, turn the client onto the clean linen and put the other side of the gown on him or her. Then finish making the other side of the bed.

23. Lower the bed to the lowest level and raise the side rails. Place a call light and other articles, such as the telephone, within the client's reach.

24. Clean up the area.

25. Remove the gloves and wash your hands.

26. Assess the client's comfort.

27. Record the procedure and other relevant information.

e. Protects the client's modesty. Prevents chilling. Provides for the client's comfort.

f. This is the "dirtiest" area and should be washed last. Decreases transmission of microorganisms.

20. Provides for the client's comfort.

21. Decreases the transmission of microorganisms. Helps to protect the client's modesty.

22. This sequence of steps allows the gown to remain clean and in contact with only clean bed linens.

23. Provides for the client's safety.

24. Decreases the transmission of microorganisms.

25. Decreases the transmission of microorganisms.

26. Provides information for planning further client care.

27. Communicates information to other members of the health care team and contributes to the legal record by documenting the care given to the client.

Example of Documentation

DATE	TIME	NOTES
12/22/93	1000	Complete bed bath given. States she is tired and wants to rest. Skin clear, dry, warm to touch, and intact. No areas of redness noted.
		L. Lorna, RN

Teaching Tips

It is important for students to allow clients to take care of as much of their personal hygiene as possible yet provide assistance as needed for those clients who are unable to bathe themselves or should not bathe themselves. At times students need assistance in making these decisions.

Home Care Variations

For clients who are homebound with family members caring for them, hygiene needs are very important. Family members may need to be taught how to bathe another person and what things to observe. If the client will be confined to bed, renting or purchasing a hospital bed will facilitate care. This also will help protect the caregivers' backs.

SKILL 10–9 PROVIDING HYGIENIC CARE OF THE GENITALIA FOR THE MALE CLIENT

Clinical Situations in Which You May Encounter This Skill

Perineal care promotes comfort, prevents infection, eliminates odor, removes drainage and secretions, and fosters healing. Clients who are incontinent, have an indwelling catheter, or have had urinary tract or rectal surgery need perineal care. This procedure may be done as part of the client's bath. Perineal care may need to be given several times a day.

In some clinical settings, personal hygiene systems are available (e.g., Hygenique, Surgigator) for perineal care. These are used with a closed supply of running water and are generally used for ambulatory clients.

Anticipated Responses

▼ The client's genitalia are clean.
▼ There is no odor.
▼ There are no signs of irritation or infection.

Adverse Responses

▼ The genitalia have an odor.
▼ Infection, irritation, swelling, redness, or discharge is present.

Materials List

Gather these materials before beginning the skill:

▼ Bath blanket or sheet
▼ Towel
▼ Washcloths
▼ Bath basin
▼ Bath thermometer
▼ Soap or other cleansing agent
▼ Irrigating bottle (optional)
▼ Waterproof pads or other linen protectors
▼ Examination gloves

▼ ACTION

1. Assess the client's previous cleaning practices.

2. Assess the client's genital area for color, odor, lesions, masses, swelling, irritation, tenderness, and discharge.

3. Review the client's chart and physician's order for any additional perineal care needed.

4. Provide the client with the opportunity to empty his bladder and bowels prior to the procedure.

5. Raise the bed to a working height.

6. Fill a bath basin one-half full of warm bath water (approximately 105° Fahrenheit).

▼ RATIONALE

1. Provides information for planning care and client teaching.

2. Provides information for planning care.

3. Provides information for planning care.

4. Provides comfort.

5. Protects your back from injury.

6. Provides comfort.

▼ *ACTION*	▼ *RATIONALE*
7. Put on gloves.	**7.** Decreases the transmission of microorganisms.
8. If the procedure is to be done in bed, replace the client's top sheet with a bath blanket and fanfold the sheets to the end of the bed. If the client's genital area is to be irrigated, place the client on a bedpan.	**8.** Protects the bed linens from becoming wet and promotes privacy.
9. Properly drape the client with a bath blanket.	**9.** Provides comfort and protects the client's modesty.
10. Help the client to spread his legs apart.	**10.** Provides adequate exposure of the area to be cleansed.
11. With a wet, warm, soapy washcloth, thoroughly wash the client's penis and scrotum (Fig. 10–16). Start at the tip of the penis at the urethral meatus and cleanse in a circular pattern. Next cleanse from the tip of the penis toward the scrotum. In an uncircumcised man, retract the foreskin (prepuce) and cleanse the penis as described above. Thoroughly yet gently cleanse the scrotum. Lift the penis and scrotum and wash back toward the anus.	**11.** Allows for the flow of dirt and microorganisms away from the client's body and from the urinary meatus (cleanest area) to the anal area (dirtiest area). Washing from clean to dirty areas prevents the spread of microorganisms. Removes smegma and other irritants that can cause pain and infection.

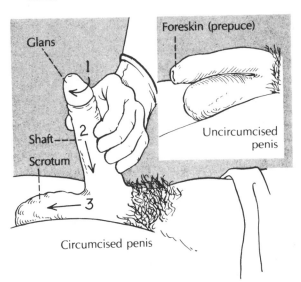

▼ **FIGURE 10–16.** Cleansing the male genitalia.

> **NOTE:** Excessive pressure on the testicles in the scrotum is painful.

Erection of the penis may occur. Cessation of cleansing usually results in loss of the erection.	Erection is a normal response to stimulation of the glans. Explaining this to the client in a matter-of-fact way may help to lessen any embarrassment he may feel.
12. Thoroughly rinse the area with clean, warm water using a clean washcloth or flush with an irrigation bottle. Be sure to rinse in the same direction as the washing was done. Dry carefully in the same direction.	**12.** Allows for removal of dirt and microorganisms that can cause odor, skin irritation, and infection. Moisture provides a good medium for the growth of bacteria.

▼ *ACTION*	▼ *RATIONALE*
The foreskin of the uncircumcised man must be pulled back into place over the glans penis after rinsing.	A foreskin that is not placed back over the glans penis will constrict the penis and may cause edema and pain.
13. Turn the client on his side, drape the buttocks area, and cleanse and dry the anal area using strokes from front to back.	13. Decreases the transmission of microorganisms and helps to promote comfort. Moisture provides a good medium for the growth of bacteria.
14. Remove the soiled linens and replace the top sheets. Lower the bed to the lowest level and raise the side rails.	14. Decreases the transmission of microorganisms. Helps to promote safety.
15. Clean up the area and the bedpan.	15. Decreases the transmission of microorganisms.
16. Remove the gloves and properly discard them.	16. Decreases the transmission of microorganisms.
17. Wash your hands.	17. Decreases the transmission of microorganisms.
18. Assess the client's comfort.	18. Provides information for planning further client care.
19. Record the procedure and other relevant information.	19. Communicates information to the other members of the health care team and contributes to the legal record by documenting the care given to the client.
20. Periodically evaluate the effectiveness of the procedure by examining the client's genital area as in step 2.	20. Provides information in order to plan appropriate care.

Example of Documentation

DATE	TIME	NOTES
5/1/93	1030	Genital area cleansed. No irritation, odor, swelling, discharge, or lesions noted. Client denies any discomfort.
		T. Graham, RN

Teaching Tips

Clients who are uncircumcised or the parents of children who are uncircumcised may need instruction about retracting the foreskin to clean under it and replacing the foreskin back over the glans penis.

Home Care Variations

The same procedure can be used to provide perineal care in the client's home.

SKILL 10–10   PROVIDING HYGIENIC CARE OF THE GENITALIA FOR THE FEMALE CLIENT

Clinical Situations in Which You May Encounter This Skill

Perineal care promotes comfort, prevents infection, eliminates odor, removes drainage and secretions, and fosters healing. Clients who have had various gynecologic procedures such as vaginal or cesarean delivery, vaginal hysterectomy, or other operations in the perineal area; are incontinent; or have an indwelling catheter need good perineal care. This procedure may be done as part of the client's bath. Perineal care may need to be given several times a day for clients in the postpartum period or clients experiencing incontinence or drainage.

In some clinical settings, personal hygiene systems are available for perineal care. These are used with a closed supply of running water and are generally used for ambulatory clients.

Anticipated Responses

▼ The client's genital area is clean.
▼ There is no odor.
▼ There are no signs of irritation or infection.

Adverse Responses

▼ The client's genitalia have an odor.
▼ Signs of infection, irritation, swelling, redness, or abnormal discharge are present.

Materials List

Gather these materials before beginning the skill:

▼ Bath blanket or sheet
▼ Towel
▼ Washcloths
▼ Irrigating bottle
▼ Cleansing solution
▼ Bath thermometer
▼ Bedpan (if the procedure is done in bed)
▼ Cotton balls and forceps (optional)
▼ Examination gloves
▼ Sanitary pad and belt (if needed)

▼ ACTION

1. Assess the client's previous genital cleansing practices.

2. Assess the client's genital area for color, odor, lesions, masses, swelling, irritation, tenderness, and discharge.

3. Review the client's chart and physician's order for any additional perineal care needs such as irrigation.

4. Provide the client with the opportunity to empty her bladder and bowels prior to the procedure.

5. Raise the bed to a working height.

6. Fill an irrigating bottle with warm (about 105° Fahrenheit) soapy water or cleansing solution. Two irrigating bottles may be needed, or the bottle may need to be refilled if the solution is to be rinsed.

7. Put on gloves.

▼ RATIONALE

1. Provides information for planning care and client teaching.

2. Provides information for planning care.

3. Provides information for planning care.

4. Provides for the client's comfort.

5. Helps prevent strain on your back.

6. Provides comfort and prevents tissue injury from water that is too hot.

7. Decreases the transmission of microorganisms.

▼ *ACTION*   ▼ *RATIONALE*

8. If the procedure is to be done in bed, replace the client's top sheet with a bath blanket. Place the bath blanket in a diamond configuration over the client and wrap the corners around the client's legs. Lift the lower corner up to expose the client's perineal area (Fig. 10–17). Fanfold the bed linens to the end of the bed.

8. Provides comfort. Helps with time and equipment management. Provides the client with a sense of modesty and dignity.

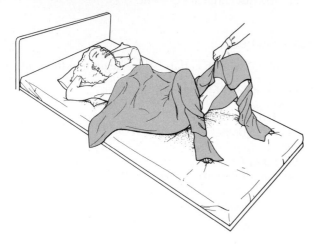

▼ **FIGURE 10–17.** Draping for hygienic care of the female genitalia.

9. Assist the client onto a bedpan.

9. Provides a solution-collecting device.

10. Help the client to spread her legs apart, and separate her labia with your nondominant hand.

10. Provides adequate exposure of the area.

11. Use your dominant hand to pour cleansing solution from front to back over the client's genital area (Fig. 10–18).

11. Allows for the flow of dirt and microorganisms away from the area of fewer organisms (urinary meatus) to the area of more organisms (anal area).

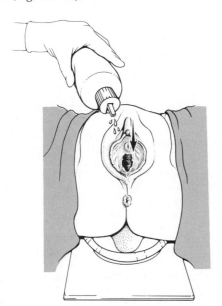

▼ **FIGURE 10–18.** Cleansing the female genitalia with solution.

▼ *ACTION* _ _ _ _ _ _ _ _ _ _ _ _ _ _   ▼ *RATIONALE* _ _ _ _ _ _ _ _ _ _ _ _ _

12. If flushing does not cleanse the area well, cotton balls or a warm wet washcloth may be used to gently wash the area from front to back beginning from the urethra to the vagina. Then wash each side of the labia (Fig. 10–19). Use a separate cotton ball or a different part of the washcloth for each wipe.

12. Allows for removal of dirt and microorganisms that can cause odor, skin irritation, and infection. Decreases the transmission of microorganisms.

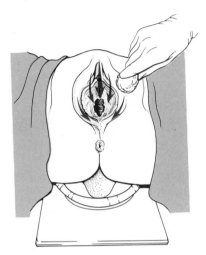

▼ **FIGURE 10–19.** Cleansing the female genitalia with cotton balls.

> **NOTE:** Be sure all skin folds are clean. Use extra washcloths if needed.

13. Rinse the client's genital area and dry from front to back with cotton balls, a dry washcloth, or a towel.

13. Some solutions can be irritating to the skin. Rinsing also provides comfort. Moisture provides a good medium for the growth of bacteria.

14. Remove the bedpan, turn the client on her side, drape the buttocks, and clean and dry the anal area by wiping from front to back.

14. Provides comfort. Decreases the transmission of microorganisms.

15. Help the client to apply a sanitary pad and belt, if needed.

15. Provides comfort. Decreases the transmission of microorganisms. The sanitary pad will collect any drainage the client may have after surgery or delivery.

16. Remove the soiled linens and replace the top sheets.

16. Decreases the transmission of microorganisms.

17. Lower the bed to the lowest level and raise the side rails.

17. Provides comfort and safety.

18. Clean up the area and bedpan.

18. Decreases the transmission of microorganisms.

19. Remove the gloves and properly discard them.

19. Decreases the transmission of microorganisms.

20. Wash your hands.

20. Decreases the transmission of microorganisms.

21. Assess the client's comfort.

21. Provides information for optimal client care.

▼ *ACTION*	▼ *RATIONALE*
22. Record the procedure and other relevant information.	**22.** Communicates information to the other members of the health care team and contributes to the legal record by documenting the care given to the client.
23. Periodically evaluate the effectiveness of the procedure by examining the client's genital area as in Step 2.	**23.** Provides information in order to plan appropriate care.

Example of Documentation

DATE	*TIME*	*NOTES*
5/1/93	1030	Perineal care with plain tap water completed. Genital area slightly reddened. No odor, swelling, discharge, or lesions noted. Client denies pain.
		D. Shipley, RN

Teaching Tips

Many clients are unaware of the importance of cleansing the genital area in a front-to-back direction. This should be strongly reinforced even for young girls.

Home Care Variations

The same technique can be used to provide perineal care in the client's home.

SKILL 10–11   TAKING CARE OF THE HANDS

Clinical Situations in Which You May Encounter This Skill

Clients may need assistance in caring for their fingernails. Nail care helps to prevent infection, stimulate circulation, and promote good hygiene.

Anticipated Responses

▼ The client's fingernails are clean, dry, and intact, without rough edges.
▼ The client's fingernails are approximately the same length as the end of the fingers.

Adverse Responses

▼ The client's fingernails have splits or tears.
▼ The client's fingernails have fungal growth beneath them.

Materials List

Gather these materials before beginning the skill:

▼ Basin
▼ Towels
▼ Washcloth
▼ Waterproof pads (two)
▼ Soap or other cleansing agent
▼ Orange stick
▼ Emery board
▼ Nail clippers (In some agencies a physician's order is needed to trim fingernails.)
▼ Nail scissors
▼ Lotion
▼ Gloves (if needed)

▼ *A C T I O N*

▼ *R A T I O N A L E*

1. Assess the condition of the client's fingernails, especially the nail color, integrity of the nails and cuticles, and angle of the nails.

2. Help the client to assume an upright position unless contraindicated.

3. Cover the bed linen with waterproof pads.

4. Place a towel on top of the client's bedside table and position the table over the client's lap.

5. Fill the basin one-half full with warm water (approximately 100° Fahrenheit).

6. Place the preferred amount of cleansing agent into the water in the basin and place the basin on the overbed table.

7. Have the client soak his or her fingers in the basin for 10 to 15 minutes. During this time, other grooming may be done, such as combing hair, soaking feet, and other bathing.

8. Put on gloves.

9. Remove the client's hands from the basin and let them rest on a towel while the basin is emptied and refilled.

10. Rinse the client's hands and dry them thoroughly with a clean, dry cloth.

11. Take one of the client's hands and use an orange stick to gently clean under each fingernail.

12. Using a washcloth or the rounded edge of an orange stick, gently push each cuticle back.

---

1. Provides information from which to plan care. Clients with circulatory and respiratory problems may require special care.

2. Allows for the most effective execution of the procedure.

3. Helps to prevent the linen from getting wet.

4. The towel helps to prevent the basin from slipping. Having the bath basin over the client's lap facilitates soaking of the client's hand.

5. This temperature is generally comfortable and soothing.

6. Promotes cleaning.

7. Soaking loosens dirt and softens nails, which makes the rest of nail care easier. Provides for the most efficient use of time.

8. Decreases the transmission of microorganisms.

9. Decreases the transmission of microorganisms. Clean water will be needed for rinsing.

10. Decreases the potential for bacterial growth.

11. Removes dirt and debris that could lead to an infection.

12. Helps prevent hangnails.

NOTE: Hangnails should be trimmed carefully with nail scissors.　　　　　Prevents trauma to the cuticle.

---

13. Using nail scissors or nail clippers, cut the fingernails straight across so that the length is just at the fingertip (Fig. 10–20).

13. Prevents trauma to the cuticle and skin.

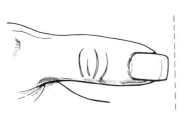

▼ **FIGURE 10–20.** Trimming the client's fingernails.

▼ _ACTION_	▼ _RATIONALE_
14. Use an emery board to smooth the edges and slightly round the corners of each fingernail.	**14.** Prevents snags.

> **NOTE:** Do not trim the nail into the side of the fingers.

15. Perform the same procedure on the client's other hand.	
16. Using lotion, massage from the fingertips to the wrists.	**16.** Moisturizes, protects, and softens the client's skin. Provides comfort.
17. Assist the client into a comfortable position.	**17.** Promotes comfort.
18. Clean up the area.	**18.** Decreases the transmission of microorganisms.
19. Remove the gloves and dispose of them properly.	**19.** Decreases the transmission of microorganisms.
20. Wash your hands.	**20.** Decreases the transmission of microorganisms.
21. Record the procedure and other relevant information.	**21.** Communicates information to the other members of the health care team and contributes to the legal record by documenting the care given to the client.

Example of Documentation

DATE	TIME	NOTES
7/27/93	1100	Hand/nail care given. Nails and hands are clear, clean, and intact. Nails trimmed and smoothed to fingertip length. Skin color is pink.
		K. Smith, RN

Teaching Tips

Emphasize to the client's family that clients who are bedridden should have their fingernails cared for and kept carefully trimmed to prevent unintentional injury to their skin.

Home Care Variations

The same procedure can be used to provide nail care in the client's home.

SKILL 10–12   PROVIDING FOOT CARE

Clinical Situations in Which You May Encounter This Skill

Clients may need assistance to care for their feet. Foot care is given for hygienic purposes, to prevent lesions to the feet, to promote circulation, and to treat diseases or problems of the feet.

Anticipated Responses

▼ The client's feet are clean, dry, and without odor or discoloration.
▼ The client's skin integrity is intact.
▼ There are no fungal growths.
▼ The client's toenails are cut straight across and are not ingrown.

Adverse Responses

▼ The client's skin integrity is compromised.
▼ There are fungal growths as in athlete's foot.
▼ The client's toenails are uncut and are too long or are cut too short.
▼ The client's toenails are ingrown.

Materials List

Gather these materials before beginning the skill:

▼ Basin
▼ Towels
▼ Washcloth
▼ Waterproof pad
▼ Soap or other cleansing agent
▼ Orange stick
▼ Emery board
▼ Nail clippers (In many agencies nurses do not clip nails or must have a physician's order to do so. Check your agency policy.)
▼ Lotion
▼ Bath powder (optional—for clients who have foot moisture)
▼ Examination gloves

▼ ACTION	▼ RATIONALE
1. Assess the reason for foot care and if the client has any underlying medical conditions that impede circulation. Specifically note areas of inflammation, lesions, edema, temperature changes, hair distribution, and texture of skin. Assess the nails for color, shape, length, texture, and capillary refill.	1. Provides information for planning care. Some conditions may require special foot care by a physician.
2. Help the client to assume a Fowler's position and place a waterproof pad under his or her feet. If the client cannot sit up, help the client to assume a comfortable position in which foot care can be given.	2. Allows for the most effective execution of the procedure. The waterproof pad will protect the client's bed linen.
3. Fill a basin one-half full with warm water (approximately 100° Fahrenheit).	3. This temperature is generally comfortable and soothing.
4. Place a cleansing agent into the water in the basin.	4. Promotes cleaning.
5. Put on gloves.	5. Decreases the transmission of microorganisms.
6. Have the client soak his or her feet in the basin for 10 to 15 minutes. During this time, other grooming may be done, such as combing the hair, soaking the fingernails, and other bathing.	6. Soaking loosens dirt and softens nails, which makes the rest of foot care easier. Provides for the most efficient use of time.
7. Use a washcloth to rub callused and dirty areas.	7. Friction helps with removal of debris.

NOTE: Avoid friction over open skin areas.   May cause trauma.

▼ *ACTION*   ▼ *RATIONALE*

8. Remove the client's washed feet from the soapy water and place them on a towel.

8. Allows the water to be changed.

9. Clean underneath the client's toenails with an orange stick.

9. Removes debris.

10. Fill the basin with fresh water and rinse the client's feet well and dry them thoroughly with a clean dry towel.

10. Allows for removal of soap and dirt. Drying decreases the potential for bacterial growth.

11. Trim the client's toenails straight across with toenail clippers (Fig. 10–21).

11. Decreases trauma. Helps prevent the formation of ingrown toenails.

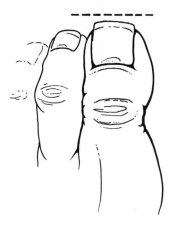

▼ **FIGURE 10–21.** Trimming the client's toenails.

> **NOTE:** Do not cut into the sides of toenails or cut too close to the skin.

12. Using an emery board, smooth the rough edges.

12. Prevents snagging of the nails.

> **NOTE:** In some agencies, nurses do not trim nails. Get a physician's order to trim the client's nails or get a podiatrist's consult for clients with circulatory disorders or diabetes mellitus.

If injuries result, the client may get an infection that may not heal.

13. With lotion, massage the client's feet by starting at the heels of each foot and working toward the toes.

13. Softens the skin. Helps the skin remain a more effective barrier to infection. Comforts the client.

> **NOTE:** Use firm pressure to avoid tickling and give special attention to reddened areas. Range-of-motion foot exercises may be done at this time.

Helps prevent footdrop.

▼ *A C T I O N*	▼ *R A T I O N A L E*
14. Help the client to assume a comfortable position.	**14.** Provides comfort.
15. Clean up the area.	**15.** Decreases the transmission of microorganisms.
16. Remove gloves and dispose of them properly.	**16.** Decreases the transmission of microorganisms.
17. Wash your hands.	**17.** Decreases the transmission of microorganisms.
18. Record the procedure and other relevant information.	**18.** Communicates information to the other members of the health care team and contributes to the legal record by documenting the care given to the client.

Example of Documentation

DATE	*TIME*	*NOTES*
8/8/93	1000	Foot care given. Skin pink, clear, dry, and intact.
		C. Durr, RN

Teaching Tips

Clients and their families need to be aware of the importance of good foot care and the consequences of neglecting it. Families should be taught how to properly trim the client's nails straight across. Diabetic clients especially need proper foot care to avoid complications.

Home Care Variations

Foot care can be provided in the client's home using the same procedure.

SKILL 10–13 PROVIDING HAIR CARE

Clinical Situations in Which You May Encounter This Skill

An ill client may need assistance with hair care. Hair care helps the client to feel refreshed and well groomed. The hair should be combed and brushed at least daily.

Clients who are confined to bed for periods of time need to have their hair washed. The hair should be washed at least every 4 to 7 days or as needed.

Anticipated Responses

▼ The client's hair is clean, dry, shiny, and untangled.
▼ The client's scalp is intact and without pediculosis or rashes.

Adverse Responses

▼ The client's scalp integrity is compromised.
▼ The client's scalp shows pediculosis or irritation.

Materials List

Gather these materials before beginning the skill:

▼ Towels (at least two)
▼ Washcloth
▼ Waterproof pads (four)
▼ Pitcher
▼ Shampoo board
▼ Shampoo
▼ Hair conditioner (if needed)
▼ Large-toothed comb (especially for long hair)
▼ Hairbrush
▼ Bucket or other water collector
▼ Hair dryer (if needed or available)
▼ Examination gloves

▼ A C T I O N	▼ R A T I O N A L E
1. Assess the condition of the client's hair and scalp.	1. Provides information for planning care. Clients may have conditions such as lice, dandruff, or an oily or dry scalp that require special shampoos.

Brushing and combing the hair

2. Obtain a clean brush and a wide-toothed comb. If necessary, clean the brush and comb in hot soapy water.	2. Brushing and combing the hair helps a person feel well groomed.
3. Raise the bed to working height. Cover the client's shoulders with a towel.	3. Raising the bed reduces back strain. Catches loose hair.
4. Divide the hair into sections. Brush or comb the sides of the client's head first. Then brush or comb the back (Fig. 10–22).	4. Facilitates grooming of the entire head.

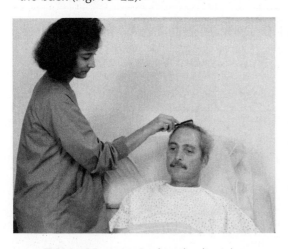

▼ FIGURE 10–22. Combing the client's hair.

5. Remove tangles by taking a small section of the tangled hair and working from the ends of the hair toward the scalp with a brush or wide-toothed comb. Application of water, vinegar, or hydrogen peroxide or conditioners to matted areas may help in removing tangles.	5. Reduces pulling and hair breakage.

▼ *ACTION* _____   ▼ *RATIONALE* _____

6. Braiding the long hair of the bedridden client may prevent future tangles. Braid the hair loosely in two or more braids. Avoid a braid at the back of the head.

6. Tight braids are uncomfortable. A single braid at the back of the head places pressure on the scalp and is uncomfortable.

Special considerations for clients with very curly hair

7. Divide the hair into small sections and brush it to remove tangles.

7. Small sections facilitate brushing hair.

8. Comb each section of hair. Work from the ends to the root of the hair shaft.

8. Prevents damage to hair and discomfort to client.

9. If the client's hair is dry, oil or petroleum jelly may be applied at the base of the hair shaft.

9. Lubricates dry hair.

10. A pick may be used in styling very curly hair. Use the pick to lift the hair away from the scalp. Then gently pat the hair to achieve a smooth rounded contour.

10. Facilitates styling hair.

Hair care for the man with a mustache and beard

11. Comb male facial hair daily using a mustache comb or regular hair comb.

11. Combing facial hair makes a person feel well groomed.

12. Periodically the beard and mustache should be shampooed with a mild shampoo.

12. Mild shampoo prevents dry skin.

Shampooing the hair of a client in bed

13. Position the bed at a comfortable level.

13. Prevents injury to your back.

14. Fill a pitcher with warm (about 110° Fahrenheit) water. Two pitchers may be needed, or the pitcher may be refilled as needed.

14. Provides comfort.

15. Lay the bed flat and position the client's head at the top of the bed.

15. Having the head of the bed flat helps to prevent water from flowing down toward the rest of the bed.

16. Place waterproof pads under the client on the top half of the bed.

16. Protects the linen from getting wet.

17. Put on gloves if the client has a condition such as pediculosis.

17. Decreases the transmission of microorganisms.

▼ *ACTION*   ▼ *RATIONALE*

18. Place a shampoo board under the client's head and position it so the client is comfortable and so the shampoo board will drain into a bucket (Fig. 10–23). A small plastic trash basket also can be used.

18. Prevents water from getting on the floor. Protects the client's eyes.

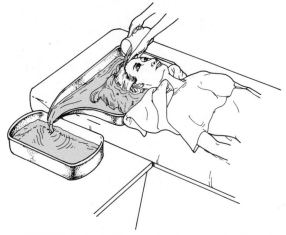

▼ **FIGURE 10–23.** Shampooing the client's hair in bed.

19. Place a bucket on an overbed table or chair and position it beneath the drain on the shampoo board.

19. The bucket needs to be positioned lower than the board in order to collect the used water.

20. Place a washcloth over the client's eyes.

20. Helps to protect the client's eyes from shampoo.

21. Carefully pour water over the client's hair until it is thoroughly wet.

21. Wet hair will help to suds the shampoo.

22. Once the hair is wet, apply a small amount of shampoo and work up a general lather.

22. Provides a chemical and mechanical action that will facilitate cleansing.

23. Starting at the anterior hairline and working toward the posterior hairline, massage all portions of the client's scalp and soap all hair.

23. Provides a systematic approach so that all hair is cleaned. Massaging stimulates circulation to the scalp.

24. With fresh warm water, rinse the hair well. Comb through the hair with your fingers and repeatedly rinse the hair until it is clean.

24. Removes all soap residue.

25. Apply conditioner (if needed).

25. Causes the hair to be more manageable.

26. Squeeze excess water from the hair.

26. Helps the hair to dry faster.

27. Wrap a bath towel around the client's head and remove the washcloth from the client's eyes.

27. Absorbs excess water.

28. Remove the towel and gently comb through the client's hair starting at the ends and working toward the scalp.

28. Removes tangles.

29. Use a hair dryer to thoroughly dry the client's hair, if possible.

29. Increases the client's comfort. Prevents chilling. Provides safety.

NOTE: All electrical equipment should be checked by maintenance personnel and should be grounded properly when in use.

▼ *ACTION*	▼ *RATIONALE*
30. Comb and style the client's hair.	**30.** Removes tangles and provides comfort and attractiveness.
31. Remove wet linens and change the client's clothes if they are wet or damp.	**31.** Decreases the transmission of microorganisms and promotes comfort.
32. Lower the bed to the lowest level and raise the side rails.	**32.** Promotes the client's safety.
33. Clean up the area, properly dispose of the bucket contents, and rinse and store the shampoo board.	**33.** Decreases the transmission of microorganisms.
34. Remove gloves if used and dispose of them properly.	**34.** Decreases the transmission of microorganisms.
35. Wash your hands.	**35.** Decreases the transmission of microorganisms.
36. Evaluate the client's comfort.	**36.** Provides information for planning further client care.
37. Record the procedure and other relevant information.	**37.** Communicates information to the other members of the health care team and contributes to the legal record by documenting the care given to the client.

Example of Documentation

DATE	TIME	NOTES
7/30/93	1400	Hair washed. Scalp integrity intact.
		B. Perry, RN

Teaching Tips

The importance of keeping the client's hair clean should be explained to the client's family. If necessary, provide a demonstration of the procedure for the family.

Home Care Variations

Improvisations with the equipment may be necessary at the client's home or the equipment may be rented from medical supply stores. The mattress should be well protected to prevent damage.

SKILL 10–14   SHAVING A CLIENT

Clinical Situations in Which You May Encounter This Skill

Shaving is most often done to remove male facial hair. Some areas of the female anatomy such as the axilla and legs may be shaved according to cultural practices. You may shave the client's arm hair before taping on an intravenous line to ease later removal of the tape. Chest hair may be shaved under electrocardiogram electrodes to enhance conduction. Finally, some areas of the body may be shaved prior to some types of operations.

This skill describes the steps of shaving the male client's facial hair; however, these principles may be applied to other situations that require shaving. Male clients who are unable to perform this type of grooming due to a mental impairment, paralysis, a cardiac condition, burns, or other limitations need to be shaved on a daily basis.

Anticipated Responses

▼ The client has a neat appearance and increased comfort.

Adverse Responses

▼ There are alterations in the client's skin integrity.

Materials List

Gather these materials before beginning the skill:

▼ Straight razor with new blade, disposable razor, or electric razor
▼ Shaving cream or soap (for straight razor)
▼ Washcloth
▼ Bath towel
▼ Washbasin
▼ After-shave or lotion (be sure to check whether the client has allergies to these and, if possible, client preference)
▼ Mirror

▼ ACTION

1. Assess whether the client is able to shave himself.

2. If the client can shave, set up the needed materials. Change the water as needed and observe for safety hazards.

3. If the client is not able to assist, ask him the steps he uses when shaving.

4. Raise the bed to working height. Help the client to assume a high-Fowler's or semi-Fowler's position unless these positions are contraindicated.

5. Place a bath towel over the client's chest and around both of his shoulders.

6. Fill the washbasin with water that is approximately 110° Fahrenheit (F) (43–44° Celsius [C]).

7. Wash your hands.

8. Place a washcloth in the basin with the water, wring it out thoroughly, and place the washcloth over the client's face with his nose and eyes uncovered for 10 to 15 seconds.

▼ RATIONALE

1. Assists in planning care.

2. Encourages the client's independence.

3. Provides for the client's participation in his care.

4. Allows for easiest access to the client's face.

5. Protects the client's bedclothes.

6. This temperature will help soften the beard and will be warm to the client, but will not burn.

7. Decreases the transmission of microorganisms.

8. Helps to soften the client's beard and facilitates shaving.

▼ *ACTION*　　　　　　　　　　▼ *RATIONALE*

9. Remove the cloth and apply shaving cream or soap evenly to the client's face over the beard area (Fig. 10–24).

9. Helps to soften the client's beard and facilitates shaving.

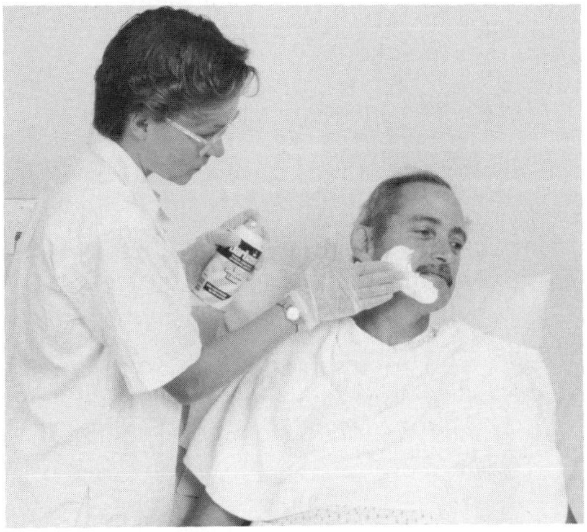

▼ **FIGURE 10–24.** Shaving the client.

10. Ask the client to indicate if the shave becomes uncomfortable.

10. Provides for the client's comfort.

11. Take a razor and begin to shave the client's neck and face as he directs, using firm, short strokes in the direction that the hair grows. Hold the razor at a 45-degree angle to the skin. Use your other hand to gently pull the client's skin taut while shaving.

11. Facilitates hair removal in a manner that decreases injury. Working in a systematic fashion increases efficiency.

NOTE: If the client is unable to direct you, start at the top of the beard on one side of his face and work down and across to the center of the face and repeat on the other side. Do not forget the area over the lip; the chin; or the neck. Avoid injured tissue areas.

Protects the client's skin integrity.

12. Dip the razor blade in the water as shaving cream and hair accumulate on the blade.

12. Increases the effectiveness of the shave while decreasing the possibility of injury.

13. After all facial hair has been removed, pour out the dirty water and refill the basin with fresh water at approximately 110° F (43–44° C).

13. Provides for the client's comfort.

14. Rinse the client's face thoroughly with a moistened warm washcloth.

14. Provides for the client's comfort.

15. Dry the client's face and apply after-shave, lotion, powder, or nothing as needed or desired. You may not be able to use anything on the client's face if he has had certain treatments or procedures (e.g., if a client is having radiotherapy to the face or neck). Lower the bed to the lowest level and raise the side rails.

15. Provides for the client's comfort and safety.

▼ *ACTION*	▼ *RATIONALE*
16. Carefully clean the razor and dispose of the blades in an appropriate container.	**16.** Decreases the transmission of microorganisms. Disposal of the blades provides for safety.
17. Place the soiled linen in a hamper.	**17.** Decreases the transmission of microorganisms.
18. Help the client to assume a comfortable position.	**18.** Promotes the client's comfort.
19. Return the rest of the cleaned equipment to the proper place.	**19.** Prepares the equipment for the next use.
20. Wash your hands.	**20.** Decreases the transmission of microorganisms.
21. Record the procedure.	**21.** Communicates to the other members of the health care team and contributes to the legal record by documenting the care given to the client.
22. Check for bleeding, especially if the client is undergoing anticoagulant therapy or has a compromised clotting system.	**22.** Clients who are undergoing anticoagulant therapy will have prolonged bleeding times and may need further intervention to stop the bleeding.

Example of Documentation

DATE	TIME	NOTES
7/22/93	1000	Client shaved. Skin pink, warm, dry, and intact. No injury or bleeding noted.
		L. Larson, RN

> **NOTE:** In some agencies a checklist is used to document this type of care.

Teaching Tips

Family members can be taught how to shave the client. This may allow the family to feel like they are "doing something" to help. Safety is a top priority and family members may need to be taught how to stop minor bleeding should it occur.

Home Care Variations

The same procedure can be used for shaving in the client's home.

SKILL 10–15 BATHING AN INFANT

Clinical Situations in Which You May Encounter This Skill

For approximately the first 2 weeks of life, an infant is given a sponge bath. This type of bath is recommended in order to give time for the umbilical cord stump to fall off and the area to heal. A tub bath can be given once the umbilical area has healed. Bathtime provides you with an excellent opportunity to inspect the integrity and cleanliness of the infant's skin. The umbilical cord can be inspected at this time for foul-smelling discharge or redness around the umbilical area.

Anticipated Responses

▼ The infant's skin is intact and clean. The umbilical area is free of any irritation or redness.

Adverse Responses

▼ The child can become chilled from undue exposure.
▼ The child may have cradle cap.
▼ The presence of infection may be evident in the umbilical area.
▼ The child may have diaper rash.

Materials List

Gather these materials before beginning the skill:

▼ Basin or small tub filled with warm water (37.8° C [100° F])
▼ Towels (at least 2)
▼ Washcloths (at least 2)
▼ Cotton balls
▼ Mild soap or cleansing agent
▼ Shirt
▼ Diaper
▼ Additional clothing such as a nightgown
▼ Baby blanket
▼ Soft-bristle brush or comb
▼ Tissue
▼ Rubbing alcohol
▼ Petroleum jelly or hydrophilic ointment
▼ Gloves

▼ ACTION

1. Review the skill in your procedure manual prior to initiation of the skill.

2. The room should be warm and free of drafts.

3. Wash your hands and put on gloves.

4. Fill the basin or small tub with warm water (37.8° C [100° F]). Test the temperature of the water with a bath thermometer or with your wrist or elbow.

5. Keep the infant clothed with a diaper and shirt, covered with a blanket, and in a supine position.

6. Begin the bath by washing each of the infant's eyes with a separate moist cotton ball. Gently wipe from the inner to the outer canthus.

7. Wash the child's external ear and behind the ear using a washcloth wrapped around your index finger. Do not use cotton swabs in the ear canal.

8. Using water only and a washcloth, gently wash the infant's face. Remove any crustations from the nares by using a twisted moist cotton ball or washcloth.

▼ RATIONALE

1. Agency guidelines for bathing an infant vary according to the institution.

2. An infant's temperature-regulating mechanisms are not completely developed.

3. Decreases the transmission of microorganisms.

4. The bath water must be tested to ensure that its temperature is warm rather than too cold, which can cause chilling, or hot, which can cause burning of the skin.

5. Prevents chilling.

6. Prevents microorganisms from entering the lacrimal ducts. Prevents irritation to the eyes.

7. Prevents possible packing of the discharge farther down the canal. Prevents damage to the eardrum.

8. Soap may irritate the infant's eyes. Moisture loosens crustations for easy removal.

▼ _A C T I O N_	▼ _R A T I O N A L E_
9. Using a mild soap, wash the infant's neck, paying particular attention to the skin folds. Sit the infant up using your arm to support the neck and shoulders. Dry the child thoroughly with a towel.	9. The skin folds are a primary site for secretions to accumulate and provide a refuge for microorganisms. Access to the skin folds is easier with the infant sitting up.
10. Place the infant in a football hold position (the infant's head is in the palm of your hand while the infant's body is supported with your forearm; see Fig. 10–25).	10. Secures the infant.

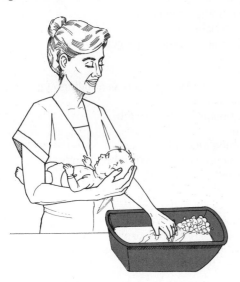

▼ **FIGURE 10–25.** Football hold.

11. Lather the infant's scalp with a mild soap or shampoo while positioning the infant's head over the basin.	11. Prevents cradle cap (a seborrheic dermatitis of the scalp consisting of thick, yellow, greasy scales).
12. Rinse the infant's scalp and hair thoroughly. Dry the scalp with a towel.	12. Soap or shampoo may irritate the scalp if either is left to dry.
13. Brush the infant's hair using a soft-bristle brush or comb.	13. Aids in removing loosened crustations.
14. Place the infant in a supine position on a towel and remove the infant's shirt and diaper. Wipe any fecal material away from the infant's perineum or buttocks area with a tissue.	14. Prevents the spread of microorganisms.
15. Cover the infant's body with a clean dry towel.	15. Prevents chilling.
16. Using a washcloth and a small amount of soap, wash the infant's arms as well as the axilla, chest, and abdomen using gentle strokes.	16. Since an infant's skin is sensitive, only a minimal amount of friction is needed to cleanse the area.
17. Rinse each body part and dry the area thoroughly with a towel. Cover the baby with the towel.	17. Prevents chilling.
18. Clean the umbilical area with soap and water. Do not wet the umbilical cord. Rinse and dry the area. Apply alcohol to the umbilical cord stump using a cotton ball.	18. Promotes drying of the stump. Prevents infection.

▼ *A C T I O N*   ▼ *R A T I O N A L E*

19. Exposing one of the infant's legs and feet at a time, wash, rinse, and dry. Cleanse between the toes.

19. Prevents chilling.

20. Place the infant on his or her stomach. Wash, rinse, and dry the baby's back. Cover the baby with a towel.

20. Prevents chilling.

21. Apply a small amount of unperfumed lotion or ointment (petroleum jelly or hydrophilic ointment) to any dry skin area.

21. Avoid baby oil because it clogs the skin pores and powders may irritate dry skin.

22. With the infant in a supine position, wash the baby girl's genitalia.
    a. Wash the skin folds of the groin area.

    a. Prevents accumulation of secretions of smegma (a cheesy, foul-smelling secretion located at the base of the labia and produced by the sebaceous glands).

    b. Gently separate the labia and wash from front to back (toward the anal area).
    You may use a portion of the washcloth or a moistened cotton ball. When using a washcloth, change the area with each wipe. When using cotton balls, change to a clean ball with each wipe.

    b. Prevents the transmission of microorganisms.

23. With the infant in a supine position, wash the baby boy's genitalia.
    a. Gently wash the penis with soap and water. In an uncircumcised male, do not forcibly retract the foreskin. If it can be retracted, wash the glans penis using a cotton ball moistened with soap and water. Dry and return the foreskin over the glans penis.
    b. In a circumcised male, gently wash the penis with plain water.

23. The foreskin may be initially too tight to be retracted.
    a. Prevents irritation and infection.

    b. Soap may irritate the area.

24. Lift the infant up by the ankles in order to expose the buttocks. Wash, rinse, and dry the child's buttocks. Apply petroleum jelly or a hydrophilic ointment to the anal area as needed.

24. Ointment helps to prevent diaper rash.

25. Apply the clean diaper. Make sure the diaper is secure. Place the top of the diaper below the umbilical area if the cord stump is still in place.

25. Prevents leakage of stool and urine. Prevents rubbing of sensitive skin areas.

26. Dress the infant in a shirt and other clothing such as a nightgown. Bundle the infant with a blanket.

26. Provides warmth and security.

27. Place the infant in a side-lying position in a crib, bassinet, or playpen.

27. Facilitates drainage from the infant's mouth. Provides a position of comfort.

28. Clean and rinse the basin. Return all of the equipment to its proper storage area. Dispose of the soiled diapers and linens in a designated receptacle.

28. Decreases the transmission of microorganisms.

29. Remove the gloves and wash your hands.

29. Decreases the transmission of microorganisms.

▼ *ACTION*   ▼ *RATIONALE*

30. Document the procedure performed, the infant's response, and any unusual findings such as impaired skin integrity, the condition of the umbilicus, or presence of cradle cap.

30. Provides information to the health care team and contributes to the legal record of the care given to the client.

Giving a tub bath

1. Proceed with steps 1 through 14 of the skill for giving a sponge bath.

1. The steps are identical prior to immersion in the tub of water.

2. Slowly immerse the infant feet first into a tub of water. The umbilical cord stump should have fallen off prior to a tub bath.

2. Decreases the startling effect.

3. Position the infant in the tub by supporting his or her head and shoulders with your arm (cradling the infant; see Fig. 10–26). Hold the infant's thigh with your hand.

3. Promotes the infant's safety. Prevents slipping and sliding of the infant while in the tub.

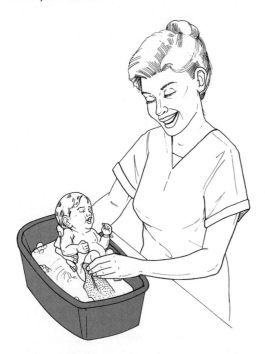

▼ **FIGURE 10–26.** Holding the infant in the tub.

4. Wash the infant with soap and rinse the infant's body beginning with the shoulders and arms down to the lower extremities. Cleanse the skin folds thoroughly.

4. Skin folds are primary sites for secretions to accumulate. A tub bath makes removal of any secretions easier.

5. Remove the infant from the tub and dry him or her thoroughly using a towel. Wrap the infant in the towel prior to dressing him or her.

5. Prevents chilling.

6. Apply a small amount of unperfumed lotion or ointment (petroleum jelly or hydrophilic ointment) to any dry skin area.

6. Avoid baby oil because it clogs the skin pores and powders may irritate dry skin.

▼ *A C T I O N*	▼ *R A T I O N A L E*
7. Follow steps 25 through 30 of the procedure for giving a sponge bath to complete the tub bath sequence.	**7.** Identical steps as those for giving a sponge bath.

Example of Documentation

Bathing an infant is usually documented on a nursing care check sheet.

Teaching Tips

You should assess the infant's skin during the bath. Remember to rinse and dry the skin thoroughly, particularly the skin folds. Keep the infant covered as much as possible to prevent heat loss.

Prior to leaving the hospital, family members should be taught to bathe the infant. Most hospitals have demonstration times when parents can practice this skill. If the infant rooms in with the mother, involve the family during bathtime; this allows time for family members to observe the infant's body parts and ask questions.

Home Care Variations

Make sure that family members understand that an infant should never be left unattended in a small tub or basin. Remind them that an infant needs to be cleansed with soap and water after each soiled diaper.

SKILL 10–16   MAKING AN UNOCCUPIED BED

Clinical Situations in Which You May Encounter This Skill

A client who is able to get out of bed usually has his or her linen changed while the bed is vacant. Linen changes help to maintain a safe, comfortable, and attractive environment.

Anticipated Responses

▼ The bed is neat and free of wrinkles.

Adverse Responses

▼ Wrinkles are beneath the client and there are signs of skin irritation or breakdown, or both.

Materials List

Gather these materials before beginning the skill:

▼ Pillowcase for each pillow
▼ Bedspread (if needed)
▼ Top sheet
▼ Drawsheet (if needed)
▼ Bottom sheet (some institutions use fitted bottom sheets)
▼ Mattress pad (if needed)
▼ Bedside chair to hold fresh linens
▼ Laundry bag (if available; if not, the used pillowcase is appropriate)
▼ Examination gloves (if the linen is soiled with bodily secretions)
▼ Waterproof pad (if needed)

▼ *ACTION* ▼ *RATIONALE*

1. Ascertain whether or not the client is able to get out of bed for this procedure.

2. Place the linen in the following order on the chair: pillow on the bottom; bedspread; blanket; top sheet; drawsheet; bottomsheet; mattress pad.

3. Put on gloves, if needed.

4. Place the bed in a high position.

5. Remove the pillow from the bed and remove the pillowcase.

6. Place the pillow on a clean chair or in another clean area.

7. Remove the linen from the bed by loosening the linen all the way around and carefully folding the linen together with soiled areas to the inside.

1. Determines whether the bed will need to be made with the client in it or not.

2. This order is efficient since the next needed piece will be on top.

3. Decreases the transmission of microorganisms.

4. Reduces the strain on your back.

5. The pillowcase can be used as a laundry bag, if needed.

6. Helps to maintain cleanliness.

7. Assists in preventing microorganisms from becoming airborne or coming into contact with your uniform.

NOTE: Be sure there are no personal items enfolded in the linens.

It is easy for articles that are important to the client (eyeglasses, dentures) to be thrown away with soiled linen.

---

8. Place these linens in the used pillowcase or laundry bag.

9. Two people may pull the mattress to the head of the bed, if necessary.

8. Decreases the transmission of microorganisms.

9. Decreases the possibility of injury.

NOTE: Use proper body mechanics.

---

10. Wipe off and dry the mattress as needed.

11. Remove your gloves and dispose of them properly.

10. Decreases the transmission of microorganisms.

11. The gloves may contaminate the clean linen. Proper disposal decreases the transmission of microorganisms.

Changing the bottom linen

12. Apply all needed clean linen to one side of the bed before proceeding to the other side by:
    a. Placing the mattress pad, if needed, on the bed and unfolding it so that it lies in the proper position.
    b. Placing the bottom sheet on top of the mattress pad so that as it is unfolded it will be in the proper position. Do not shake the sheets to open them.
       i. The bottom of the bottom sheet should be even with the mattress end.
       ii. Have the center fold in the center of the bed.
       iii. Fanfold the top fold of the bottom sheet to the center of the bed.

12. Provides for efficient use of your energy.

    a. Mattress pads assist in promoting client comfort.

    b. Prevents microorganisms from becoming airborne.

       i. It is most efficient to work from the foot to the head of the bed.

       iii. It is most efficient to complete one side before going to the other.

▼ *ACTION* _ ▼ *RATIONALE* _ _ _ _ _ _ _ _ _ _ _ _ _

c. Tucking in the bottom sheet at the head of the bed using the miter technique. To miter the corners:
 i. Standing diagonally, face the head of the bed.
 ii. Place the hand that is closest to the bed under the mattress corner and lift.

c. Mitered corners hold the linen firmly in proper position.

NOTE: Work with your palms down.

Working with your palms down prevents injury to your knuckles and jewelry.

---

iii. With your free hand, pull the extra sheet over and under the uplifted mattress (Fig. 10–27A).

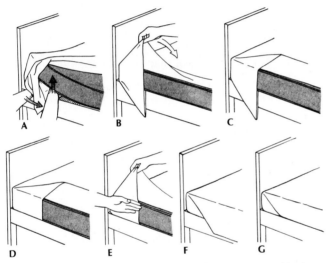

▼ **FIGURE 10–27.** Mitering the corners of an unoccupied bed.

iv. Turn and face the side of the bed.
 v. Lift the side edge of the sheet to make a triangle to the head of the bed. The side edge will hang at a right angle to the bed (Fig. 10–27B).
 vi. Fold the upper part of the sheet back on the bed by making a crease along the mattress top edge (Fig. 10–27C).
 vii. Tuck the lower hanging portion of the sheet under the mattress (Fig. 10–27D).
 viii. With your thumb down on your palm, place the back side of one hand firmly against the tucked-in portion of the sheet at the head of the bed (Fig. 10–27E).
 ix. With your free hand, pick up the sheet corner lying on the bed and bring it down over the hand on the mattress (Fig. 10–27F).
 x. Face the side of the bed.
 xi. Tuck the side edge of the sheet under the mattress down the whole side of the mattress (Fig. 10–27G).

▼ *ACTION* _ _ _ _ _ _ _ _ _ _ _ _ _ _ _ _ ▼ *RATIONALE* _ _ _ _ _ _ _ _ _ _

d. Placing the drawsheet on the bed so that it is in the middle of the bed by:
   i. Identifying the center fold and placing it in the center.
   ii. Fanfolding the rest of the drawsheet to the center of the bed.

d. A drawsheet is used to lift, move, and turn clients more easily while they are in bed.

13. Go to the other side of the bed and repeat the miter process for the bottom sheet.

NOTE: Pull the sheet so that it fits snugly. Tuck the drawsheet in securely.

Helps the linen to stay in place and assists in client comfort.

Changing the top linen

14. Open the clean top sheet with the center fold in the center of the bed. Align the top of the sheet with the top of the mattress.

14. Allows for proper placement of the bed linens.

15. Do the same with the blanket and the bedspread, if used.

15. Allows for proper placement of the bed linens.

16. Cuff the bedspread under the blanket. Then cuff the top sheet over the bedspread and blanket.

16. Makes a neater looking bed. Helps maintain the linen placement.

17. Tuck the top linens under the foot of the mattress:
   a. Stand at the foot of the bed and face diagonally to the opposite corner.
   b. Lift the mattress corner with your closest hand.
   c. With your other hand, tuck all of the linens under the mattress.
   d. You may make a toe pleat by placing a horizontal fold in the top sheet and top covers about 1 foot from the bottom of the mattress (Fig. 10–28).

17. Holds top linens in place.

d. Allows extra space for the client's feet, preventing plantar flexion.

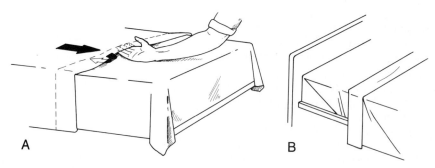

A   B

▼ FIGURE 10–28. Making a toe pleat on an unoccupied bed.

▼ _ACTION_ _ _ _ _ _ _ _ _ _ _ _ _ _ _ _   ▼ _RATIONALE_ _ _ _ _ _ _ _ _ _ _ _

18. Place a clean pillowcase on the pillow using the following technique:

  a. Grasp the closed end of the pillowcase in the middle (Fig. 10–29*A*).
  b. With your free hand, open the pillowcase and invert it over your hand that is holding the other end (Fig. 10–29*B*).
  c. Grasp the pillow end with your hand holding the pillowcase (Fig. 10–29*C*) and use your other hand to pull the case down over the pillow (Fig. 10–29*D*).

18. This method of changing the pillowcase prevents contact of pillow with your uniform, thus reducing transmission of microorganisms.

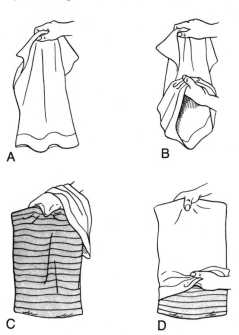

▼ **FIGURE 10–29.** Placing a clean pillowcase on a pillow.

19. Place the pillow in the top center of the bed.

19. The pillow will be in place for the client.

20. Place the bed into the low position and make the call light accessible to the client. Raise the side rails if needed.

20. Provides for the client's safety.

21. Straighten the client's room by putting soiled linens in the proper area.

21. Assists in preventing the transmission of microorganisms.

22. Wash your hands.

22. Decreases the transmission of microorganisms.

23. Record the procedure.

23. Communicates to the other members of the health care team and contributes to the legal record by documenting the care given to the client.

24. Assess the client's comfort.

24. Provides information useful for planning future care.

Example of Documentation

Many patient care areas have checklists for this type of daily activity (Fig. 10–30). Be sure the linen change is noted appropriately whether or not a checklist is used.

Date:	11 - 7 SHIFT	7 - 3 SHIFT	3 - 11 SHIFT
DIET — Type Diet:			
Amt. Consumed		Breakfast 25% __ 50% __ 75% __ 100% __ Lunch 25% __ 50% __ 75% __ 100% __	Dinner 25% __ 50% __ 75% __ 100% __
Supplement / Snack			
Tube Feeding Route	Nasog. ____ Gastr. ____ Jejun ____	Nasog. ____ Gastr. ____ Jejun ____	Nasog. ____ Gastr. ____ Jejun ____
Residual Checked	0000 ____ Amt. ____ 0400 ____ Amt. ____ 0100 ____ Amt. ____ 0500 ____ Amt. ____ 0200 ____ Amt. ____ 0600 ____ Amt. ____ 0300 ____ Amt. ____ 0700 ____ Amt. ____	0800 ____ Amt. ____ 1200 ____ Amt. ____ 0900 ____ Amt. ____ 1300 ____ Amt. ____ 1000 ____ Amt. ____ 1400 ____ Amt. ____ 1100 ____ Amt. ____ 1500 ____ Amt. ____	1600 ____ Amt. ____ 2000 ____ Amt. ____ 1700 ____ Amt. ____ 2100 ____ Amt. ____ 1800 ____ Amt. ____ 2200 ____ Amt. ____ 1900 ____ Amt. ____ 2300 ____ Amt. ____
Enteral / IVAC Pump			
Solution & Rate			
HYGIENE — Type Bath: Bed ____ Tub ____ Shower ____	Partial ____ Self ____ Complete ____ Refused ____	Partial ____ Self ____ Complete ____ Refused ____	Partial ____ Self ____ Complete ____ Refused ____
Linen Change	Yes ____ No ____ Refused ____	Yes ____ No ____ Refused ____	Yes ____ No ____ Refused ____
Mouth Care	Self ____ Complete ____ Assisted	Self ____ Complete ____ Assisted	Self ____ Complete ____ Assisted
Hair Care	Yes ____ No ____ Self ____ Nurses or Other ____	Yes ____ No ____ Self ____ Nurses or Other ____	Yes ____ No ____ Self ____ Nurses or Other ____
Catheter Care	Yes ____ No ____ NA ____	Yes ____ No ____ NA ____	Yes ____ No ____ NA ____
Stockings Knee ____ Thigh ____	Yes ____ Removed ____ No ____ Reapplied ____ NA ____	Yes ____ Removed ____ No ____ Reapplied ____ NA ____	Yes ____ Removed ____ No ____ Reapplied ____ NA ____
ACTIVITY — Activity and Tolerance	Ambulatd Distances _____ BRP ____ Dangle ____ Bedrest ____ Chair ____ Length of time in chair: ____15 min. ____30 min. or longer	Ambulatd Distances _____ BRP ____ Dangle ____ Bedrest ____ Chair ____ Length of time in chair: ____15 min. ____30 min. or longer	Ambulatd Distances _____ BRP ____ Dangle ____ Bedrest ____ Chair ____ Length of time in chair: ____15 min. ____30 min. or longer
Range of Motion	Physical Therapy ____ Nurses or Other ____	Physical Therapy ____ Nurses or Other ____	Physical Therapy ____ Nurses or Other ____
Siderails Up	All ____ Left ____ Right ____ NA ____	All ____ Left ____ Right ____ NA ____	All ____ Left ____ Right ____ NA ____
Bed Position	Down ____ Locked ____	Down ____ Locked ____	Down ____ Locked ____
Call Light in Reach	Yes ____ No ____	Yes ____ No ____	Yes ____ No ____
Restraints	Vest Yes __ Wrist Rt __ Ankle Rt __ No __ Lt __ Lt __	Vest Yes __ Wrist Rt __ Ankle Rt __ No __ Lt __ Lt __	Vest Yes __ Wrist Rt __ Ankle Rt __ No __ Lt __ Lt __
Other			
TREATMENTS & ETC — Telemetry / Monitor Rhythm	Yes ____ No ____	Yes ____ No ____	Yes ____ No ____
Suction Machine	Yes ____ No ____	Yes ____ No ____	Yes ____ No ____
T-Pump	Yes ____ No ____	Yes ____ No ____	Yes ____ No ____
Egg Crate / Sheep Skin	Yes ____ No ____	Yes ____ No ____	Yes ____ No ____
Packs / Compresses Site / Desc. / Supplies Used	Hot ____ Cold ____ Other _____	Hot ____ Cold ____ Other _____	Hot ____ Cold ____ Other _____
Wound Care Site / Desc. / Supplies Used	Decubitus ____ Surgical ____ Drains ____ Other _____	Decubitus ____ Surgical ____ Drains ____ Other _____	Decubitus ____ Surgical ____ Drains ____ Other _____

OTHER

Patient Instructions		Discharge Planning:	
Time		Time	

NOTE:

RN Signature _____	RN Signature _____	RN Signature _____
LPN Signature _____	LPN Signature _____	LPN Signature _____
Nursing Assistant Signature _____	Nursing Assistant Signature _____	Nursing Assistant Signature _____

▼ **FIGURE 10–30.** Checklist on which to note linen change.

Teaching Tips

Good body mechanics should be used during this procedure to prevent a back injury.

Home Care Variations

There are no variations in making the bed at home. You may need to teach home caregivers how to place and use a drawsheet to facilitate moving the bedridden client. Encourage hygiene and proper use of body mechanics when making the bed.

SKILL 10–17 MAKING AN OCCUPIED BED

Clinical Situations in Which You May Encounter This Skill

The client who is confined to bed requires linen changes while in bed. Linen changes help to maintain a safe, comfortable, and attractive environment.

Anticipated Responses

▼ The client's bed is free of wrinkles.
▼ The client is not injured as a result of the bed being changed.

Adverse Responses

▼ Wrinkles are beneath the client and there are signs of skin irritation or breakdown, or both.

Materials List

Gather these materials before beginning the skill:

▼ Pillowcase for each pillow
▼ Bedspread
▼ Top sheet
▼ Drawsheet (if needed)
▼ Bottom sheet (some institutions use fitted bottom sheets)
▼ Mattress pad (if needed)
▼ Bath blanket or sheet
▼ Bedside chair to hold fresh linens
▼ Laundry bag (if available; if not, the used pillowcase is appropriate)
▼ Examination gloves (if there is drainage of body secretions on the sheets)
▼ Waterproof pads (if needed)

▼ ACTION	▼ RATIONALE
1. Ascertain how much the client can assist.	1. If the client cannot assist, another nurse will be needed to help turn the client.
2. Place the linen in the following order on the chair: pillow on the bottom; bedspread; blanket; top sheet; drawsheet; bottom sheet; mattress pad.	2. This order is efficient since the next needed piece will be on top.
3. Put on gloves, if needed.	3. Decreases the transmission of microorganisms.
4. Place the bed in a high position. Lower side rails on your side of the bed.	4. Reduces the strain on your back and allows access to the client.
5. Loosen the top linen at the foot of the bed.	5. Facilitates removal of the linen.
6. Place a bath blanket over the client and ask him or her to hold onto the bath blanket while the rest of the top linen is folded carefully down to the end of the bed, pulled out from under the bath blanket, and off of the bed.	6. Protects the client's modesty.

▼ _ACTION_ _ _ _ _ _ _ _ _ _ _ _ _ _ _ _ ▼ _RATIONALE_ _ _ _ _ _ _ _ _ _ _ _ _ _ _

7. Place soiled linens in a laundry bag or pillowcase. Fold the blanket or bedspread, if not soiled, for reuse. Leave one pillow under the client's head.

7. Decreases the spread of microorganisms. Pillow promotes comfort.

NOTE: Make sure that none of the client's possessions are folded in any linens removed from the client's bed.

It is easy for articles important to the client (e.g., eyeglasses, dentures) to be thrown away with soiled linen.

---

8. Get extra help to move the mattress to the head of the bed, if needed.

8. Decreases the possibility of injury. Helps keep the linens in place and the client comfortable.

NOTE: Use proper body mechanics.

---

9. Move the pillow to the far side of the bed and pull up the side rail on that side.

9. Provides space to work. Provides for the client's safety.

10. Help the client to turn to a side-lying position. Sometimes extra assistance is needed to help the client maintain this position.

10. Leaves the opposite side of the bed empty. Decreases the possible strain to your back.

Changing the bottom linen

11. Start the bottom linen change from the side of the bed that is empty by lowering the side rail.

11. Allows access to the bed for the linen change.

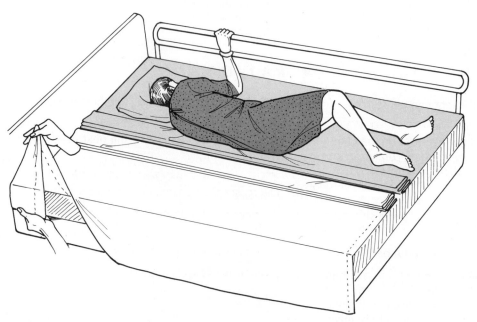

▼ FIGURE 10–31. Changing the bottom linen of an occupied bed.

▼ *A C T I O N* _ | ▼ *R A T I O N A L E* _ _ _ _ _ _ _ _ _ _ _ _ _ _

12. Loosen the soiled linen on the empty side of the bed and roll it up against or slightly under the client's back. Make the linen roll as flat as possible.

12. Provides space for application of clean linen. Provides for the client's comfort when he or she rolls back over the linen roll to the other side of the bed.

13. Wipe off and dry the mattress as needed.

13. Decreases the transmission of microorganisms.

14. Apply all needed clean linen to this side of the bed before proceeding to the other side by:
  a. Placing a mattress pad, if needed, on the bed and unfolding it so that it lies in the proper position.
  b. Folding one-half of the pad so that it lies under the soiled linen.

14. Provides for efficient use of your energy and the client's energy.

  b. Mattress pads provide for the client's comfort.

NOTE: If the soiled linen is wet, use a waterproof pad between the soiled and clean linens

Decreases the contamination of the clean linens.

---

  c. Placing the bottom sheet on top of the mattress pad so that as it is unfolded it will be in the proper position.
    i. The bottom of the bottom sheet should be even with the mattress end.
    ii. Have the center fold in the center of the bed.
    iii. Fanfold the rest of the sheet to the center of the bed on top of the mattress pad and under the soiled linen (or barrier) (Fig. 10–31).
  d. Tucking in the bottom sheet at the head of the bed using the miter technique. To miter the corners:
    i. Stand diagonally and face the head of the bed.
    ii. Place your hand that is closest to the bed under the mattress corner and lift.

    i. It is most efficient to work from the foot to the head of the bed.
    ii. Provides for even distribution of the sheet.

    iii. It is most efficient to complete one side before going to the other.

  d. Mitered corners hold the linen firmly in the proper position.

NOTE: Work with your hands palm down.

Working with the palms down prevents injury to your knuckles and jewelry.

---

    iii. With your free hand, pull the extra sheet over and under the uplifted mattress (see Fig. 10–27*A*).
    iv. Turn and face the side of the bed.
    v. Lift the side edge of the sheet to make a triangle to the head of the bed. The side edge will hang at a right angle to the bed (see Fig. 10–27*B*).
    vi. Fold the upper part of the sheet back on the bed by making a crease along the top edge of the mattress (see Fig. 10–27*C*).
    vii. Tuck the lower hanging portion of the sheet under the mattress (see Fig. 10–27*D*).

    iii. Working with the palms down protects your knuckles and jewelry.

▼ *ACTION*   ▼ *RATIONALE*

       viii. With your thumb down on your palm, place the back side of one hand firmly against the tucked-in portion of the sheet at the head of the bed (see Fig. 10–27 E).

        ix. With your free hand, pick up the sheet corner that is lying on the bed, and bring it down over your hand on the mattress (see Fig. 10–27 F).

         x. Face the side of the bed.

        xi. Tuck the side edge of the sheet under the mattress down the whole side of the mattress (see Fig. 10–27 G).

    e. Placing the drawsheet so that it is in the middle of the bed by:

        i. Identifying the center fold and placing it in the center.

       ii. Fanfolding the rest of the drawsheet to the center of the bed over the bottom sheet and under the soiled linen (or barrier).

    f. If any waterproof pads are to be used, placing them fanfolded on top of the drawsheet.

e. A drawsheet is used to lift, move, and turn clients while they are in bed.

15. Help the client to roll back onto the side facing you.

15. Provides access to the other side of the bed.

16. Raise the side rail next to the client before moving to the other side.

16. Provides for the client's safety.

17. Move to the other side of the bed and lower the side rail.

17. Dirty linen will be accessible for removal.

18. Remove the soiled linen by carefully pulling the linens off of the bed and rolling the soiled areas to the inside. Place the linen in a laundry bag.

18. Decreases the transmission of microorganisms.

19. Wipe off and dry the mattress.

19. Decreases the transmission of microorganisms.

20. While making sure the bath blanket covering the client is not caught in the clean linen, carefully pull the clean linens into place on the empty side of the bed.

20. Protects the client's modesty and provides comfort.

21. Repeat the miter process for this side of the bottom sheet, or tuck the fitted ends around the mattress. Pull the sheet so that it fits snugly without wrinkles.

22. Tuck in the drawsheet by grasping the excess linen in your hands with the knuckles up and pull snugly, tucking in the middle, then the top, and the bottom of the drawsheet.

22. Provides for the client's comfort.

23. The client may roll into a supine position on the bed, if he or she wishes.

23. Provides for the client's comfort without task interference.

Changing the top linen

24. Open the clean top sheet with the center fold in the center of the bed.

24. Provides for an even distribution of the top sheet.

25. Ask the client to hold the top sheet or tuck it around the client's shoulders.

25. Keeps the top sheet in place as the bath blanket is removed.

▼ *ACTION* ▼ *RATIONALE*

26. Stand at the foot of the bed, grasp the soiled bath blanket under the top sheet, and carefully pull the soiled linen off the bed, leaving the top sheet in place.

26. Protects the client's modesty.

27. Open the blanket and then the bedspread over the top sheet, cuff the bedspread under the blanket, and cuff the top sheet over the bedspread and blanket.

27. Makes for a neater looking bed and helps maintain the linen placement.

28. Tuck the top linens under the foot of the mattress:
    a. Stand at the foot of the bed and face diagonally to the opposite corner.
    b. Ask the client to dorsiflex his or her feet before you tuck in the linen.
    c. Lift the mattress corner with your closest hand.
    d. With your other hand, tuck all of the linens under the mattress at one time.

    a. Uses your energy efficiently.

    b. Provides room for free movement of the client's feet. Tight linens can cause footdrop.

29. Carefully remove the pillow from under the client's head, remove the soiled pillowcase, and put on a new pillowcase by:
    a. Grasping the closed end of the pillowcase in the middle.
    b. Opening the pillowcase with your free hand and inverting it over the hand holding the other end.
    c. Grasping the pillow end with your hand holding the pillowcase and using your other hand to pull the case down over the pillow.

    a. Uses your energy efficiently.

30. Replace the pillow under the client's head.

30. Provides for the client's comfort.

31. Raise the side rails.

31. Provides for the client's safety.

32. Straighten the client's room by putting soiled linens in the proper area.

32. Assists in preventing the transmission of microorganisms.

33. Remove the gloves and discard them.

33. Decreases the transmission of microorganisms.

34. Place the client in a comfortable position.

34. Provides for the client's comfort.

35. Assess the client's comfort.

35. Provides you with information useful for the client's optimal wellness.

36. Place the bed into the low position and make the call light accessible to the client.

36. Provides for the client's safety.

37. Wash your hands.

37. Decreases the transmission of microorganisms.

38. Record the procedure.

38. Communicates to the other members of the health care team and contributes to the legal record by documenting the care given to the client.

39. Periodically evaluate the client's comfort, and whether the linen requires further adjustments.

39. Provides for the client's hygiene and comfort.

Example of Documentation

Many patient care areas have checklists for this type of daily activity. Be sure the linen change is noted appropriately whether or not a checklist is used.

Teaching Tips

A complete linen change while the client is bedridden offers you the opportunity to assess the client's physical status and to perform other skills, such as a back rub or chest percussion, if appropriate.

Good body mechanics should be used during this procedure to prevent injury to your back. Additional help may be needed.

Home Care Variations

Family members of bedridden clients often need to be taught the most efficient way of changing a bed. Conservation of linens by reusing unsoiled linens may be taught, as well as using drawsheets to conserve time and energy for turning and moving the client.

SKILL 10–18 MAKING A SURGICAL BED

Clinical Situations in Which You May Encounter This Skill

A surgical bed is made for clients who are returning from operations or other procedures. These clients must be moved to their bed from another bed, table, or stretcher, usually without their help.

Anticipated Responses

▼ The linens on the bed do not obstruct the efficiency of transferring the client to the bed.

Adverse Responses

▼ The linens on the bed obstruct the efficiency of the moving process.

Materials List

Gather these materials before beginning the skill:

▼ Pillowcase for each pillow
▼ Bedspread (if needed)
▼ Top sheet
▼ Drawsheets (two)
▼ Bottom sheet (some institutions use fitted bottom sheets)
▼ Mattress pad (if needed)
▼ Bedside chair to hold fresh linens
▼ Laundry bag (if available; if not, the used pillowcase is appropriate)
▼ Gloves (if the linen is soiled with bodily secretions)
▼ Waterproof pad

▼ ACTION

1. Review the surgery or procedure schedule to determine whether it is necessary to make a surgical bed.

2. Place the linens in the following order on the chair: one drawsheet; pillow case; bedspread; blanket; top sheet; second drawsheet; bottom sheet; mattress pad.

3. Raise the bed to its highest position and lower the side rails.

4. Follow steps 3 to 18 of Skill 10–16.

5. Do not place the pillow on the bed, but place it in an easily accessible place.

6. Grasp the top of the top sheet and bedspread and fanfold these linens to the very bottom of the bed.

▼ RATIONALE

1. Provides for planning.

2. This order is efficient since the next needed piece will be on top.

3. Provides for the best use of body mechanics.

5. The client's type of operation may preclude the use of a pillow.

6. Prevents obstruction by the top sheets when moving the client onto the bed.

▼ *ACTION*	▼ *RATIONALE*
7. Leave the bed in the high position with the side rails down.	7. Leaves the bed in the correct position for transferring clients with proper body mechanics.
8. With assistance, arrange the bed and furniture in the room to allow free passage of the stretcher.	8. Provides easy access to the bed and facilitates transferring the client.
9. Straighten the client's room by putting the soiled linens in the proper area. Place loose articles in a safe place.	9. Assists in preventing the transmission of microorganisms.
10. Place a pole for an intravenous line at the head of the bed.	10. Clients often return to their room after an operation with an intravenous line.
11. Place tissues, an emesis basin, a towel, and a washcloth at the bedside.	11. Nausea and vomiting are side effects of anesthesia and pain medications.
12. Wash your hands.	12. Decreases the transmission of microorganisms.
13. Record the procedure.	13. Communicates to the other members of the health care team and contributes to the legal record by documenting the care given to the client.

Example of Documentation

Many patient care areas have checklists for this type of daily activity. Be sure the linen change is noted appropriately whether or not a checklist is used.

Teaching Tips

The purpose of the surgical bed should be explained to the client's family or significant others.

Home Care Variations

The same procedure can be used to prepare the bed in the home for the client's arrival.

References

Crosby, C. (1989). Method in mouth care. *Nursing Times*, 35 (85), 38–41.

de Wit, S. C. (1994). Promoting hygiene. In V. Bolander (Ed.), *Basic Nursing* (3rd ed.). Philadelphia: W.B. Saunders.

Dudjak, L. A. (1987). Mouth care for mucositis due to radiation therapy. *Cancer Nursing*, 3 (10), 131–140.

Harrell, J., et al. (1992). Bedmaking in the coronary care unit. *Heart and Lung*, 21 (3), (abstract), 297.

Lawson, K. (1989). Oral-dental concerns of the pediatric oncology patient. *Issues in Comprehensive Pediatric Nursing*, 12, 199–206.

Trenter, P., and Creason, N. (1986). Nurse administered oral hygiene: Is there a scientific basis? *Journal of Advanced Nursing Science*, 11 (3), 323–331.

CHAPTER 11

Promoting Rest and Sleep

Difficulty resting and sleeping is a commonly heard complaint in the hospital setting. There are many nonpharmacologic methods that can be used to assist the individual in resting and sleeping. These include:

▼ Avoiding the use of stimulants such as cola, tea, coffee, and nicotine before bedtime.
▼ Establishing a regular bedtime.
▼ Incorporating regular exercise into the daily routine.
▼ Avoiding the use of alcohol.
▼ Developing a sleep routine or ritual such as listening to quiet music, reading, praying, meditating, or taking a warm bath.

In the hospital setting, a back massage may help a person relax before sleeping. A back rub or massage is the purposeful manipulation of muscles and tissues to promote relaxation and improve circulation.

SKILL 11–1   GIVING A BACK RUB (BACK MASSAGE)

Clinical Situations in Which You May Encounter This Skill

Clients may experience musculoskeletal aches for a variety of reasons, including prolonged bed rest and tension. At times back rubs are used to induce or enhance relaxation. Back rubs also may be used to stimulate circulation in the client's back.

The back rub can preclude the client's use of sleep-inducing medication. At other times it can be used as an adjunctive therapy to induce sleep. It also provides an opportunity for you to assess the skin on the client's back. A minimum of 4 to 6 minutes is needed to provide an adequate back rub, so you should not appear hurried.

Some clients are hypersensitive to touch and may experience a tickling sensation that causes increased muscle tension. Using firm strokes may help prevent this. You should clearly communicate to the client the reason for the back rub and what will occur during the procedure. The client's modesty should be protected.

Anticipated Responses

▼ The client experiences increased relaxation and comfort and decreased muscle tension.
▼ There are no signs of skin breakdown on the client's back.

Adverse Responses

▼ The client remains tense or unable to sleep.
▼ There are signs of skin breakdown on the client's back.

Materials List

Gather these materials before beginning the skill:

▼ Lotion or powder (make sure the client is not allergic to them)
▼ Sheet or bath blanket for drape
▼ Pillows
▼ Examination gloves (if needed)

▼ ACTION

1. Check the client's diagnosis to make sure there is no contraindication for the procedure.

2. Before beginning the back rub, allow the client the opportunity to empty his or her bladder and complete other hygiene measures.

3. Wash your hands.

4. Raise the bed to a position that is comfortable for you. Lower the side rail on your side.

5. Ask the client to lie in a comfortable prone position with his or her back bare from head to buttocks. Usually, the client's arms are raised and the client's head is turned to one side. Drape the client's genitalia, legs, and front of his or her torso with a bath blanket, sheet, or towel. If the client is unable to assume a prone position, turn him or her onto one side.

▼ RATIONALE

1. Clients with conditions such as skin lesions or who have had a recent back operation or trauma such as fractured ribs may not be allowed to have a back rub.

2. Provides for client comfort.

3. Decreases the transmission of microorganisms.

4. Prevents strain on your back.

5. Allows for the most comfort and relaxation. Draping protects the client's modesty and dignity.

▼ *ACTION*   ▼ *RATIONALE*

6. Make sure your hands are warm and relaxed by holding them under warm water or by rubbing them together.

6. Warmth will aid relaxation. Cold may cause tensing.

7. Place 1 to 2 teaspoons of lotion in your hands. Warm the lotion with your hands or warm the bottle of lotion in warm water before pouring it. Powder may be used instead of lotion, if desired. (Use caution with powder around the client's face.)

7. Reduces irritating friction between the client's back and your hands. Also allows for lubrication of the client's skin. Powder can irritate the client's respiratory tract.

8. Put the palmar surface of your hands on the client's back for a few seconds before beginning the massage.

8. Allows for the gradual trespass into the client's personal space.

9. a. Start stroking the base of the client's spine and, using firm strokes, move your hands upward toward the client's shoulders (Fig. 11–1).

9. a. Covers the area to be rubbed. Lets the client know where the massage will be.

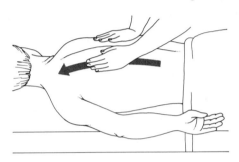

▼ **FIGURE 11–1.** Stroking.

b. Rotate your hands outward from the client's spine down toward the buttocks, massaging the client's whole back with firm, smooth, even strokes.

b. Short, uneven, light strokes are uncomfortable and ineffective. All areas of the back should be massaged to be most effective. Strokes that are light may initiate a tickling response that will produce muscle tension.

c. Use your thumb to stroke the client's cervical vertebrae up to the occipital area.

▼ *ACTION*　　　　　　　　　　　　　　▼ *RATIONALE*

10. Kneading (Fig. 11–2):
  a. Press down on the client's skin with your palm. Then pick up the tissue with your thumb and the first three fingers of your hand, and knead one side of the back and then the other side, beginning along the gluteal area and working up to the shoulders, deltoids, and upper arms. (This kneading stroke is called pétrissage or foulage.) Switch your hands smoothly if one or the other becomes tired.

  b. At times a scissor-like stroke using the flat sides of your hands may be performed up and down both sides of the client's back. (This stroke is called tapotement.)

a. Kneading muscle fibers helps relieve tension in the client's muscles and increases circulation.

b. Increases skin circulation.

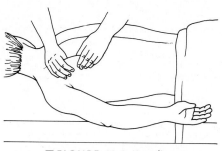

▼ **FIGURE 11–2.** Kneading.

11. Friction (Fig. 11–3): Using the tips of your second and third fingers, exert friction in a small circular motion using gentle pressure around the client's bony prominences such as the sacrum, scapula, and trochanter. Do not massage skin lesions or injured tissue.

11. Increases the client's circulation.

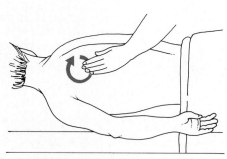

▼ **FIGURE 11–3.** Exerting friction.

▼ ACTION	▼ RATIONALE
12. End the back rub with long strokes up the length of the client's back. Gradually reduce the pressure as you move your hands.	**12.** Increases the client's comfort and relaxation.
13. Remember to follow these general guidelines: Keep both of your hands on the client's back at all times. Use overlapping strokes to cover the area.	**13.** Increases the client's comfort and relaxation. Decreases the tickling sensation.
14. Remove gloves if worn and wash your hands.	**14.** Decreases the transmission of microorganisms.
15. Lower the bed to the lowest level and raise the side rails.	**15.** Provides for client safety and comfort.
16. Provide the client with easy access to a signal light and other comfort items.	**16.** Provides for client safety and comfort.
17. After the back rub, assist the client into another position and assess his or her comfort level.	**17.** Allows for effectiveness of the procedure and maintenance of the client's comfort.
18. Record the procedure and other relevant information.	**18.** Communicates the information to the other members of the health care team and contributes to the legal record by documenting the care given to the client.

Example of Documentation

DATE	TIME	NOTES
11/10/93	2110	Back rub given. Client states he is relaxed and hopes to sleep without the aid of "sleeping pill" tonight.
		S. Smart, RN

Teaching Tips

Encouraging the client to use other relaxation techniques will further enhance the relaxation produced by this skill. Encourage the client to empty his or her bladder and finish other tasks before receiving the back rub as this will allow him or her to go to sleep once the back rub is completed.

Home Care Variations

Bedridden clients especially need comfort measures. This procedure also provides for position changes and skin assessment. Family members can be taught this skill easily and it may boost their confidence if they are feeling overwhelmed with many other technical tasks.

Reference

Hudacek, S. S. (1994). Promoting rest and sleep. In V. Bolander (Ed.), *Basic nursing* (3rd ed.). Philadelphia: W. B. Saunders.

CHAPTER 12

Relieving Pain and Applying Heat and Cold Therapy

- -

You should use both pharmacologic and nonpharmacologic measures to relieve a client's pain or discomfort. With a physician's order, you may administer narcotic and nonnarcotic medications to relieve pain. Drugs can be administerd intermittently on an as needed (PRN) basis, or continuously using a patient-controlled analgesia (PCA) pump.

Nonpharmacologic measures may be taken exclusively in certain situations or in combination with medications to relieve pain. When properly carried out, nonpharmacologic measures such as progressive muscle relaxation are very effective in reducing discomfort.

One of the oldest nursing measures to reduce pain and promote healing is the application of heat. Applying heat results in vasodilation and increased capillary permeability. These vascular changes promote circulation, provide local warmth due to increased blood flow, bring nutrients to injured areas, aid the inflammatory process, and remove waste products from the injured area. Heat also results in muscle relaxation and reduction of joint stiffness and contractures.

You may use either moist or dry heat applications. Moist heat can be applied with sitz baths and soaks or compresses and hot packs. Dry heat can be applied with a hot water bottle, heating pad, aquathermia pad, or disposable heat pack.

The application of cold results in vasoconstriction and decreased capillary permeability. These vascular changes reduce bleeding, edema, and inflammation. Cold also decreases conduction of nervous impulses and results in anesthesia. Application of cold also can produce systemic cooling.

You may use either moist or dry applications of cold. Moist cold may be applied in the form of cool compresses or tepid sponge baths. Dry cold may be applied with ice bags, ice collars, and dry cold packs.

You must use care when applying heat or cold to prevent injury to the client's tissues. Frequent assessment of the client's skin during the therapy and correct application of the heat or cold are essential.

- -

- -

OVERVIEW OF RELATED RESEARCH

GIVING A SITZ BATH

LaFoy, J., and Geden, E.A. (1989). Postepisiotomy pain: Warm versus cold sitz bath. *Journal of Obstetric, Gynecologic, and Neonatal Nursing*, 18 (5), 399–403.

Heat and cold have been used as therapeutic treatments for a long time. The authors studied whether warm or cold sitz baths would be more effective in treating postepisiotomy pain. The findings indicated no difference between the two groups on any of the measures. Edema appeared to be lessened more with cold; however, warm sitz baths did not seem to increase swelling. Based on these findings, the investigators suggested that the client be given the option of deciding which temperature to use, unless contraindications exist.

PROVIDING RELAXATION THERAPY

Miller, K. M. (1987). Deep breathing relaxation—A pain management technique. *AORN Journal*, 45 (2), 484–488.

Miller reviewed the psychologic and physiologic changes that occur during pain and some methods used to evaluate pain, including the effects and benefits of relaxation exercises for patients after operations. A clinical pilot study using deep breathing relaxation as part of pain management care was presented. The results revealed a statistically significant drop in all of the patients' physiologic responses and a decrease in 11 of 15 patients' verbal reports of postoperative pain.

Munro, B. H., et al. (1988). Effect of relaxation therapy on postmyocardial infarction patients' relaxation. *Nursing Research*, 37, 231–235.

The purpose of this study was to determine the effect of relaxation therapy on physical (blood pressure, heart rate, and aerobic conditioning level) and psychosocial factors in 30 male patients who had had a myocardial infarction. This group experienced a statistically significant decrease in diastolic blood pressure. Relaxation therapy did not significantly affect either heart rate or psychosocial functioning.

APPLYING HEAT AND COLD

Hill, P. D. (1989). Effects of heat and cold on the perineum after episiotomy/laceration. *Journal of Obstetric, Gynecologic, and Neonatal Nursing*, 18 (2), 124–129.

This study was conducted to determine the effect of heat and cold (warm perineal pack, cold perineal pack, or warm sitz bath) on the perineum after delivery. Ninety subjects, 30 in each treatment group, participated in the study. Postpartum healing of the perineum before and after exposure to one of the three treatments was evaluated with the Redness Edema Ecchymosis Discharge Approximation (REEDA). No statistically significant differences were found in the REEDA score among the groups before and after treatment.

SKILL 12–1   GIVING A SITZ BATH

Clinical Situations in Which You May Encounter This Skill

A sitz bath involves immersing the client's perineum and pelvic area in warm water. It benefits clients who have pelvic areas that are swollen and painful due to trauma such as vaginal hysterectomy, childbirth, and hemorrhoidectomy. The warmth from the water aids the inflammatory process and promotes comfort and healing.

Anticipated Responses

▼ The client has an increased level of comfort in the affected area.
▼ A decrease in the amount of swelling may be noted.

Adverse Responses

▼ The client experiences an increase in the level of discomfort in the affected area.
▼ The client experiences a continued increase in the amount of swelling or in the size of any hematomas that may be present.
▼ The client experiences new or increased bleeding that is unexpected.

Materials List

Gather these materials before beginning the skill:

▼ Sitz bath (some hospital units have a built-in sitz bowl) or a disposable sitz bath (Fig. 12–1)
▼ Bath thermometer
▼ Towel
▼ Sanitary pads, if needed

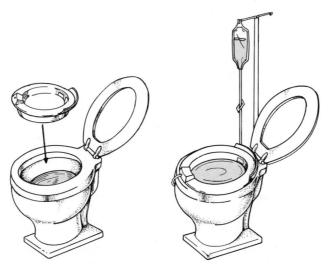

▼ **FIGURE 12–1.** Disposable sitz bath.

▼ _A C T I O N_	▼ _R A T I O N A L E_
1. Check the client's chart to ascertain the type of trauma the perineum has sustained and to make sure there are no contraindications to the procedure.	1. Alerts you to the client's condition and helps to provide for the client's safety.
2. Wash your hands.	2. Decreases the transmission of microorganisms.

3. Prepare the sitz bath for the client:
  a. With a unit sitz bath by:
    i. Thoroughly cleaning the bowl with a disinfectant and rinsing well.
    ii. Placing clean towels around the seat.
 	
  b. With a portable sitz bath by:
    i. Placing the bowl on the toilet.
    ii. Following the manufacturer's instructions for proper setup.
	i. Decreases the transmission of microorganisms.
	ii. Provides comfort for the client's buttocks. Also, prevents the client from slipping on the wet surface of the seat.

4. Fill either sitz bath bowl so that it is one-third to one-half full. The water temperature should be between 100 and 105° Fahrenheit. Some models of sitz baths continuously drain and refill. (If instructions are provided, follow them carefully.)	4. Prevents spillage of the water, which can be a safety hazard. This water temperature will not burn the client, yet will relax the immersed body part.
5. Help the client to undress and immerse the affected part of the body in the water. Drape exposed body parts.	5. Prevents chilling.
6. Assess the client's comfort. If you are unable to stay with the client during the procedure, provide an emergency call light.	6. Provides you with information useful for the client's optimal wellness. Provides for the client's safety. Clients may become dizzy from the warmth of the water and the position.
7. Generally, the client is allowed to soak for 15 to 20 minutes.	7. Promotes relaxation of the immersed part of the body.

▼ *ACTION*	▼ *RATIONALE*
8. During this time, check on the client frequently. You may need to refill the bath with more warm water.	**8.** Provides for the client's safety. Clients may become dizzy from the warmth of the water and the position. Keeping the water warm increases the effectiveness of the treatment.
9. At the end of the allotted time, assist the client from the bath and help to dry him or her. Reposition the client's clothes and sanitary pads or dressings (if needed).	**9.** Provides for the client's safety.
NOTE: If contact with body fluids is a possibility, you should wear gloves.	Decreases the possibility of transmission of microorganisms.
10. Help the client to get into bed and assess his or her comfort.	**10.** Provides information useful for the client's optimal wellness.
11. Empty and clean the sitz bath with a disinfectant and rinse well. Allow the portable sitz bath to dry before putting it away. Dispose of towels and gloves in proper containers.	**11.** Decreases the transmission of microorganisms.
12. Wash your hands.	**12.** Decreases the transmission of microorganisms.
13. Record the procedure and other relevant information.	**13.** Communicates the information to the other members of the health care team and contributes to the legal record by documenting the care given to the client.

Example of Documentation

DATE	TIME	NOTES
1/20/93	1000	100° F sitz bath provided for client for 15 minutes. No change noted in perineal skin color, edema, or discharge from 8 A.M. assessment. Client states she voided without difficulty during the sitz bath. Bladder area is soft to palpation and is not distended.
		S. Smart, RN

Teaching Tips

Encourage the client to empty his or her bladder prior to using the sitz bath. If the client has been having trouble defecating after a hemorrhoidectomy, the sitz bath can be very beneficial. At times the first postoperative bowel movement occurs while the client is using the sitz bath. Let the client know that this is normal. Do not allow the client to sit in the feces and be sure the sitz bath is thoroughly cleaned and disinfected before further use. Encourage the client to use relaxation techniques during the procedure to increase comfort.

Home Care Variations

Emphasize that the water temperature must be checked before the client uses the sitz bath to prevent burns. Skin areas that have been traumatized may not accurately detect that the water is too hot and resultant burns may occur. The sitz bath must be cleaned thoroughly and dried between uses and must not be shared with other family members.

SKILL 12–2   TEACHING PROGRESSIVE MUSCLE RELAXATION

Clinical Situations in Which You May Encounter This Skill

Progressive muscle relaxation (PMR) technique can be used for clients who are experiencing stress, pain, or anxiety, or who require calmness, relaxation, or comfort.

Until the client gains experience in this technique, he or she may feel some impatience. As positive benefits are gained, the impatience usually disappears.

Since relaxation can enhance the effects of sedatives, antihypertensive medications, and insulin, you should observe the client for possible alterations in dosage that may be needed.

Anticipated Responses

▼ The client experiences decreased feelings of stress, anxiety, and pain and increased feelings of calmness, comfort, and relaxation.

Adverse Responses

▼ The client's level of stress, anxiety, or pain does not decrease.

Materials List

Gather these materials before beginning the skill:

▼ One or more mental focal points (tape, focus object, word, etc.)

▼ *A C T I O N*

1. Determine the nature of the client's illness.

2. Prior to beginning the procedure, ask the client to wear comfortable clothes and to empty his or her bladder.

3. Ask the client to lie in a comfortable position in bed or to sit comfortably in a chair. The environment should be quiet.

4. Ask the client to close his or her eyes and focus on a muscle group, such as the muscles in the lower arms and hands. Ask the client to:
   a. Tense these muscles by consciously tightening the forearm muscle and making a fist.
   b. Note the sensation when the muscles are tense.
   c. Hold the tenseness for 5 to 7 seconds.
   d. Relax the muscles in the hand and forearm.
   e. Concentrate on the different sensations between tenseness and relaxation.
   f. Duplicate the procedure with other major muscle groups throughout the body. It is best to start with the muscle groups in the upper part of the body and work down.

▼ *R A T I O N A L E*

1. Allows for individualized client care.

2. Provides for the client's comfort.

3. Sets the proper stage.

4. Closing the eyes encourages concentration.

   a–f. PMR techniques help the client to differentiate between tenseness and relaxation. Clients who are in pain have increased autonomic nervous system (ANS) activity that further increases tension and pain. When clients are taught to relax, the pain cycle is broken. Choosing a systematic approach is most effective.

▼ *ACTION* ▼ *RATIONALE*

5. Explain to the client that while practicing PMR, he or she should incorporate slow, rhythmic, deep breathing.

5. Deep breathing has a calming effect.

NOTE: Clients should be cautioned not to hyperventilate. Also, clients with respiratory problems should minimize or eliminate the deep breathing exercises. Normal depth of breathing should be used.

Dizziness may occur. Respiratory problems may be exacerbated by deep breathing.

---

6. Encourage the client to continue this procedure for 15 to 20 minutes.

6. Allows the client time to practice the technique and gain its benefits.

7. When the client wishes to end the exercise, he or she should:
   a. Concentrate just on rhythmic breathing for a minute.
   b. Open his or her eyes slowly.
   c. Stretch, as if awakening from sleep.
   d. Move around until he or she feels alert.

7. Helps the client to return to normal activity gradually and to retain some benefits of relaxation.

8. The client should be informed that for the best results he or she should practice the PMR exercises at least twice a day for 15 to 20 minutes.

8. Immediate results are unlikely, as PMR is a learned behavior.

9. Encourage the client's progress and help him or her to find the time needed to practice. Explain that distracting thoughts are likely to happen, but that they are normal. The client should try to ignore them and go on.

9. Assists the client in health-seeking behaviors.

10. If the client is having difficulty with the procedure, an audiotape of the procedure may be beneficial.

10. Helps the client to learn the procedure.

11. Record the procedure and other relevant information.

11. Communicates the information to the other members of the health care team and contributes to the legal record by documenting the care given to the client.

12. Evelute the client's comfort and determine if further interventions are needed.

12. Provides for optimal client care.

Example of Documentation

DATE	TIME	NOTES
1/20/93	1900	PMR technique taught to client. Client states he is interested in learning ways to control his pain without drugs. States his pain level was a 3/10 after the technique as compared to a 6/10 before the technique. States he does not want pain medication at this time. Was encouraged to practice at least twice daily.
		S. Smart, RN

Teaching Tips

It is helpful to clients and students if they have practiced the technique and feel comfortable with it.

Home Care Variations

Clients need to be encouraged to continue to practice this technique at home, preferably twice a day. Outside influences may take precedence over the practice and the client may experience increased pain. The client must find a quiet place and practice the technique as if it were a prescribed medication. Family members also need to be made aware of the importance of PMR.

SKILL 12–3   MONITORING A PATIENT-CONTROLLED ANALGESIA PUMP

Clinical Situations in Which You May Encounter This Skill

Patient-controlled analgesia (PCA) pumps are used for clients who have postoperative, acute, or chronic pain and are able to participate consciously in controlling their analgesia. A PCA pump is an analgesic administration system that is designed to facilitate optimal serum analgesic levels during a therapeutic course.

A thorough reading of the manufacturer's instructions is necessary for proper operation of the PCA pump. The following definitions are also helpful:

▼ Loading dose—The initial dose of medication that is to be infused. This dose is usually greater than the following doses.
▼ PCA dose—The volume (milliliters) of medication that is to be given in each infusion.
▼ Delay (lock-out) interval—The minimum prescribed time in minutes during which medication may not be infused.
▼ Basal rate—Prescribed milliliters per hour of a continuous infusion rate.
▼ Maximum hourly limit—The total volume that can be infused in a certain time period (pumps vary from 1–4 hr).
▼ Bolus dose (incremental)—This may be the loading dose. Some manufacturers define this as the PCA dose.
▼ Attempts—Number of times the client pushes the button to try to receive an infusion of medication.
▼ Injections—Number of times the client received an infusion of medication. Usually a ratio of attempts to injections is given on the pump display.
▼ Total dose—The volume of medication the client received within the time interval evaluated.

> **NOTE:** PCA pumps infuse narcotics and must be accounted for accurately according to Food and Drug Administration policy. The narcotics in the pumps are usually under double locks just like other narcotics.

Anticipated Responses

▼ The client is free of pain, denies nausea, and is rested.
▼ The client feels more personal control.
▼ The client tolerates moving.
▼ The client coughs and deep breathes well.
▼ The number of attempts does not greatly exceed the number of administered doses of medication.
▼ The number of attempts and the number of administered doses of medication decrease as the time from the procedure increases.

Adverse Responses

▼ The client continues to have unrelieved pain and nausea and is not able to rest.
▼ The client feels less control.
▼ The client is not tolerant of movement and does not cough and deep breathe well.
▼ The number of attempts greatly exceeds the number of administered doses of medication.
▼ The number of attempts and the number of administered doses stay the same or increase over time.

Materials List

Gather these materials before beginning the skill:

▼ PCA pump and instructions for its use
▼ Materials called for in the pump instructions (such as intravenous [IV] tubing, key for the pump, and stand for the pump)
▼ A patent, well-functioning primary IV or epidural line
▼ Properly prepared medication from the physician's order sheet
▼ Naloxone hydrochloride (Narcan) 0.4 mg at the client's bedside (usually for clients undergoing epidural infusion)

▼ ACTION	▼ RATIONALE
1. Assess the physician's order for the drug, dosage, and other parameters such as lock-out intervals and maximum dose.	1. PCA pumps require a physician's order.
2. Assess the client's knowledge about the procedure and the reasons for it.	2. Provides you with information from which to plan the client's care.
3. Assess the client's level of consciousness.	3. The client should be able to operate the pump.
4. Assess the IV site and its patency.	4. The IV is the access route. Prevents inaccurate administration of the medication. Infiltrated IVs cause serious tissue injury.
5. Set the primary IV infusion for the prescribed fluid and rate.	5. Maintains a patent system.
6. Check the client's identification band before preparing and administering the medication.	6. Ensures that you are giving the medication to the correct person.
7. Prepare the medication and place the narcotic infuser in the pump. Be sure the syringe is properly placed.	7. Loads the machine for use. Prevents inaccurate administration of the medication.
8. Flush the PCA pump tubing. Connect the PCA tubing to the patient's IV line with an 18-gauge needle inserted into an injection port. Tape all connections.	8. Prevents an air embolus. Prevents accidental disconnection. Allows the IV system to be primed with medicated solution.
9. Set the various medication dials to their lowest settings.	9. Provides for the client's safety.
10. Follow the set-up instructions for the PCA pump model being used (see "Teaching Tips"). Follow the physician's orders for the loading dose, PCA dose, delay time, and 1-hour maximum dose. (Some agencies have standing orders for these settings.)	10. Allows for the safest, most effective care.
11. After the loading dose has been injected, give the client the "button" with which to administer the medication and be sure he or she knows how to use it.	11. Provides the means of administering the medication.
12. Reinforce previous instructions. (Continuous infusion of medication may be ordered until the client is able to participate in the procedure. You would program this continuous infusion into the PCA pump.)	12. The client may have been drowsy from previous medication. The client should have instructions reinforced until he or she is alert enough to remember them.
13. Provide other postoperative care as needed.	13. Provides total care.

▼ ACTION	▼ RATIONALE
14. Frequently evaluate the client's condition, including pain relief, level of consciousness, blood pressure, heart rate, and respiratory rate. (Remember: narcotics are being administered.)	**14.** Provides information needed for further care.
15. Evaluate the patency of the IV system and the PCA system.	**15.** Helps to ensure correct functioning of the systems.
16. Review the manufacturer's instructions concerning changing the syringe, obtaining medication administration history from the pump, and alarm descriptions.	**16.** Allows for safe, efficient nursing care.
17. Record the procedure in the client's record and on the appropriate controlled substance records.	**17.** Communicates to the other members of the health care team and contributes to the legal record by documenting the care given to the client.

Example of Documentation

DATE	TIME	NOTES
7/18/93	1300	Client arouses easily. Oriented × 3. BP = 136/86. AP = 96. RR = 20. PCA pump initiated. Loading dose of 4 mg morphine sulfate (MSO$_4$) given. Pump set to deliver 1 mg MSO$_4$ with a delay time of 15 minutes. Maximum hourly limit of 4 mg MSO$_4$.
		H. White, RN

(Some agencies have PCA infusion records that also must be maintained.)

Teaching Tips

Explain to the client or the client's family, or both, the purpose of the PCA pump and that it is designed to provide optimal pain relief. The client should also understand that you will be checking the pump for accuracy and the client's response to the pump at frequent intervals. Families need to be reminded it is "patient-controlled," not "family-controlled." They should not press the button for the client, as they can overmedicate the client.

Home Care Variations

The same procedure is used in the home setting. The family caregiver should be taught the proper techniques to care for the pump and administer the medication.

SKILL 12-4 APPLYING MOIST HEAT

Clinical Situations in Which You May Encounter This Skill

Heat is often applied to reduce swelling and inflammation. Heat also can be used to promote pain relief, increase circulation, promote healing, reduce muscle spasms, and soften exudates.

Anticipated Responses

▼ Heat is applied without causing further trauma to the client's skin.

Adverse Responses

▼ The client's skin shows signs of burns or heat intolerance such as redness, blisters, or further swelling.

Materials List

Gather these materials before beginning the skill:

▼ 4- × 4-inch gauze strips or towels (clean or sterile as required by the procedure) for making the moist compress
▼ Sterile basin (if the procedure requires sterile technique)
▼ Bath basin
▼ Bath thermometer
▼ Sterile isotonic saline or tap water
▼ Disposable heat pack or aquathermia pad
▼ Clean or sterile towels for drying the treated area
▼ Sterile gloves (if there is a wound)
▼ Waterproof pads (two)
▼ Petroleum jelly (optional)
▼ Tape or ties

> **NOTE:** If there is no open wound, this is a clean procedure and does not require the use of sterile isotonic saline or sterile technique. If an open wound is present, use sterile technique and sterile supplies.

▼ _ACTION_

1. Assess the client's skin at the affected site for any areas of redness, breakdown, or scar tissue.

2. Determine the diagnosis of the client's condition and any history of diabetes mellitus or impairments in sensation.

3. Check the physician's order and the reason for the warm compress.

4. Wash your hands.

5. Warm the container of sterile saline or tap water by placing it in a bath basin filled with hot tap water. Sterile saline should be warmed to 105 to 113° Fahrenheit. If you are using a commercial compress, follow the manufacturer's directions for heating the compress.

6. Place a waterproof pad under the body area that needs the warm compress.

7. A thin layer of petroleum jelly may be placed on the client's skin in the area to be treated. Do not put petroleum jelly on an open wound or use with oxygen therapy.

▼ _RATIONALE_

1. Provides baseline data with which to compare future assessments. Since scar tissue may be heat sensitive, this area should be avoided, if possible, when the compress is applied.

2. Sensation is often impaired in the diabetic. Persons with impairments in sensation may not be able to tell if the compress is too hot. The risk of burns is greater with moist heat than with dry heat. The medical diagnosis may alert you to other problems.

3. A physician's order is required. The reason for the compress should be explained to the client.

4. Decreases the transmission of microorganisms.

5. Sterile saline is used to prevent any contamination of the wound. A temperature above 113° F will cause further injury.

6. Protects the client's bed and clothing.

7. Helps protect the client's skin from heat injury.

▼ _ _A C T I O N_ _ _ _ _ _ _ _ _ _   ▼ _R A T I O N A L E_ _ _ _ _ _ _ _ _

8. Pour the sterile saline into the sterile basin. Soak a 4- × 4-inch piece of gauze or a towel, wring out the excess water, and place it on the affected area (Fig. 12–2). Wear gloves if there is any drainage of the client's body fluids. Wear sterile gloves if there is an open wound.

8. A sterile basin is used to prevent further contamination. Excess saline may increase the chance of burns.

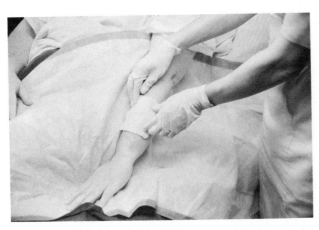

▼ **FIGURE 12–2.** Applying moist heat.

9. Wrap the area with a waterproof pad or apply a disposable heat pack or aquathermia pad.

9. Maintains or holds in the heat.

10. Check the client's skin periodically for signs of heat intolerance.

10. Signs of intolerance may include redness, blisters, or further swelling.

11. If it is tolerated, leave the compress in place for approximately 20 minutes and then remove it.

11. Application of moist heat for a longer period of time may damage the client's skin and may predispose the client to edema formation from circulatory congestion.

12. Dry the affected area with sterile towels if there is an open wound and with clean towels if there is no open wound.

12. The client may feel chilled when the warm compress is removed. He or she will need to have the area completely dried to prevent further chilling.

13. Properly dispose of all single-use equipment.

13. The basins and thermometer can be used again. Proper disposal of all other equipment decreases the transmission of microorganisms.

14. Clean the bath basin and thermometer. Return the sterile basin to the appropriate place for resterilization.

14. Decreases the transmission of microorganisms and gets the equipment ready for use again.

15. Remove gloves if they were worn and wash your hands.

15. Decreases the transmission of microorganisms.

16. Reassess the condition of the client's skin.

16. The condition of the client's skin and any signs of heat sensitivity should be assessed and documented.

17. Record the procedure. Note the condition of the client's skin and the length of the application.

17. Communicates the findings to the other members of the health care team and contributes to the legal record by documenting the care given to the client.

Example of Documentation

DATE	TIME	NOTES
11/9/93	0930	IV discontinued. Area red and swollen. Warm moist compress applied for 20 minutes. No signs of heat intolerance.
		R. Walker, RN

Teaching Tips

Explain the procedure and the purpose of the procedure to the client or the client's family member, or both. Explain the danger of leaving the hot compress in place for too long.

Home Care Variations

The client can use towels instead of 4- × 4-inch gauze strips if a sterile dressing is not needed. A home health care nurse may need to assist the client in obtaining other equipment. The client can test the temperature of the water on his or her forearm instead of purchasing a bath thermometer.

SKILL 12–5 APPLYING DRY HEAT

Clinical Situations in Which You May Encounter This Skill

Dry heat is often applied to reduce swelling and inflammation. Heat also can be used to promote pain relief, increase circulation, promote healing, and reduce muscle spasms. Dry heat can be applied with a hot water bottle, disposable heat pack, heating pad, or aquathermia pad.

Any equipment used to apply dry heat may injure the client if the client is unable to perceive discomfort due to decreased feeling, decreased sensorium, sedation, or agitation; the client cannot be left alone safely; or the client alters the controls of the heating pad or aquathermia pad.

Diabetics or clients with vascular disease should not use dry heat without specific orders to do so from the physician.

Anticipated Responses

▼ Heat is applied without causing further trauma to the client's skin.
▼ Swelling or inflammation, or both, are reduced.

Adverse Responses

▼ The client's skin shows signs of burns or heat intolerance such as redness, blisters, or further swelling.

Materials List

Gather these materials before beginning the skill:

▼ Aquathermia pad, heating pad, or hot water bottle
▼ Bath thermometer (for hot water bottle and aquathermia pad)
▼ Protective cover (for hot water bottle)

▼ *A C T I O N*

1. Assess the affected site for any areas of redness, breakdown, or scar tissue.

▼ *R A T I O N A L E*

1. Provides baseline data with which to compare future assessments. Since scar tissue may be heat sensitive, this area should be avoided, if possible, when the heat is applied.

▼ *A C T I O N*

▼ *R A T I O N A L E*

2. Determine the diagnosis of the client's illness and any history of diabetes mellitus or impairments in sensation.

2. Sensation may be impaired in the person with diabetes. Persons with impairments in sensation may not be able to tell if the heat is too hot. The medical diagnosis may alert you to other problems. For example, heat should not be used over a malignancy or over an area of potential hemorrhage.

3. Check the physician's order and the reason for the heat application.

3. A physician's order is required. The reason for the heat application should be explained to the client.

4. Wash your hands.

4. Decreases the transmission of microorganisms.

5. If using a hot water bottle:
   a. Check the temperature of the heated tap water with a bath thermometer before filling the hot water bottle.
   b. Fill the hot water bottle two-thirds full. Expel any remaining air from the bottle and close it.
   c. Check for leaks.
   d. Wrap the bottle in a towel or protective cover and place it on the affected area (Fig. 12–3).

   a. A safe range to prevent burns is 115 to 125° Fahrenheit (F) for adults and 105 to 115° F for children.
   b. Makes the bottle lighter and easier to mold to the client's body.
   c. Excess water may increase the chance of burns.
   d. The hot water bottle is wrapped to prevent injury to the client's skin.

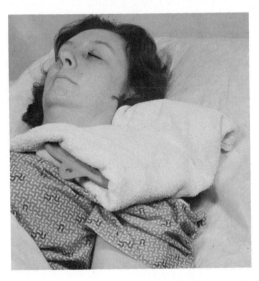

▼ **FIGURE 12–3.** Applying dry heat with a hot water bottle.

6. If using a disposable heat pack:
   a. Activate the pack according to the manufacturer's directions.
   b. Wrap the pack in a towel and place it on the affected area.
   c. Discard the pack after treatment.

   a. When the pack is activated, it will heat automatically.
   b. The pack is wrapped to prevent injury to the client's skin.
   c. The pack cannot be used again.

7. If using a heating pad:
   a. Place the flannel cover on the heating pad.
   b. Instruct the client not to lie on the heating pad.

   c. Turn the switch on to low and place the heating pad on the affected area.

   a. Prevents injury to the client's skin.
   b. When the client lies on the heating pad, hot spots that may burn the client can be created.
   c. The client's skin may be more sensitive to the heat than he or she is aware of. The temperature can be increased if necessary.

▼ *ACTION*	▼ *RATIONALE*
d. Instruct the client not to increase the heat level.	d. Burns can result.
8. If using an aquathermia pad:	
a. Fill the control unit to the line with distilled water.	a. Distilled water prevents the formation of mineral deposits that will damage the equipment.
b. Turn the unit on and check the temperature of the heated water after several minutes with a bath thermometer.	b. The proper temperature of the water is 105° F.
c. Check the unit, pad, and tubing for leaks.	c. If there is a leak in any of the equipment, it should be exchanged. The leak is a safety hazard for both you and the client.
d. Place a towel on or around the affected area. Apply the aquathermia pad and secure it with tape if it is wrapped around an extremity.	d. A towel should be used between the pad and the client's skin to prevent injury to the skin.
9. Check the client's skin periodically for signs of heat intolerance.	**9.** Signs of intolerance may include redness, blisters, and further swelling.
10. If it is tolerated, leave the pad in place for approximately 20 minutes and then remove it.	**10.** A longer application may damage the skin.
11. Return the aquathermia pad to the appropriate place for cleaning and decontamination.	**11.** The aquathermia pad should be turned off and saved for further use.
12. Properly dispose of the remaining equipment.	**12.** Decreases the transmission of microorganisms.
13. Wash your hands.	**13.** Decreases the transmission of microorganisms.
14. Reassess the condition of the client's skin.	**14.** The condition of the client's skin and any signs of heat sensitivity should be assessed and documented.
15. Record the procedure. Note the condition of the client's skin and the length of the heat application.	**15.** Communicates the findings to the other members of the health care team and contributes to the legal record by documenting the care given to the client.

Example of Documentation

DATE	TIME	NOTES
11/9/93	0930	Left forearm red and swollen. Aquathermia pad applied for 20 minutes. No signs of heat intolerance.
		R. Walker, RN

Teaching Tips

When applying heat, you should explain to the client the purpose of the heat therapy and that it should be used only for short intervals. If symptoms worsen, the therapy should be discontinued and the physician should be contacted. Also, explain the signs of heat intolerance and tell the client that if the signs develop, the therapy should be discontinued and the physician should be contacted.

Home Care Variations

Heat therapy can be used in the client's home. The client should be given instructions for proper usage and taught the signs of heat intolerance.

SKILL 12–6   APPLYING COLD

Clinical Situations in Which You May Encounter This Skill

Cold is often applied to reduce bleeding and inflammation. Cold also can be used to promote pain relief and prevent swelling. Cold can be applied with an ice bag, ice collar, or disposable cold pack.

Anticipated Responses

▼ Cold is applied without causing further trauma to the client's skin.

Adverse Responses

▼ The client's skin shows signs of cold intolerance such as pallor, mottling, or numbness.
▼ The client's skin is red because the cold application has been left in place too long.

Materials List

Gather these materials before beginning the skill:

▼ Ice bag, ice collar with ice, or disposable cold pack
▼ Towel

▼ ACTION	▼ RATIONALE
1. Assess the client's skin color and sensation at the application site.	1. Provides baseline data with which to compare future assessments.
2. Determine the diagnosis of the client's illness and any history of circulatory impairment.	2. Cold causes vasoconstriction and can cause tissue damage in persons with impaired circulation.
3. Check the physician's order and the reason for the application of cold.	3. A physician's order is required. The reason for the application of cold should be explained to the client.
4. If using an ice bag: a. Fill the bag three-fourths full with ice. Expel the remaining air from the bag and close the bag. Check for leaks. b. Wrap the bag in a towel or protective cover and place it on the affected area.	a. Makes the bag lighter and easier to mold to the client's body. b. The bag is wrapped to prevent injury to the client's skin.
5. If using an ice collar: a. Fill the collar three-fourths full with ice. Expel the remaining air from the collar and close it. Check for leaks.	a. Makes the collar lighter and easier to mold to the client's body.

▼ *ACTION*   ▼ *RATIONALE*

b. Place the collar in a protective cover and place it around the client's neck (Fig. 12–4).

b. The collar is wrapped to prevent injury to the client's skin.

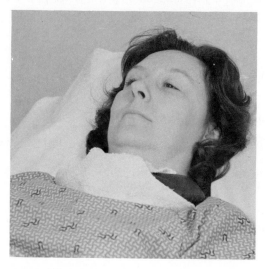

▼ **FIGURE 12–4.** Applying cold with an ice collar.

6. If using a disposable cold pack:
   a. Activate the pack according to the manufacturer's directions.
   b. Wrap the pack in a towel and place it on the affected area. (Some packs have their own cover on one side.)
   c. Discard the pack after the treatment.

a. When the pack is activated, it will become cold.
b. Prevents injury to the client's skin.

c. The pack cannot be used again.

7. Check the client's skin periodically for signs of cold intolerance.

7. Signs of intolerance include pallor, mottling, or numbness of the skin.

8. If it is tolerated, leave the cold application in place for approximately 30 minutes.

8. A longer application may damage the client's skin. Reflex vasodilatation occurs after 20 to 30 minutes, thereby negating the therapeutic effect of the cold.

9. Reassess the condition of the client's skin.

9. The condition of the client's skin should be assessed and any signs of cold intolerance should be documented.

10. Record the procedure. Note the condition of the client's skin and the length of the application.

10. Communicates the findings to the other members of the health care team and contributes to the legal record by documenting the care given to the client.

Example of Documentation

DATE	TIME	NOTES
11/9/93	1330	Upon admission, Mr. Z. was noted to have a left sprained wrist. Disposable cold pack applied for 30 minutes. No signs of cold intolerance.
		R. Sims, RN

Teaching Tips

When applying cold therapy, explain to the client the purpose of the cold therapy and the signs of cold intolerance. If signs of cold intolerance develop or the symptoms necessitating the cold therapy increase, the therapy should be discontinued and the physician should be contacted.

Home Care Variations

Cold therapy can be used in the client's home. The client should be given instructions for proper usage and taught the signs of cold intolerance.

SKILL 12–7   GIVING A TEPID SPONGE BATH

Clinical Situations in Which You May Encounter This Skill

A tepid sponge bath can be given when a client's body temperature is elevated (fever). As the client's body is sponged with tepid water, heat is lost through evaporation. There are several methods that can be used to give a tepid sponge bath. These include: covering the client's body with a bath blanket or large sheet moistened with tepid water, sponging each body part separately, and placing the client's body in a tub of tepid water. Sponge baths are most frequently used with infants and children.

Anticipated Responses

▼ The client's body temperature is reduced.

Adverse Responses

▼ The client may become chilled, which can cause the body temperature to further elevate.

Materials List

Gather these materials before beginning the skill:

▼ Basin or tub
▼ Tepid water
▼ Bath thermometer
▼ Bath blanket or large sheet
▼ Washcloths
▼ Towels
▼ Waterproof pads
▼ Thermometer
▼ Gloves
▼ Alcohol (optional)

▼ ACTION	▼ RATIONALE
1. Review the procedure manual for your agency protocol for giving a tepid sponge bath.	1. Some agencies require that a particular method be used. Some agencies require a physician's order, whereas others view the skill as an independent nursing decision.
2. Assess the client's temperature, pulse, and respiration. Observe the client for signs and symptoms of a fever (pale and warm skin, general malaise, muscle aches, restlessness, headache, confusion, and delirium).	2. Provides you with baseline data to be used when evaluating the client's response to the treatment.
3. Explain the procedure to the client or his or her parents, or both.	3. Informing the client contributes to an increase in participation and a decrease in his or her anxiety level.
4. Position the bed at a comfortable working level for you.	4. Protects your back from strain.
5. Wash your hands and put on gloves.	5. Decreases the transmission of microorganisms.

▼ ACTION	▼ RATIONALE
6. Remove the client's clothing and place a bath blanket over him or her.	**6.** Ensures privacy and protects modesty.
7. Place waterproof pads under the client.	**7.** Protects the linen from soiling.
8. Fill a basin with tepid water (27 to 37° C [80–98.6° F]). Check the water temperature with a bath thermometer.	**8.** Tepid water prevents chilling. Alcohol sponges are used infrequently because they can irritate the skin and cause nausea.
9. Immerse the washcloths in tepid water. Place the tepid compresses on the client's forehead, groin, and axilla for 20 to 30 minutes.	**9.** Transfer of heat is more effective when compresses are placed on areas with large superficial blood vessels such as the groin and axillary area.
10. If you are using a tub, immerse the client into the tepid tub water for 20 to 30 minutes. Support the head and shoulders of an infant or young child (see Skill 10–15).	**10.** Immersion into a tub promotes more effective heat loss.
11. Gently sponge the client's face and each extremity for 5 minutes. Then sponge his or her back and buttocks for 5 to 10 minutes. Pat dry each body part with a towel after sponging.	**11.** Promotes a decrease in temperature within a safe time frame. Minimizes the chance of chilling.
12. Monitor the client's responses to the treatment. Monitor the client's temperature, pulse, and respirations every 10 minutes throughout the treatment.	**12.** Evaluates the effectiveness of the treatment. Prevents a sudden decrease in temperature. Arrhythmias can result as a complication due to a change in blood flow during heat loss.
13. When the client's body temperature is slightly above normal, the treatment may be discontinued.	**13.** Prevents the temperature from becoming subnormal.
14. Replace the client's clothing and cover him or her with a light sheet.	**14.** Maintains the person's body temperature. Excessive clothing and covering can result in a temperature elevation.
15. Replace any soiled linen and remove the equipment used.	**15.** Prevents transmission of microorganisms.
16. Lower the bed to a safe height.	**16.** Promotes the client's safety.
17. Remove the gloves and wash your hands.	**17.** Prevents transmission of microorganisms.
18. Document the treatment performed, the client's vital signs, response to the treatment, and any complications.	**18.** Provides information to the health care team regarding the client's response to the treatment. It also contributes to the legal record of care given to the client.
19. Take the client's vital signs every 1 to 2 hours until the client has stabilized after the treatment.	**19.** Provides data of a possible reelevation of temperature.

Examples of Documentation

DATE	TIME	NOTES
5/31/94	0800	T = 104° F, P = 100, R = 28 Tepid sponge bath given to client for 30 minutes. Vital signs monitored every 10 minutes and recorded on a graph. Client tolerated treatment without complications. Temperature returned to 99° and sponge bath discontinued. *M. Smith, RN*

Teaching Tips

Washcloths should be moist rather than dripping wet. You should use slow gentle motions when sponging the client. Strong brisk motions increase the metabolism of tissue and heat production.

Home Care Variations

Since infants and young children can suddenly develop a high fever, it is important to teach family members how to give a tepid sponge bath at home. You should emphasize that the infant's head and shoulders need to be supported when the child is being sponged in a tub. This support can be a family member's arm or a towel or sheet folded and placed under the infant's head and shoulders. It is also important to emphasize the safety of the child. No infant or child should be left unattended in the tub. The child's temperature should be taken before and 20 to 30 minutes after immersion in the tub.

SKILL 12–8   USING A HYPOTHERMIA OR HYPERTHERMIA BLANKET

Clinical Situations in Which You May Encounter This Skill

A client's temperature may be unusually high (hyperthermia) or unusually low (hypothermia). The physician may order a hypothermia blanket to lower or a hyperthermia blanket to raise the client's temperature. These blankets are mechanically operated and can be set to heat or cool. The manufacturer's directions should be followed and the client's temperature should be closely monitored.

Anticipated Responses

▼ The client's temperature is raised or lowered to the desired level.

Adverse Responses

▼ The client's temperature is raised or lowered too rapidly.
▼ The client's temperature is raised or lowered too much.

Materials List

Gather these materials before beginning the skill:

▼ Hypothermia or hyperthermia blanket with machine and thermometer probe
▼ Thermometer (if a thermometer probe is not provided with the machine and blanket)

▼ ACTION	▼ RATIONALE
1. Check the client's temperature and vital signs.	1. Provides baseline data for future comparisons to determine the effectiveness of the treatment.
2. Check the physician's order for the desired body temperature.	2. You may not legally complete the treatment without an order.
3. Explain the procedure to the client or the client's family, or both.	3. Explanations help to allay anxiety.
4. Check to make sure the plug is not frayed and is grounded.	4. Helps to ensure the client's safety.
5. Add the solution to the machine. Follow the manufacturer's directions for the type and amount of solution to use.	5. The solution will either be heated or cooled by the machine for the desired effect.
6. Place the blanket on the client's bed, cover it with a sheet, and connect it to the machine.	6. Helps to protect the client's skin.
7. Insert the temperature probe if one is available and tape it to the client's buttocks.	7. Allows for constant monitoring of the client's temperature.
8. Set the machine to the desired temperature and turn it on.	8. Allows the blanket to begin cooling or warming the client.
9. Check the client's temperature every 15 minutes and turn the machine off when the temperature is within several degrees of the desired temperature.	9. The temperature will continue to drift down or up once the machine is turned off. The temperature is checked frequently to determine if it is being raised too rapidly.
10. Periodically check the client's temperature with a glass thermometer.	10. Helps to determine the accuracy of the temperature probe.
11. Check the client's vital signs every 30 minutes and observe for shivering if the blanket is being used to cool the client.	11. Shivering increases the client's metabolic rate and can increase heat production.
12. Turn the client every 1 to 2 hours and assess his or her skin.	12. The skin can be damaged from the effects of heat and cold.
13. Record the procedure. Note the length of time needed to raise or lower the temperature and all of the temperature recordings and vital signs.	13. Communicates to the other members of the health care team and contributes to the legal record by documenting the care given to the client.

Example of Documentation

DATE	TIME	NOTES
3/6/94	0800	Temperature 103.8° F rectally. Placed on cooling blanket.
3/6/94	0815	Temperature 103.2° F rectally.
3/6/94	0830	Temperature 103° F rectally.
3/6/94	0845	Temperature 102.8° F rectally.
3/6/94	0900	Temperature 102.6° F rectally.
3/6/94	0915	Temperature 102.2° F rectally.
3/6/94	0930	Temperature 100.8° F rectally.
3/6/94	0945	Temperature 100.4° F rectally.
3/6/94	1000	Temperature 100° F rectally. Cool blanket turned off. No signs of shivering. Vital signs stable.
		S. Smith, RN

Teaching Tips

The purpose of the blanket and the procedure should be explained to the client or his or her family members, or both. Explain that you will be monitoring the client's temperature every 15 minutes. Ask the client or his or her family member to notify you if the client starts to shiver.

Home Care Variations

These blankets are not usually used in the home. However, you may need to talk to the family about alternative methods of raising or lowering the client's temperature.

References

Clark, L. A. (1994). Facilitating relief from pain. In V. Bolander (Ed.), *Basic nursing* (3rd ed.). Philadelphia: W. B. Saunders.

Hill, P. D. (1989). Effects of heat and cold on the perineum after episiotomy/laceration. *Journal of Obstetric, Gynecologic, and Neonatal Nursing*, 18 (2), 124–129.

LaFoy, J., and Geden, E. A. (1989). Postepisiotomy pain: Warm versus cold sitz bath. *Journal of Obstetric, Gynecologic, and Neonatal Nursing*, 18 (5), 399–403.

Miller, K. M. (1987). Deep breathing relaxation—A pain management technique. *AORN Journal*, 45 (2), 484–488.

Munro, B. H., et al. (1988). Effect of relaxation therapy on postmyocardial infarction patients' relaxation. *Nursing Research*, 37, 231–235.

Shannon, M. L. (1994). Caring for persons with wounds. In V. Bolander (Ed.), *Basic nursing* (3rd ed.). Philadelphia: W. B. Saunders.

CHAPTER 13

Administering Blood Products

Blood transfusion involves administration of whole blood or blood products such as platelets, plasma, or packed red blood cells (RBCs). Whole blood is administered to replace blood volume lost during surgery or due to trauma or hemorrhage. Blood products are administered to replace selected blood components such as RBCs in the anemic client or platelets and plasma in the individual who needs clotting factors to treat bleeding disorders.

You have the primary responsibility for correctly administering blood and monitoring the client for possible adverse reactions during the transfusion (see Table 13–1 on page 393). A febrile nonhemolytic blood reaction is the most common type of transfusion reaction. Febrile reactions occur due to an antigen-antibody reaction to the white blood cells (WBCs) or platelets in the blood product. Signs and symptoms occur during the administration or up to 6 hours after the administration and include fever and chills.

An allergic urticarial transfusion reaction usually occurs during the transfusion and represents an allergy to an antigen in the plasma of the blood. The most common sign is a rash.

Hemolytic transfusion reactions can be either immediate or delayed. An immediate hemolytic reaction occurs because of blood type (ABO) incompatibility and can be life threatening. Signs and symptoms occur during the first 5 to 15 minutes of the transfusion and include facial flushing, urticaria, fever and chills, lumbar pain, headache, abdominal cramps, nausea and vomiting, dyspnea, tachycardia, hypotension, hematuria, and oliguria, which may progress to anuria. A delayed hemolytic reaction occurs 10 or more days after the transfusion due to an RBC antigen incompatibility. The primary signs are a decreasing hemoglobin level and a low-grade fever.

An anaphylactic transfusion reaction can also be life threatening. This type of allergic transfusion reaction occurs rarely. The signs and symptoms occur after the infusion of only a few milliliters of blood and include bronchospasm and cardiovascular and respiratory failure.

When a transfusion reaction occurs, you should discontinue the transfusion immediately and keep the intravenous (IV) line open with normal saline. Both the physician and the blood bank should be notified of the reaction. Monitor the client's vital signs. A urine specimen may be collected to assess for hematuria. A blood specimen may be ordered to assess for hemolysis. The blood bag with any remaining blood and the tubing should be returned to the blood bank. Lastly, you should be prepared to carry out emergency resuscitation measures if needed.

SKILL 13–1 ADMINISTERING WHOLE BLOOD AND PACKED RED BLOOD CELLS

Clinical Situations in Which You May Encounter This Skill

Whole blood may be administered to clients who are chronically anemic or to clients who have lost 2 or more units (1,000 ml or more) of blood during surgery, through trauma, or because of a disease process. Whole blood restores blood volume and replenishes the oxygen-carrying capacity in a patient who has had a massive hemorrhage. Whole blood also can supply coagulation factors. Each unit of whole blood contains 500 ml.

Packed red blood is prepared by removing the plasma from whole blood. When the plasma is removed, the sodium and potassium content is reduced. Packed RBCs replenish the blood's oxygen-carrying capacity while minimizing the risk of fluid overload in clients with severe anemia, slow blood loss, or congestive heart failure. They are also administered to burn patients who are experiencing hyperkalemia. Each unit of packed RBCs contains 250 ml of packed RBCs. State requirements and hospital policies vary, but an informed consent from the patient may be required prior to administration of blood products.

If a client experiences a reaction (fever, chills, rash, dyspnea, or shock) to the blood administered, the transfusion should be discontinued immediately and the physician should be notified. The client should be placed in a supine position with the legs elevated and vital signs monitored at least every 15 minutes, according to the severity of the reaction. The intravenous (IV) line should be kept open with normal saline, and the blood bag and administration set should be returned to the hospital laboratory for analysis. According to the type of the client's reaction and hospital policy, a urine specimen may be collected and blood may be drawn for analysis.

If blood is to be administered rapidly, the physician may order the blood warmed and administered through a blood pump.

Anticipated Responses

▼ The whole blood or packed cells are infused within 4 hours (the usual time is 2–3 hr), the client's hemoglobin increases, and the vital signs are stable.
▼ If platelets are administered, the client's platelet count increases and the likelihood of spontaneous bleeding decreases.

Adverse Responses

▼ The client has a reaction to the blood (see Table 13–1, p. 393).

Materials List

Gather these materials before beginning the skill:

▼ Blood administration set (Y-type [Fig. 13–1] or straight)
▼ Plasma transfer set (if administering packed RBCs)
▼ 19-gauge (or larger) IV angiocatheter or butterfly needle at insertion site
▼ 250–500 ml 0.9% normal saline (NaCl)
▼ Blood product ordered
▼ Examination gloves
▼ Blood warmer (optional)
▼ Blood pump (optional)
▼ Alcohol swabs
▼ 18-gauge needle (if piggybacking into the existing IV line)
▼ Adhesive tape (if piggybacking into the existing IV line)
▼ Plastic bags (to return used blood bag to laboratory)

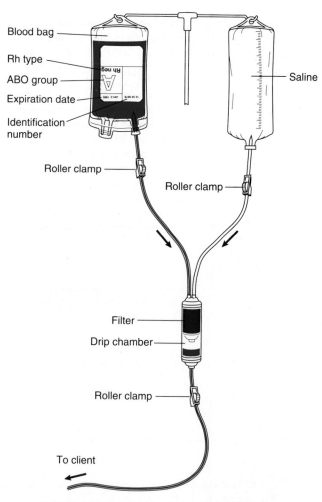

▼ FIGURE 13–1. Y-tubing blood administration set.

▼ *A C T I O N* ───────────── ▼ *R A T I O N A L E* ──────

1. Review the physician's order for the type of blood to be administered, the client's transfusion history, and the reason for the transfusion.

2. If required, obtain informed consent from the client.

3. Assess the client's vital signs and record them in the client's chart.

4. Obtain the blood from a blood bank. No more than 20 minutes should elapse from the time the blood is obtained from the blood bank to the time infusion is begun.

5. a. In the presence of the laboratory personnel, verify on the laboratory slip attached to the unit of blood the client's name, hospital number, blood identification number, blood type, blood unit number, and blood unit expiration date.
   b. Sign the laboratory records.

6. Return to the hospital unit and, with a licensed person, check the crossmatch slip for the client's name, room number, physician, blood type, donor number, and arm band number.

7. With the other licensed person, check the blood bag for blood type, donor number, arm band number, and expiration date.

8. In the client's room with the other licensed person, check the blood with the client's arm band for name, room number, and arm band number.

9. Both nurses should sign the crossmatch slip.

10. Return to the medicine preparation room.

11. If administering whole blood, gently invert the bag several times.

1. A physician's order is required. Reviewing the reason for the transfusion will allow you to monitor the client for expected responses. Reviewing the client's transfusion history will clue you in to prior reactions and potential reactions.

2. Hospital procedure may require that informed consent be obtained prior to initiation of the procedure.

3. Initial vital sign assessment gives you a baseline from which to compare vital signs taken during and after the transfusion.

4. Blood is stored in the blood bank under controlled conditions. Bacterial growth is facilitated when administration is delayed.

5. a. Verifies that the client receives the correct blood and that the expiration date has not passed.

   b. Signing verifies that blood products were released to nursing personnel.

6. This is a safety precaution to verify that the client is receiving the correct blood product.

7. This is a safety precaution to verify that the client is receiving the correct blood product.

8. Verifies that the right client is receiving the right blood product. Serious life-threatening reactions could occur if the wrong person received the blood.

9. Contributes to the legal record by documenting the care given to the client.

10. After the blood is checked, it is prepared for administration.

11. Blood will separate when left standing. Inverting the bag will mix the blood. Shaking is avoided because damage could occur to the blood cells.

Administering whole blood with Y-tubing

12. a. Don examination gloves.

   b. Close all clamps on the Y-tubing.

   c. Insert one spike of Y-tubing into the normal saline.

   d. Open the clamp to the normal saline and prime the tubing.

12. a. Reduces the risk of transmission of microorganisms.
   b. The clamps prevent the tubing from becoming filled with air and normal saline when the tubing is inserted into the normal saline.
   c. The normal saline will infuse through one spike and the blood will infuse through the other spike.
   d. Priming removes air from the tubing.

▼ _ _A C T I O N_ ▼ _ _R A T I O N A L E_ _ _ _ _ _ _ _ _ _ _ _ _ _ _ _ _

e. Open the clamp on the spike for blood, allow the saline to prime the tubing, and close the clamp.

f. Insert the Y-tubing into the blood bag.

g. Take the prepared blood and normal saline to the client's room.

13. a. If the client has an IV line, assess the catheter size, patency, and whether any signs of infiltration are present.

b. If the client does not have an IV line in place, perform a venipuncture (preferably with an 18- or 19-gauge needle).

| **NOTE:** See Skill 19–1. |

14. Start the infusion of normal saline at a KVO (keep vein open) rate to ascertain the patency of the line before beginning the infusion of blood. If using an existing line, infuse approximately 50 ml of saline to flush the line before beginning the infusion of blood.

15. Start the infusion of blood at a keep-open rate for 15 minutes and observe the client for signs of a reaction.

16. If there are no signs of a reaction after 15 minutes, increase the flow to the prescribed rate.

Administering whole blood or packed red blood cells with a straight blood administration set

12. a. Ensure that the client has an IV line of normal saline infusing.
    b. Close the clamp on the straight tubing.

13. Don disposable gloves.

14. a. Insert the spike into the port on the blood product and fill the drip chamber approximately halfway.
    b. Place an 18-gauge needle on the distal end of the IV tubing.

    c. Prime the tubing with blood and close the clamp.
    d. Piggyback the blood into the port most proximal to the IV insertion site.

    e. Secure the needle with adhesive tape.
    f. Open the clamp to the blood and infuse the blood at a KVO (keep vein open) rate for the first 15 minutes.

e. Priming removes air from the tubing.

g. The saline and blood are ready for administration.

13. a. If the catheter is smaller than 19-gauge, the blood may lyse as it passes through the catheter. A larger catheter should be inserted. If there are signs of infiltration or if the line is not patent, a new IV line should be started.

14. Blood should be mixed only with normal saline. A chance of incompatibility exists between the blood and other IV solutions. Blood should never be mixed with medications because the mixture would complicate the determination of the source of an adverse reaction.

15. Reactions most commonly occur during the first 15 minutes.

16. Whole blood should be infused within 2 to 4 hours. Packed cells should be infused over an hour.

12. a. Blood products are compatible only with normal saline.
    b. Prevents air from entering the tubing.

13. Decreases the transmission of microorganisms from the blood products to you.

14. a. Overfilling of the drip chamber will not allow clear visibility for counting the drops.

    b. The viscosity of the blood will impede the flow rate if a smaller needle is used. Furthermore, lysis of the cells could occur.
    c. Priming removes air from the tubing.

    d. Allows the transfusion to be discontinued without further infusion of blood products in the IV line.
    e. Prevents the needle from becoming dislodged.
    f. Most blood reactions occur within the first 15 minutes of administration.

▼ _ACTION_ _____ ▼ _RATIONALE_ _____

15. Remove the disposable gloves.

15. Prevents contamination of vital-sign equipment with blood.

16. Regulate the flow rate to infuse the blood product at the prescribed rate.

16. Whole blood should infuse within 2 to 4 hours. Packed red blood cells should infuse over an hour.

17. Record the vital signs on the client's chart or a flow sheet.

17. Communicates to the health care team and contributes to the legal record by documenting the care given to the client.

18. Assess the client's vital signs every 15 minutes for 1 hour, then every 30 minutes until the blood has infused completely.

18. Documents any changes in the client's vital signs that would alert you to a transfusion reaction.

19. When the infusion is completed, flush the IV tubing with normal saline.

19. Removes blood from the IV line to prevent hemolysis in the tubing.

20. Don disposable gloves.

20. Decreases the transmission of microorganisms from the blood to you.

21. Disconnect the blood bag from the tubing and dispose of the tubing according to agency guidelines.

21. Proper disposal prevents transmission of microorganisms.

22. Complete the crossmatch slip with the date and time the transfusion was completed.

22. The slip should accompany the empty bag back to the blood bank.

23. Double-bag the blood bag and return it to the laboratory with one copy of the completed crossmatch slip.

23. Double-bagging prevents transmission of microorganisms.

24. Place the original crossmatch slip on the client's chart.

24. The original slip provides documentation of the blood that was administered.

25. Record the procedure. Note the type and amount of blood product given and the client's response to the transfusion.

25. Communicates to the health care team and contributes to the legal record by documenting the care given to the client.

T ABLE 13–1. Nursing Responses to Transfusion Reactions

Type of Reaction	Signs and Symptoms	Nursing Actions
ABO incompatibility	Flushing, urticaria headache, lumbar pain, fever, chills, nausea, vomiting, hypotension, tachycardia, dyspnea	Discontinue blood. Maintain intravenous line with normal saline. Send remaining blood to laboratory for analysis. Assess vital signs. Obtain urinalysis for presence of Hgb, RBCs, and urobilinogen. Monitor urine output (insert indwelling urinary catheter if needed).
Febrile reaction	Fever, chills	Discontinue blood. Maintain intravenous line with normal saline. Send remaining blood to laboratory for analysis. Monitor vital signs and urine output. Treat reaction with antipyretics. For subsequent transfusions use leukocyte-poor blood to prevent future febrile reactions.
Allergic reaction	Pruritus, urticaria	Slow blood transfusion for mild reactions. Stop transfusion if reaction is severe. Monitor vital signs. Treat mild reaction with antihistamines. Epinephrine may be used for severe reactions. For subsequent transfusions, use washed RBCs to prevent future allergic reactions.
Delayed hemolytic reaction	May be asymptomatic fall in hematocrit	Monitor hematocrit.

Example of Documentation

DATE	TIME	NOTES
10/19/93	0900	V/S = 116/60, 90, 16, 98.4. One unit of whole blood started at 5 ml per minute.
		S. Williams, RN
	0905	V/S = 118/62, 90, 17, 98.4.
		S. Williams, RN
	0910	V/S = 114/64, 88, 16, 98.4.
		S. Williams, RN
	0915	V/S = 116/68, 86, 16, 98.4.
		S. Williams, RN
	0930	V/S = 120/68, 84, 15, 98.4.
		S. Williams, RN
	1000	V/S = 122/70, 82, 16, 98.4.
		S. Williams, RN
	1030	V/S = 122/72, 82, 16, 98.4.
		S. Williams, RN
	1100	V/S = 120/74, 80, 16, 98.6. 500 ml whole-blood transfusion completed. No evidence of chills, fever, pain, nausea, dyspnea, or wheezing. Normal saline infusing at KVO.
		S. Williams, RN

Special Considerations

Using a blood-warming device

Because cold blood can lead to hypothermia, especially in the newborn, hospital policy may indicate that a blood-warming device should be used. The blood-warming device maintains the blood at a constant temperature of 98.6° Fahrenheit (F) (37° Celsius).

To use either a blood-warming coil or a dry-heat warmer:

1. Plug in the device.
2. Prepare the client and the blood product.
   a. Use a straight-line set for the blood-warming coil.
   b. Use a Y-type set for the dry-heat warmer.
3. Flush the line with normal saline to clear the line of air.

Then, to use a blood-warming coil:

4. Turn on the machine.
5. Remove the coil from the sterile wrapper (use sterile technique).
6. Close the clamps.
7. Attach the male adapter on the blood line to the female adapter on the blood-warming coil.
8. Attach an 18-gauge needle to the distal end of the coil.
9. Immerse the coil in a basin of 98.6° F water. (Do not immerse adapters in the water or the water may enter the tubing and contaminate the blood.)
10. Open the clamp and allow the blood to fill the tubing.
11. Proceed with the straight-line administration of the blood product.
12. After administering the blood product, flush the coil with normal saline to remove any blood in the tubing.
13. Replace the blood-warming coil after 24 hours.

To use a dry-heat warmer:

4. Insert the warming bag into the blood warmer.

5. Attach the bottom lead to the blood line and the top lead to the line leading to the client.

6. Secure the warming bag on the support pins (the bag must be flat against the back panel) and secure the pins.

7. Close the blood warmer and secure the latch.

8. Turn the dry-heat warmer on.

9. Allow the blood to warm for at least 2 minutes to warm the blood to 98.6° F. (Do not open the door to the warmer until the transfusion is completed.)

10. Open the clamp to the saline line.

11. Open the main flow clamp to the blood-warming bag so that the blood-warming bag is filled with saline solution.

12. Close the main flow clamp and release the chamber when the saline is in the top lead chamber.

13. Remove the adapter cover on the top lead.

14. Open the top lead.

15. Open the clamp.

16. Expel any air from the line.

17. Proceed with the administration of the blood product as with the Y-set.

Administering blood using a pressure cuff or positive-pressure set

Pressure pumps are used to administer blood when rapid administration of the blood is necessary. The pressure cuff is a sleeve that is placed over the unit of blood. The cuff is inflated (as with a blood pressure cuff) up to, but not to exceed, 300 mmHg. Greater pressure will result in hemolysis of the blood. The positive-pressure set contains a built-in pressure chamber and increases the delivery rate of the blood through gravity when manual pressure is applied.

To use a pressure cuff:

1. Place the unit of blood into the pressure cuff through the center opening.

2. Hang the unit of blood on the IV pole.

3. Turn the screw on the pressure cuff counterclockwise.

4. Compress the pressure bulb to inflate the pressure cuff to the desired pressure.

5. Turn the screw to maintain the pressure. Frequently check the pressure. As the unit of blood deflates, the pressure will decrease and slow the flow rate.

To use a positive-pressure administration set:

1. Open the flow clamps on the administration set.

2. Compress and release the pump chamber to force or pump the blood from the bag into the client. Allow the chamber to completely fill before compressing again.

Teaching Tips

The purpose of the blood administration and the procedure should be explained to the client and the client's family. The client should be told the symptoms to observe during the blood administration and to report them immediately.

Home Care Variations

When blood transfusions are needed at home, the visiting nurse can collect a blood sample in the client's home for type and crossmatch. Informed consent is obtained after transfusion information has been shared with the client. The nurse then applies an identification bracelet to the client's arm and completes an information sheet that contains the client's identification bracelet number. After the sample is collected, the nurse attaches labels that contain the client's name, identification number, and the date to it. After the type and crossmatch are completed, the visiting nurse makes an appointment with the client for the transfusion. The nurse picks up the blood, checks it, and transports it in a container with an appropriate coolant. The procedure for infusion is the same as the one described above.

SKILL 13–2 ADMINISTERING PLATELETS AND FRESH FROZEN PLASMA

Clinical Situations in Which You May Encounter This Skill

Fresh frozen plasma (FFP) and derivatives of plasma such as platelets are given for a variety of reasons. For example, platelets (mixed with approximately 50 ml of plasma) are given to correct platelet counts below 10,000 per cubic millimeter. Low platelet counts can occur with hematologic diseases such as leukemia and aplastic anemia, and in clients receiving chemotherapy. Usually, 4 or more units of platelets are required to control or prevent bleeding in an adult.

FFP may be given to a client who has a massive hemorrhage until whole blood is available or to treat a client with a Factor V deficiency. The plasma acts as an intravascular volume expander to maintain circulatory volume. FFP also may be used to treat hypoproteinemia and hypoalbuminemia.

If the client has a reaction to the plasma or platelets, place the client in a supine position, elevate the lower extremities 20 to 30 degrees, and administer oxygen. The physician also may order additional fluids, epinephrine, and corticosteroids.

Anticipated Responses

▼ If platelets are administered, the client's platelet count increases.
▼ Bruising, oozing from a wound, or other signs of a low platelet count are improved therapeutically.
▼ If plasma is administered, the client's intravascular volume increases and the blood pressure rises.

Adverse Responses

▼ The client has a reaction to the transfusion.

Materials List

Gather these materials before beginning the skill:

▼ Unit of FFP or platelets
▼ Venipuncture set (optional)
▼ Alcohol swab
▼ Component drip set
▼ 250–500 ml normal saline
▼ 18- to 20-gauge needle
▼ Adhesive tape
▼ Examination gloves

▼ ACTION

1. Review the physician's order for the type of blood product ordered, the amount, and the client's previous transfusion history.

2. Obtain a signed informed consent from the client.

3. Obtain the blood product from the blood bank. Obtain the FFP at least 20 minutes before the transfusion.

4. Identify the client by asking him or her to state his or her name and by examining the arm band.

▼ RATIONALE

1. Ensures that the correct blood product is given. Reviewing transfusion history allows for careful evaluation of potential reactions.

2. Because of the risks associated with transfusions of blood products, informed consent is required by most state laws and institutions.

3. FFP takes at least 20 minutes to thaw. FFP must be given within 4 hours of thawing because it contains no preservatives.

4. Ensures that the right blood product is given to the right client.

▼ _ A C T I O N _ _ _ _ _ _ _ _ _ _ | ▼ _ R A T I O N A L E _ _ _ _ _ _ _ _

5. Don examination gloves.

5. Decreases the transmission of microorganisms.

6. If the client has an existing IV line, carefully assess it for patency and for signs of infiltration. If the client does not have an IV line, perform a venipuncture with an 18- to 20-gauge IV catheter. (See Skill 19–1).

6. Blood products should be given through an 18- to 20-gauge needle to avoid lysis of the cells. If signs of infiltration are present or if the IV line is not patent, a new one should be started.

7. Start an infusion of normal saline.

7. Blood products should be infused only with normal saline.

8. Obtain baseline vital signs (blood pressure, temperature, pulse, and respiratory rate) and record them.

8. Provides a basis for comparison with subsequent vital signs.

Administering an FFP with a blood administration set

9. a. Prepare the plasma for administration by:
   i. Spiking the plasma bag with the blood administration set tubing.
   ii. Attaching the needle to the other end of the tubing.
   iii. Priming the tubing with the plasma.
 b. Wipe the port on the primary administration set that is most proximal to the IV insertion site with an alcohol swab and insert the needle from the plasma administration set into the port.
 c. Close the clamp on the saline infusion.
 d. Adjust the flow rate on the plasma to the prescribed rate.

   i. Allows plasma to flow from bag into administration set.
   ii. The plasma will be piggybacked into the IV tubing.
   iii. Priming removes the air from the tubing.
 b. Swabbing and friction on surfaces remove surface microorganisms.

 c. The saline should not infuse with the plasma.
 d. The rate is carefully regulated to give the plasma within the given time.

Administering platelets with a component drip set

9. a. Prepare the platelets for administration by:
   i. Pulling back the tabs on the bag of platelets to open the port.
   ii. Closing the clamp on the administration set.

   iii. Inserting the administration set spike into the port on the platelets.
   iv. Compressing the drip chamber so that platelets completely cover the filter.
   v. Attaching the needle to the other end of the tubing.
   vi. Priming the tubing with platelets.
 b. Wipe the port on the primary administration set that is most proximal to the IV insertion site with an alcohol swab and insert the needle from the platelet administration set into the port.
 c. Close the clamp on the saline infusion.
 d. Open the flow clamp on the platelet administration set to allow the platelets to flow in as rapidly as possible.

   i. Exposes port, allowing administration set access into bag.
   ii. Prevents air and platelets from entering the tubing.

   v. The platelets will be piggybacked into the IV tubing.

 b. Swabbing and friction on surfaces help to remove microorganisms.

 c. The saline should not infuse with the platelets.
 d. Platelets should be administered over a 10-minute period to avoid clumping and loss of activity.

▼ *ACTION*	▼ *RATIONALE*
10. When the unit of plasma or platelets has infused, restart the normal saline to flush the line with 20 to 30 ml of saline.	**10.** Flushing the line with saline will prevent occlusion of the line.
11. Restart the original IV solution and adjust the flow rate according to the physician's orders.	**11.** Maintains patency of the line.
12. Record the procedure. Note the amount of the blood product administered, the duration of the transfusion, the vital signs, and the client's tolerance of the procedure.	**12.** Communicates to the other members of the health care team and contributes to the legal record by documenting the care given to the client.

Example of Documentation

DATE	*TIME*	*NOTES*
10/19/93	0900	Vital signs = 110/60, 88, 18, 98.4. 4 units (240 ml) of platelets administered. No signs of bleeding or reaction noted.
		S. Williams, RN

Teaching Tips

Instruct the client to report any signs of bleeding, itching, swelling, shortness of breath, dizziness, or chest pain. The client also should be told the anticipated duration of the transfusion. To avoid any anxiety on the client's part, explain to the client the rationale for taking vital signs frequently.

Home Care Variations

The blood should be cross-checked very carefully prior to taking it to the client's home. Plan carefully for the administration of the blood products as they must be administered within 4 hours of obtaining them from the blood bank. If the client has a history of a reaction to a transfusion, he or she is a poor candidate for home transfusion therapy.

SKILL 13–3   ADMINISTERING AUTOTRANSFUSION THERAPY

Clinical Situations in Which You May Encounter This Skill

Autotransfusion, or autologous transfusion, is the reinfusion of the client's own blood after collection, filtration, and anticoagulation. The advantage of autotransfusion is that the danger of transmitting blood-borne diseases (hepatitis and acquired immunodeficiency syndrome, for example) from the blood donor to the recipient is eliminated, religious objections to blood transfusions may be overcome, and the transfusion is compatible with the client's blood. The blood used in autotransfusions also contains more normal levels of electrolytes and ammonia than those found in stored blood.

Autotransfusions may be used if the client has a rare blood type or does not need to risk isoimmunization. They may be used preoperatively, at scheduled intervals prior to elective surgery; immediately prior to surgery through hemodilution; intraoperatively, through the salvage of blood from the operative site; or postoperatively, after cardiac surgery, traumatic chest or abdominal injury, or orthopedic surgery.

If blood is donated preoperatively, the client must be free of bacteremia, and the hemoglobin must be at least 11 gm/dl. Adequate hydration should be maintained before and immediately after the donation of blood to avoid hypovolemia. Hypovolemic reactions more commonly occur in the client who is older or underweight. Normal saline may be administered intravenously during donation if the client becomes hypovolemic or experiences hypotension, sweating, dizziness, or nausea.

Sepsis, malignancy, and contamination of the blood from urine, infective tissue, or ruptured bowels are contraindications for autotransfusion. If a wound site is more than 4 hours old, autotransfusion is not attempted from the wound site because of potential infection. If the client receives eight or more autologous transfusions that have been mixed with the anticoagulant preservative citrate-phosphate-dextrose-adenine (CPDA-1), inadequate clotting or thrombocytopenia may develop. If the client develops inadequate clotting times, anticipate administering fresh frozen plasma and platelets.

Blood collected intraoperatively and postoperatively is usually reinfused within 4 hours. However, hospital policies may differ and may dictate that the blood be reinfused every hour.

The procedure for performing autotransfusion differs according to the type of autotransfusion performed and the specific equipment used. For example, blood may be reinfused as whole blood or the cells may be washed to remove the plasma and debris, mixed with isotonic saline, and reinfused as packed cells. The specific manufacturer's guidelines should be consulted for the specific procedure to be used. This chapter will describe the procedure for orthopedic drainage and reinfusion of blood using a cell saver (Solcotrans).

Adverse Responses

▼ The client's blood becomes septic and the client develops symptoms such as tachycardia, elevated temperature, and malaise.
▼ The client develops hypocalcemia, hyperkalemia, or citrate toxicity.
▼ The client develops inadequate clotting times.
▼ The client develops hemolysis.
▼ The client has respiratory difficulty from microemboli.

Materials List

Gather these materials before beginning the skill:

▼ Cell saver (Solcotrans) system
▼ Anticoagulant solution
▼ Bed rail hanger
▼ Standard blood infusion set
▼ 40-micron microaggregate blood transfusion filter
▼ Hand bulb with safety valve for reinfusion under pressure or standard hand bulb with manometer
▼ Portable intermittent suction device (Gomco) or wall suction
▼ Hemostat
▼ Examination gloves
▼ Anticoagulant (as specified by the physician)
▼ IV pole

Anticipated Responses

▼ The client's blood is collected and returned to the client.
▼ The client remains free of infection.
▼ Hemoglobin and coagulation levels remain or return to within normal limits.

▼ ACTION

1. Review the physician's orders to determine whether gravity drainage or suction is needed; the procedure performed on the client; and hemoglobin, hematocrit, and other pertinent laboratory data.

2. Assess and record the client's vital signs and the amount and type of bleeding from the wound.

3. Using aseptic technique, inject the anticoagulant into the injection port on the line attached to the yellow port.

▼ RATIONALE

1. Provides input into the type of equipment needed and pertinent assessment data.

2. This information will provide a basis for comparison.

3. The anticoagulant will prevent the blood from clotting. Aseptic technique will prevent the transmission of microorganisms.

▼ *ACTION*   ▼ *RATIONALE*

4. Hang the Solcotrans unit on the bed rail with the yellow end up.
   a. Make sure the yellow clamp on the collection line and the red clamp on the suction line are open.
   b. Record the client's name, hospital number, and time collection was begun on the Solcotrans unit.

       b. Provides pertinent identifying information.

5. a. For gravity collection, leave the red clamp open.
   b. For vacuum drainage, set the wall regulator to a low setting (less than 100 mmHg) and connect the suction line to the white connector. If wall suction is ordered and is not available, attach the suction line to low Gomco suction.

   5. a. Vents the system to allow for drainage of fluid.

       b. Excessive pressure may cause hemolysis of the blood cells.

6. Regularly assess for continuous drainage in the unit; the client's vital signs; neurologic status; signs of bruising, bleeding, or dyspnea; and urine output.

   6. Provides continuing data of the client's status. An excessive loss of blood is prevented by the air filter that will not allow fluids to pass. If the filter becomes wet from overfilling the unit or placing a partially filled unit on its side, further drainage will automatically shut off.

7. Periodically gently agitate the Solcotrans unit.

   7. Ensures proper mixing of the anticoagulant with the blood as the blood enters into the unit.

8. When the unit is filled:
   a. Close the red slide clamp.

       a–b. The clamps are closed to prevent the blood from escaping.

   b. Close the yellow slide clamp.
   c. Using a hemostat, compress the evacuator tube near the sleeve connector.

9. Don examination gloves.

   9. Decreases the transmission of microorganisms.

10. Using aseptic technique:
    a. Disconnect the evacuator tube at the sleeve connector.
    b. Disconnect the red slide clamp below the suction line.

    10. Aseptic technique prevents the transfer of microorganisms.

11. If further collection is desired:
    a. Instill anticoagulant into the port on the line attached to the yellow port (use aseptic technique).

        a. The anticoagulant keeps the blood from coagulating before it is reinfused.

    b. If no further collection for reinfusion is indicated, attach the evacuator tube from the drainage device to the sleeve connector and release the hemostat. Use aseptic technique.

▼ *A C T I O N* ▼ *R A T I O N A L E*

Performing reinfusion

12. Review the physician's order to determine the amount of blood to be reinfused.	**12.** Ensures that the appropriate amount of blood product is reinfused.
13. Position the container unit with the yellow cap in an upward position.	
14. Don disposable gloves.	**14.** Decreases the transmission of microorganisms.
15. Using aseptic technique, remove the white injection port connector and evacuator tube from the yellow port.	
16. Insert a 40-micron microaggregate blood transfusion filter into the yellow port.	**16.** Filters debris from the blood.
17. Attach a standard blood infusion set to the filter tubing.	
18. Open the yellow slide clamp.	
19. Remove the white Luer-Lok.	**19.** Allows air to enter the space between the blood bag and the outer shell.
20. Apply pressure with a standard hand bulb attached to the white luer connector.	**20.** Facilitates venting of air from the blood bag.
21. Invert the container on an IV pole with the red cap at the top.	
22. Review the physician's orders to determine the rate for reinfusion.	**22.** The reinfusion rate must be prescribed by the physician.
23. Reinfuse the client's blood either by gravity flow or under pressure by the hand bulb attached to the white luer-lock connector.	
24. Record the client's response to the transfusion (vital signs, signs of excessive clotting time, mentation).	**24.** Communicates to the other members of the health care team and contributes to the legal record by documenting the care given to the client.
25. Monitor hourly output and report urine output of less than 30 ml per hour.	**25.** If hypovolemia develops, urinary output will decrease.
26. Monitor the client's hematocrit, hemoglobin, and serum creatine levels and report abnormalities.	**26.** If unwashed blood is used, hemolysis may develop.
27. Observe for signs of hypocalcemia, hyperkalemia, or citrate toxicity.	**27.** If more than 8 units are transfused, these signs and symptoms may develop.
28. Assess the client's neurologic and pulmonary status hourly. Report any changes in mentation, chest pain, or dyspnea.	**28.** Microemboli can occur as a result of transfused hemolytic cell debris or platelet clumping.

Example of Documentation

DATE	*TIME*	*NOTES*
10/19/93	0800	V/S = 98/60, 110, 24, 97.6. Blood draining slowly through tubing. Client drowsy, but oriented and arousable.
		S. Williams, RN
	1100	300 ml blood in Solcotrans container. Drainage discontinued.
		S. Williams, RN

Teaching Tips

Teach the client the reasons for the autotransfusion and which side effects to report. Caution the client to report any signs of dizziness, dyspnea, or bleeding.

References

Porth, C. (1990). *Pathophysiology: Concepts of altered health states* (3rd ed.). Philadelphia: J. B. Lippincott.

CHAPTER 14

Meeting Nutritional Needs

Good nutrition is essential to maintaining a healthy body. Poor nutrition results from a diet that is inadequate in calories or nutrients. As a nurse you care for clients who may not eat adequately for many reasons, including anorexia, anomalies or diseases of the gastrointestinal (GI) tract, and coma. Along with registered dietitians, you should assess your client's nutritional status and provide assistance in maintaining optimal nutrition.

Nutrition may be provided by the enteral or parenteral route. Enteral nutrition is used when the client has a functional GI tract. This type of nutrition may include high-calorie supplements to a regular diet. Enteral nutrition also may include tube feedings of commercial or home-mixed formulas instilled in nasogastric, gastric, or jejunal tubes. Tube feedings are used when the client cannot or will not swallow food but has a GI tract that is able to absorb nutrients.

Parenteral nutrition is used when enteral nutrition is not adequate or possible. Parenteral nutrition includes the administration of a hypertonic solution by hyperalimentation, or total parenteral nutrition (TPN). The TPN solution contains glucose, amino acids, vitamins, minerals, electrolytes, and other additives prescribed by a physician. Insulin is a common additive. The TPN solution is infused into a large central vein such as the superior vena cava via a central intravenous line. Intravascular infusions of lipids also may be administered along with the TPN solutions.

OVERVIEW OF RELATED RESEARCH

ASSISTING WITH BREAST-FEEDING

Auervach, K. G. (1990). Sequential and simultaneous breast pumping: A comparison. *International Journal of Nursing Study,* 27 (3), 257–265.

Breast-feeding mothers are often concerned about maintaining an adequate milk supply during periods of separation from the baby. Twenty-six women were asked to pump milk from their breasts on four separate occasions with an electric intermittent vacuum pump. They used one of three possible regimens on each occasion: 5-minute sequential pumping; unlimited sequential pumping; or unlimited simultaneous pumping. The results indicated that in both limited and unlimited pumping sessions, the simultaneous double-pumping option obtained higher mean milk volumes. Differences in milk fat concentrations were not statistically significant between simultaneous breast pumping and sequential pumping. The mothers' preferred pumping regimens were related to an increase in the mean milk volumes obtained.

Kearney, M. H., Cronenwett, L. R., and Barrett, J. A. (1990). Breast-feeding problems in the first week of postpartum. *Nursing Research,* 39 (2), 90–95.

Problems that occur in the first days of breast-feeding have been associated with women weaning their infants by 1 month postpartum. Prenatal and perinatal variables commonly found to predict breast-feeding duration were examined in 128 families for association of breast-feeding problems in the first week postpartum. The families were assigned randomly to one of two groups: a group in which bottle-feedings would be avoided in weeks 2 to 6 postpartum and a group in which approximately one bottle per day would be given during the same period. Statistical analysis revealed that bottle use in the hospital, lower satisfaction with the first breast-feeding, and group assignment were slightly predictive of breast-feeding problems. The negative effect of hospital bottle use was greater for women in the bottle-restricted group than for women in the planned-bottle group.

Lindenberg, C. S., Artola, R. C., and Jimenez, V. (1990). The effect of early postpartum mother–infant contact and breastfeeding promotion on the incidence and continuation of breastfeeding. *International Journal of Nursing Studies,* 27 (1), 179–186.

Eighty percent of the world's infants live in third world countries where breast-feeding is a critical factor in infant health and survival. Three maternity hospitals' practices regarding postpartum mother–infant contact and breast-feeding promotion were studied to examine their influence on the incidence and continuation of breast-feeding among 375 urban Nicaraguan primigravida women in poor health. Mother–infant pairs were assigned to one of three groups: complete separation throughout hospitalization with usual breast-feeding promotion; a 45-minute mother–infant contact period immediately after birth with usual breast-feeding promotion followed by complete separation until discharge; and continuous postpartum contact until discharge with standard breast-feeding promotion. Results indicated that breast-feeding was initiated with 87% of the infants, but only 54% of the mothers continued breast-feeding for at least 4 months. There was a significant relationship between rooming-in and standard breast-feeding promotion and the continuation of breast-feeding. The findings suggest that postpartum mother–infant contact practices combined with standard breast-feeding promotion may influence the initial choice to breast-feed, but these practices alone are not enough to prolong breast-feeding.

HELPING THE ADULT TO EAT

Kotodny, V., and Malek, A. M. (1991). Improving feeding skills. *Journal of Gerontological Nursing,* 17 (6), 20–24.

Nurses are challenged to refine their feeding skills as they assist elderly residents in maintaining nutritional status, independence, and dignity. Twenty-two staff members (9 registered nurses, 9 certified nursing assistants, 3 orderlies, and 1 unit aide) completed a 20-item multiple-choice knowledge questionnaire to assess knowledge and attitudes toward feeding the elderly. A mean score of 63% was obtained with no relationship between mean scores and the length of time the respondents had worked in nursing or whether they worked full time or part time or were casual staff. It was concluded that the staff members lacked knowledge of feeding principles and required assistance in refining their feeding skills; consideration should be given to factors other than full-time status and seniority as assignments are made for residents who require specialized feeding techniques; and the staff members did not understand certain feeding principles such as the importance of sitting to ensure that the food is presented to the resident from below the mouth. Staff education programs were developed as a result of the study.

FEEDING TUBES

Beckstrand, J., et al. (1990). The distance to the stomach for feeding-tube placement in children predicted from regression on height. *Research in Nursing and Health,* 13, 411–420.

Data were collected from archival sources regarding 30 children with nasally inserted feeding tubes and 77 children with orally inserted feeding tubes. The purpose of the study was to determine if Strobel, Byrne, Ament, and Euler's regression coefficients could predict accurately the esophageal length necessary for nasogastric tube insertion. The equations for oral nasogastric tubes performed the best and could be used in children 1 month to 4 years of age. Prediction equations should account for gender differences in older children.

Crocker, K. S., et al. (1986). Microbial growth in clinically used enteral delivery systems. *American Journal of Infection Control,* 14, 255–256.

This prospective study was done to compare microbial contamination during a 4-hour hang time with the microbial contamination during the hang time of a prefilled 1,000-ml pouch. The hang times of the 1,000-ml prefilled pouch ranged from 8 to 24 hours. Nineteen clients were involved in the study, with a total of 57 days of continuous feeding. Samples of formula were obtained at 0-, 4-, 8-, 12-, and 24-hour intervals from a specifically adapted administration tubing. A 61% overall contamination rate was found. The findings indicated that contamination of enteral formulas is common. Environmental contamination by the caregiver is the most likely source of contamination.

Eisenberg, P., Metheny, N., and McSweeney, M. (1989). Nasoenteral feeding-tube properties and the ability to withdraw fluid via syringe. *Applied Nursing Research*, 2 (4), 168–172.

The purpose of this study was to determine if the ability to withdraw fluid is affected by the diameter (No. 8, 10, or 12 French) of the tube and the type of material (polyurethane or silicone). The volume aspirated was affected significantly by the tube diameter and the type of material. The largest aspirated mean volumes were from the polyurethane tube. Furthermore, larger aspirated mean volumes were obtained from the No. 10 French tubes than from the No. 8 French or No. 12 French tubes.

Metheny, N. A., Eisenberg, P., and McSweeney, M. (1988). Effect of feeding-tube properties and three irrigants on clogging rates. *Nursing Research*, 37, 165–169.

This study was conducted to determine the effect of feeding-tube properties (diameter and material, polyurethane or silicone) and irrigant (cranberry juice, cola, and water) on clogging rates. The polyurethane tube was found to be superior to the silicone tube in terms of clogging rates. There was no significant difference in clogging rate in relation to tube diameter. Both cola and water were considerably better as irrigants.

Metheny, N. A., et al. (1990). Effectiveness of the auscultatory method in predicting feeding-tube location. *Nursing Research*, 39, 262–267.

The purpose of this study was "to determine the extent to which sounds generated by air insufflations through feeding tubes could be used to predict where the tubes' ports ended in the GI tract (esophagus, stomach, or proximal small intestine), and to differentiate between gastric and respiratory placement"

(p. 262). Either tubes were inserted using fluoroscopy or placement of tubes was confirmed with an abdominal x-ray. One hundred and fifteen usable tape recordings were made of a series of air insufflations. Tube location was classified correctly for 34.4% of the tapes. Thus, the findings of this study suggest that the auscultatory method is not effective in predicting feeding-tube location.

Metheny, N. A., Spies, M., and Eisenberg, P. (1988). Measures to test placement of nasoenteral feeding tubes. *Western Journal of Nursing Research*, 10, 367–383.

The purposes of this descriptive study were "(1) to describe the frequency with which nurses reported being able to: (a) aspirate at least 5 milliliters of fluid from each tube and (b) adequately measure gastric retention in patients with large-bore and small-bore feeding tubes; (2) to describe the frequency with which nurses were able to predict proper placement of nasoenteral tubes by testing the patient's ability to speak; and (3) to describe the frequency with which nurses were able to predict proper placement of nasogastric tubes by epigastric auscultation of 10 milliliters of air insufflated through the tube." Data were collected from 20 clients with nasogastric tubes and 55 clients with nasointestinal tubes.

Nurses were able to aspirate 5 ml of gastric contents in 45% of attempts in clients with small-bore nasogastric tubes, 33% of attempts in clients with small-bore nasointestinal tubes, and 79% of attempts in clients with large-bore nasogastric tubes. Collapse of the tube was the most commonly cited reason for failure to aspirate gastric contents. Nurses were able to measure gastric retention adequately in 90% of the clients with large-bore tubes and in 48% of the clients with small-bore tubes.

If the tube was placed correctly, all clients were able to speak unless the client was comatose, aphasic, or had an endotracheal or tracheostomy tube. Air was heard in the epigastric region 16 of 34 times when x-ray films demonstrated that the tube was somewhere other than in the stomach. Of these 16 instances, 11 tubes were in the duodenum, 3 tubes were in the jejunum, and 2 tubes were in the esophagus. There was no difference in the amount of fluid aspirated when the tube was in the correct place or when it was displaced.

The findings indicated that collapse of the flexible small-bore tubes occurred more frequently than collapse of the large-bore tubes; this can prevent adequate assessment of placement and gastric retention in clients with small-bore tubes.

Metheny, N. A., Spies, M., and Eisenberg, P. (1986). Frequency of nasoenteral tube displacement and associated risk factors. *Research in Nursing and Health*, 9, 241–247.

Metheny, Spies, and Eisenberg examined the frequency of spontaneous tube displacement and associated risk factors in 105 clients. The clients had either a weighted nasogastric tube, an unweighted nasointestinal tube, or a weighted nasointestinal tube. Clients with weighted nasogastric tubes had a significantly greater frequency of tube displacement when they were coughing or when they had a decreased level of consciousness. Clients with unweighted nasointestinal tubes had a significantly greater frequency of displacement during coughing and while experiencing upper airway obstruction. Clients with weighted nasointestinal tubes did not have a significantly greater frequency of tube displacement in relation to risk factors.

Mickschl, D. B., et al. (1990). Contamination of enteral feedings and diarrhea in patients in intensive care units. *Heart and Lung*, 19, 362–370.

Data were collected from 36 critically ill adults to determine the effects of the contamination of feeding solutions on the incidence of diarrhea. Feedings were administered by an aseptic or routine protocol. Enteral feeding solutions were cultured for the first 4 days. Contamination was significantly greater for the patients fed by the routine protocol. The patients who received the feeding solution via the routine protocol had more days of diarrhea. However, receipt of contaminated formula did not affect the incidence of diarrhea significantly.

Petrosino, B. M., Meraviglia, M., and Becker, H. (1987). Mechanical problems with small-diameter enteral feeding tubes. *Journal of Neuroscience Nursing*, 19, 276–280.

Petrosino, Meraviglia, and Becker investigated the extent of mechanical problems with small-diameter feeding tubes and the procedures used to care for the tubes. A survey form was sent to 200 hospitals to obtain the data. Fifty-eight percent of the hospitals that responded reported a significant occurrence of mechanical problems. Problems reported were slowing of the flow rate or complete occlusion of the small-diameter tube. Thirty-one percent had a written procedure for irrigation of the tubes. Of these, 57% used water, 14% used cranberry juice, and 9% used cola for irrigation. ▪

SKILL 14–1 BOTTLE-FEEDING THE INFANT

Clinical Situations in Which You May Encounter This Skill

Infants in the newborn nursery or infants hospitalized for illnesses who are not being breast-fed should be bottle-fed. An infant usually continues to take oral nutrition from a bottle until approximately the age of 12 months. An infant also may need to be bottle-fed oral solutions for diagnostic tests such as a barium swallow.

The amount and number of feedings depend on the age of the baby. A newborn infant has a limited stomach capacity and may take only 1 ounce of formula at a feeding. After the newborn period the infant needs approximately 24 ounces of formula each day. The amount of formula given at each feeding increases as the intervals lengthen between feedings and the number of feedings decreases. The newborn may average six to 10 feedings each 24 hours. By the time the child is 1 year old, the number of feedings per 24 hours decreases to approximately three.

Anticipated Responses

▼ The infant sucks the oral nutrition from the bottle, is relaxed, satisfied, and sleepy after the feeding, and gradually gains weight.

Adverse Responses

▼ The infant fusses or cries after the feeding.
▼ The infant chokes on the oral feedings and aspirates the fluids.

Materials List

Gather these materials before beginning the skill:

▼ Bottle
▼ Nipple
▼ Oral nutrition (ready-to-use powdered or concentrated formula mixed to the correct dilution, an oral electrolyte maintenance solution, or other liquid nutrition as ordered by the physician)

▼ ACTION

1. Check the physician's order for the type of oral feeding and the amount indicated.

2. If the infant is in the hospital, ask the parent if the infant usually takes a bottle or is breast-fed.

3. If the infant is a newborn, assess the mother's experience with bottle-feeding.

4. Wash your hands.

5. Ascertain that the formula is at room temperature by shaking a few drops on your inner wrist. The formula should not feel too warm or too cool.

6. Pick the infant up from the bassinet or crib.

▼ RATIONALE

1. The type and amount of feedings vary, depending on the age and diagnosis of the infant's condition.

2. If the infant is usually breast-fed, he or she may resist the bottle. If possible, the mother should continue to breast-feed. It may be necessary to have the mother pump her milk and leave it for the infant.

3. If the mother has no experience with bottle-feeding, she should be taught how to bottle-feed her infant correctly.

4. Decreases the transmission of microorganisms.

5. Feedings that are cold may increase intestinal peristalsis. Feedings that are too hot may burn the baby's GI tract.

6. Holding the infant provides him or her with feelings of security and promotes normal psychologic development.

▼ *A C T I O N* _____ ▼ *R A T I O N A L E* _____

7. Sit in a chair and
   a. Hold the infant upright in the bend of your elbow; or

   b. Hold the infant in a football hold by supporting the infant's back and head with your hand and forearm. The body of the infant will be held securely between your elbow and waist; or
   c. If the infant cannot be taken from the bassinet, use one hand to support the infant in a low Fowler's or semi-Fowler's position.

8. Place a bib or clean cloth under the infant's chin.

9. Insert the nipple of the bottle into the infant's mouth, above the tongue. Be sure the bottle is at a 45-degree angle and the nipple is filled with the formula.

10. While the infant feeds (Fig. 14–1), observe closely for respiratory distress.

a. The infant should be in a semi-Fowler's position to prevent aspiration of fluid and reflux of fluid into the eustachian tubes.

b. The football hold leaves one of your hands free while still supporting the infant's head and body.

8. The bib absorbs any formula dripped from the infant's mouth and protects your clothing.

9. Prevents air from being swallowed by the infant.

10. Respiratory distress can occur if the infant aspirates the formula.

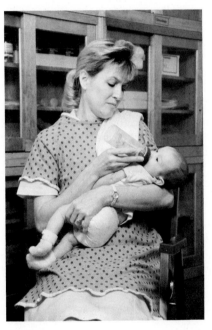

▼ **FIGURE 14–1.** Bottle-feeding an infant.

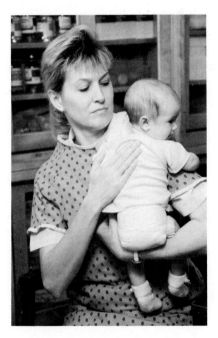

▼ **FIGURE 14–2.** Burping an infant.

11. About halfway through the feeding, burp (bubble) the infant (Fig. 14–2) by:

   a. Placing a clean cloth over the part of your uniform that will be next to the infant's mouth.
   b. Sitting the infant on your lap with his or her chin supported with one of your hands, or Placing the infant prone over your lap, or Supporting the infant in an upright position on your shoulder.

11. Babies often swallow air, which expands the stomach and leaves less room for oral nutrition. Abdominal distention can result from swallowing air excessively.
   a. Protects your uniform from any formula regurgitated by the infant.
   b. The sitting position is preferred because the infant's responses can be observed.

▼ *ACTION*	▼ *RATIONALE*
c. Gently rubbing your other hand in a circular motion over the infant's back until the infant burps (about 5 min); or Gently patting the infant's back just below the scapular area.	c. Relaxes the infant. Air in the stomach rises to the cardiac sphincter and can be expelled by the infant. Air or bubbles in the lower part of the stomach rise to the top of the stomach and can be expelled by the infant.
12. Resume the feeding until the bottle is empty or until the infant stops sucking or falls asleep.	12. When full, the infant stops sucking or falls asleep.
13. Burp the infant at the end of the feeding.	13. The infant needs to expel any air in the stomach to decrease flatus and gastric distention.
14. Check to see if the baby's diaper needs changing.	14. Because of the gastrocolic reflex, young infants often have bowel movements during or shortly after feedings.
15. Return the infant to the crib or bassinet. Place the infant on his or her side.	15. If the infant regurgitates, aspiration of gastric contents is less likely in this position than in other positions. The cardiac sphincter is on the left side of the stomach. In the right side-lying position, air is likely to rise to the top of the stomach and be expelled with less regurgitation of the formula than in other positions.

> **NOTE:** If the infant often regurgitates after a feeding, place him or her in the right side-lying position.

16. If the infant is placed in a crib, raise the side rails.	16. Prevents the infant from falling out of the crib.
17. Record the amount and type of oral nutrition and the infant's response to the feeding.	17. Communicates to the other members of the health care team and contributes to the legal record by documenting the care given to the client.

Example of Documentation

DATE	TIME	NOTES
10/18/93	0830	30 ml formula taken vigorously. No regurgitation. Placed on left side. *S. Williams, RN*

Teaching Tips

This is an appropriate time to discuss with the child's parents the types, amounts, and methods of preparation of oral nutrition appropriate for the age of the infant. Let the parents practice preparing the formula and correctly positioning the infant for a feeding while you are there. The parents should hold the infant rather than prop the bottle. Teach the parents about management of regurgitation, hiccups, constipation, and introduction of solid foods.

Home Care Variations

Parents may warm a refrigerated bottle by placing it in a pan of warm water or by running warm water from the faucet over the bottle. The bottle should not be placed in a microwave oven for warming because of uneven heat distribution that may result in overheating of the formula and injury to the infant.

If city water is used to mix with powdered or concentrated formula, sterilizing bottles is usually unnecessary.

Washing bottles in a dishwasher is preferable to washing them by hand because high temperatures generated in the dishwasher destroy most harmful bacteria.

An infant who regurgitates formula after a feeding may be placed in a low Fowler's position in an infant seat following the feeding. Caution parents not to leave a baby unattended in an infant seat.

SKILL 14-2   ASSISTING WITH BREAST-FEEDING

Clinical Situations in Which You May Encounter This Skill

A client who has chosen to breast-feed her infant needs assistance and education to ensure a successful and positive experience. Although an infant's sucking action is instinctive, breast-feeding is a learned process for the mother. Usually a woman decides during pregnancy to breast-feed her infant, so that is the best time to introduce information. However, you may need to clarify information in the postpartum period, when the client may express myths and misinformation.

You should ensure that the mother wears a supportive nursing brassiere at all times, including while she sleeps. Nursing bras are available at most department stores. The bras have a flap in the cup that unhooks to expose the breast for feeding the infant. The bra should be washed daily.

Afterbirth pains, which occur with involution of the uterus as the infant sucks and cause oxytocin to be released, are not experienced by the first-time mother, but are with subsequent births. If the client experiences afterbirth pains, reassure her that they are normal and that they will continue only for a few days. Administer a mild analgesic 30 minutes before the infant is put to the breast.

Sore nipples may discourage the mother. The client may have heard of many home remedies for treating sore nipples, such as applying egg whites, salad oil, or cocoa butter. However, these remedies as well as creams and lotions should be avoided. The breast milk has a physiologic substance with bacteriostatic qualities that should be left on the nipples to dry between feedings. The mother may feel that she did not adequately "toughen" her nipples during pregnancy. She should be reassured that prenatal "toughening" does little to prevent nipple discomfort in the postpartum period. Also, stimulation of the nipples during pregnancy is not recommended because doing so releases oxytocin, which can cause uterine contractions. Limiting the duration of feedings does little to prevent nipple soreness and only postpones the onset of sore nipples and leads to painful engorgement.

Nipple shields do more harm than good. Thick rubber breast shields may reduce the mother's milk supply and promote improper sucking. If the mother has inverted nipples, a thin silicone shield may be used at the beginning of each feeding until the nipple everts.

If the client complains of sore nipples, observe the infant breast-feeding. Often the infant does not have the nipple and areola completely in his or her mouth and is biting, nibbling, or chewing the nipple. Other causes also should be investigated, such as improper positioning of the infant at the breast, breaking suction improperly, improper or excessive pumping of the breast, thrush, or lack of nipple exposure to light and air.

Engorgement of the breast is not only painful to the mother, but it also can lead to mastitis. Engorgement can be prevented and easily corrected. The easiest method of avoiding engorgement is to allow the infant to nurse frequently and soon after delivery. For example, the infant should breast-feed without restrictions in the first 48 hours postpartum. Because 75% of the milk taken by the infant is replaced within 2 hours of emptying the breast, the infant should not wait too long to breast-feed again or the breast will become overfilled and the nipples will be difficult to grasp. If the mother's breasts become engorged, the mother should be taught to apply warm compresses to the breasts and gently hand express some milk to soften the nipples before offering the breast to the infant. There is no place in the early postpartum period for rigid scheduling for the breast-fed infant.

Frequent feedings during the first several weeks postpartum may cause the mother to feel that her milk is inadequate in quantity and quality. The mother needs reassurance that breast milk is easily digested (and almost 100% utilized) by the infant. The infant has an adequate intake per day if he or she is wetting 6 to 8 diapers per day.

The infant should be offered both breasts at each feeding. The cream or fat content of the breast milk is higher in the hindmilk, so feedings should begin on alternate breasts.

Questions about the introduction of solid foods may arise. Stress that the American Academy of Pediatrics recommends that no solids be introduced for 4 to 6 months.

The mother may mistake the breast-fed infant's soft, runny stool for diarrhea. Explain to the mother that the consistency of the stool is such because of high utilization of the breast-milk nutrients. Also stress that the main characteristic of a diarrhea stool is a foul odor caused by bacteria. Breast milk stools do not have a foul odor, but rather have a "sweet" odor.

Emotional and psychologic support is essential for the mother to have a positive experience with breast-feeding. You should stress that breast-feeding is the natural and ideal nutrition for the infant. Verbal reassurances as well as nonverbal communication through your facial expressions must convey positive support.

In the hospital setting, ensure that favorable conditions are present to convey a positive experience for the client who is breast-feeding. For example, the facility should have photos or paintings of nursing mothers. In the postpartum period, there should be no separation of the breast-feeding infant and the mother. The hospital staff should be educated about the needs of the breast-feeding infant and the mother. No samples of formula should be given to the mother upon her discharge from the hospital. The American Academy of Pediatrics describes giving formula to the mother as "tacit discouragement of breast-feeding."

Anticipated Responses

▼ The mother holds the baby so that he or she is facing her. The infant holds the nipple and areola of the

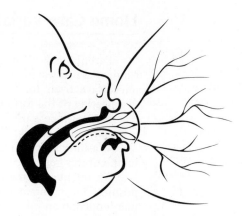

▼ **FIGURE 14–3.** Breast-feeding an infant.

breast between his or her tongue and hard palate (Fig. 14–3). As the infant begins to suck, the mother experiences a "let-down" or "ejection" reflex. After about 3 weeks of the infant receiving only breast milk for nourishment (no juice, formula, etc.), the mother will have established a milk supply that meets the demands of her infant.

▼ The infant has 6 to 8 wet diapers per day. The infant gains weight, grows appropriately, and is satisfied after feedings.

Adverse Responses

▼ The mother's breasts become engorged.
▼ The mother's nipples become sore.

Materials List

Gather these materials before beginning the skill:

▼ Clean diaper
▼ Burping cloth (clean cloth diaper)

▼ ACTION

1. Change the infant's diaper, if necessary.

2. Ask if the mother has ever breast-fed an infant before and what her experience was like.

3. Position the mother for comfort:
   a. Side-lying with a pillow behind her back, or

▼ RATIONALE

1. The infant may have voided or had a bowel movement since the previous feeding.
   Changing the diaper promotes the infant's comfort and prevents soiling of the mother's clothes as the infant is held closely.

2. Discussing previous experiences gives you an opportunity to dispel any misconceptions, address any questions or beliefs, and discuss what the client can expect. If the client has breast-fed successfully before, she still may have questions and need support.

   a. This position is often comfortable for the client after a cesarean section. Pressure on the suture line is reduced.

▼ *ACTION*   ▼ *RATIONALE*

    b. Sitting upright with her arms supported.

4. Position the infant:
    a. Across the mother's chest or with pillows in the mother's lap. Place the infant on his or her side and at the level of the mother's nipples, with his or her legs around her waist. The infant's head should be supported in the crook of the mother's arm.

    b. Lying next to the mother. With the mother in a side-lying position, place the infant on a folded blanket next to the mother at the level of her nipple.

    b. Lessens the mother's fatigue and promotes the breast-feeding process.

    a. This position allows the mother to see her infant and easily use one hand to support her breast with four fingers underneath and her thumb on top. With her hand in the correct position, she can use her index finger to gently pull down on the infant's chin to open his or her mouth or roll out the lower lip.

    b. The blanket elevates the infant to the level of the mother's nipple and allows the mother to remain in a comfortable position. In this position, the mother can feed the infant from the other breast by shifting further to the side.

NOTE: Caution the mother not to fall asleep as the infant breast-feeds.

Nipples can be damaged with periods of sustained negative pressure.

---

    c. In the "football hold." Place the infant on a pillow at the mother's side, facing the breast with his or her mouth at the nipple level. Have the mother bring the infant to the breast while she supports his or her head.

5. Help the infant to grasp the mother's nipple properly by eliciting the rooting reflex: gently stroke the infant's cheek (on the side near the mother's breast) softly toward the infant's lips.

6. Allow the infant to suck on the first breast for approximately 10 to 15 minutes.

7. Help the mother to break the infant's suction: insert a finger into the infant's mouth so the negative pressure is released.

8. Ensure that the mother burps or bubbles the infant between feedings from each breast or at least every 15 minutes.

9. Help the mother to reposition herself and the baby so the infant can breast-feed from the other breast.

10. At the completion of the feeding, check the baby's diaper for soiling.

11. Position the infant on his or her side for sleep.

12. Encourage the mother to rest between feedings while the infant sleeps.

    c. Supporting the infant's head while he or she is in this position prevents the infant from extending his or her back and arching off the breast.

5. The rooting reflex is present at birth. As the cheek is touched or stroked, the infant instinctively turns his or her head in that direction.

6. The breast is emptied after about 10 minutes.

7. Pulling the infant off the mother's breast without relieving the suction can damage the mother's nipples.

8. Although the breast-fed infant who properly sucks takes in little air, a small amount of air is ingested. Burping the infant helps to expel the air, facilitates the infant's comfort, and allows more space for the ingestion of milk.

9. The infant should breast-feed from both breasts at each feeding to remove all the hindmilk.

10. The infant often has a bowel movement during or soon after the feeding because of stimulation of the gastrocolic reflex.

11. Positioning the infant on his or her side minimizes the chance of aspiration if any milk is expelled with eructations.

12. If the mother is fatigued, the milk supply may decrease.

▼ ACTION	▼ RATIONALE
13. Encourage the mother to expose her nipples to air to allow the breast milk to dry on the nipples.	13. Breast milk has a physiologic substance with bacteriostatic qualities that should be left on the nipples to dry between feedings.
14. In the client's chart, record the breast-feeding. Note the length of the feeding and any difficulties encountered.	14. Communicates the findings to the other members of the health care team and contributes to the legal record by documenting the care given to the client.

Example of Documentation

DATE	TIME	NOTES
2/25/93	0800	Infant breast-fed on both breasts. Mother reported strong sucking by infant. Infant asleep on right side in bassinet near mother's bedside.
		S. Williams, RN

Teaching Tips

The mother should be encouraged to feed the infant on demand and not to expect a rigid schedule to be followed by the infant. The mother can be reassured that the infant is taking adequate amounts of milk if the infant is wetting a diaper 6 to 8 times per day. Teach the mother the difference between a diarrhea stool and the stool of a breast-fed infant.

Teach the mother the importance of a nutritious diet that will supply her caloric needs and provide enough calories to sustain an adequate milk supply. In general, the mother should continue her prenatal vitamins while breast-feeding and should consume an additional 2,000 calories per day above her normal intake. The additional calories are needed to produce breast milk, which has 20 calories per ounce. Additional fluids should be consumed (at least 3,000 ml per day) to ensure adequate hydration. If the mother has an 8-ounce glass of fluid at each of the infant's feedings, fluid intake should be adequate.

Encourage the mother to limit caffeine in drinks and nicotine in cigarettes as these may stimulate the infant and disturb his or her sleep. If the mother notices that foods such as chocolate, cabbage, or onions cause gas in the infant, she should avoid ingesting them because they will be secreted in the breast milk.

Alcohol consumption should be limited or avoided. The alcohol is secreted in the breast milk and will sedate the infant.

The mother should check with her physician before taking any over-the-counter drugs. If an antibiotic is prescribed for the mother, she should notify the physician that she is breast-feeding. Drugs taken by the mother pass into the breast milk and are then ingested by the infant.

If the mother experiences leaking of milk from her breasts between feedings, she may be advised to breast-feed the infant more frequently. Also, she may wear breast shields that do not have a plastic liner. The plastic liner may cause an increase in bacterial growth on the nipples.

Home Care Variations

The mother should be educated as noted above. The mother who experiences any difficulties needs emotional support from you.

Encourage the mother to call when problems arise. Frustrations can be avoided, and the experience of breast-feeding can be a positive one for the entire family.

SKILL 14–3   HELPING THE ADULT TO EAT

Clinical Situations in Which You May Encounter This Skill

An adult needs assistance to eat with a spoon or fork anytime chewing and swallowing of food are possible but self-feeding is limited or not possible because the client is blind, has had a cerebrovascular accident (CVA or stroke) and has paralysis, is elderly and fatigues easily, or has bilateral orthopedic appliances (casts, for example) on the arms.

Choking can be a hazard for the paralyzed client. If the client chokes, quickly turn him or her to the side, place one finger in his or her mouth, and sweep any food out of the mouth. If the food is not visible, perform the Heimlich maneuver. (See Skill 3–3.)

Anticipated Responses

▼ The client is hungry, accepts the spoon-feeding or fork-feeding, and is satisfied after eating.
▼ The client's weight is stable or, if indicated, increases.

Adverse Responses

▼ The client refuses feedings or loses weight.
▼ The client chokes on the food.

Materials List

Gather these materials before beginning the skill:

▼ Spoon or fork
▼ Food
▼ Straw
▼ Clean cloth
▼ Supplies to provide oral hygiene
  Toothbrush
  Toothpaste
  Cup
  Water

▼ ACTION	▼ RATIONALE
1. Make sure the client can swallow and has a gag reflex. Ask the client to swallow or test for the gag reflex by touching the back of the client's throat with a cotton swab. Assess for gagging.	1. Decreases the chance of aspiration of the food or fluids into the bronchus.
2. Ask the client about food allergies or food intolerances.	2. Food allergies or intolerances can lead to symptoms such as nausea and vomiting, diarrhea, colic in infants, or urticaria.
3. Wash your hands.	3. Decreases the transmission of microorganisms.
4. Place the client in a semi-Fowler's or high-Fowler's position if he or she must remain in bed or assist the client in getting to a chair. If the client cannot sit or elevation of his or her head is contraindicated, assist the client in assuming a side-lying position.	4. Decreases the chance of aspiration.
5. Place a clean cloth over the client's chest.	5. Protects the client's clothing.
6. Provide or assist with oral hygiene by brushing the client's teeth or encouraging the client to rinse his or her mouth with peroxide and water or mouthwash.	6. Removes debris and any bad tastes so the client can taste the food being offered.
7. Put in the client's dentures if needed.	7. Facilitates eating.
8. Help the client to wash his or her hands and face.	8. Prevents transmission of microorganisms from the hands to the mouth.
9. Place the tray on the overbed table and place it within easy reach of the client.	9. Helps the client to feed himself or herself, if possible.

▼ ACTION

▼ RATIONALE

10. If needed, sweeten the client's tea, open a carton of milk, place a straw in the beverage, cut up the food, etc.

10. Assists clients who are weak or who lack manual dexterity.

11. Identify and describe the foods to the client. If you are helping a blind client to eat, describe the food on the plate as though you were telling time (12 o'clock, 3 o'clock, etc.).

11. Permits the client to identify any foods that he or she dislikes and the order in which he or she would like to eat the food.

12. Allow the client to choose which foods he or she prefers to eat first.

12. Encourages the client's independence and decision making.

13. Make sure that the food is not too hot by ensuring that steam is not rising from the food. Cold food should be served cold. Warn the client if the food is hot or cold.

13. Excessively hot food could cause thermal injuries.

14. Place one spoonful or forkful of food into the client's mouth above his or her tongue (Fig. 14–4).

14. Prevents choking and aspiration.

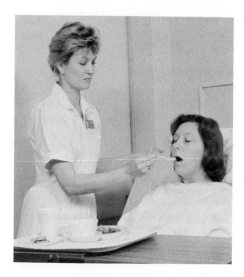

▼ FIGURE 14–4. Feeding an adult.

15. Allow the client to chew and swallow the food before offering another spoonful or forkful.

15. Prevents overfilling of the client's mouth with food, which can cause choking.

16. Talk to the client while you are feeding him or her.

16. Makes mealtime more pleasant for the client.

17. Allow the client to drink liquids with a straw.

17. The client can take the amount desired.

18. Very patiently continue to offer the client food until he or she indicates that he or she does not want any more.

18. If you appear rushed, the client may not finish eating.

19. After completion of the feeding, provide oral hygiene for the person.

19. Removes any remaining food from the client's mouth.

20. Wash the client's hands and face.

20. Helps the client to feel clean after eating.

21. Remove the tray from the client's room.

22. Record the amount and types of food eaten and any difficulties encountered.

22. Communicates to the other members of the health care team and contributes to the legal record by documenting the care given to the client.

Example of Documentation

DATE	TIME	NOTES
10/20/93	0830	Assisted client to high-Fowler's position. Accepted three-fourths of breakfast.
		S. Williams, RN

Teaching Tips

This is an excellent time to discuss nutrition with the client. Help the client to select menu items for the next day. Also, encourage the client to be as independent as possible.

SKILL 14–4   HELPING THE CHILD TO EAT

Clinical Situations in Which You May Encounter This Skill

Until about 1 year of age, infants are unable to feed themselves with utensils and need to be fed with a spoon. Older children who are unable to feed themselves (children with bilateral upper-extremity orthopedic appliances or cerebral palsy, for example) also need to be fed by another person.

Choking is a hazard for a child who has paralysis or a decreased gag reflex and for debilitated children. If an infant chokes, quickly turn him or her upside down and briskly strike between his or her scapulas with your hand. If an older child chokes, turn the child on his or her side, open the mouth, and sweep with your finger to remove the food. If the food is not visible, perform the Heimlich maneuver. (See Skill 3–3.)

Anticipated Responses

▼ The child accepts the food on the spoon or fork and gains weight at an appropriate rate.

Adverse Responses

▼ The child refuses the food, spits it out, or chokes on the food.

Materials List

Gather these materials before beginning the skill:

▼ Feeding utensils (spoon or fork)
▼ Food
▼ Bib
▼ Warm moist washcloth
▼ Infant seat or high chair

▼ *ACTION*

▼ *RATIONALE*

1. Assess the child's developmental level:
   a. Birth to 6 months: The infant should take only formula or breast milk. The tongue protrusion reflex that makes spoon-feeding difficult is present until 4 months of age.
   b. Age 5 to 6 months: The infant puts his or her hands in the mouth and tries to pick up objects using sweeping movements with a cupped hand. The baby is able to chew soft foods (such as mashed bananas).
   c. Age 7 to 8 months: The baby picks up objects and foods. He or she is able to pick up and eat crackers unassisted.
   d. Age 9 to 12 months: The child uses a pincer grasp to pick up foods. Finger foods cut into small bite-sizes are appropriate.
   e. Age 12 to 18 months: The child is able to hold a spoon in his or her hand and attempts to eat with utensils. There is much spilling of food from the spoon.
   f. By age 2 to 3 years: The child is able to feed himself or herself with a spoon or fork with minimal spilling.

2. Wash your hands.

3. Help the child to wash his or her hands and face with a warm washcloth.

4. Place the food in an unbreakable bowl or on an unbreakable plate. Put liquids in an unbreakable cup.

5. Place the infant in an infant seat in a semi-Fowler's position; place the child in an upright position in a high chair. The infant or child also may be held in your lap while you feed him or her (Fig. 14–5). If an upright position is contraindicated, position the child on his or her side.

1. Determines the appropriate foods and methods of feeding for the developmental level of the child.

2. Decreases the transmission of microorganisms.

3. Prevents the transmission of microorganisms from the hands to the mouth.

4. Avoids breakage of plates or cups if the child pushes them onto the floor.

5. The upright position helps to facilitate eating and prevents choking.

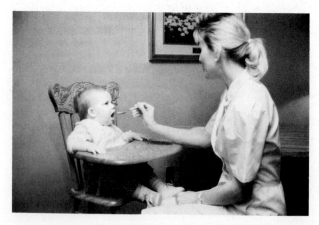

▼ FIGURE 14–5. Positioning a child for feeding.

6. Place the bib around the child's neck to cover the chest area and secure the ties or snaps at the back of his or her neck.

6. Protects the child's clothing.

▼ *ACTION*	▼ *RATIONALE*
7. Make sure the environment is relaxed and free of distractions.	7. Babies from the age of 8 months are easily distracted.
8. Offer the child food beginning with the less sweet items and going to the sweet items last.	8. The child may refuse less sweet items if sweet ones are eaten first.
9. Place the food in the infant's or child's mouth above the tongue.	9. Facilitates swallowing.
10. If the infant spits out any of the food, wipe it off his or her lips or chin with the spoon and place it in the infant's mouth again.	10. If the protrusion reflex is still present, the infant's tongue will eject food when he or she swallows.
11. Continue to feed the infant or child until the food is gone or until the child is no longer interested in eating and seems satisfied.	
12. While feeding the child, talk to him or her.	12. Encourages socialization and verbalization and makes mealtime pleasant.
13. At the conclusion of the meal, wash the child's hands with a washcloth.	13. Removes any food from the child's hands.
14. Record the amount and types of foods fed to the child.	14. Communicates to the other members of the health care team and contributes to the legal record by documenting the care given to the client.

Example of Documentation

DATE	TIME	NOTES
10/20/93	1230	Placed in high chair. Ate all of meat, vegetables, and fruit with assistance.
		S. Williams, RN

Teaching Tips

This is an excellent time to discuss nutrition, growth and development, and cooking safety with the child's parents. For example, foods must be cut into very small bites for young children to prevent choking. Never hold a child while cooking foods on the stove top and always turn the handles of cooking pots to the back of the stove.

Home Care Variations

Encourage parents not to leave a child unattended if the child is eating finger foods. Also, parents should serve foods and drinks in nonbreakable plastic containers.

SKILL 14–5 INSERTING A NASOGASTRIC TUBE

Clinical Situations in Which You May Encounter This Skill

A nasogastric tube for feeding may be inserted in clients who are comatose, who have had head or neck surgery, or who have mechanical ventilation. Nasogastric tubes should be inserted cautiously in persons with myocardial infarction, aortic aneurysm, esophageal varices, thrombocytopenia, or esophageal cancer and stenosis. Have suction equipment available in case the person vomits during the procedure.

Small-bore flexible feeding tubes are nasogastric tubes that are often inserted for clients who require continuous-drip tube feedings. The continuous-drip feeding enhances absorption and decreases the chance of diarrhea. The flexible feeding tube often has a weighted tip and is long enough to allow passage through the pylorus into the duodenum.

A large-bore nasogastric tube may be inserted and connected to suction to withdraw fluids and gas from the stomach. This procedure is often done in clients who have had GI tract surgery.

Anticipated Responses

▼ The nasogastric tube is inserted into the client's stomach without meeting an obstruction.
▼ The feeding tube is positioned correctly.

Adverse Responses

▼ The tube is passed into the client's bronchus or is coiled in the mouth or at the back of the throat.

Materials List

Gather these materials before beginning the skill:

▼ Examination gloves
▼ Nasogastric tube
▼ Water-soluble lubricant
▼ Hypoallergenic tape and safety pin to secure the tube
▼ Towel
▼ Waterproof pad
▼ Emesis basin
▼ Basin of ice chips to stiffen the rubber tube, if necessary
▼ Basin of warm water to soften the stiff plastic tube, if necessary
▼ Glass of water with a straw (for a conscious person)
▼ Tissues
▼ Guidewire (for use with a flexible feeding tube)
▼ 30-ml catheter-tipped syringe
▼ Stethoscope
▼ Flashlight or penlight
▼ Toothbrush and toothpaste or lemon and glycerin swabs
▼ Suction equipment (will be needed in case client vomits)
▼ Clamp
▼ Pump (if the client is to receive continuous feedings)
▼ Feeding-tube plug

▼ ACTION	▼ RATIONALE
1. Determine the reason for the tube (feeding or decompression).	1. Different-sized tubes are usually used for feeding and decompression. The reason for the tube should be explained to the client or the client's parent.
2. Assess the client's level of consciousness and his or her ability to understand your explanations and directions.	2. If possible, the client should assist with insertion.
3. Assess the client's ability to move and maintain desired positions.	3. Another person may be needed to maintain the client's position.
4. Raise the client's bed to a comfortable working height.	4. Assists in preventing strain on your back.
5. Raise the client to a high-Fowler's position and tilt the client's head back. If this is not possible, insert the tube with the client in either the side-lying or supine position.	5. This position makes insertion of the tube easier, facilitates swallowing of water, and facilitates downward movement of the tube through the GI tract.

▼ *ACTION* _ _ _ _ _ _ _ _ _ _ _ _ | ▼ *RATIONALE* _ _ _ _ _ _ _ _ _ _

6. Stand on the right side of the bed if you are right-handed.

6. Makes insertion easier.

7. Examine the client's naris with a penlight for obstructions or deformities.

7. Attempts to introduce a tube into an obstructed naris or previously fractured nose with a deviated septum may cause the client to experience discomfort and unnecessary trauma. Insert the tube through the client's mouth if the nares are obstructed.

8. Measure the distance you will need to insert the tube by measuring from the tip of the person's nose to the earlobe and then from the nose to the xiphoid process (Fig. 14–6).

8. This is the approximate distance that the tube should be inserted to reach the stomach.

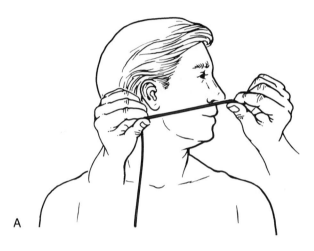

A

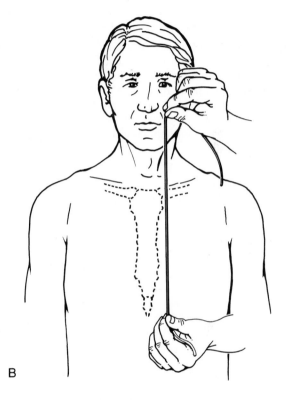

B

▼ **FIGURE 14–6.** Measuring from the tip of the nose to the earlobe (*A*) and from the nose to the xiphoid process (*B*).

9. Use tape to mark this distance on the tube.

9. The tape mark will remind you of the distance to insert the tube.

10. Coil the tube around your fingers.

10. It is easiest to insert a curved tube.

11. Place a waterproof pad under the client's chin and across his or her chest.

11. Helps to protect the client's clothing.

12. Place an emesis basin beside the client.

12. Insertion of the tube may stimulate vomiting.

13. Put on gloves.

13. When there is a chance of coming into contact with bodily secretions, gloves should be worn to prevent the possible transmission of microorganisms.

14. Lubricate the end and approximately 4 inches of the tube with water-soluble lubricant.

14. Water-soluble lubricant makes insertion of the tube easier by reducing friction between the nasopharyngeal mucous membranes and the tube. An oil-based lubricant should not be used since it can cause pneumonia if inhaled.

▼ *ACTION* ▼ *RATIONALE*

15. If you are inserting a flexible feeding tube, insert the guidewire.

15. Facilitates insertion of the feeding tube. The guidewire is not used for large-bore tubes.

16. Ask the client to slightly flex his or her neck.

16. Makes insertion of the tube easier.

17. Gently insert the tube into a naris and ask the client to swallow as the tube is slowly advanced to the nasopharynx.

17. Swallowing facilitates passage of the tube.

18. If the client gags as the tube reaches the nasopharynx, stop a moment and allow the client to rest. If the client continues to gag, inspect the posterior portion of his or her mouth to see if the tube has coiled there. If the tube is coiled, withdraw the tube until it is no longer coiled and try to advance it again.

18. The tube may stimulate the gag reflex. Allowing the client to rest may prevent vomiting. If the tube is coiled in the back of the client's mouth, it will not advance downward.

19. Ask the client to swallow sips of water or crushed ice and advance the tube several inches each time the client swallows until you reach the tape mark. If you meet frank resistance, stop and do not force the tube. Also stop if there are signs of respiratory distress such as excessive gasping, coughing, or cyanosis and immediately withdraw the tube several inches.

19. Swallowing will assist the tube to pass through the esophageal sphincter.
Forcing the tube can cause trauma to the tissue. The tube may be in the person's trachea.

20. Check to ensure that the tube is in the stomach by:
a. Injecting approximately 5 to 10 cc of air with a catheter-tipped syringe and auscultating over the epigastric area for the sound of air ("swooshing sound") entering the stomach (Fig. 14–7);

a. If the tube is in the person's stomach, a swooshing sound is heard as air enters the stomach. If no air is heard, the tube may be in the client's lungs.

> **NOTE:** Because of the small diameter of flexible feeding tubes, this test is not a reliable indicator with small-bore tubes.

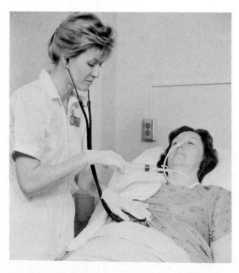

▼ **FIGURE 14–7.** Auscultating over the client's epigastric area.

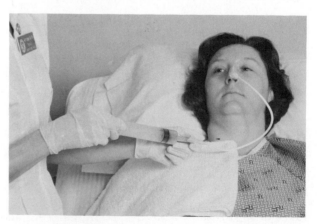

▼ **FIGURE 14–8.** Aspirating gastric contents into a syringe.

b. Aspirating the gastric contents into a syringe (the most reliable of the four methods) (Fig. 14–8);

b. If the tube is in the person's stomach, you should be able to aspirate the gastric contents. If you are not successful in aspirating the gastric contents, the tube may be in the lungs. You may want to check the aspirate with pH test tape. Gastric contents should be acidic.

▼ *ACTION* _____   ▼ *RATIONALE* _____

c. Placing the end of the tube in a glass of water and watching for bubbles; and

d. Asking the person to speak.

c. If the tube is in the lungs, you should see bubbles each time the client breathes.

d. If the tube is separating the vocal cords, the person will not be able to speak.

21. Secure the tube to the client's nose with nonallergenic tape. Make sure the skin on the person's nose is clean and dry. Cut a 3- to 4-inch strip of tape and cut it up the center 1 to 1.5 or 2 inches. Place the solid portion on the nose and wrap the ends tightly around the tube.

21. Taping the tube to the nose helps to keep it from slipping out or being pulled out. Dry, clean skin facilitates adhesion of the tape to the nose.

22. Connect the distal end of the tube to suction, or insert a tube plug. Most nasogastric tubes are connected to low intermittent suction.

22. Connecting the tube depends on the purpose for which the tube was inserted. If the tube is not connected to suction, the tube is plugged to keep the gastric contents from draining out the open end. Placement of the flexible feeding tube is checked by x-ray before the tube is connected to tube feeding.

23. Place adhesive tape around the point where the tube is to be pinned to the gown, insert the pin through the tape tag, and pin it to the gown (Fig. 14–9). Leave slack in the tubing to allow the client to move in bed.

23. Pinning the tube to the gown assists in keeping the tube from being pulled out.

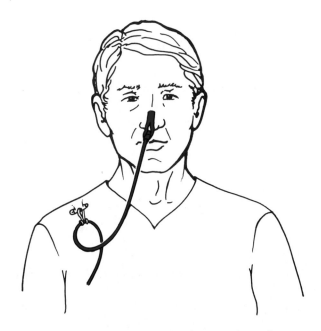

▼ **FIGURE 14–9.** Nasogastric tube secured to a client.

24. Clean the tube of any remaining lubricant and provide for the client's oral hygiene.

24. Oral hygiene and cleansing promote the client's comfort and sense of well-being.

NOTE: Oral hygiene should be performed frequently while the tube is in place.

▼ *ACTION*	▼ *RATIONALE*
25. Remove the gloves and wash your hands.	**25.** Decreases the transmission of microorganisms.
26. Record the procedure.	**26.** Communicates to the other members of the health care team and contributes to the legal record by documenting the care given to the client.

Example of Documentation

DATE	*TIME*	*NOTES*
11/15/93	1000	Flexible feeding tube inserted. X-ray done for placement. Dr. M. called and stated that tube is in place. Tube connected to pump and one-fourth strength Isocal started at 30 ml per hour.
		T. White, RN

Teaching Tips

Explain the purpose of the tube and the procedure to the client or the client's family. If the tube is inserted for decompression, explain to the client that he or she will not be allowed to drink while the tube is in place. To facilitate the client's cooperation during insertion, establish a signal for the person to use to tell you to wait a minute.

Home Care Variations

Periodically assess the family member's ability to check the placement of the tube, check residual gastric contents, and administer tube feedings (if ordered). Check the family member's knowledge regarding the length of time that the tube feeding can hang.

SKILL 14–6 COLLECTING A GASTRIC SPECIMEN

Clinical Situations in Which You May Encounter This Skill

A gastric specimen may be collected to determine pH or to check for the presence of occult blood. A pH analysis of gastric contents is done to determine the degree of acidity of secretions present in the stomach. Tests of pH also may be done on vomit. The pH is normally between 1.5 and 3.5. A guaiac test of gastric specimens may be done to determine the presence of blood.

Gastric contents are normally greenish in color. The appearance of gastric contents that contain blood varies depending on how recent the bleeding occurred and how active the bleeding is. The color may range from bright red to dark brown and the gastric contents may look like coffee grounds.

Anticipated Responses

▼ The client is able to tolerate insertion of the nasogastric tube.
▼ The gastric secretions have their characteristic greenish color and there are no signs of bleeding.
▼ The pH is normal.

Adverse Responses

▼ The client has difficulty tolerating insertion of the nasogastric tube.
▼ The pH is outside the normal range.
▼ The color of the gastric secretions is abnormal.
▼ The gastric secretions contain blood.

Materials List

Gather these materials before beginning the skill:

▼ 60-ml catheter-tipped syringe
▼ pH test paper
▼ Guaiac test paper and developer
▼ 1-ml syringe
▼ Examination gloves
▼ Emesis basis
▼ Watch

▼ ACTION	▼ RATIONALE
1. Determine the reason for the test.	1. The reason should be explained to the client.
2. Put on your gloves.	2. Gloves should be worn whenever there is possible contact with blood or body fluids to prevent the transmission of microorganisms.
3. Position the client in Fowler's position.	3. Facilitates placement of the nasogastric tube, and aids in preventing aspiration of gastric contents into the stomach.
4. Insert the nasogastric tube if it is not already present. (Refer to Skill 14–5 regarding insertion of nasogastric tubes if necessary.)	4. Gastric secretions are obtained by aspirating the specimen from the client's stomach via a nasogastric tube.
5. Using a 60-ml syringe, withdraw 10 ml of gastric secretions and place the fluid in an emesis basin.	5. Most nasogastric tubes require a catheter-tipped syringe to withdraw gastric secretions.
6. Observe the gastric secretions for color and for the presence of blood.	6. These data should be charted.

Assessing the pH of gastric contents

7. Using a 1-ml syringe, apply one drop of gastric secretions to the pH test paper.	7. Only a small amount of gastric contents is needed for the pH analysis.
8. Wait 30 seconds.	8. Adequate time is needed for the test to develop properly.
9. Compare the pH paper with the color chart to determine the results.	9. The color chart provides a scale for determining results.

Assessing for the presence of occult blood

10. Using the 1-ml syringe, apply one drop of the gastric contents to the occult blood test paper.	10. Only a small amount of the gastric contents is needed to perform the test.
11. Apply two drops of the guaiac developer over the sample and one drop between the positive and negative control monitors.	11. Developer will react with the gastric sample if there is blood present.
12. Wait 60 seconds and compare the color to the control monitors.	12. Blue color indicates a positive test.
13. Reconnect the nasogastric tube to the suction or clamp as indicated, or if the tube was inserted solely to collect the gastric specimen, withdraw the tube.	13. Returns the equipment to functional status.

▼ ACTION	▼ RATIONALE
14. Dispose of soiled equipment in an appropriate container.	14. Proper disposal decreases the transmission of microorganisms.
15. Wash your hands.	15. Decreases the transmission of microorganisms.
16. Explain the results to the client.	16. Keeps the client informed of his or her health status and allows the client to actively participate in his or her care.
17. Help the client to assume a position of comfort.	17. Promotes the client's comfort.
18. Offer mouth care to the client.	18. Provides for hygiene and removes any distasteful or odorous secretions from the client's mouth.
19. Record the procedure and results in the client's record.	19. Communicates the findings to the other members of the health care team, and contributes to the legal record by documenting the care given to the client.

Example of Documentation

DATE	TIME	NOTES
1/2/94	0800	10 ml gastric contents aspirated from NG tube. pH 2.5.
		C. Lammon, RN

Teaching Tips

Explain the procedure and the purpose of the test to the client or his or her family, or both.

Home Care Variations

This procedure is not usually performed in the client's home.

SKILL 14–7   REMOVING A NASOGASTRIC TUBE

Clinical Situations in Which You May Encounter This Skill

The nasogastric tube is removed when suction or tube feeding is no longer required.

Anticipated Responses

▼ The tube is removed.

Adverse Responses

▼ Removal of the tube stimulates gagging.

Materials List

Gather these materials before beginning the skill:

▼ Examination gloves
▼ Towel and washcloth
▼ Waterproof pad
▼ Toothbrush and toothpaste or lemon and glycerin swab
▼ Emesis basin
▼ Feeding-tube plug

▼ *A C T I O N*_____   ▼ *R A T I O N A L E*_____

▼ **ACTION**	▼ **RATIONALE**
1. Check the physician's order.	**1.** The tube should not be removed without an order.
2. Raise the client to a Fowler's position and tilt the client's head back.	**2.** This position facilitates removal of the tube and decreases the chance of aspiration if the client vomits.
3. Place a waterproof pad under the client's chin and across his or her chest.	**3.** The pad helps to protect the client's clothing. The tube also may be placed in the pad for disposal.
4. Place the emesis basin by the client.	**4.** Manipulation of the tube may induce gagging and vomiting.
5. Put on gloves.	**5.** When there is a chance of coming into contact with bodily secretions, gloves should be worn to prevent the possible transmission of microorganisms.
6. Stop the tube feeding or the suction, disconnect the tube from the suction or tube feeding, and insert the plug into the distal end of the tube.	**6.** Prevents spillage of gastric secretions or tube feeding.
7. Gently remove the tape from the person's nose.	**7.** Facilitates removal of the tube.
8. Have the client take a deep breath.	**8.** Facilitates removal of the tube.
9. Withdraw the tube with one hand in a slow continuous motion and hold the waterproof pad with the other hand to collect the tube.	**9.** Removing the tube in one motion prevents gagging and excessive discomfort. The waterproof pad prevents the dirty tube from soiling the client or the bed.
10. Provide oral hygiene for the client.	**10.** Oral hygiene promotes the client's comfort and sense of well-being.
11. Properly dispose of the equipment.	**11.** Decreases the transmission of microorganisms.
12. Remove the gloves and wash your hands.	**12.** Decreases the transmission of microorganisms.
13. Record the procedure.	**13.** Communicates to the other members of the health care team and contributes to the legal record by documenting the care given to the client.

Example of Documentation

DATE	TIME	NOTES
11/15/93	0930	Tube feeding stopped and flexible feeding tube removed. Oral hygiene administered.
		T. White, RN

Teaching Tips

Tell the client or the client's family why the tube feeding is being discontinued. Explain that you will need to measure all intake to determine if the client is taking enough nutrition in by mouth.

Home Care Variations

Dispose of soiled equipment in a sealed plastic bag.

SKILL 14–8 ADMINISTERING A CONTINUOUS-DRIP TUBE FEEDING

Clinical Situations in Which You May Encounter This Skill

Tube feedings may be administered through oral or nasal tubes or gastrostomy or jejunostomy tubes. Feedings may be administered by the intermittent-drip or continuous-drip method. The continuous-drip method is the most commonly used method of tube feeding. The incidence of diarrhea and absorption problems is considered to be lowest with continuous-drip tube feedings. Although tube feedings can be given by gravity alone, electronic feeding pumps are often used to maintain a constant flow rate. Placement of the tube and the residual volume of the tube feeding should be checked every 4 hours after the feeding has begun.

Anticipated Responses

▼ The tube feeding is administered without vomiting or aspiration.
▼ The client shows a steady weight gain or stable weight indicative of adequate nutrition.
▼ No signs of fluid and electrolyte imbalances are seen.

Adverse Responses

▼ The client develops vomiting or diarrhea or aspirates.
▼ The client exhibits a weight loss.
▼ The client shows signs of fluid and electrolyte imbalances.

Materials List

Gather these materials before beginning the skill:

▼ 60-ml syringe
▼ Bottle of tube-feeding solution
▼ Pump for tube feeding
▼ Tubing for pump and administration set tubing
▼ IV pole
▼ Stethoscope
▼ Waterproof pad
▼ Overbed table
▼ Examination gloves

▼ _ACTION_

1. Check the physician's order for the type and rate of flow of the tube feeding.

2. Assess the client's weight since the tube feeding was begun.

3. Assess the client's electrolyte values.

4. Check the date on the last tubing change for the administration set and pump tubing.

5. Place the equipment on the overbed table.

6. Close the clamp on the administration set tubing.

7. Connect the tubing of the administration set to the bottle of tube-feeding solution and hang the bottle on the IV pole.

8. Insert the pump tubing into the pump, connect the administration set tubing to the pump tubing, and prime the tubing by opening the clamp and turning on the pump.

9. Close the clamp and turn off the pump.

10. Place a waterproof pad under the client's chin and across his or her chest.

11. Raise the head of the bed 30 to 45 degrees.

▼ _RATIONALE_

1. Many different types of tube feedings are available. Flow rates vary according to the age and condition of the client.

2. The weight is a good indication of whether the tube feeding is appropriate and adequate.

3. Early detection of electrolyte imbalances is crucial.

4. The tubing should be changed every 24 hours to prevent bacterial growth.

5. The equipment should be within easy reach.

6. Prevents spillage of the tube-feeding solution.

7. The tube feeding flows from the bottle through the administration set to the pump.

8. Air must be removed to prevent gastric distention.

9. Prevents the spillage of tube-feeding solution.

10. Helps to protect the client's clothing.

11. Elevating the head of the bed helps to prevent reflux and aspiration of the feeding.

▼ _A C T I O N_ ▼ _R A T I O N A L E_ _ _ _ _ _ _ _ _ _ _ _ _ _ _ _ _

12. Put on gloves.

13. Check the tube placement and residual gastric contents every 4 hours. Check to ensure that the tube is in the person's stomach by:
   a. Injecting approximately 5 to 10 cc of air with a catheter-tipped syringe and auscultating over the epigastric area for the sound of air ("swooshing sound") entering the stomach (see Fig. 14–7);

   b. Aspirating the gastric contents into a syringe (see Fig. 14–8). This is the most reliable placement check. Note the amount of gastric contents you are able to aspirate. This is the "residual" amount. Return the residual contents to the stomach.

   c. Placing the end of the tube in a glass of water and watching for bubbles; and
   d. Asking the person to speak.

14. Attach the pump tubing to the nasogastric tube, set the flow rate on the pump, and turn on the pump (Fig. 14–10).

12. When there is a chance of coming into contact with bodily secretions, gloves should be worn to prevent the possible transmission of microorganisms.

   a. If the tube is in the stomach, a "swooshing" sound is heard as air enters the stomach. If no air is heard, the tube may be in the person's lungs. Because of the small diameter of flexible feeding tubes, this test is not a reliable indicator with small-bore tubes.
   b. If the tube is in the person's stomach, you should be able to aspirate the gastric contents. If you are not successful in aspirating the gastric contents, the tube may be in the lungs. A residual of more than 50% of the previous hour's intake indicates delayed emptying of the stomach. Notify the physician. Return the gastric contents to the person's stomach to prevent fluid and electrolyte imbalances.
   c. If the tube is in the lungs, you should see bubbles each time the client breathes.
   d. If the tube is separating the person's vocal cords, the person will not be able to speak.

14. Once the correct placement is determined, the tube feeding may be started.

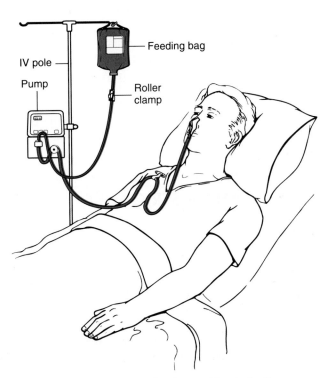

▼ **F I G U R E 14–10.** Continuous-drip tube feeding.

▼ ACTION	▼ RATIONALE
15. Observe the flow of the tube feeding.	**15.** Observation is necessary to ensure that the solution is flowing properly.
16. Remove and properly dispose of the equipment.	**16.** Decreases the transmission of microorganisms.
17. Remove the gloves and wash your hands.	**17.** Decreases the transmission of microorganisms.
18. Record the procedure. Note the tube placement check, the amount and type of tube feeding, the flow rate of the feeding, and how the client tolerated the procedure.	**18.** Communicates the findings to the other members of the health care team and contributes to the legal record by documenting the care given to the client.

Example of Documentation

DATE	TIME	NOTES
11/15/93	1000	Nasogastric tube placement checked. 30 ml of residual obtained and returned. Administration set and pump tubing changed. 240 ml of half-strength Isocal infusing at 60 ml per hour. No symptoms of distress.
		T. White, RN

Teaching Tips

Talk with the client or the client's family member regarding the need for the tube feeding and normal daily dietary requirements.

Home Care Variations

Periodically check the family member's knowledge of how to check the tube position and residual and how to administer a continuous-drip tube feeding. Check that the tube-feeding solution is being properly stored. Check the pump for frayed wires or damage. The intermittent-drip method may be preferred for feeding in the client's home. With this method, a prescribed amount of feeding is given periodically using a tube-feeding drip set and adjusting the rate as tolerated by the client. Usually the feeding is given every 4 to 6 hours over 30 minutes to 1 hour.

SKILL 14–9   IRRIGATING A NASOGASTRIC TUBE

Clinical Situations in Which You May Encounter This Skill

An irrigation of a nasogastric tube is performed when the tube is no longer patent, is draining sluggishly, or the tube-feeding solution does not flow in properly. An irrigation is contraindicated for the client who has had gastric surgery.

Anticipated Responses

▼ Patency is maintained or restored to the tube.

Adverse Responses

▼ Patency cannot be restored to the tube.

Materials List

Gather these materials before beginning the skill:

▼ Irrigation set containing a 60-ml syringe and basin
▼ Normal saline for irrigation (decompression tubes) or water (feeding tubes)
▼ Stethoscope
▼ Glass of water
▼ Rubber-shod forceps or clamp (for nasogastric tube)
▼ Nasogastric plug or cap (for tubing connected to the nasogastric tube)
▼ Waterproof pad
▼ Overbed table
▼ Examination gloves

▼ *ACTION*	▼ *RATIONALE*
1. Determine the client's diagnosis and the reason for the tube.	1. If the client has had gastric surgery, the tube should not be irrigated.
2. Check the physician's order for the irrigation and type of irrigant to be used.	2. Helps to ensure that the proper irrigant is used. You may need to obtain a physician's approval for the irrigation.
3. Place the equipment on the overbed table.	3. The equipment should be within easy reach.
4. Raise the client to a Fowler's position.	4. Decreases the chance of aspiration if the client vomits.
5. Place a waterproof pad under the client's chin and across his or her chest.	5. Helps to protect the client's clothing.
6. Put on gloves.	6. When there is a chance of coming into contact with bodily secretions, gloves should be worn to prevent the possible transmission of microorganisms.
7. Check to ensure that the tube is in the stomach by: a. Injecting approximately 5 to 10 cc of air with a catheter-tipped syringe and auscultating over the epigastric area for the sound of air ("swooshing sound") entering the stomach;	a. If the tube is in the stomach, a "swooshing" sound is heard as air enters the stomach. If no air is heard, the tube may be in the person's lungs. Because of the small diameter of flexible feeding tubes, this test is not a reliable indicator with small-bore tubes.
b. Aspirating the gastric contents into a syringe; this is the most reliable placement check.	b. If the tube is in the person's stomach, you should be able to aspirate the gastric contents. If you are not successful in aspirating the gastric contents, the tube may be in the client's lungs.
c. Placing the end of the tube in a glass of water and watching for bubbles; and	c. If the tube is in the person's lungs, you should see bubbles each time the client breathes.
d. Asking the person to speak.	d. If the tube is separating the vocal cords, the person will not be able to speak.

▼ *ACTION* _____   ▼ *RATIONALE* _____

8. Disconnect the nasogastric tube from the feeding or suction, and clamp it shut (Fig. 14–11A). Insert the nasogastric plug or cap on the connecting tubing or clamp it shut.

8. The clamp and cap prevent spillage of either tube-feeding solution or gastric contents.

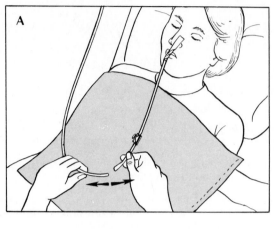

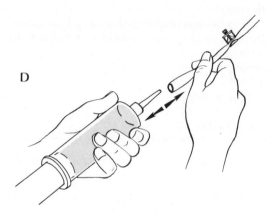

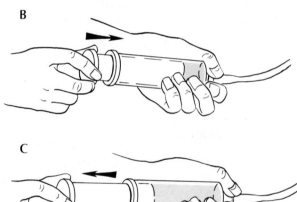

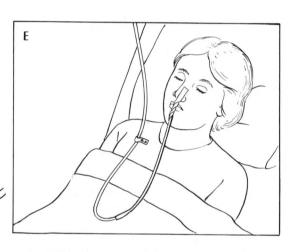

▼**FIGURE 14–11.** Irrigating a nasogastric tube.

9. Pour saline for the irrigation into a basin, draw up 30 ml of saline into a syringe, unplug the tube, insert syringe into nasogastric tube, and inject it slowly into the nasogastric tube (Fig. 14–11B).

9. The saline should flush the tube so that it becomes patent.

10. Withdraw the irrigating solution by pulling back on the syringe plunger (Fig. 14–11C).

10. Assesses the patency of the tube.

NOTE: Only inject the saline through the large port of a double-lumen tube. Only air should be injected through the pigtail of a double-lumen tube.

The tube does not function properly if the irrigant is instilled through the pigtail.

NOTE: If frank resistance is met, do not force the irrigant through the tube. Ascertain whether the tube is kinked.

Use of force can cause trauma to the mucosa. If the tube is kinked, the irrigant will not go through the tube.

▼ *ACTION*	▼ *RATIONALE*
11. Continue to instill and withdraw fluid several times until fluid flows freely.	**11.** Keep up with the total amount of fluid instilled because this total should be subtracted from the total gastric output.
12. Clamp the nasogastric tube and disconnect the syringe (Fig. 14–11*D*).	**12.** Prevents the spillage of gastric contents.
13. Reconnect the tube to the suction or feeding tube and release the clamp (Fig. 14–11*E*).	**13.** Restores the equipment to its original function and maintains a closed system.
14. Properly dispose of the equipment.	**14.** Decreases the transmission of microorganisms.
15. Remove the gloves and wash your hands.	**15.** Decreases the transmission of microorganisms.
16. Record the procedure. Note the position of the client, the tube placement check, and the patency of the tube following the irrigation.	**16.** Communicates the findings to the other members of the health care team and contributes to the legal record by documenting the care given to the client.

Example of Documentation

DATE	TIME	NOTES
11/15/93	0900	Nasogastric tube sluggishly removing contents via suction. Placement checked and tube irrigated with 60 ml of saline. Suction functioning well.
		R. Reed, RN

Teaching Tips

Explain the procedure and the purpose of the irrigation to the client or the client's family. Ask the client to tell you if he or she feels that the tube is not functioning properly.

Home Care Variations

If irrigations are to be performed at home, check the family member's knowledge of the irrigation procedure.

SKILL 14–10 PROVIDING SITE CARE FOR A GASTROSTOMY TUBE, PERCUTANEOUS ENDOSCOPIC GASTROSTOMY TUBE, OR JEJUNOSTOMY TUBE

Clinical Situations in Which You May Encounter This Skill

A gastrostomy is a surgically created temporary or permanent stoma that allows tube feedings to be introduced directly into the stomach by way of a gastrostomy tube.

A percutaneous endoscopic gastrostomy (PEG) tube is one of the latest techniques for placement of a feeding gastrostomy tube. It is a nonsurgical procedure in which a tract is created between the stomach and the skin of the upper abdominal wall and a catheter is inserted via endoscopy.

A jejunostomy is a surgically created stoma that allows tube feedings to bypass the stomach and be placed directly into the jejunum. Jejunal feedings result in a higher incidence of dumping syndrome and diarrhea and make adequate nutrition more difficult to ensure than with gastrostomy or PEG tube feedings.

Gastric or jejunal feeding tubes (Fig. 14–12) may be inserted in clients who have an impairment of deglutition, dysphagia from a tumor, chronic aspiration, or an altered level of consciousness or who require long-term alimentation. There are few complications from these tubes. The most common complication is wound infection. Others may include leakage around the tube, skin redness and irritation, an ileus, the tube being pulled out, or the tube becoming blocked. Leakage around the tube can occur because of improper positioning of the client during tube feeding or because of tube-feeding solution being infused too rapidly. Tube migration, gastric leakage, or an allergic reaction to a cleansing agent can lead to skin redness and irritation. The most common causes for the tube becoming blocked are inadequate flushing of the tube and the administration of medications through the tube. Ideally only liquid medications should be administered through the tube. If tablet medications are used, they should be crushed well and mixed with water.

The procedure for administering tube-feeding solution through the gastric or jejunal tube is the same as that for administering tube-feeding solution through a nasogastric or flexible feeding tube. The feeding may be given continuously or intermittently (see Skill 14–8).

Anticipated Responses

▼ The client's skin around the insertion site is in good condition without signs of irritation or infection.
▼ There is no leakage of tube-feeding solution or gastric secretions from the insertion site.
▼ The tube-feeding solution infuses easily.

Adverse Responses

▼ The tube is occluded.
▼ There are signs of irritation or infection at the insertion site.
▼ No bowel sounds are present.
▼ The tube has migrated outward or inward.

Materials List

Gather these materials before beginning the skill:

▼ Stethoscope
▼ Hydrogen peroxide
▼ 4- × 4-inch gauze pads
▼ Gloves
▼ Drain sponges (a 4 × 4 can be cut if a drain sponge is not available)
▼ Tape
▼ Washcloth
▼ Towel
▼ Bath basin containing warm water
▼ Antimicrobial soap

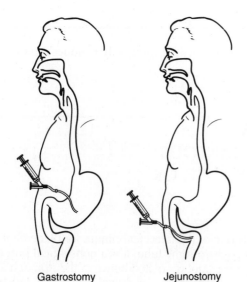

Gastrostomy   Jejunostomy

▼ FIGURE 14–12. Gastrostomy and jejunostomy sites.

▼ *A C T I O N* _____ | ▼ *R A T I O N A L E* _____

1. Assess the client's abdomen for the presence of bowel sounds.

   1. Decreased or absent bowel sounds are indicative of an ileus.

2. Put on gloves and remove the dressing (if present).

   2. Gloves prevent transmission of microorganisms.

3. Inspect the skin around the insertion site for redness, swelling, irritation, purulent drainage, or gastric leakage.

   3. Infection at the insertion site is the most common complication. Gastric leakage can cause skin irritation.

4. Inspect the tube for migration in or out. (A mark is usually made on the tube with an indelible marker at the point of exit either at the time of insertion or when the client returns to the floor.)

   4. Migration of the tube outward can cause leakage of gastric secretions. Migration of the tube inward can cause gastric outlet obstruction.

5. Cleanse the skin around the tube with peroxide using a spiral motion.

   5. Decreases the chance of infection at the insertion site.

6. Cleanse the skin around the tube with an antimicrobial soap using a spiral motion.

   6. Decreases the chance of infection at the insertion site.

7. Rinse the skin well and pat the area dry.

   7. Soap residue can irritate the skin. Rubbing the skin dry can cause irritation.

8. Apply a new dressing to the tube site (if needed) (Fig. 14–13).

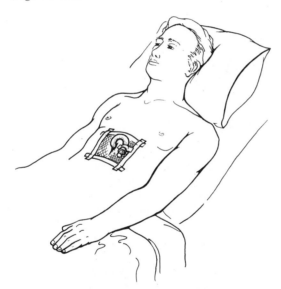

▼ **FIGURE 14–13.** Applying a new dressing to the tube site.

9. Record the procedure. Note the presence or absence of bowel sounds, the condition of the skin around the tube, whether or not the tube has migrated in or out, and the presence or absence of gastric leakage.

   9. Communicates the findings to the other members of the health care team and contributes to the legal record by documenting the care given to the client.

Example of Documentation

DATE	TIME	NOTES
6/18/93	0915	Skin around PEG tube cleansed with hydrogen peroxide and soap. No signs of irritation, infection, tube migration, or gastric leakage.
		J. Smith, RN

Teaching Tips

The purpose of the tube should be explained to the client and his or her family and they should be taught how to assess the skin, how to cleanse the skin, the signs and symptoms to report of either skin infection or tube malfunction, and how to administer tube feedings. Both skin care and tube feeding should be demonstrated for the client or the client's family.

Emphasize to the family the importance of checking the residual before each feeding if intermittent feedings are being done or every 4 hours for continuous feedings. If the residual is greater than 50% of the previous hour's intake, the tube feeding should be delayed for 1 hour and the residual should be rechecked. If a consistently high residual is observed, the physician should be notified. The feeding rate or schedule may need to be altered.

Time should be allowed for a return demonstration by the client or the client's family. Return demonstrations allow time for further questions to be answered and any additional teaching to be done.

Home Care Variations

Skin care should be provided in the client's home. Peroxide and an antimicrobial soap are usually used for cleansing for the first 3 weeks after insertion. Then, soap and water can be used for cleansing.

SKILL 14–11   ASSISTING WITH INSERTION OF A CENTRAL VENOUS CATHETER FOR ADMINISTRATION OF TOTAL PARENTERAL NUTRITION

Clinical Situations in Which You May Encounter This Skill

Total parenteral nutrition (TPN) is a form of nutritional support that is intended to supply complete nutrient requirements. TPN involves the administration of a hypertonic solution of calories, protein, fluid, electrolytes, vitamins, and trace elements through a central venous line. The central venous line is placed into the superior vena cava via the jugular or subclavian vein (Fig. 14–14).

TPN is indicated for clients who cannot tolerate oral or tube feedings, refuse oral feedings, should not be fed, or who are malnourished and unable to

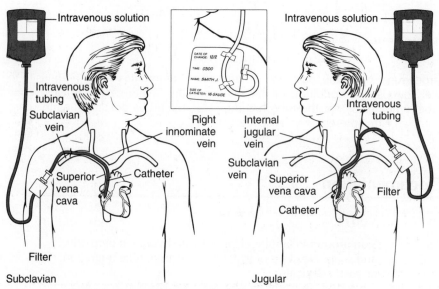

▼ **FIGURE 14–14.** Jugular and subclavian venous line placement.

consume enough calories to maintain an appropriate nutritional status and normal nitrogen balance. These clients may have severe burns, ulcerative colitis, an enteric fistula, metastatic cancer, a paralytic ileus, or anorexia nervosa.

When a central venous line is inserted, a pneumothorax can result if the catheter penetrates the pleural lining of the lungs. This adverse response is most common following subclavian vein insertion. X-rays should be made following insertion to verify correct placement of the catheter. If pneumothorax is suspected, the client will exhibit labored breathing and chest pain. Abnormal breath sounds will be heard upon auscultation.

The client may develop metabolic complications from TPN. These complications include hyperglycemia, osmotic diuresis, and hyperosmolar nonketotic coma. Most complications can be prevented or quickly averted by close monitoring of laboratory values such as glucose (blood and urine), electrolytes, blood urea nitrogen, protein, and urinalysis.

Table 14–1 outlines nursing measures to prevent complications of TPN.

Anticipated Responses

▼ The client receives the parenteral nutrition and maintains the appropriate weight and anabolic state through a positive nitrogen balance.

Adverse Responses

▼ The client develops a pneumothorax, sepsis, air embolus, thrombophlebitis, or osmotic diuresis.
▼ The client develops a metabolic complication such as hyperglycemia.

Materials List

Gather these materials before beginning the skill:

For insertion of a central venous line:
▼ Masks (for you and the physician)
▼ Sterile gloves
▼ Sterile gown (for the physician)
▼ Sterile drape or sterile towels
▼ Antiseptic solution
▼ Swabs (1 package sterile)
▼ Sterile 4- × 4-inch gauze strips (6 packages)
▼ Tape
▼ Skin anesthetic (lidocaine)
▼ Sterile 3-ml syringe with 25-gauge needle
▼ Sterile 10-ml syringe
▼ Bag or bottle of D_5W or normal saline
▼ IV administration set
▼ Two sterile intravenous (subclavian) catheters with stylets (one is extra in case of contamination of the first catheter)
▼ Suture kit
▼ Transparent occlusive dressing or 4 × 4 gauze and Elastoplast tape
▼ Tincture of benzoin

For administration of TPN:
▼ 1,000-ml bag of TPN
▼ IV administration set (macrodrip)
▼ Extension tubing
▼ Filter
▼ Infusion pump
▼ Skin preparation kit (optional): Excessive hair should be removed to prepare the skin and remove the tape)

TABLE 14–1. Nursing Measures to Prevent Complications of Total Parenteral Nutrition (TPN) Administration

Possible Complication	Nursing Actions	Possible Complication	Nursing Actions
Infection	• Use sterile technique when inserting an intravenous (IV) catheter. • Use sterile technique for dressing, tubing, and IV solution changes. • Do not allow TPN solution to hang more than 24 hours. • Do not administer medications or other IV fluids in the TPN IV line.	Dehydration due to osmotic diuresis	• Maintain a proper rate of infusion by using an infusion control device. • Monitor intake and output. • Monitor daily weights. • Assess for signs and symptoms of dehydration.
Pneumothorax	• Teach the client to perform Valsalva's maneuver during insertion of the catheter. • Place the client in Trendelenburg's position during insertion to dilate the vein. • Obtain a chest x-ray film after insertion is completed.	Blood glucose changes	• Begin TPN infusions slowly and gradually increase the rate to the ordered rate of infusion. • Administer insulin as ordered to control the client's blood glucose. • Do not suddenly discontinue TPN as this may cause hypoglycemia. • Maintain a steady infusion rate. • Monitor the client's blood glucose at least every 6 hours by finger stick.
Air embolism	• Take precautions to prevent air from entering the IV tubing, especially during tubing changes. • If air bubbles are seen in the IV tubing, use a sterile syringe to withdraw them before they are infused into the circulatory system.		

▼ *A C T I O N*   ▼ *R A T I O N A L E*

1. Assess the client's nutritional and hydration status by obtaining his or her weight and observing the skin turgor, mucous membranes, and intake and output record. Assessment of output also should include GI suction, emesis, stools, urine, and wound. For dehydration, assess for a depressed periorbital area, decreased urine output, diarrhea, emesis, diaphoresis, and dry skin. For fluid excess, assess for ascites, peripheral edema, edematous periorbital areas, sudden weight gain, and moist rales in the chest.

1. Provides a baseline for future comparison.

2. Assess the client's ability to hold his or her breath and tolerate Trendelenburg's position.

2. The client is asked to hold his or her breath as the catheter is inserted into the subclavian vein. Trendelenburg's position is used to increase dilatation of the veins and slightly increase positive pressure in the central veins, thus reducing the risk of an air embolus.

3. Prepare a 250-ml bottle or bag of D_5W by:
   a. Inserting the spiked end of the IV tubing into the bag or bottle;
   b. Hanging the bag of IV fluids on the IV pole;
   c. Opening the roller clamp and allowing the fluid to flow through the tubing; and
   d. Closing the roller clamp and replacing the plastic cap on the end of the tubing.

3. Fluid should be prepared and ready to attach to the central venous line as soon as it is inserted to prevent occlusion of the line.
   b. Fluid flows by gravity.

4. Prepare the TPN infusion by:
   a. Inserting the spiked end of the IV tubing into the bottle or bag of TPN fluids;

   b. Attaching the infusion tubing to the pump administration set;
   c. Placing the pump administration set in an IV pump according to the manufacturer's directions;
   d. Attaching the tubing from the pump to the filter and extension tubing;

   e. Priming the tubing and pump with TPN fluids; and
   f. Closing the clamp on the tubing and replacing the protective cap on the end of the IV and fluids.

   a. TPN should be ready to connect to the central venous line as soon as correct placement has been determined.
   b. Fluid flows from the bottle into the pump.
   c. The pump tubing is inserted differently for different brands of pumps.
   d. Fluid flows from the pump through the filter and extension tubing to the client. Extension tubing provides for greater client mobility.
   e. Removes air from the tubing and prevents an air embolus.
   f. Prevents contamination of the tubing and fluids.

5. Take and record the client's vital signs.

5. Provides baseline data for later comparison.

6. Place the client in Trendelenburg's position. If this position cannot be tolerated, place the client in the supine position.

6. Facilitates insertion of the catheter.

7. a. For subclavian insertion, place a rolled bath blanket under the client's shoulders.
   b. For jugular insertion, place a rolled bath blanket under one of the client's shoulders (opposite from the insertion site).

7. a. Increases venous distention.

   b. Extends the client's neck and increases visibility of the jugular veins.

8. Turn the client's head away from the insertion site.

8. Extends the client's neck for increased visibility of the insertion site and reduces the transmission of microorganisms from the client's respiratory tract.

▼ _ACTION_ _ _ _ _ _ _ _ _ _ _ _ _ _ _ _ _ _ _

▼ _RATIONALE_ _ _ _ _ _ _ _ _ _ _ _ _ _ _

9. Shave the client's neck or clavicle area if excessive hair is present.

9. Reduces microorganisms and reduces discomfort when the tape is removed.

10. Don a mask and sterile gloves.

10. Decreases the transmission of microorganisms.

11. Using a swab, cleanse the client's skin with antiseptic solution using a circular motion from the innermost part of the circle to the outermost part.

11. Reduces the number of microorganisms on the skin. A circular motion prevents recontamination of the site with microorganisms.

12. Remove the gloves and discard them in a waste receptacle.

12. Decreases the transmission of microorganisms.

13. Open a package of sterile gloves for the physician without contaminating them.

13. This is a sterile procedure.

14. After the physician dons the gloves, open the package of sterile towels or a sterile drape for the physician to drape the client.

14. The physician cannot touch nonsterile objects with sterile gloves.

15. Open a sterile 3-ml syringe for the physician.

15. This will be used to administer the local anesthetic.

16. Swab the rubber stopper on the local anesthetic with alcohol.

16. Removes microorganisms.

17. Invert the bottle and hold it firmly as the physician withdraws the anesthetic.

17. Holding the bottle in this position allows the physician to withdraw the anesthetic and maintain sterility of the gloves.

18. As the physician injects the local anesthetic, open the packages containing the catheter and the 10-ml syringe. The physician will insert the catheter.

19. Explain to the client what the physician is doing.

19. Simple explanations help to reduce apprehension and anxiety.

20. As the physician removes the stylet from the catheter, have the client perform Valsalva's maneuver (the client should hold his or her breath and bear down as though having a bowel movement).

20. The Valsalva maneuver increases intrathoracic pressure and prevents air from entering the IV tubing as it is connected to the catheter.

21. Quickly connect an IV line of D₅W to the central venous line.

21. Maintains a flow of fluid through the line and prevents occlusion.

22. Open a suture kit for the physician.

22. The catheter usually is sutured into place to avoid displacement or accidental removal.

23. After the physician sutures the catheter to the client's skin, apply a sterile dressing to the insertion site by:
    a. Donning sterile gloves.

    b. Asking the client to abduct his or her arm and turn his or her head away from the insertion site.
    c. Applying tincture of benzoin to the surrounding skin and allowing the area to air-dry (about 1 min).
    d. Looping the tubing and applying the dressing directly on top.

23. The dressing serves as a barrier to microorganisms.

    a. Decreases the transmission of microorganisms.
    b. This movement stretches the skin so that movement is possible after the dressing is applied.
    c. Tincture of benzoin protects the skin and promotes the adhesion of the tape to the skin.

    d. Looping the tubing assists in preventing a direct pull on the tubing at the insertion site.

24. Remove the gloves and discard them in a receptacle.

24. Decreases the transmission of microorganisms.

25. Prepare the client for x-ray confirmation of the placement of the catheter.

25. Most institutions require x-ray confirmation of placement before starting the TPN.

▼ *ACTION*	▼ *RATIONALE*
26. Complete the label to be applied to the dressing with your name, as well as the date and time and the size of the catheter.	**26.** Provides information that other nurses will need to plan the next dressing change.
27. Disconnect the D_5W and connect the TPN.	**27.** After x-ray confirmation of the placement of the central venous line, the TPN can be hung and the D_5W can be discontinued.
28. Set the rate on the infusion device for the TPN.	**28.** The device should deliver the TPN at the rate set.
29. Record the procedure. Note the date, time of insertion, size and location of the catheter, and the type of fluids infusing.	**29.** Communicates to the other members of the health care team and contributes to the legal record by documenting the care given to the client.
30. Evaluate the client for signs of air emboli, pneumothorax, sepsis, and hyperglycemia.	**30.** Dyspnea, tachycardia, apprehension, cough, hypotension, chest pain, temperature, chills, nausea, vomiting, and general malaise may indicate air emboli, pneumothorax, or sepsis. Hyperglycemia may be detected by evaluating the client's urine for sugar or by testing the client's blood sugar with a chemical reagent strip.
31. As the TPN is infusing, monitor it to ensure that the solution does not run dry. If this occurs, hang a bag of $D_{10}W$ until another bag of TPN can be hung.	**31.** The TPN contains concentrated sugars, and the client's pancreas is excreting insulin to maintain a normal glucose level. If the TPN is stopped abruptly, the client can experience sudden hypoglycemia.
32. Check the hospital policy for tubing changes with TPN.	**32.** Policies differ for tubing changes, from each time a new bag is hung to every 24 hours.

Example of Documentation

DATE	TIME	NOTES
10/30/93	1300	Central venous line inserted into left clavicle area per Dr. Jones. Sutured in place with 4.0 nylon. Sterile dressing applied and 250 ml D_5W infusing at 100 ml per hour per infusion pump.
		S. Williams, RN
	1330	Catheter placement checked per x-ray. 1,000 ml TPN infusing at 175 ml per hour. Vital signs stable.
		S. Williams, RN

Teaching Tips

Ensure that the client understands the importance of sterile technique during the insertion of the catheter and the importance of maintaining an intact dressing.

Home Care Variations

The client or family member must be taught how to change a sterile dressing and how to administer and maintain TPN fluids. Teach the client to check his or her urine for sugar and acetone and to report abnormalities immediately. The client should weigh himself or herself daily at the same time in the same clothes. Stress to the client that a weight gain of more than 0.5 kg (1.1 lb) per day may indicate excessive fluid intake and should be reported.

SKILL 14–12 PROVIDING SITE CARE FOR A CENTRAL VENOUS CATHETER

Clinical Situations in Which You May Encounter This Skill

Site care should be performed every 24 to 48 hours (depending on hospital policy) for a client who has a central venous catheter in place. More frequent dressing changes are necessary if the dressing becomes soiled or wet.

Anticipated Responses

▼ The dressing is changed using sterile technique.
▼ There is no evidence of infection or inflammation.

Adverse Responses

▼ The site has signs of infection or inflammation.

Materials List

Gather these materials before beginning the skill:

▼ Sterile gloves (2)
▼ Antiseptic solution (10% acetone and betadine solution)
▼ Betadine ointment
▼ Sterile cotton swabs (1 package)
▼ 4- × 4-inch gauze (precut), or 4- × 4-inch gauze and sterile scissors to cut the gauze, or transparent occlusive dressing, or 4- × 4-inch gauze and tape
▼ Tincture of benzoin
▼ Tape
▼ Paper bag for soiled dressing

▼ *A C T I O N*	▼ *R A T I O N A L E*
1. Review the client's chart for the date of the catheter insertion and the last dressing change, and the condition of the site at the last dressing change or time of insertion.	1. Provides a basis from which to make comparisons.
2. Help the client to assume supine or semi-Fowler's position.	2. Facilitates changing of the dressing.
3. Ask the client to turn with his or her face away from the insertion site. (Check your agency policy. Some hospitals require that the client also wear a mask.)	3. Reduces the transmission of microorganisms from the client's upper respiratory tract to the catheter insertion site.
4. Open the sterile supplies on a clean overbed table. (See Skill 1–9.)	4. The sterile field should be set up prior to beginning the procedure. Once you have put on sterile gloves, nonsterile items cannot be touched.
5. Remove the dressing from the insertion site and put it in the paper bag.	5. Decreases the transmission of microorganisms.
6. Assess the insertion site for signs of infection, such as redness, tenderness, or swelling.	6. Direct visibility of the area is possible when the dressing is removed.
7. Wash your hands.	7. Decreases the transmission of microorganisms.
8. Don sterile gloves.	8. Decreases the transmission of microorganisms to the insertion site.
9. Cleanse the skin around the insertion site by: a. Holding the tubing in one hand up off the client's skin.	a. Prevents recontamination from the catheter.

▼ *ACTION*

▼ *RATIONALE*

b. Using sterile 4- × 4-inch gauze pads soaked in Betadine, cleanse the skin in a circular motion moving from the innermost circle (next to the insertion site) to the outermost part of the circle (Fig. 14–15). Discard the 4- × 4-inch gauze pads after each circular movement on the client's skin.

b. Using an outward motion prevents reintroduction of microorganisms onto the site that was previously cleansed.

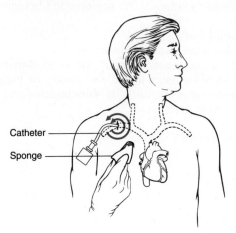

Catheter

Sponge

▼ **FIGURE 14–15.** Cleansing the skin around the catheter insertion site.

NOTE: Take care not to pull the catheter from the insertion site.

---

c. Using sterile 4- × 4-inch pads soaked in acetone, cleanse the skin in a circular motion, moving from the innermost area to the outermost area.

c. The acetone cleanses and defats the skin, removes tape, and destroys the cell walls of bacteria.

10. Cleanse the proximal tubing:
   a. Use a 4- × 4-inch pad with Betadine solution and clean the catheter from the insertion site in a circular motion to the outer distal port.
   b. Allow the Betadine solution to remain on the catheter until it air-dries or at least 30 seconds.

a. Decreases the transmission of microorganisms from the catheter to the client.

b. Decreases the transmission of microorganisms from the catheter to the client.

11. Apply Betadine ointment to the site with a cotton swab.

11. Betadine ointment assists in decreasing microorganisms at the insertion site.

12. Examine the tubing connections and ensure that all connections are secured.

12. Connections can become loose with turning and manipulation.

13. Remove your gloves.

13. Gloves used for cleansing the site and tubing are considered contaminated.

14. Don a new pair of sterile gloves.

14. Decreases the transmission of microorganisms.

15. Apply a sterile occlusive dressing (4- × 4-inch pads with Elastoplast or transparent dressing) by:

15. The sterile dressing protects the insertion site and surrounding skin from contamination with airborne microorganisms.

▼ *ACTION* _____ | ▼ *RATIONALE* _____

a. Asking the client to abduct his or her arm and turn his or her head away from the insertion site

b. Applying tincture of benzoin to the surrounding skin and allowing the area to air-dry (about 1 min).

c. Looping the tubing and applying the dressing directly over the tubing.

16. Remove the gloves and discard them in a receptacle.

17. Label the dressing with your name, the date and time of the dressing change, and the gauge of the needle (see Fig. 14–14).

18. Record the procedure. Note the date and time and the description of the site.

a. This movement will stretch the skin so that movement is possible after the dressing is applied.

b. Tincture of benzoin protects the skin and promotes adhesion of the tape to the skin.

c. Looping the tubing assists in preventing a direct pull on the tubing at the insertion site.

16. Decreases the transmission of microorganisms.

17. Provides information necessary to plan the next site care.

18. Communicates to the other members of the health care team and contributes to the legal record by documenting the care given to the client.

Example of Documentation

DATE	TIME	NOTES
11/30/89	1300	Site care and dressing change of central venous catheter using sterile technique. Site slightly red—no swelling or temperature change in skin noted. TPN running at 150 ml per hour.
		S. Williams, RN

Teaching Tips

Dressing changes provide an opportunity to teach the client about infection and the importance of sterile technique during dressing changes. Teach the client to report any signs of infection immediately.

Home Care Variations

To change a dressing in the client's home, follow the same procedure as described above. Dispose of the soiled materials in a plastic bag or other nonpenetrable bag.

Teach the client the adverse signs and symptoms of infection, thrombosis, air embolism, and displacement. These should be reported immediately. For infection, the client must report fever; chills; redness, drainage, swelling, pain, or tenderness at the site; tachypnea; and diaphoresis. The home health nurse also should monitor the client's blood work for an elevated leukocyte count, hypotension, or shock in severe cases.

For symptoms of thrombosis, the client should report edema of the arm or catheter insertion site, neck pain, and jugular vein distention. Symptoms of an air embolus should be taught to another person in the client's home. These symptoms include confusion, pallor, lightheadedness, tachycardia, tachypnea, hypotension, anxiety, and unresponsiveness.

The client should be taught to observe the site during dressing changes for displacement. Leaking of fluid from the insertion site or pain or discomfort as the fluids are infused may indicate displacement of the catheter; this must be reported immediately.

References

Auervach, K. G. (1990). Sequential and simultaneous breast pumping: A comparison. *International Journal of Nursing Study*, 27 (3), 257–265.

Beckstrand, J., et al. (1990). The distance to the stomach for feeding-tube placement in children predicted from regression on height. *Research in Nursing and Health*, 13, 411–420.

Boortz, M. E. (1994). Administering intravenous therapy. In V. Bolander (Ed.), *Basic nursing* (3rd ed.). Philadelphia: W. B. Saunders.

Crocker, K. S., et al. (1986). Microbial growth in clinically used enteral delivery systems. *American Journal of Infection Control*, 14, 255–256.

Eisenberg, P., Metheny, N., and McSweeny, M. (1989). Nasoenteral feeding-tube properties and the ability to withdraw fluid via syringe. *Applied Nursing Research*, 2 (4), 168–172.

Kearney, M. H., Cronenwett, L. R., and Barrett, J. A. (1990). Breast-feeding problems in the first week of postpartum. *Nursing Research*, 39 (2), 90–95.

Kotodny, V., and Malek, A. M. (1991). Improving feeding skills. *Journal of Gerontological Nursing*, 17 (6), 20–24.

Lindenberg, C. S., Artola, R. C., and Jimenez, V. (1990). The effect of early postpartum mother-infant contact and breastfeeding promotion on the incidence and continuation of breastfeeding. *International Journal of Nursing Studies*, 27 (1), 179–186.

Metheny, N. A., Eisenberg, P., and McSweeney, M. (1988). Effect of feeding-tube properties and three irrigants on clogging rates. *Nursing Research*, 37, 165–169.

Metheny, N. A., et al. (1990). Effectiveness of the auscultatory method in predicting feeding-tube location. *Nursing Research*, 39, 262–267.

Metheny, N. A., Spies, M., and Eisenberg, P. (1988). Measures to test placement of nasoenteral feeding tubes. *Western Journal of Nursing Research*, 10, 367–383.

Metheny, N. A., Spies, M., and Eisenberg, P. (1986). Frequency of nasoenteral tube displacement and associated risk factors. *Research in Nursing and Health*, 9, 241–247.

Mickschl, D. B., et al. (1990). Contamination of enteral feedings and diarrhea in patients in intensive care units. *Heart and Lung*, 19, 362–370.

Petrosino, B. M., Meraviglia, M., and Becker, H. (1987). Mechanical problems with small-diameter enteral feeding tubes. *Journal of Neuroscience Nursing*, 19, 276–280.

Worthington-Roberts, B. S., and Koester, P. W. (1994). Meeting nutritional needs. In V. Bolander (Ed.), *Basic nursing* (3rd ed.). Philadelphia: W. B. Saunders.

CHAPTER 15

Meeting Bowel Elimination Needs

Assistance with elimination needs is indicated whenever a client experiences an alteration in his or her normal elimination pattern. Common alterations in elimination include constipation, fecal impaction, excessive flatulence, diarrhea, and the presence of an ostomy. In addition to providing assistance in resolving these elimination problems, you should teach the client how to maintain healthy bowel function. A diet high in fiber, adequate intake of liquids, regular exercise, and timely responsiveness to the urge to defecate should be stressed as important factors that promote normal elimination.

OVERVIEW OF RELATED RESEARCH

OSTOMY

Coe, M., and Kluka, S. (1988). Concerns of clients and spouses regarding ostomy surgery for cancer. *Journal of Enterostomal Therapy, 15,* 232–239.

Data were collected by interviewing 20 clients and their spouses to determine their concerns. Nine categories of concerns were identified. They were acceptance, adaptation, body image, cancer, equipment, family, need for information, pain, and the surgical procedure. Forty-eight different concerns were identified. An example of the concerns included wanting to be involved in the learning, being able to resume sex, feeling alone, odor, change in body appearance, and paying for medical supplies.

Gloeckner, M. R. (1984). Perceptions of sexual attractiveness following ostomy surgery. *Research in Nursing and Health, 7* (2), 87–92.

Gloeckner's study investigated the effect of ostomy surgery on clients' (n = 40) sexual attractiveness. Data were collected by a tape-recorded interview in the subjects' homes. No difference according to type of ostomy was found. Significant

differences were found in sexual attractiveness before surgery, 1 year after surgery, and at the time of the interview. Clients who had management problems with their ostomy viewed themselves as less attractive than clients who did not experience management problems.

Hedrick, J. K. (1987). Effects of ET nursing intervention on adjustment following ostomy surgery. *Journal of Enterostomal Therapy, 14* (6), 229–239.

A study was done by Hedrick to determine the effects of nursing intervention by enterostomal therapists (ETs) on the client's adjustment following ostomy surgery. Data were collected from 40 clients, 20 of whom received nursing intervention from an ET while hospitalized and 20 of whom did not receive nursing intervention from an ET. The clients had either a permanent colostomy, ileostomy, or ileal conduit. Adjustment was measured by using the Maklebust Ostomy Adjustment Scale. A significant difference in the two groups was reported, which indicated increased client adjustment for clients who received nursing interventions from an ET.

Kelman, G., and Minkler, P. (1989). An investigation of quality of life and self-esteem among individuals with ostomies. *Journal of Enterostomal Therapy, 16* (1), 4–11.

The purpose of the study was to examine the relationship between quality of life and self-esteem in individuals (n = 50) with ostomies. Quality of life was measured by Padilla and Grant's Quality of Life Index and self-esteem was measured by Rosenberg's Self-Esteem Scale. A significant relationship was found between quality of life and self-esteem. Overall, the subjects had a positive self-esteem and viewed their quality of life as good.

Kobza, L. (1983). Impact of ostomy upon the spouse. *Journal of Enterostomal Therapy, 10* (2), 54–57.

Kobza conducted a descriptive study to determine the needs of the spouses of ostomy clients (n = 20). Data were collected using a semistructured interview. Needs expressed by the spouses related to information, support, and being needed.

SKILL 15–1 ADMINISTERING AN ENEMA

Clinical Situations in Which You May Encounter This Skill

An enema may be administered to relieve constipation and intestinal flatus, stimulate defecation, and prepare the bowel for surgery or diagnostic tests. There are three types of enemas: cleansing, oil-retention, and return-flow. The cleansing enema is used to treat constipation, facilitate removal of a fecal impaction, or empty the bowel for diagnostic procedures or surgery. An oil-retention enema is usually administered to lubricate or soften the feces and promote expulsion. The third kind of enema, the return-flow (Harris flush), is administered to relieve gaseous distention.

Enema solutions may be hypotonic, isotonic, or hypertonic. The most common hypotonic solution is tap water, whereas the most common isotonic solution is physiologic saline. Large amounts (750–1,000 ml) are instilled when administering a hypotonic or an isotonic enema.

Fluid and electrolyte disturbances may occur as a result of enema administration. Infants or people with cardiac or kidney disease are especially prone to fluid

imbalance. When a hypotonic solution is used, fluid flows out of the bowel into the surrounding tissue because there is less osmotic pressure in the solution than in the interstitial tissues. Repeated hypotonic enemas can result in hypokalemia and water intoxication. Symptoms of water intoxication include dizziness, sweating, pallor, and difficulty in breathing. A hypertonic solution causes water to be drawn from the cells and into the colon. Dehydration may occur from the shift of fluid into the colon.

If the solution is instilled too rapidly or is too hot, the client may complain of abdominal cramping from the increased stimulation of reflex peristalsis. The enema will not be retained and will not produce the anticipated results.

Other adverse effects can occur as a result of vagus nerve stimulation. The vagus nerve is part of the parasympathetic nervous system that innervates the gastrointestinal tract and major organs such as the heart. Manipulation of the rectal area and distention of the bowel from the enema solution stimulate the vagus nerve and may initiate a parasympathetic response such as myocardial infarction, cardiac dysrhythmia, or a decreased pulse rate. Clients with cardiac disease are particularly at risk. Therefore, administer enemas cautiously to clients with cardiac problems.

If the enema tubing is not inserted carefully or the fluid is instilled under high pressure, perforation of the bowel wall is possible. Thus, the tubing should never be forced during insertion.

Anticipated Responses

▼ Bulk stool, usually dark brown in color, is evacuated from the client's colon.
▼ The fluid from the enema irrigation is returned.

Adverse Responses

▼ Stool is not evacuated from the client's colon.
▼ The client complains of abdominal cramping.
▼ The enema solution is not returned.
▼ The client's pulse rate decreases or cardiac dysrhythmias occur, or both.
▼ The client's bowel wall is perforated or there is trauma to the tissue.

▼ The client experiences symptoms of fluid or electrolyte imbalances.
▼ The client exhibits signs of congestive heart failure or cerebral edema.

Materials List

Gather these materials before beginning the skill:

▼ Waterproof pad
▼ Bedpan
▼ Enema administration kit
▼ Enema solution
▼ Examination gloves
▼ Water-soluble lubricant (if the tubing tip is not prelubricated)
▼ Toilet tissue
▼ Towel and washcloth
▼ Bath basin with warm water
▼ IV pole
▼ Retention catheter (optional, for incontinent clients)

▼ ACTION	▼ RATIONALE
1. Ascertain the reason the enema is ordered.	1. You will need to explain to the client the purpose for the enema.
2. Review the physician's order for the type and amount of solution and the number of times the enema should be administered.	2. You may not legally complete the treatment without an order.
3. Check the diagnosis of the client's medical condition, and the client's other health problems and vital signs.	3. Alerts you to potential problems that could occur as a result of the enema administration. You should avoid giving an enema if the client has a history of ulcerative colitis or regional enteritis.
4. Warm the enema solution to 105° Fahrenheit (40.5° centigrade).	4. A solution that is too cool could cause intestinal cramping. A solution that is too hot could burn the client's intestines.
5. Check the temperature of the solution with a bath thermometer.	5. A solution that is too cool could cause intestinal cramping. A solution that is too hot could burn the client's intestines.
6. Close the clamp on the enema bag tubing and add enema solution to the bag.	6. The clamp is closed to prevent spilling of the solution.
7. Prime the tubing by opening the clamp and allowing the solution to flow through the entire length of the tubing.	7. The tubing is primed to remove the air from the tubing. Introduction of air into the intestinal tract may produce abdominal cramping.
8. Close the clamp after all of the air is removed from the tubing.	8. Prevents leakage of the solution.
9. Lubricate the end of the tubing with a water-soluble lubricant.	9. The lubricant will ease insertion and decrease rectal irritation.
10. Screen the client by closing the door and curtains around the bed.	10. Provides privacy for the client.
11. Raise the client's bed to a comfortable height.	11. Reduces the strain placed on your back.

▼ *ACTION*   ▼ *RATIONALE*

12. Place the enema solution bag on the IV pole approximately 12 to 18 inches above the client.

12. The enema fluid should flow in by gravity. Raising the container higher than 18 inches will cause the solution to flow too rapidly and could cause abdominal cramping and distention.

13. Place the client in a left Sims' position.

13. The enema solution should flow by gravity in the natural direction of the colon.

> **NOTE:** Cleansing enemas should not be administered to a client who is seated on the toilet.

> **NOTE:** The knee-chest position is recommended for administration of a hypertonic solution.   Distributes the solution throughout the colon.

14. Drape the client and place a waterproof pad under the client's hips and buttocks.

14. Draping protects the client's privacy and the pad protects the bed.

15. Put on gloves.

15. When there is a chance of coming into contact with feces, gloves should be worn to prevent the possible transmission of microorganisms.

16. Separate the client's buttocks and insert the enema tubing 2 inches (0.5–1 inch for a child) into the client's rectum with the tip pointing in the direction of the client's umbilicus (Fig. 15–1). Do not force the tube.

16. Separating the client's buttocks allows visualization of the rectal orifice. The length of the tubing to be inserted varies depending on the client's size. Forcing the tube could perforate the client's bowel wall.

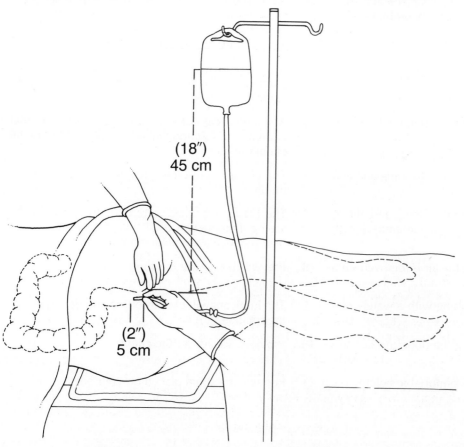

(18")
45 cm

(2")
5 cm

▼ **FIGURE 15–1.** Administering an enema.

▼ *ACTION*   ▼ *RATIONALE*

NOTE: For the incontinent client, a retention catheter can be inserted and the balloon can be inflated.

The retention catheter with the balloon prevents backflow of the enema solution.

---

17. Ask the client to breathe deeply.

17. Deep breathing facilitates insertion of the tube by promoting relaxation of the rectal sphincter.

18. Release the clamp and allow the solution to flow in slowly.

18. Infusing the solution too rapidly can cause cramping and distention.

NOTE: If the client complains of cramping, stop the flow of solution by closing the tubing clamp and instruct the client to breathe slowly through the mouth for approximately 1 minute. Gently massage the client's abdomen over the splenic and hepatic flexures. Then resume the flow of enema solution.

Breathing through the mouth will help the client to relax.

---

19. Administer the appropriate amount of solution (infants: 150–250 ml; small child (18 mo–5 yr): 250–350 ml; larger child (5–12 yr): 300–500 ml; adolescent (>12 yr): 500–750 ml; and adult: 500–750 ml).

19. The amount of solution varies with the size and age of the client.

20. Clamp the tubing and remove it from the client's rectum after the appropriate amount has infused.

20. Clamping prevents leakage of any more solution from the tube.

21. Ask the client to retain the solution for at least 5 minutes.

21. Promotes peristalsis and more complete evacuation.

22. Hold together the buttocks of an infant, small child, or anyone else who is unable to retain the solution.

22. Helps the client to retain the solution.

NOTE: For an oil-retention enema, the solution should be held for 1 hour.
NOTE: Some enemas (e.g., medicated or nutritive enemas) should never be evacuated.

---

23. Place the client in a sitting position on a bedpan or assist him or her in getting to the bathroom.

23. An upright, sitting position facilitates defecation by gravity.

24. Stay with the client and observe for syncope, decreased heart rate, and cardiac dysrhythmias.

24. Vagal stimulation can occur from distention of the bowel.

25. Instruct the client or the child's parent not to flush the toilet.

25. Observation of the results of the enema is necessary for accurate charting.

26. Observe the feces for amount, color, consistency, and odor.

26. You will need to chart the results. If the client has poor results, it may be necessary to administer additional solution.

▼ *ACTION*	▼ *RATIONALE*
27. Cleanse the client's rectal area with toilet tissue or a washcloth and warm water.	**27.** Fecal material is caustic to the skin. Washing the client's rectal area decreases skin irritation and prevents the spread of microorganisms. The client is cleansed from front to back to prevent contamination of the urinary meatus with *Escherichia coli,* the organism primarily responsible for urinary tract infections. Thorough drying prevents excoriation of the skin and discourages growth of microorganisms.
28. Properly dispose of or store the equipment.	**28.** Prevents the transmission of microorganisms.
29. Remove the gloves and wash your hands.	**29.** Decreases the transmission of microorganisms.
30. Return the client's bed to the lowest position.	**30.** Reduces the potential of injury from falls.
31. Assess the results of the enema and how well the client tolerated the procedure.	**31.** Provides data necessary for charting.
32. Record the procedure. Note the type and amount of solution administered, the amount of solution returned, and the results.	**32.** Communicates to the other members of the health care team and contributes to the legal record by documenting the care given to the client.

Example of Documentation

DATE	*TIME*	*NOTES*
10/12/93	0930	650 ml normal saline enema administered. Retained for 5 minutes. Moderate amount of soft, formed, brown stool returned.
		S. Smith, RN

Teaching Tips

The purpose of the enema should be explained to the client or the client's family member, or both. You should explain to the client that breathing through his or her mouth will help to relax the abdominal muscles as the enema tubing is inserted and the fluid is instilled.

This is a good time to discuss normal elimination patterns with the client or the client's family member. The client should be told that not all persons have a bowel movement every day and that this is normal. The client should not use enemas routinely to stimulate defecation. Enemas should be used only when the client is constipated.

If the enema is being administered because of constipation, measures to prevent constipation should be discussed. If possible, the client should increase fluid intake, bulk in the diet, and exercise.

Home Care Variations

Enemas may be administered in the client's home. A hook can be attached to the wall or the doorway to hang the enema bag. The hook should be approximately 12 to 18 inches above the level of the client's intestines. Enema equipment should be cleaned, dried, and stored for future use.

SKILL 15–2   ADMINISTERING A PREPACKAGED ENEMA

Clinical Situations in Which You May Encounter This Skill

A prepackaged enema may be administered to the client to relieve constipation and intestinal flatus and to prepare the lower colon for diagnostic examination.

Fluid and electrolyte disturbances may occur as a result of enema administration. Prepackaged enemas are hypertonic solutions. Hypertonic solutions can cause water to be withdrawn from the cells and dehydration may result.

Adverse effects also can occur as a result of vagus nerve stimulation. The vagus nerve is part of the parasympathetic nervous system that innervates the gastrointestinal tract as well as major organs such as the heart. Manipulation of the rectal area may stimulate the vagus nerve and initiate a parasympathetic response such as cardiac dysrhythmia or a decreased pulse rate.

Anticipated Responses

▼ Bulk stool, usually dark brown in color, is evacuated from the client's colon and flatus is relieved.

Adverse Responses

▼ The client is unable to defecate.
▼ The client has a decreased pulse or a cardiac dysrhythmia.

Materials List

Gather these materials before beginning the skill:

▼ Prepackaged enema
▼ Waterproof pad
▼ Bedpan or toilet
▼ Toilet tissue
▼ Water-soluble lubricant
▼ Examination gloves
▼ Bath basin with warm water
▼ Towel and washcloth

▼ ACTION	▼ RATIONALE
1. Review the physician's order for the type of enema to be given.	1. You may not legally complete the treatment without the order.
2. Check the client's medical diagnosis and the client's other health problems and vital signs.	2. Alerts you to potential problems that could occur as a result of the enema administration.
3. Screen the client by closing the door and curtains around the bed.	3. Provides privacy for the client.
4. Raise the bed to a comfortable height.	4. Reduces the strain placed on your back.
5. Place the client in a left Sims' position.	5. Facilitates the flow of the enema solution by gravity in the natural direction of the colon.
6. Put on gloves.	6. When there is a chance of coming into contact with feces, gloves should be worn to prevent the possible transmission of microorganisms.
7. Drape the client and place a waterproof pad under the client's hips and buttocks.	7. Draping protects the client's privacy and the pad protects the bed.
8. Remove the cap on the enema tip and check the tip for adequacy of lubrication.	8. Prelubricated tips may dry with the passage of time.
9. If necessary, add additional water-soluble lubricant.	9. Lessens irritation to the client's rectal tissues and eases insertion.
10. Expel excess air by gently squeezing the container.	10. Air leads to distention without any therapeutic effect.

▼ *ACTION*   ▼ *RATIONALE*

11. Separate the client's buttocks and insert the enema tip 1 to 2 inches (Fig. 15–2).

11. Inserting the tip toward the client's umbilicus decreases the chance of scraping the client's rectal wall.

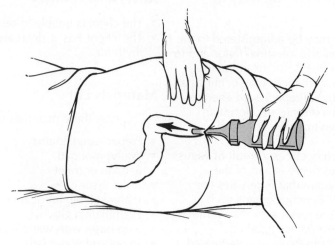

▼ **FIGURE 15–2.** Administering a prepackaged enema.

12. Squeeze and roll the enema container toward the client's rectum until all of the solution is administered.

12. Rolling the container dispenses the solution into the intestines.

13. Remove the container and ask the client to retain the solution for 5 to 10 minutes.

13. Promotes peristalsis and more complete evacuation.

14. Hold together the buttocks of an infant, small child, or anyone else who is unable to retain the solution.

14. Facilitates retention of the enema solution.

15. Place the client in a sitting position on a bedpan or assist him or her in getting to the bathroom.

15. An upright, sitting position facilitates defecation by gravity.

16. Stay with the client and observe for syncope, decreased heart rate, and cardiac dysrhythmias.

16. Vagal stimulation can occur from distention of the bowel.

17. Instruct the client or the child's parent not to flush the toilet.

17. Observation of the feces is necessary for accurate charting.

18. Observe the results. Note the amount, color, consistency, and odor of the stool.

18. Record the results in the client's chart. If the client has poor results, it may be necessary to administer a different type of enema.

19. Cleanse the client's rectal area from front to back with toilet tissue or a washcloth and warm water.

19. Fecal material is caustic to the skin. Washing the client's rectal area decreases skin irritation and prevents the spread of microorganisms. The client is cleansed from front to back to prevent contamination of the urinary meatus.

20. Properly dispose of the equipment.

20. Prevents the transmission of microorganisms.

21. Remove the gloves and wash your hands.

21. Decreases the transmission of microorganisms.

22. Return the client's bed to the lowest position.

22. Reduces the potential of injury from falls.

23. Assess the results of the enema and how well the client tolerated the procedure.

23. Provides data for charting.

▼ *ACTION*

▼ *RATIONALE*

24. Record the procedure in the client's chart. Note the amount, color, and consistency of the stool and the client's ability to tolerate the procedure.

24. Communicates the findings to the other members of the health care team and contributes to the legal record by documenting the care given to the client.

Example of Documentation

DATE	TIME	NOTES
10/12/93	0930	Enema administered. Moderate amount of brown, soft, formed stool returned.
		S. Smith, RN

Teaching Tips

The purpose of the enema should be explained to the client or the client's family member, or both. You should explain to the client that breathing through his or her mouth will help to relax the abdominal muscles as the enema tubing is inserted and the fluid is instilled.

This is a good time to discuss normal elimination patterns with the client or the client's family member. The client should be told that not all persons have a bowel movement every day and this is normal. The client should not use enemas routinely to stimulate defecation. Enemas should be used only when the client is constipated.

If the enema is being administered because of constipation, measures to prevent constipation should be discussed. If possible, the client should increase fluid intake, bulk in the diet, and exercise.

Home Care Variations

Prepackaged enemas may be administered in the client's home without altering the procedure.

SKILL 15–3   REMOVING A FECAL IMPACTION

Clinical Situations in Which You May Encounter This Skill

A fecal impaction is an extension of constipation that may develop when a client is on prolonged bed rest, has not had a bowel movement for a prolonged period of time, or has had a barium test. When a fecal impaction forms, it may be removed manually. This procedure may be uncomfortable and embarrassing for the client.

Vagus nerve stimulation may occur as a result of manipulation of the rectal area. The vagus nerve is part of the parasympathetic nervous system that innervates the gastrointestinal tract as well as major organs such as the heart. Manipulation of the rectal area may stimulate the vagus nerve and initiate a parasympathetic response such as a cardiac dysrhythmia or decreased pulse rate.

Anticipated Responses

▼ The client's fecal impaction is removed.
▼ The client's abdomen is soft and not distended.

Adverse Responses

▼ You are unable to reach all of the impaction.
▼ The client has a decreased pulse rate or cardiac dysrhythmia, or both.

Materials List

Gather these materials before beginning the skill:

▼ Examination gloves
▼ Waterproof pad
▼ Water-soluble lubricant
▼ Bedpan
▼ Towel and washcloth
▼ Basin of warm soapy water

▼ *A C T I O N*	▼ *R A T I O N A L E*
1. Determine when the client last had a bowel movement, if there is any liquid seepage of stool from the rectum, and the presence of abdominal distention.	1. The longer the client has not had a bowel movement the more likely he or she is to have a fecal impaction. Abdominal distention and the seepage of stool from the rectum are symptoms of a fecal impaction.
2. Assess the client's vital signs.	2. Provides baseline data to determine if vagus nerve stimulation occurred.
3. Check the client's chart for a physician's order to remove the impaction and check the agency's policy manual.	3. A physician's order is usually required. In some institutions, only a physician can remove an impaction.
4. Screen the client by closing the door and curtains around the bed.	4. Provides privacy for the client.
5. Raise the bed to a comfortable height.	5. Reduces the strain placed on the your back.
6. Place the client in a left Sims' position.	6. Allows you to palpate the colon for a fecal mass.
7. Drape the client and place a waterproof pad under the client's hips and buttocks.	7. Draping protects the client's privacy and the pad protects the bed.
8. Place a bedpan beside the client.	8. The fecal material that is removed will be placed in the bedpan.
9. Put on gloves.	9. When there is a chance of coming into contact with feces, gloves should be worn to prevent the possible transmission of microorganisms.
10. Generously lubricate your index finger.	10. The lubricant eases insertion and lessens irritation to the client's rectal area.
11. Separate the client's buttocks and gently insert your index finger into the anal canal toward the umbilicus.	11. Allows you to palpate along the natural curve of the colon wall.
12. Check to see if you can feel a fecal mass. If a mass is present, work your finger around and attempt to break it up. You may need to ask the client to bear down to push the fecal mass within your reach. Remove the feces in small pieces and place them in the bedpan.	12. In order to feel the fecal mass, it is necessary to move your finger in all directions. The impaction feels like a hardened mass. It is easiest and least traumatic to the client to remove the mass in pieces.
13. Wash the client's rectal area with soap and water. Rinse and dry the area.	13. Fecal material is caustic to the skin. Washing the rectal area promotes the client's sense of well-being.
14. Return the client's bed to the lowest position.	14. Reduces the potential of injury from falls.
15. Properly dispose of the equipment.	15. Prevents the transmission of microorganisms.
16. Remove the gloves and wash your hands.	16. Decreases the transmission of microorganisms.
17. Assess the client's vital signs and tolerance of the procedure.	17. Determines if there were any adverse effects from vagus nerve stimulation.

▼ *ACTION*	▼ *RATIONALE*
18. Record the procedure in the client's chart. Note the amount, color, odor, and consistency of the stool.	**18.** Communicates the findings to the other members of the health care team and contributes to the legal record by documenting the care given to the client.

Example of Documentation

DATE	*TIME*	*NOTES*
10/12/93	0930	No bowel movement for 1 week. Large fecal mass felt during digital examination. Fecal mass was removed digitally.
		S. Smith, RN

Teaching Tips

Measures to prevent constipation should be discussed with the client or the client's caregiver, or both. Unless contraindicated, the client should increase his or her fluid intake and bulk in the diet.

Immobile clients are prone to impactions. If the client is immobile, the physician may need to be consulted regarding the use of stool softeners.

Home Care Variations

Fecal impactions can be removed in the client's home. A thorough assessment should be performed prior to the procedure to ascertain any cardiac abnormalities. This procedure should be performed with caution for any client with prior cardiac abnormalities.

SKILL 15–4 INSERTING A RECTAL TUBE

Clinical Situations in Which You May Encounter This Skill

Formation of excessive amounts of flatus in the lower gastrointestinal tract occurs any time peristalsis is decreased or absent and the flatus cannot be eliminated by the client. A rectal tube may be inserted to facilitate the client's passage of excessive flatus.

Anticipated Responses

▼ Flatus is removed successfully.

Adverse Responses

▼ The client's abdomen remains distended.

Materials List

Gather these materials before beginning the skill:

▼ Rectal tube:
  Adults: size 22–32 French
  Infants: size 12 French
  2- to 6-year-olds: size 12–14 French
  6- to 12-year-olds: size 14–18 French
  Adolescents: size 22–30 French
▼ Water-soluble lubricant
▼ Examination gloves
▼ Waterproof pad
▼ Towels (2) and washcloth
▼ Tape
▼ Plastic bag
▼ Rubber band

▼ *ACTION*

▼ *RATIONALE*

1. Assess the client's abdomen for distention.

2. Check the client's chart for a physician's order.

3. Screen the client by closing the door and curtains around the bed.

4. Raise the bed to a comfortable height.

5. Place the client in a left Sims' position.

6. Drape the client and place a waterproof pad under the client's hips and buttocks.

7. Put on gloves.

8. Generously lubricate the tip of the rectal tube.

9. Separate the client's buttocks and gently insert the tip of the tube 4 inches into the anal canal toward the umbilicus for an adult, 2 to 3 inches for a child, and 1 to 1.5 inches for an infant. If the tube slips out, you may tape it to one buttock. Do not force the tube if you meet resistance.

10. Instruct the client to remain in a side-lying position.

11. Place the open distal end of the rectal tube in a plastic bag and close it with a rubber band (Fig. 15–3).

1. Determines the need for the rectal tube.

2. A physician's order is required.

3. Provides privacy for the client.

4. Reduces the strain placed on your back.

5. Allows for easier insertion of the tube.

6. Draping protects the client's privacy and the pad helps to protect the bed from any seepage of feces.

7. When there is a chance of coming into contact with feces, gloves should be worn to prevent the possible transmission of microorganisms.

8. Eases insertion and lessens irritation to the client's rectal area.

9. Allows the tube to be inserted in the natural direction of the colon. If you force the tube, you could perforate the client's colon.

10. If the client turns, the tube may be dislodged.

11. The plastic bag will fill with air as flatus is passed and will allow you to see if flatus has been expelled.

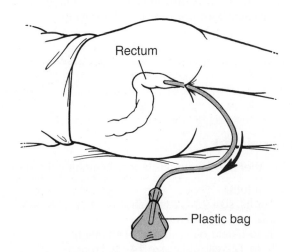

Rectum

Plastic bag

▼ FIGURE 15–3. Inserted rectal tube with plastic bag attached.

▼ *ACTION*	▼ *RATIONALE*
12. Leave the tube in place for 20 to 30 minutes and then remove it.	**12.** If the tube is left in place longer, it will irritate the client's rectal mucosa.
13. Wash the client's rectal area with warm soapy water. Rinse and dry the area.	**13.** Fecal material is caustic to the skin. Washing the rectal area promotes the client's sense of well-being.
14. Remove the gloves and wash your hands.	**14.** Decreases the possible transmission of microorganisms.
15. Return the client's bed to the lowest position.	**15.** Reduces the potential of injury from falls.
16. Properly dispose of the equipment.	**16.** Prevents the transmission of microorganisms.
17. Assess the client for relief of distention.	**17.** Chart whether the client's abdomen is distended.
18. Record the procedure in the client's chart. Note whether the client experienced relief from the distention.	**18.** Communicates the findings to the other members of the health care team and contributes to the legal record by documenting the care given to the client.

Example of Documentation

DATE	TIME	NOTES
10/12/93	0930	Complaining of abdominal pain. Abdominal distention noted. No. 24 French rectal tube inserted and left in place for 20 minutes. Abdominal distention relieved.

S. Smith, RN

Teaching Tips

If a rectal tube is to be used in the client's home, the client's caregiver should be taught the procedure. Measures to reduce formation of flatulence should be discussed with the client. Instruct the client to avoid chewing gum, drinking carbonated beverages, eating rapidly, and drinking with a straw. These activities increase air swallowing and will predispose the client to development of flatulence. Also instruct the client to avoid gas-forming foods such as beans, cabbage, radishes, onions, cauliflower, and cucumbers.

Home Care Variations

A rectal tube can be used in the client's home without any alteration of the procedure.

SKILL 15–5 ASSISTING WITH THE USE OF INCONTINENT BRIEFS

Clinical Situations in Which You May Encounter This Skill

Incontinent briefs are indicated for clients who are experiencing incontinence of urine or feces while bedridden or ambulatory. You should check the client every 2 hours for soiling of the briefs.

Anticipated Responses

▼ The briefs contain the urine or feces, or both, without leakage.
▼ The client's skin is intact with no signs of irritation from the material used in the briefs or from contact with urine or stool.

Adverse Responses

▼ There is leakage of urine or feces, or both, around the briefs.
▼ The client complains of itching or the area of skin touched by the briefs is irritated.
▼ The client experiences skin breakdown.

Materials List

Gather these materials before beginning the skill:

▼ Disposable adult briefs (diapers)
▼ Washcloth(s)
▼ Towel
▼ Mild soap
▼ Lukewarm water in a bath basin
▼ Waterproof pad(s)
▼ Powder, if desired and appropriate for the client's skin type
▼ Skin protectors (optional)
▼ Examination gloves

▼ ACTION

1. Review the client's chart to determine the reason for the briefs.

2. Assess the client's knowledge and feelings about the procedure and the reason for it.

3. Close the door and draw the bedside curtains around the client.

4. Put on gloves.

5. Place the bed in a high position.

6. Place a towel or waterproof pad under the client's hips.

7. Carefully remove the soiled briefs and discard them in an appropriate receptacle.

8. Using clean, warm water and mild soap, gently cleanse the area covered by the briefs. Rinse and dry the client's skin well. Be sure the areas hidden in the folds of the skin are cleansed.

9. Inspect the client's perineum and surrounding skin areas for any areas of irritation.

10. If ordered, use a protective ointment, medication, or skin barrier over the clean area.

▼ RATIONALE

1. Allows you to prepare for the procedure.

2. This is especially important for the first time the briefs are used, as the client may have many negative feelings about their use.

3. Provides privacy.

4. Decreases the transmission of microorganisms.

5. Reduces the strain on your back.

6. Prevents soiling of clean linen.

7. Decreases the transmission of microorganisms.

8. Incontinence causes skin irritation and breakdown. Prevention includes keeping the skin clean and dry.

9. If skin irritation is undetected and untreated, skin breakdown can occur.

10. Areas of irritation that go untreated can lead to pressure sores.

▼ *A C T I O N*   ▼ *R A T I O N A L E*

> **NOTE:** Apply powder or ointment before putting the briefs on the client. Brief tapes should not come in contact with powders and ointments.
>
> Powder and ointment cause the tapes to lose their sticky properties.

11. If the waterproof pad is soiled, remove and discard it at this time. If it is not soiled, it can be removed when the procedure is finished.

11. Prevents contamination of the clean briefs with excrement.

12. Place a pair of clean open briefs with the tapes at the top back of the briefs under the client. The tapes should border the client's waist. The soft inner lining should be next to the client's skin.

12. Provides the best fit. Briefs that are too loose leak urine and feces. Briefs that are too tight are uncomfortable and may compromise circulation.

13. Bring the front of the briefs up between the client's legs and place the top front of the briefs at the level of the client's waist.

13. See step 12.

14. Remove the gloves and dispose of them properly.

14. If the gloves are not removed, the tapes on the briefs will stick to the gloves.

15. Open the tapes and fasten one side of the briefs and then the other (Fig. 15–4).

15. See above.

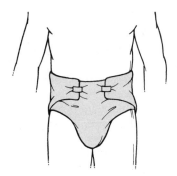

▼ **FIGURE 15–4.** Adult incontinent briefs.

> **NOTE:** Two to three fingers should be able to fit between the briefs and the client's skin.
>
> The briefs should fit snugly but not be binding.

16. Remove the waterproof pad if it has not been removed already.

16. Provides for a clean, comfortable bed.

17. Assess the client's comfort and other needs.

17. Provides for the client's optimal wellness.

18. Lower the bed to its lowest position.

18. Provides for the client's safety.

19. Wash your hands.

19. Decreases the transmission of microorganisms.

20. Record the procedure.

20. Communicates to the other members of the health care team and contributes to the legal record by documenting the care given to the client.

Example of Documentation

DATE	TIME	NOTES
10/28/93	1000	Client's briefs changed. Skin area under briefs cleansed. Skin area intact. No areas of redness noted.
		D. Walker, RN

Teaching Tips

The purpose of using briefs should be explained to the client or the client's family, or both. Explain that the client should not remain in the briefs if they become soiled. Good hygienic care should be stressed since skin irritation and breakdown could occur.

Home Care Variations

Family members should be educated about the importance of good skin care for the client and the damage skin breakdown can cause physically, emotionally, and financially.

SKILL 15–6 DIAPERING AN INFANT

Clinical Situations in Which You May Encounter This Skill

Infants and young children lack voluntary control of their bowel and bladder activity and therefore require diapers for elimination. Voluntary control of the anal sphincter usually occurs around 18 to 24 months of age. Control of bowel movements, however, involves psychologic readiness as well as physical readiness and may not be completed until the end of the second year. Bladder control, including nighttime control, may not be completely achieved until 4 to 5 years of age. During periods of illness, children who have been toilet trained may regress and have toileting accidents. Avoid shaming the child should this occur.

Cloth or disposable diapers may be used for diapering the infant at home. In clinic settings and hospitals, disposable diapers are used to prevent the spread of infection and eliminate the need for laundering the diapers.

NORMAL STOOL PATTERNS FOR SELECTED DEVELOPMENTAL STAGES

First 36 hours after birth	Meconium stool: Sticky, greenish black stool composed of intrauterine debris such as bile pigments, epithelial cells, fatty acids, mucus, blood, and amniotic fluid.
Third day after birth	Transitional stool: Greenish brown to yellowish brown stool that occurs with the initiation of feeding. A transitional stool is less sticky in consistency than a meconium stool.

Fourth day after birth	Milk stool: The milk stool varies with the method of infant feeding. In breast-fed infants, the milk stool is yellow to golden in color, pasty in consistency, and has an odor similar to sour milk. Breast-fed babies have more stools than bottle-fed babies, with a frequency ranging from one stool every other day to six stools per day. The stools of bottle-fed infants are pale yellow to light brown and are firmer in consistency than those of breast-fed babies. The bottle-fed infant's stool has a more offensive odor than that of the breast-fed infant and the stools are less frequent. Bottle-fed babies are somewhat more prone to constipation than breast-fed infants are.
First year of life	Because of the child's immature digestive processes, the stool may contain recognizable pieces of solid fibrous foods such as peas, carrots, and corn. Diets high in roughage may lead to loose bulky stools. Bowel evacuation is still under involuntary control.
Fourteen to 18 months of age	Myelination of the spinal cord is complete and voluntary control of bowel movements is possible.
Eighteen to 24 months of age	Toilet training is under way during this time. Fibrous foods are digested more completely and stools are more like adult stools.
Childhood	Variables such as food and fluid intake, exercise patterns, responsiveness to defecation urge, stress level, and medications affect the stool pattern and characteristics.

NORMAL URINATION PATTERNS FOR SELECTED DEVELOPMENTAL STAGES

Newborn	The kidney of a newborn is unable to concentrate urine, so the urine is colorless, odorless, and has a specific gravity of about 1.008. The total volume of urine per 24 hours ranges from 200 to 300 ml. The bladder has a small capacity and involuntarily empties after approximately 15 ml of urine accumulates, which results in 20 or more voidings per 24 hours.
First year	The renal system is still immature and predisposes the child to rapid loss of body fluids and dehydration during illness. These children void less frequently than newborns because of an increase in the bladder capacity.
Second year	The mature renal system is capable of conserving body fluids during stress and the risk of dehydration is decreased. Urine characteristics are similar to those of an adult.

Anticipated Responses

▼ The infant's anal and perineal area is clean and dry.
▼ The infant's skin is free of diaper rash and skin break-down.

Adverse Responses

▼ The diapers leak, soiling the bedding and the child's clothing.
▼ The infant has diaper rash.

Materials List

Gather these materials before beginning the skill:

▼ Disposable diaper or cloth diaper with diaper pins
▼ Disposable cleansing wipes or wash basin, soap, washcloth, and towel
▼ Skin barrier cream of choice
▼ Examination gloves

▼ ACTION

1. Wash your hands.

2. Put on examination gloves.

3. Place the child on a firm surface such as a changing table. Keep your hands on the child and do not turn away from him or her at any time.

4. Remove the soiled diaper and assess the contents of the diaper for unusual appearance or odor.

5. Discard the soiled diaper in a container designated for blood or body secretions.

6. Assess the infant's skin in the diaper area for redness, rash, or excoriation.

7. Cleanse the infant's skin with disposable wipes or a wet soapy washcloth. If you are using a washcloth, be sure to rinse the soap from the child's skin and pat the area dry.

8. Apply a protective barrier cream to the diaper area if desired.

9. Apply the new diaper securely.

10. Remove the soiled gloves and wash your hands.

11. Record the characteristics of the bowel or bladder elimination.

▼ RATIONALE

1. Reduces the transmission of microorganisms.

2. Protects your hands from contact with bodily secretions.

3. Prevents injury from falls.

4. Unusual characteristics may indicate a gastrointestinal or urinary disorder.

5. Prevents the transmission of microorganisms from one client to another.

6. Contact with urine or feces can irritate the skin. Early detection and treatment are necessary to prevent further skin breakdown and infection.

7. Removes feces and urine from the skin. Soap residue and moisture can irritate the skin and lead to breakdown.

8. Protects the skin from contact with urine and feces.

9. Prevents accidental soiling.

10. Prevents the transmission of microorganisms.

11. Communicates the findings to the other members of the health care team and contributes to the legal record by documenting the care given to the client.

Example of Documentation

DATE	TIME	NOTES
1/1/90	0830	Diaper soiled with small amount of soft, pasty, yellowish brown stool. No signs of redness or skin irritation noted. Skin care given and barrier cream applied to the diaper area before applying new diaper.
		C. Lammon, RN

Teaching Tips

When teaching the new mother about hygiene, you should discuss the application of diapers and explain the importance of keeping the infant clean and dry. Explain that urine and feces cause skin irritation and breakdown.

SKILL 15–7 CARING FOR A STOMA

Clinical Situations in Which You May Encounter This Skill

Clients who have undergone permanent colostomies (ileostomy; cecostomy; ascending, transverse, descending, or sigmoid colostomy) or temporary (double-barrel or loop) colostomies have one or two stomas on their abdominal wall (Fig. 15–5)

through which fecal material passes into a collection bag worn over the stoma (Fig. 15–6). Since fecal drainage is caustic to the skin, clients with abdominal stomas need meticulous skin care to prevent skin excoriation. Initially the appliance (collection bag) is usually changed every other day. After the initial period, the appliance can be left in place as long as there is no leakage and the skin is in good condition.

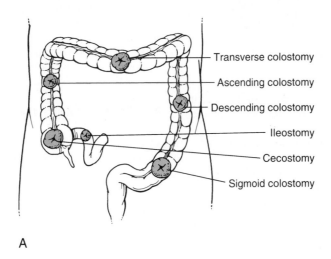

- Transverse colostomy
- Ascending colostomy
- Descending colostomy
- Ileostomy
- Cecostomy
- Sigmoid colostomy

A

Double-barrel colostomy

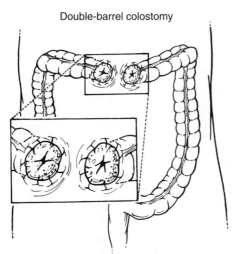

Loop colostomy

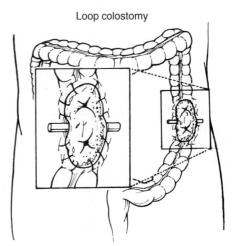

B

▼ **FIGURE 15–5.** Stoma sites in the abdominal wall for permanent colostomies (*A*). Stoma sites for temporary colostomies (*B*) can be located anywhere along the colon.

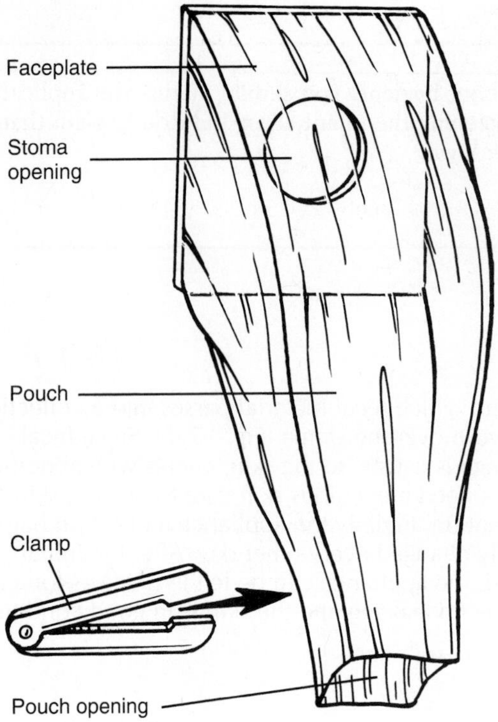
Faceplate
Stoma opening
Pouch
Clamp
Pouch opening

▼ **FIGURE 15–6.** Ostomy collection bag.

Changing the appliance too frequently can cause skin irritation. The appliance should be changed any time there is leakage.

Ostomy surgery causes emotional stress for the client. The client may grieve over the loss of normal body function and feel unclean, undesirable, and unable to lead a normal life. You should provide support for the client and help the client and his or her family to learn to care for the ostomy.

Anticipated Responses

- ▼ After a demonstration of skin care and bag changes, the client is able to perform these skills.
- ▼ Skin integrity and control of odor are maintained.
- ▼ Stool is expelled into the bag.

Adverse Responses

- ▼ The client refuses to look at the stoma or accept the need to learn about stoma care.
- ▼ The client's skin is excoriated.

Materials List

Gather these materials before beginning the skill:

- ▼ 4- × 4-inch gauze pads
- ▼ Scissors
- ▼ Examination gloves
- ▼ Ostomy appliance
- ▼ Skin barrier
- ▼ Stoma measuring guide
- ▼ Waterproof pad
- ▼ Clamp
- ▼ Basin of warm soapy water
- ▼ Towel and washcloth
- ▼ Plastic bag
- ▼ Toilet paper
- ▼ 4- × 4-inch gauze pad soaked in alcohol

▼ *ACTION*	▼ *RATIONALE*
1. Determine the type of ostomy that the client has.	**1.** Since the consistency of fecal drainage varies with the type of ostomy, this will alert you to the type of fecal drainage to be expected.
2. Assess the client's readiness to learn about ostomy care.	**2.** The client's ability to learn is affected by the readiness to learn.
3. Screen the client by closing the door and curtains around the bed.	**3.** Provides privacy for the client.
4. Raise the client's bed to a comfortable working height.	**4.** Reduces the strain on your back.
5. Place the client in either a supine or sitting position.	**5.** The sitting position allows the client to observe the procedure.
6. Position the client's gown above the stoma.	**6.** Provides an unobstructed work area.
7. Fold a waterproof pad around the edge of the gown.	**7.** Protects the gown.
8. Put on gloves.	**8.** When there is a chance of coming into contact with feces, gloves should be worn to prevent the possible transmission of microorganisms.

▼ *A C T I O N*	▼ *R A T I O N A L E*
9. Explain each of the steps to the client.	**9.** Teaches the client about the procedure.
10. Gently massage the client's proximal intestine toward the stoma.	**10.** Stimulates peristalsis to move the fecal material near the stoma into the bag.
11. Empty the ostomy appliance into the bedpan (Fig. 15–7). Observe the color, consistency, and odor of the feces.	**11.** Prevents spilling of the feces when the appliance is removed.

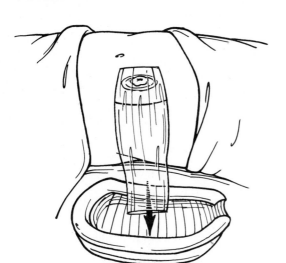

▼ **FIGURE 15–7.** Draining an ostomy appliance into a bedpan.

12. Loosen the skin barrier with a 4- × 4-inch pad soaked in alcohol.	**12.** The alcohol will loosen the adhesive on the back of the bag.
13. Support the client's skin and gently remove the barrier and bag by pulling it diagonally away from your hand.	**13.** There will be less pulling and skin irritation when the appliance is removed diagonally.
14. Place toilet paper over the stoma.	**14.** Prevents soiling from leakage.
15. Place the used appliance in a plastic bag and discard it.	**15.** Prevents the spread of microorganisms.
16. Wash the skin around the stoma with warm water and a mild soap and the stoma with clear water.	**16.** Prevents skin irritation and removes any feces and mucus that may have collected. Feces are caustic to the skin.
17. Rinse the area and pat it dry.	**17.** Rubbing can irritate the skin. Wetness will cause skin excoriation and breakdown.
18. Assess the color, moisture, and protrusion of the stoma and the condition of the surrounding skin.	**18.** It is easiest to fit an appliance over a protruding stoma. The stoma should be pink or red and moist. A dark color can indicate poor circulation and necrosis. The client also may develop dermatitis or a yeast infection of the skin around the stoma.

▼ _A C T I O N_   ▼ _R A T I O N A L E_

19. Measure the stoma with the stoma measuring guide, trace the size on the skin barrier, and cut out the hole (Fig. 15–8).

19. The skin barrier should fit snugly around the stoma to prevent skin breakdown and leakage.

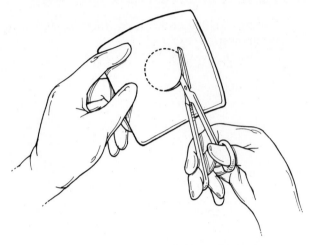

▼ **FIGURE 15–8.** Cutting a hole in a skin barrier.

20. Trace a circle one-eighth to one-quarter inch larger than the size of the stoma on the back of the appliance and cut out the hole.

20. The appliance should fit snugly around the stoma since the feces are caustic to the skin.

21. Prepare the barrier and the appliance as a unit by removing the paper from the adhesive surface of the appliance and positioning the appliance over the skin barrier.

21. It is easiest to apply the barrier and appliance as a unit.

22. Gently smooth the barrier to remove all air bubbles.

22. A good seal is necessary to prevent leakage of feces onto the skin.

23. If the stoma borders are irregular, fill in the irregularities with skin paste.

23. Further protects the skin and prevents the feces from undermining the skin barrier and the appliance.

24. To apply the unit, remove the paper from the adhesive side of the skin barrier and apply it around the stoma, positioning it so the bag hangs in a dependent position (Fig. 15–9).

24. If the bag is not in a dependent position, the force of gravity will loosen the bag.

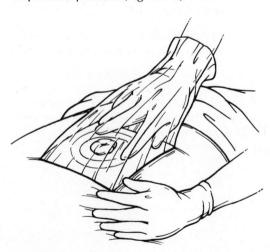

▼ **FIGURE 15–9.** Positioning the appliance over a stoma.

▼ _A C T I O N_

▼ _R A T I O N A L E_

25. Attach the dependent edge first.

25. Prevents leakage before the entire appliance is attached.

26. Smooth down the skin barrier around the stoma.

26. Provides a good seal.

27. If needed, add odor controller (chlorophyll, activated charcoal, or vanilla) to the bag.

27. The client may be embarrassed by any odor.

28. Close the end of the appliance with a clamp.

28. Feces will drain out the open end.

29. Place 1-inch waterproof tape around the outer edges of the appliance in a picture frame fashion.

29. Makes the appliance more secure.

30. Cover the client and remove the contaminated equipment.

30. Assists in maintaining the client's privacy and promotes his or her sense of well-being.

31. Remove the gloves and wash your hands.

31. Prevents the spread of microorganisms.

32. Return the client's bed to the lowest position.

32. Reduces the potential of injury from falls.

33. Assess the appliance to determine whether it adheres smoothly to the client's skin and whether it is leaking.

33. Leakage causes skin irritation.

> **NOTE:** If the appliance leaks, it should be reapplied.

34. Ask the client if he or she has any questions about the procedure.

34. Questions should be answered immediately to help the client retain the information.

35. Record the procedure. Note the appearance of the skin and stoma and the color, amount, and consistency of the feces.

35. Communicates the findings to the other members of the health care team and contributes to the legal record by documenting the care given to the client.

> **NOTE:** The technique may vary with the type of appliance used.

Example of Documentation

DATE	TIME	NOTES
10/17/93	1000	Sigmoid colostomy appliance changed. Stoma pink, moist, flush with the skin. Skin intact with no redness. Moderate amount of brown, formed feces in the bag.
		S. Williams, RN

Teaching Tips

The client should understand the consistency of drainage to be expected from the ostomy. Dietary modifications needed to prevent diarrhea, flatus, and constipation and to control odor should be discussed with the client or the client's caregiver. Foods such as beer, lettuce, and fruit may cause diarrhea. Medications such as diuretics and antibiotics also may cause diarrhea. Cabbage, onions, and beans are gas-forming foods that should be avoided. A decreased fluid intake and the use of sedatives can lead to constipation. A diet containing figs and prunes can help to alleviate or prevent constipation. Yogurt and buttermilk can be added to the diet to control odor.

Home Care Variations

Ostomy care can be performed in the client's home. Used ostomy bags can be placed in a sealable plastic bag for disposal.

SKILL 15–8   CARING FOR A CONTINENT ILEOSTOMY

Clinical Situations in Which You May Encounter This Skill

A continent ileostomy is usually created for clients with ulcerative colitis following a total colectomy. An internal reservoir for collection of feces is created from the terminal ileum and an outlet valve is created from intussuscepted ileum. A catheter is inserted into the pouch through the outlet valve approximately three times per day to eliminate gas and drain feces.

Anticipated Responses

▼ The client learns to do the procedure.
▼ Feces are drained and gas is eliminated from the pouch.

Adverse Responses

▼ The client has difficulty learning the procedure.
▼ The skin is excoriated.

Materials List

Gather these materials before beginning the skill:

▼ Red Robinson catheter (size 28 French)
▼ Water-soluble lubricant
▼ Examination gloves
▼ 50-ml catheter-tipped syringe
▼ Normal saline for irrigation
▼ 4- × 4-inch gauze pad
▼ Tape
▼ Washcloth and towel
▼ Soap

▼ ACTION	▼ RATIONALE
1. Assess the client's readiness to learn the procedure.	1. The client's ability to learn is affected by his or her readiness to learn.
2. Position the client on a toilet or bedside commode. If the client cannot get up, a bedpan may be placed by the client in the bed.	2. The feces will drain into the toilet, bedside commode, or bedpan.
3. Put on gloves.	3. When there is a chance of coming into contact with feces, gloves should be worn to prevent the possible transmission of microorganisms.
4. Remove the ostomy dressing and dispose of it in a proper receptacle.	4. A dressing is used to cover the continent ileostomy since there is no fecal drainage.
5. Generously lubricate 3 inches of the catheter.	5. Makes insertion of the catheter easier and more comfortable for the client.
6. Place the distal portion of the catheter into the toilet, bedside commode, or bedpan.	6. As soon as the catheter is inserted, feces will begin to drain out of its distal end.

▼ *ACTION* ▼ *RATIONALE*

7. Gently insert the catheter at a downward angle into the stoma for approximately 2 inches or until you meet resistance.

7. When the catheter meets resistance, it has reached the outlet valve.

8. Instruct the client to take a deep breath. Insert the catheter through the outlet valve into the pouch (Fig. 15–10).

8. Deep breathing will relax the client and will facilitate passage of the catheter.

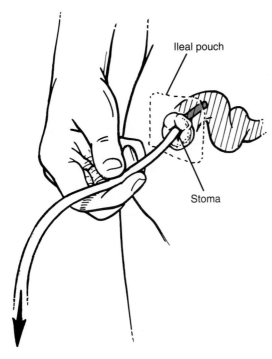

Ileal pouch

Stoma

▼ **FIGURE 15–10.** Inserting a catheter into an ileostomy pouch.

9. Drain all of the contents from the pouch. If the drainage is expelled sluggishly, use a 50-ml catheter-tipped syringe and irrigate the catheter with 30 to 50 ml of normal saline.

9. The pouch should be emptied completely.

10. Clean the stoma and surrounding skin with warm soapy water.

10. Feces are caustic to the skin. Washing also helps to prevent skin irritation and promote the client's sense of well-being.

11. Rinse the area and pat dry.

11. A warm, moist environment could lead to the growth of microorganisms. Rubbing irritates the skin.

12. Place a clean 4- × 4-inch gauze pad over the stoma and secure it with tape.

12. Helps to protect the stoma from irritation.

13. Properly clean and dispose of the equipment. Store any clean equipment that can be reused.

13. Prevents the transmission of microorganisms.

14. Remove the gloves and wash your hands.

14. Decreases the possible transmission of microorganisms.

15. Ask the client if he or she has any questions about the procedure.

15. Questions should be answered immediately to help the client retain the information.

16. Record the procedure. Note the amount of feces drained from the pouch.

16. Communicates the findings to the other members of the health care team and contributes to the legal record by documenting the care given to the client.

Example of Documentation

DATE	TIME	NOTES
10/17/93	1000	Continent ileostomy pouch drained of 100 ml of liquid, brown feces. Client instructed on the procedure. Stoma pink and moist. Clean 4 × 4 applied over the stoma.
		S. Williams, RN

Teaching Tips

The client should be taught the procedure and have the opportunity to practice. Several sessions may be required before the client is comfortable with the procedure.

Home Care Variations

The client can be taught to perform the procedure at home using this same technique.

SKILL 15–9　PERFORMING A COLOSTOMY IRRIGATION

Clinical Situations in Which You May Encounter This Skill

A colostomy irrigation is usually performed daily for clients with a descending or sigmoid colostomy to train the intestines to empty at the same time every day and to prevent fecal spilling between irrigations. An irrigation also may be performed to cleanse the bowel before surgery or diagnostic procedures.

Since the drainage from an ileostomy and some other types of colostomies is liquid to semisolid and regularity cannot be established, irrigations for these types of colostomies are not performed on a routine basis.

The client's presurgical bowel pattern affects the response to regulation. Therefore, it is important to determine the client's previous bowel pattern. Not all persons have a bowel movement every day, and the time of day varies. If the client is able to regulate his or her bowel pattern with irrigation, it is not necessary for him or her to wear a pouch. Irrigations should not be initiated until peristalsis has returned.

A cone is the preferred device for an irrigation. The cone limits the depth of insertion and decreases the chance of bowel perforation. If the client is unable to achieve good results with a cone, a tube with a backflow prevention device or a catheter can be used. The chance of perforation of the bowel wall is greater with the tube and the catheter.

Anticipated Responses

▼ Feces are successfully removed from the colon.
▼ All of the water used for the irrigation is returned.

Adverse Responses

▼ There is retention of the irrigation water.
▼ The client complains of cramping.

Materials List

Gather these materials before beginning the skill:

▼ Waterproof pad (if performed at the bedside)
▼ Clip
▼ Irrigation set with irrigation sleeve (Fig. 15–11)
▼ Irrigation bag
▼ Cone-shaped irrigation tip (Fig. 15–12)
▼ Water-soluble lubricant
▼ Belt
▼ IV pole
▼ Plastic bag
▼ Washcloth and towel
▼ Basin of warm soapy water
▼ Ostomy appliance
▼ 1,000 ml of water for irrigation
▼ Examination gloves
▼ Bath thermometer

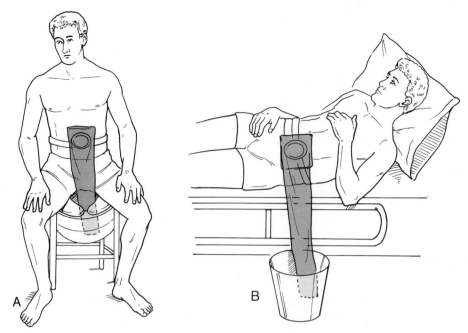

▼ **FIGURE 15–11.** Colostomy irrigation sleeve used (*A*) with a bedside commode and (*B*) with a container by the client's bed.

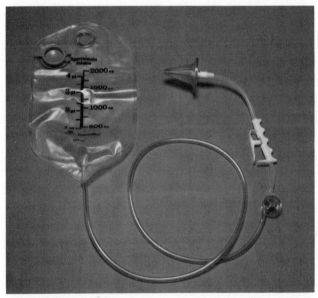

▼ **FIGURE 15–12.** Cone-shaped irrigation tip.

▼ *ACTION*	▼ *RATIONALE*
1. Check the physician's order for irrigation.	**1.** A physician's order is necessary to begin an irrigation. If the client has a double-barrel colostomy, the order should indicate which portion (distal or proximal) is to be irrigated.
2. Determine the type of ostomy that the client has.	**2.** The consistency of fecal drainage varies with the location of the ostomy.
3. Ask the client the time of day it will be best for him or her to irrigate at home and, if possible, schedule the irrigation at this time.	**3.** Helps the client to establish a pattern for elimination.

▼ *ACTION*	▼ *RATIONALE*
4. Assess the client's readiness to learn the procedure.	4. The client's ability to learn is affected by his or her readiness to learn.
5. Close the door and the curtains around the bed if the procedure is to be done in the bed or at the bedside.	5. Provides privacy for the client.
6. Warm the water for irrigation to 104° Fahrenheit or 40° centigrade and fill the irrigation bag with 500 to 1,000 ml.	6. If the solution is too cool, intestinal cramping may occur. If the solution is too warm, it can burn the client's intestinal mucosa.
7. Check the temperature with a bath thermometer.	7. A solution that is too cool can cause intestinal cramping and a solution that is too hot can burn the intestine.
8. Hang the bag at the client's shoulder-level and clear the air from the tubing.	8. The solution should flow in by gravity. Raising the container higher could cause abdominal cramping and distention.
9. Clear the air from the tubing by opening the clamp and allowing the solution to flow through the length of the tubing.	9. Air will distend the client's intestines and may produce abdominal cramping.
10. Close the clamp after all of the air is removed.	10. Prevents leakage of the solution.
11. Position the client on the toilet, bedside commode, or beside a bedpan if he or she is unable to get out of bed.	11. The solution and feces should flow into the toilet, bedside commode, or bedpan.
12. Put on gloves.	12. When there is a chance of coming into contact with feces, gloves should be worn to prevent the possible transmission of microorganisms.
13. Empty the ostomy appliance into the bedpan.	13. Prevents spilling of feces when the appliance is removed.
14. Observe the amount, color, consistency, and odor of the feces.	14. This information is necessary for accurate charting.
15. Loosen the skin barrier with a 4- × 4-inch gauze pad soaked in alcohol.	15. Alcohol loosens the adhesive on the back of the appliance.
16. Loosen the upper inner aspect of the skin barrier and appliance and gently pull diagonally away from the skin to remove them.	16. There will be less pulling and skin irritation when the appliance is removed diagonally.
17. Assess the stoma and the surrounding skin. Observe for dark discoloration of the stoma and redness or breakdown of the surrounding skin.	17. The stoma should be pink or red and moist. A dark color can indicate poor circulation and necrosis.
18. Place the used appliance in a plastic bag and discard it.	18. Helps to prevent the spread of microorganisms.
19. Place a belt around the client and attach the irrigation sleeve.	19. The belt is used to hold the irrigation sleeve in place.
20. Place the distal end of the sleeve into the toilet, bedside commode, or bedpan if the client is confined to the bed.	20. The irrigation sleeve is placed in the toilet, bedside commode, or bedpan to drain any solution that may leak as the irrigation fluid is instilled and so the feces and irrigation solution can drain into the toilet at the end of the irrigation procedure.
21. Lubricate the cone with a water-soluble lubricant.	21. Makes insertion easier and more comfortable for the client.

▼ _ACTION_	▼ _RATIONALE_
22. Insert the cone through the top opening of the irrigation sleeve and into the stoma. Do not force the cone into the stoma.	**22.** The cone directs the irrigation fluid into the intestine.
23. Release the clamp on the tubing and let the water flow slowly into the intestines. If cramping occurs, stop the flow and let the client rest. Then slowly resume the flow. The water should flow in over 15 minutes.	**23.** Cramping may occur from infusion that is too rapid or too much pressure.
24. Remove the cone, fold down the top of the irrigation sleeve, and secure it with a clip.	**24.** Prevents spilling of feces on the client's skin. Fecal material is caustic to the skin.
25. Check that the distal end of the sleeve is still in the toilet, commode, or bedpan.	**25.** The sleeve is placed so that the feces and irrigation solution can drain.
26. Have the client remain on the toilet for 15 minutes.	**26.** It takes 15 minutes for most of the feces and irrigation solution to drain.
27. Clamp the bottom of the sleeve for 1 hour. The client may ambulate or return to bed.	**27.** A 1-hour time period is necessary to collect the remainder of the feces and irrigation solution. Ambulation stimulates peristalsis.
28. Remove the irrigation sleeve, empty it, and rinse.	**28.** The irrigation sleeve is cleaned so that it can be reused.
29. Wash the stoma and the skin around the stoma with warm soapy water. Rinse and dry the area.	**29.** The area is cleansed to prevent skin irritation.
30. Remove the gloves and wash your hands.	**30.** Prevents the spread of microorganisms.
31. Apply the clean appliance.	**31.** See Skill 15–7.
32. Ask the client if he or she has any questions about the procedure.	**32.** Questions should be answered immediately to help the client retain the information.
33. Record the procedure in the client's chart. Note the amount, color, odor, and consistency of the feces.	**33.** Communicates the findings to the other members of the health care team and contributes to the legal record by documenting the care given to the client.

Example of Documentation

DATE	TIME	NOTES
10/17/93	1000	Sigmoid colostomy irrigated with 500 ml of water. Moderate amounts of soft, brown, formed feces were returned. Stoma pink and moist. Procedure explained.

S. Williams, RN

Teaching Tips

Explain to the client that the irrigations need to be done at the same time every day to establish a regular bowel evacuation time. The client and his or her family member should have a good understanding of the procedure. If the client is sick and unable to perform the irrigation, the family member can perform the irrigation.

Home Care Variations

Colostomy irrigations are done in the same manner in the client's home. A meat thermometer can be used instead of a bath thermometer to check the water temperature. A hook on which to hang the irrigation bag can be attached to the bathroom wall or door.

References

Coe, M., and Kluka, S. (1988). Concerns of clients and spouses regarding ostomy surgery for cancer. *Journal of Enterostomal Therapy*, 15, 232–239.

Daly, J. (1994). Meeting bowel elimination needs. In V. Bolander (Ed.), *Basic nursing* (3rd ed.). Philadelphia: W. B. Saunders.

Gloeckner, M. R. (1984). Perceptions of sexual attractiveness following ostomy surgery. *Research in Nursing Health*, 7 (2), 87–92.

Hedrick, J. K. (1987). Effects of ET nursing intervention on adjustment following ostomy surgery. *Journal of Enterostomal Therapy*, 14 (6), 229–239.

Kelman, G., and Minkler, P. (1989). An investigation of quality of life and self-esteem among individuals with ostomies. *Journal of Enterostomal Therapy*, 16 (1), 4–11.

Kobza, L. (1983). Impact of ostomy upon the spouse. *Journal of Enterostomal Therapy*, 10 (2), 54–57.

CHAPTER 16

Meeting Urinary Elimination Needs

The urinary system plays a major role in ridding the body of waste products and maintaining fluid and electrolyte balance. When a client experiences an alteration in urinary elimination, assistance from the health care team is needed. Common alterations include urinary retention, urinary incontinence, oliguria or anuria, polyuria, and dysuria. When assisting with urinary elimination needs, take care to provide privacy and to protect the client's dignity.

OVERVIEW OF RELATED RESEARCH

Classen, D. C., et al. (1991). Prevention of catheter-associated bacteriuria: Clinical trial of methods to block three known pathways of infection. *American Journal of Infection Control*, 19 (3), 136–142.

This study examined the use of preconnected sealed catheters, daily catheter care, and disinfection of the urinary drainage bag outflow tube in the prevention of urinary tract infections in 606 patients. One group of patients (n = 300) received daily catheter care and disinfection of the urinary drainage bag outflow tube. The second group of patients (n = 306) did not receive either of these treatments. Both groups had preconnected sealed catheters inserted. There was no statistically significant difference in the rate of bacteriuria in the two groups. Thus, these measures did not decrease the rate of urinary tract infections in these patients.

Classen D. C., et al. (1991). Daily meatal care for prevention of catheter-associated bacteriuria: Results using frequent applications of polyantibiotic cream. *Infection Control and Hospital Epidemiology*, 12 (3), 157–162.

This study examined the use of a polyantibiotic cream in the prevention of catheter-associated urinary infections in 747 patients. The cream was applied three times a day to the urethral meatus–catheter interface. There was no significant difference in the rate of infection between the two groups.

Dodds, P., and Hans, A. L. (1990). Distended urinary bladder drainage practices among hospital nurses. *Applied Nursing Research*, 3 (2), 68–69.

The purpose of this study was to examine distended urinary bladder drainage practices by nurses (n = 149) who were employed on surgical, medical, and maternity units. The majority of the nurses (97%) palpated for bladder distention prior to catheterizing the patient. Further assessments by 72 nurses included ascertaining the time of the patient's last voiding, examining patient intake and output, and examining the patient's uterine fundus. Fifty-seven percent of the nurses limited the amount of urine drained after catheterization to between 750 and 1,000 ml.

Ehrenkranz, N. J., and Alfonso, B. C. (1991). Failure of bland soap handwash to prevent hand transfer of patient bacteria to urethral catheters. *Infection Control and Hospital Epidemiology*, 12 (11), 654–662.

This study compared the use of a bland soap handwash and an isopropyl alcohol hand rinse in preventing hand transfer of patient bacteria to urethral catheters by health care workers. A significant difference was found between the two methods of hand cleansing. There was a failure rate of 92% for the bland soap handwash and 17% for the alcohol hand rinse.

SKILL 16–1   MEASURING URINARY OUTPUT

Clinical Situations in Which You May Encounter This Skill

Urinary output is measured for clients who are receiving parenteral fluids or total parenteral nutrition. It also may be measured for clients after surgery; clients with cardiac or renal disease, endocrine imbalance, or head injury; clients who have a urinary drainage system in place; or clients who are receiving medications such as diuretics or steroids. The normal output for adults is 1,200 to 1,700 ml per day or 50 to 70 ml per hour.

Clients who are dehydrated or clients with diseases in which there is an increased secretion of antidiuretic hormone and aldosterone may have a decreased output. Oliguria occurs if the output falls to 500 ml per day or less or is less than 25 ml per hour. Output is increased for clients with diseases in which there is a decreased secretion of antidiuretic hormone and aldosterone. The client taking diuretics also may have an increased output.

Anticipated Responses

▼ The client has a normal urinary output.
▼ The client's bladder is not distended.

Adverse Responses

▼ The urinary output is decreased.
▼ The urinary output is increased.
▼ The client's bladder is distended.

Materials List

Gather these materials before beginning the skill:

▼ 1,000-ml graduated container, toilet specimen container ("hat"), or urinal
▼ Intake and output sheet
▼ Pen
▼ Examination gloves

▼ *ACTION*

▼ *RATIONALE*

1. Assess the client's ability to learn.

2. Put on gloves.

3. Collect the client's urine.
   a. To obtain urine from a bedpan, pour the urine into a graduated container and read the level.
   b. To obtain urine from a toilet specimen container, read the level on the graduated strip inside the container.
   c. To obtain urine from a urinal, read the level on the graduated side of the urinal.
   d. To collect urine from a catheter drainage bag, place the graduated container below the drainage bag outflow tubing.
      i. Detach the outflow tubing from the protective cover on the bag and place the outflow tubing into the container without touching the sides of the container.

      ii. Open the clamp on the outflow tubing and allow all of the urine to drain from the bag into the graduated container.
      iii. When the bag is empty, clamp the outflow tubing.
      iv. Return the outflow tubing to the protective cover.

4. To read the amount, place the graduated container with the urine on a level surface in the bathroom or utility room for soiled articles.

5. Assess the color, odor, and clarity of the urine.

6. Empty the urine into the toilet.

7. Rinse the measuring device and return it to storage.

8. Remove the gloves and wash your hands.

9. Record the amount of urine on the output side of the intake and output sheet. Record the color, odor, and clarity of the urine in the progress notes.

10. If the urine was emptied from an indwelling catheter bag, ensure that the outflow tubing is closed and the tubing from the catheter to the drainage bag is not kinked but is hanging freely.

1. If the client is able to learn, he or she can be taught to measure and record his or her own urinary output.

2. Gloves should be worn to prevent the possible transmission of microorganisms when there is a chance of coming in contact with any body fluid.

   a. The graduated container provides an acceptable measurement.
   b. The graduated strip provides an acceptable measurement.

   c. The graduated side of the urinal provides an acceptable measurement.

      i. The outflow tubing is used to drain the urine into the container. If the outflow tubing touches the side of the container, it is contaminated and microorganisms can migrate into the client's bladder.
      ii. The urine can be measured accurately in the graduated container.

      iii. Prevents loss of urine from the drainage bag.
      iv. Prevents contamination by microorganisms.

4. The urine container is placed on a level surface so that the fluid level is even and an exact reading can be obtained.

5. Provides pertinent data for charting.

6. Proper disposal decreases the transmission of microorganisms.

7. The container is clean and ready for use the next time it is needed.

8. Decreases the possible transmission of microorganisms.

9. Communicates the findings to the other members of the health care team and contributes to the legal record by documenting the care given to the client. Allows members of the health care team to compare the client's output and intake.

10. These measures assist in the continued proper functioning of the catheter.

Example of Documentation

See Table 16–1. Record any abnormalities in the nurses' notes.

TABLE 16–1. Intake and Output Sheet

Date: 10/18/93	Intake				Output			
Time	PO	NG	IV	Other	Urine	Bowel	Emesis	Other
0700–1500	600	—	150	—	725	× $\overset{.}{1}$	—	—
1500–2300								
2300–0700								
24-hour totals								
Total intake _____					Total output _____			

Teaching Tips

The purpose of measuring urinary output and the importance of measuring the output accurately should be explained to the client and the client's family. If the urine output is too low and the client's fluid intake is not restricted, you should explain to the client the importance of an adequate fluid intake.

Home Care Variations

Urinary output can be measured in the client's home using the same procedure.

SKILL 16–2 ASSISTING THE CLIENT WITH A BEDPAN OR FRACTURE PAN

Clinical Situations in Which You May Encounter This Skill

A bedpan is usually used for clients who are unable to get to the bathroom or bedside commode. Most bedpans are made of plastic, but some are made of stainless steel. A fracture pan is a different type of bedpan that is used for the client who is unable to turn to the side or who is immobilized or uncomfortable on a regular bedpan. Most fracture pans are made of plastic. The fracture pan is smaller and more shallow than a regular bedpan (Fig. 16–1).

Anticipated Responses

▼ The client is able to use the bedpan to urinate or defecate.

Adverse Responses

▼ The client is unable to use the bedpan because of uncomfortable positioning or embarrassment.

Materials List

Gather these materials before beginning the skill:

▼ Bedpan
▼ Toilet tissue
▼ Washcloth and towel
▼ Soap
▼ Bath basin with warm water
▼ Examination gloves

Regular bedpan

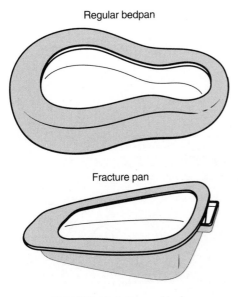

Fracture pan

▼ **FIGURE 16–1.** Types of bedpans.

▼ *ACTION*	▼ *RATIONALE*
1. Assess the client's mobility and ability to assist with using a bedpan.	1. If the client is immobile, a fracture pan is needed. You may need to ask for another nurse to assist you if the client is immobile or has difficulty moving.
2. Check the physician's order for any restrictions in movement and the diagnosis of the client's medical conditions.	2. Movement may be restricted. For example, a client with a spinal cord injury should not sit until his or her spine has been stabilized.
3. Screen the client by closing the door and the curtains around the bed.	3. Provides privacy for the client.
4. Raise the client's bed to a comfortable height.	4. Reduces the strain placed on your back.
5. Position the client's bed flat and the client on his or her back.	5. Facilitates placement of the bedpan.
6. Fold the top linen down and across the client's abdomen. Raise the client's gown and fold it across his or her abdomen.	6. Prevents the linen and gown from becoming soiled and provides access for you to slide the bedpan under the client.
7. Instruct the client to flex his or her knees and push with the feet to lift the hips. If a trapeze is in place, have the client pull on it to help raise his or her hips.	7. The client should assist as much as possible in lifting his or her hips to prevent unnecessary strain on your back.

▼ *ACTION*   ▼ *RATIONALE*

8. Support the client's hips with one hand and slide the bedpan under his or her buttocks from the side (Fig. 16–2).

8. This support helps to prevent strain on the client's hips.

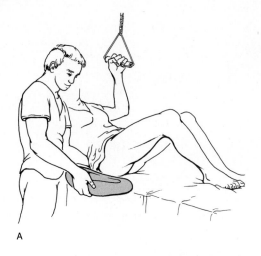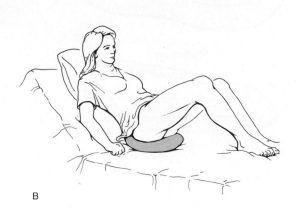

A   B

▼ **FIGURE 16–2.** Supporting the client's hips while positioning the bedpan (A). The bedpan in place (B).

9. If the client is unable to assist, roll him or her to one side.

9. Lessens the strain on your back.

10. Place the bedpan against the client's buttocks and roll him or her back onto the bedpan (Fig. 16–3). Place pressure on the bedpan to keep it under the client when he or she turns. This may require another person's assistance.

10. If the bedpan is placed against the client's buttocks, it will be in the proper position when the client rolls back.

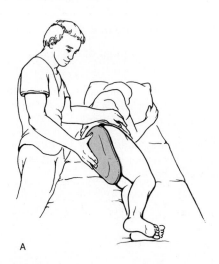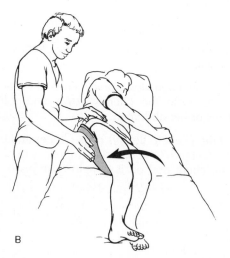

A   B

▼ **FIGURE 16–3.** Placing the bedpan against the client's buttocks (A) and turning the client back onto the bedpan (B).

11. Cover the client with the top linen.

11. Prevents exposure of the client.

12. If permitted, raise the client to a sitting position (see Fig. 16–2B).

12. An upright position facilitates defecation and urination.

13. Place the call light within the client's reach. Instruct the client not to put toilet paper in the bedpan if the output is to be measured or if a specimen is needed.

13. The call light gives the client a feeling of security and enables the client to call you quickly if assistance is needed.

▼ _ACTION_	▼ _RATIONALE_
14. To remove the bedpan, put on gloves and repeat Steps 5 to 7.	**14.** Gloves should be worn to prevent the possible transmission of microorganisms when there is a chance of coming into contact with any body fluid.
15. If necessary, help the client to cleanse his or her perineal area. Remember to cleanse from the pubic area to the anal area.	**15.** Cleanse from the pubic area to the anal area to prevent contamination of the pubic area with fecal material (i.e., _Escherichia coli_).
16. Replace the client's gown and top linens.	**16.** Helps the client to maintain privacy.
17. Offer the client a clean wet washcloth and towel to cleanse his or her hands.	**17.** Provides comfort for the client and prevents the spread of microorganisms.
18. Assess the client's urine or feces for the color, amount, consistency, and presence of any abnormal constituents.	**18.** These data are necessary for charting.
19. Empty the bedpan into the toilet and clean it. If the client's output is being measured, note the amount.	**19.** Proper cleaning decreases offensive odors and prevents the growth and spread of microorganisms.
20. Remove the gloves and wash your hands.	**20.** Prevents the possible transmission of microorganisms
21. Return the clean, dry bedpan to the bedside table.	**21.** The bedpan is clean and ready for use the next time it is needed.
22. Record the results. Note the amount, color, and consistency of the urine or feces.	**22.** Communicates the findings to the other members of the health care team and contributes to the legal record by documenting the care given to the client.

Example of Documentation

DATE	TIME	NOTES
10/18/93	0900	Voided 120 ml clear yellow urine. No blood, pus, or sediment noted.
		S. Williams, RN

Teaching Tips

The importance of emptying and cleaning the bedpan after each use should be stressed to the client's caregiver. The caregiver also should be encouraged to give the client a washcloth to wash his or her hands after using the bedpan and the caregiver should wash his or her hands after handling the bedpan.

Home Care Variations

Bedpans can be used in the home of any client who is confined to bed.

SKILL 16–3 ASSISTING THE MALE CLIENT WITH A URINAL

Clinical Situations in Which You May Encounter This Skill

A urinal is used for male clients who are unable to ambulate to the toilet or whose intake and output are being measured. Unless contraindicated, the client should stand beside the bed.

Anticipated Responses

▼ The client is able to urinate into the urinal successfully.

Adverse Responses

▼ The client is unable to urinate into the urinal.

Materials List

Gather these materials before beginning the skill:

▼ Urinal
▼ Washcloth and towel
▼ Examination gloves

▼ ACTION	▼ RATIONALE
1. Check the physician's order regarding restrictions in the client's movement.	1. Lets you know if the client is allowed to stand.
2. Screen the client by closing the door and the curtains around the bed.	2. Provides privacy for the client.
3. Put on gloves.	3. Gloves should be worn to prevent the possible transmission of microorganisms when there is a chance of coming into contact with any body fluid.
4. For the client confined to the bed: a. Fold the top linen down and across the client's abdomen. Raise the client's gown and fold it across his abdomen. b. Place the urinal between the client's legs with the bottom portion of the urinal resting on the bed. The handle side should be on top away from the bed. If necessary, place the client's penis into the urinal (Fig. 16–4).	a. Prevents the linen and gown from being soiled and provides access for you to place the urinal. b. This position makes it easier for the client to use the urinal and helps to prevent spilling.

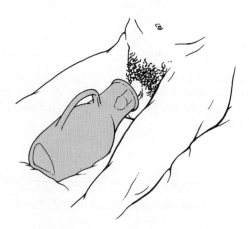

▼ FIGURE 16–4. The urinal in place.

5. If the client is able to stand, help him to assume a standing position beside the bed and hand him the urinal. Stay with the client if necessary.	5. This is the normal position for a man and it facilitates the male client's ability to urinate.

▼ *ACTION*	▼ *RATIONALE*
6. Place the call light within the client's reach.	**6.** The call light gives the client a feeling of security and enables him to call you quickly if assistance is needed.
7. Assess the color and amount of urine and the presence of any sediment in the urine.	**7.** These data are necessary for charting.
8. Remove the urinal, empty it, and rinse it out. If the client's output is being measured, note the amount.	**8.** Proper cleaning decreases offensive odors and prevents the growth and spread of microorganisms.
9. Help the client to clean himself. Offer a clean washcloth to the client for him to wash his hands.	**9.** Promotes a sense of well-being.
10. Return the clean dry urinal to the bedside area.	**10.** The urinal is ready for the next time that it is needed.
11. Remove the gloves and wash your hands.	**11.** Prevents the possible transmission of microorganisms.
12. Record the results. Note the color, amount, and odor of the urine.	**12.** Communicates the findings to the other members of the health care team and contributes to the legal record by documenting the care given to the client.

Example of Documentation

DATE	TIME	NOTES
10/18/93	0930	Voided 90 ml of clear yellow urine. No sediment noted.
		S. Williams, RN

Teaching Tips

The importance of emptying and cleaning the urinal after each use should be stressed to the client's caregiver. The caregiver also should be encouraged to give the client a washcloth to wash his hands after using the urinal and the caregiver should wash his or her hands after handling the urinal.

Home Care Variations

Urinals can be used in the home of any client who is confined to bed. Instruct the person's family to rinse the urinal well after each use.

SKILL 16–4   INSERTING AN INDWELLING CATHETER

Clinical Situations in Which You May Encounter This Skill

A retention (indwelling) catheter (Fig. 16–5) facilitates continuous drainage of urine. A retention catheter may be inserted into a client prior to an operation or delivery of a baby to maintain an empty bladder. It also may be inserted into clients who are unable to void spontaneously because of anesthesia, surgery, trauma, or a disease process. It is used to instill medications, splint the urethra, or obtain an accurate measurement of urinary output of clients with renal or cardiac disease, burns, or shock.

This is a sterile procedure and surgical asepsis should be used. The most common complication of a catheterization is a urinary tract infection.

Anticipated Responses

▼ You use sterile technique to insert the catheter without contamination or trauma to the client.
▼ Urine flows through the catheter into the drainage bag.

A. Single lumen

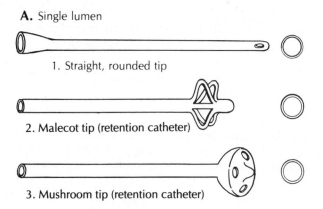

1. Straight, rounded tip

2. Malecot tip (retention catheter)

3. Mushroom tip (retention catheter)

B. Double lumen (Retention catheter with rounded tip)

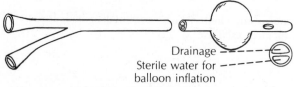

Drainage
Sterile water for
balloon inflation

C. Triple lumen (Retention catheter with coude tip)

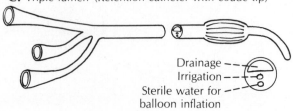

Drainage
Irrigation
Sterile water for
balloon inflation

▼ **FIGURE 16–5.** Types of indwelling catheters.

Adverse Responses

▼ The catheter meets an obstruction and cannot be inserted. This may occur in the male client because of hypertrophy of the prostate.
▼ There is no drainage of urine.
▼ The catheter is inserted into the client's vaginal orifice instead of the urinary meatus.

Materials List

Gather these materials before beginning the skill:

▼ Sterile prepackaged catheter insertion kit containing:
    Indwelling catheter:
        Adult female: size 14–16 French
        Adult male: size 18–20 French
        Infant or child: size 8–10 French
    Gravity drainage bag
    Prefilled syringe containing sterile water
    Cotton balls
    Disinfectant solution
    Sterile gloves
    Small waterproof pad
    Fenestrated drape
    Forceps
    Water-soluble lubricant
▼ Disposable waterproof linen protector
▼ Washcloth and towel
▼ Tape
▼ Soap and basin of warm water
▼ Adequate light source

▼ *A C T I O N*

▼ *R A T I O N A L E*

1. Check the client's chart for a physician's order and the reason for the catheterization.

2. Assess the client's ability to follow directions and cooperate.

3. Screen the client by closing the door and the curtains around the bed.

4. Raise the bed to a comfortable working height.

5. Position the client. A female client should be placed in the dorsal-recumbent position with her feet spread apart. The male client should be placed in the supine position with his legs together. Raise the client's penis and scrotal sac to rest on top of his legs.

6. a. For the female: Place the drape over the client in a diamond configuration with one corner over each knee and one corner over the perineum. One corner is then wrapped securely around each of the client's feet (Fig. 16–6).

1. A physician's order is required. The reason for the catheter should be explained to the client.

2. It may be necessary for another nurse to assist you if the client is uncooperative or unable to assist.

3. Protects the client's privacy.

4. Protects your back from strain.

5. These positions facilitate visibility of the urinary meatus.

6. Alllows you to expose the client's perineal area while covering the rest of the body.

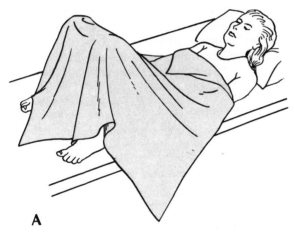

A

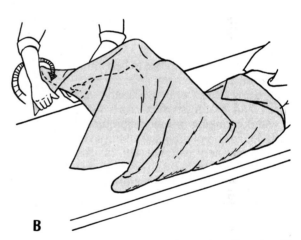

B

▼ **FIGURE 16–6.** Draping for catheterization of the female client. The drape is placed over the client in a diamond configuration *(A)* and corners are wrapped securely around the client's feet *(B)*.

b. For the male: Cover the client's chest with a folded sheet and place a towel under his penis (Fig. 16–7).

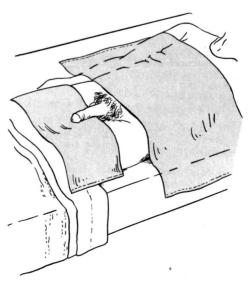

▼ **FIGURE 16–7.** Draping for catheterization of the male client.

▼ *ACTION*

▼ *RATIONALE*

7. Place a waterproof pad under the client's buttocks.

7. Prevents the bed linens from becoming soiled.

8. Wash the client's genital area with warm water and soap. Rinse and dry the area.

8. Removes secretions and feces.

9. Using sterile technique, open the sterile prepackaged catheter insertion kit.
   a. For the female: Open the kit on the bed between the client's feet.
   b. For the male: Place the overbed table over the bed at the level of the client's knees and open the kit on the overbed table.

9. The inside of the wrapper becomes your sterile working field.

10. Remove the sterile pad, open it at the corners so as not to contaminate the pad, and place it between female client's legs under the perineal area. For the male client, place the pad on the client's thighs.

10. The pad becomes an extension of the sterile work area.

11. Remove the sterile gloves from the package and put them on using sterile technique (see Skill 1–7).

11. Sterile technique prevents the introduction of microorganisms into the urinary tract, which is normally sterile.

12. Remove the fenestrated drape and place it over the client's genital area so that only the genitalia are exposed. Do not move the drape once it has touched the client's skin. Prevent your gloved hands from touching the client's skin.

12. The drape provides minimal exposure of the client. The client's skin is contaminated and if your gloved hands touch the skin they will become contaminated. If moved, the drape also will become contaminated.

13. Open the disinfectant solution and pour it over the cotton balls.

13. Cotton balls are used to cleanse the urinary meatus.

14. Attach the prefilled syringe to the balloon port. Test the balloon by filling it with the sterile water in the syringe. Then deflate the balloon. Retain the solution for inflating the balloon once the catheter is inserted into the bladder.

14. The syringe is used to inflate the balloon around the catheter tip inside the bladder. Testing the balloon prior to insertion ensures that it is free of leaks.

15. Open the water-soluble lubricant and lubricate the tip of the catheter approximately 2 inches for a female client and the entire length of the catheter to the bifurcation for a male client.

15. The lubricant decreases friction between the catheter and the urinary meatus during catheter insertion. The female urethra is approximately 2 inches long and the male urethra is approximately 6 inches long.

▼ *ACTION*

▼ *RATIONALE*

16. a. For the female: Using the thumb and forefinger (or forefinger and middle finger) of your nondominant hand, spread the person's labia (Fig. 16–8). The labia should not be allowed to close during the procedure. If the labia do close, you should stop the procedure and start over at this step.

16. a. Closing the labia causes contamination once the perineal cleansing has begun.

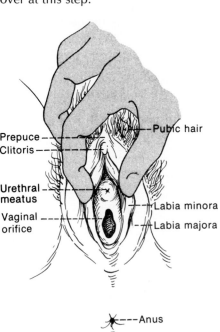

Prepuce
Clitoris
Pubic hair

Urethral meatus

Labia minora
Vaginal orifice
Labia majora

Anus

▼ **FIGURE 16–8.** Spreading the labia.

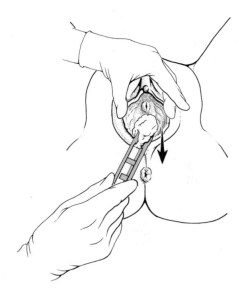

▼ **FIGURE 16–9.** Cleansing the meatus with one downward stroke.

b. For the male: Use your nondominant hand to position the client's penis perpendicular to his body.

17. Grasp the forceps in your dominant hand and pick up a cotton ball containing disinfectant solution.
  a. For the female: Using a separate cotton ball for each stroke, cleanse each side of the meatus with one downward stroke (Fig. 16–9). Then cleanse from the meatus to the rectum with one stroke. Do not let the labia come together.
  b. For the male: Cleanse the penis using a circular motion from the meatus to the base of the penis (Fig. 16–10). Retract the foreskin on the uncircumcised male. The meatus and penis should be cleansed several more times with a new, sterile disinfectant-soaked cotton ball each time.

17. The area around the meatus is cleansed to prevent contamination of the catheter by microorganisms.

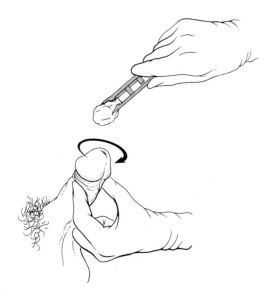

▼ **FIGURE 16–10.** Cleansing the penis using a circular motion.

▼ _A C T I O N_   ▼ _R A T I O N A L E_

18. Visualize the urinary meatus, which may be near or in the anterior vaginal orifice in elderly or multiparous clients. Use of a flashlight or lamp may be necessary in order to locate the meatus on the female client.

18. The meatus may be difficult to locate on some female clients and extra light may be necessary.

19. Lift the lubricated tip of the catheter and gently insert it into the meatus. Ask the client to take a deep breath while you insert the catheter. The labia should still be spread with your nondominant hand (Fig. 16–11). For the male, the foreskin should still be retracted and the penis should be held firmly and perpendicular to the client's body (Fig. 16–12).

19. When the client takes a deep breath, it will help to relax the urinary meatus. Since gentle pressure may cause an erection, the penis is held firmly but not tightly. If the penis is held tightly, pressure collapses the urethra and prevents advancement of the catheter. If the male has an erection, stop the procedure until there is a nonerectile state. You should start the procedure again at the beginning.

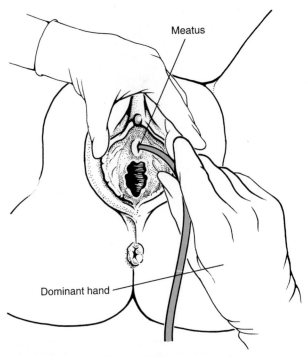

Meatus

Dominant hand

▼ **FIGURE 16–11.** Holding the labia apart with the nondominant hand while inserting the catheter tip into the meatus.

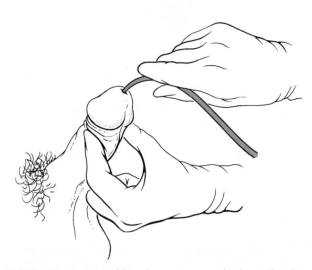

▼ **FIGURE 16–12.** Holding the penis perpendicular to the client's body for catheterization.

20. Insert the catheter 2 to 3 inches for adult females until urine begins to flow. Then insert another inch. Insert the catheter to the bifurcation of the catheter for adult males. Take care not to touch the perineal hair or skin as the catheter is advanced. If obstruction is encountered, do not force the catheter.

20. The female's urethra is approximately 2 inches long. Inserting the catheter to 3 inches plus an additional inch prevents possible trauma to the urethral wall when the balloon is inflated. The male's urethra is approximately 6 inches long or longer. In the male the catheter is inserted to the bifurcation to prevent possible trauma to the urethral wall when the balloon is inflated. Hair or skin could contaminate the catheter. Forcing the catheter can cause trauma, bleeding, and possible scar formation that can lead to strictures and obstruction of the urethra.

▼ _A C T I O N_   ▼ _R A T I O N A L E_

21. Inject the sterile water according to the amount specified on the balloon port. Figure 16–13 shows correct catheter placement with the balloon inflated.

21. Prevents the catheter from slipping out. If the client complains of pain, aspirate the fluid and insert the catheter a little farther and attempt to inflate the balloon again. Since overfilling can cause rupture of the balloon, use only the amount specified.

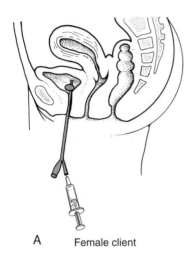
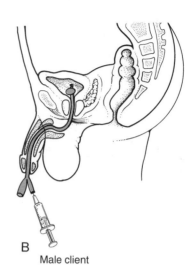

A   Female client   B   Male client

▼ **FIGURE 16–13.** Catheter with the balloon inflated in the bladder.

22. Gently tug on the catheter with your nondominant hand.

22. Ensures that the catheter is securely in the bladder.

23. Disconnect the syringe.

24. Return the foreskin on the uncircumcised male.

24. Prevents impairment of circulation to the penis. Failure to return the foreskin can lead to swelling of the penis and complications.

25. If it is not connected already, connect the drainage bag to the catheter and attach it to the frame of the bed. The bag should be below the level of the client's bladder and the tubing should be between the side rails and the mattress. Extra tubing should be coiled on the bed and a short piece should be run directly to the bag. The tubing should have no obstructions, kinks, or dependent loops.

25. The drainage bag is positioned below the level of the client's bladder to prevent reflux of urine through the drainage tube and back into the bladder. Dangling tubing may impede the flow of urine.

26. Remove the gloves and wash your hands.

26. Prevents the possible transmission of microorganisms.

▼ *A C T I O N*　　　　　　　　　▼ *R A T I O N A L E*

27. Tape the catheter tubing to the thigh of the female client (Fig. 16–14) or to the abdomen or upper thigh of the male client (Fig. 16–15).

27. The catheter is taped to prevent any tension from being placed on the catheter inside the bladder. Also, the slipping of the catheter in and out of the urethra can cause contamination. The catheter is taped to the male's abdomen or upper thigh to prevent pressure, breakdown, scarring, and stricture at the penile-scrotal angle.

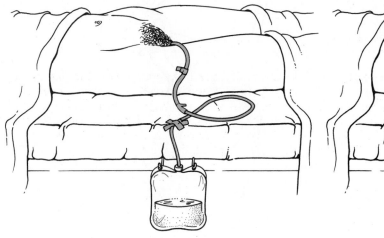

▼ **FIGURE 16–14.** The catheter tubing attached to a collection bag and taped to the bed and the female client's leg.

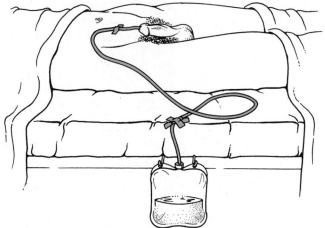

▼ **FIGURE 16–15.** The catheter tubing taped to the abdomen of the male client.

28. Cleanse the client and make him or her comfortable.

28. Increases the client's sense of well-being.

29. Remove and properly dispose of the contaminated equipment.

29. Prevents the transmission of microorganisms.

30. Return the client's bed to the lowest position.

30. Reduces potential injury to the client from falls.

31. Determine that urine is draining through the catheter into the bag and note the color and the presence of any sediment.

31. These data are necessary for charting.

32. Record the procedure. Note the time, date, catheter size, number of milliliters of sterile water in the balloon, whether urine was draining into the tubing and bag, the color of the urine, and the presence of any sediment.

32. Communicates the findings to the other members of the health care team and contributes to the legal record by documenting the care given to the client.

Example of Documentation

DATE	TIME	NOTES
10/18/93	1100	Unable to void 3 hours after surgery. Bladder palpable above the symphysis pubis. Number 16 French retention catheter inserted. Balloon inflated with 10 ml sterile water. Output = 400 ml clear yellow urine. *S. Williams, RN*

Teaching Tips

The purpose of the catheter and the procedure should be explained to the client and the client's caregiver. The client should be taught to always keep the catheter below the level of the bladder to prevent reflux and to make sure that the tubing does not become kinked or crimped. The client or caregiver should be told to report problems such as a catheter that is not draining urine or not draining adequate amounts of urine; cloudy or foul-smelling urine; or the presence of blood in the urine. Instruct the client to drink plenty of fluids (unless contraindicated) and to cleanse well after defecation. Also tell the client that he or she can move around with the catheter in place.

Home Care Variations

Many clients are discharged from the health care facility with an indwelling urinary catheter. The catheter should be changed at prescribed intervals. A visiting nurse, home health care nurse, or hospice nurse may be contacted to make visits to the home to check functioning of the catheter and to change the catheter at the prescribed intervals. However, the client and his or her caregiver should learn how to care for the catheter. Demonstrate how to perform hygienic care of the perineum or penis, how to empty the bag, and where to store the equipment.

SKILL 16–5 PROVIDING HYGIENIC CARE FOR A CLIENT WITH AN INDWELLING CATHETER

Clinical Situations in Which You May Encounter This Skill

Hygienic care should be performed at least twice daily for a client who has an indwelling catheter to prevent catheter-associated urinary tract infections. Microorganisms in the perineal area could cause a urinary tract infection.

Anticipated Responses

▼ The client's urinary meatus is cleansed and no signs of irritation or infection are noted.

Adverse Responses

▼ There are signs of irritation around the client's urinary meatus.
▼ There is vaginal drainage or discharge.

Materials List

Gather these materials before beginning the skill:

▼ Basin of warm water
▼ Waterproof pad
▼ Towel and washcloth
▼ Examination gloves
▼ Soap

▼ ACTION	▼ RATIONALE
1. Determine the length of time the catheter has been in place. Check the agency policy for how often the catheter can remain in place without being changed.	1. If the catheter has been in place for several days, it may need to be changed.
2. Ask if the client is having any pain from the catheter.	2. Pain could indicate a urinary tract infection.
3. Screen the client by closing the door and the curtains around the bed.	3. Provides for the client's privacy.
4. Put on gloves.	4. Gloves should be worn to prevent the possible transmission of microorganisms when there is a chance of coming into contact with any body fluid.

▼ A C T I O N	▼ R A T I O N A L E
5. Raise the client's gown and fold it across the client's abdomen.	5. Provides access to perineal area and prevents gown from being soiled.
6. Position the client. A female client should be placed on a bedpan with her feet spread apart. The male client should be placed in the supine position.	6. These positions facilitate visibility of the urinary meatus. The bedpan makes cleansing easier and more thorough for the female client.
7. Drape the client.	7. Decreases exposure and decreases client embarrassment.
8. Slide a waterproof pad under the hips of the female client or next to the male client.	8. Keeps the bed linen dry.
9. Use warm soapy water to cleanse around the client's urinary meatus and the catheter itself. Retract the foreskin on the uncircumcised male and cleanse the area. Then return the foreskin to its normal position.	9. Removes any drainage or feces that could enter the meatus and lead to a urinary tract infection. Failure to return the foreskin can lead to swelling of the penis and complications.
10. Do not manipulate the catheter tubing any more than necessary.	10. Movement of the catheter could cause organisms to enter the urinary tract.
11. Rinse and dry the client's perineum.	11. A warm, moist environment could lead to further growth of microorganisms.
12. Observe for any signs of irritation or trauma, secretions, or incrustation on the catheter. If these are noted, check the client's temperature for an elevation.	12. The catheter may need to be changed, repositioned, and retaped. These signs also can indicate a urinary tract infection.
13. Remove the waterproof pad and fold down the client's gown and top linens.	13. Helps the client to maintain privacy.
14. Remove the gloves and wash your hands.	14. Prevents the possible transmission of microorganisms.
15. Check that the tubing is properly positioned.	15. Promotes drainage of the urine through the tubing.
16. Note the color of the urine and the presence of any sediment.	16. The urine will appear cloudy and may contain sediment if the client has a urinary tract infection. These data are also necessary for charting.
17. Record the procedure in the client's chart.	17. Communicates the findings to the other members of the health care team and contributes to the legal record by documenting the care given to the client.

Example of Documentation

DATE	TIME	NOTES
10/18/93	1030	Perineal area cleansed with warm soapy water. No signs of irritation noted. Catheter draining clear, yellow urine.
		S. Williams, RN

Teaching Tips

The purpose of catheter care, the procedure, and the necessity for daily catheter care should be explained. The client's family or caregiver should be instructed to report any signs of irritation, infection, or drainage in the client's perineal area.

Home Care Variations

The same procedure can be used to provide catheter care in the client's home. The client's family or caregiver can be taught to provide catheter care.

SKILL 16–6 REMOVING AN INDWELLING CATHETER

Clinical Situations in Which You May Encounter This Skill

The indwelling retention catheter is removed when it is no longer needed, has been in place for a prolonged period of time and needs changing, or becomes obstructed with clots.

Anticipated Responses

▼ The balloon is deflated and the catheter is removed.

Adverse Responses

▼ The balloon does not deflate.
▼ The tip of the catheter contains crusts.

Materials List

Gather these materials before beginning the skill:

▼ Syringe (check the balloon portal to determine the size of the syringe needed)
▼ Waterproof pad
▼ Examination gloves
▼ Basin of warm soapy water
▼ Washcloth and towel
▼ 1,000-ml graduated container
▼ Bedpan

▼ *ACTION*	▼ *RATIONALE*
1. Check the client's chart for an order to discontinue the catheter.	1. A physician's order is required.
2. Determine the length of time that the catheter has been in place.	2. The client's bladder tone may be decreased if the catheter has been in place for a long period of time. Measures to help the client to void may be needed.
3. Screen the client by closing the door and the curtains around the bed.	3. Protects the client's privacy.
4. Put on gloves.	4. Gloves should be worn to prevent the possible transmission of microorganisms when there is a chance of coming into contact with any body fluid.
5. Raise the client's gown and fold it across the client's abdomen.	5. Provides access to perineal area and prevents gown from being soiled.
6. Position the client. A female client should be placed in the dorsal-recumbent position with her feet spread apart. The male client should be placed in the supine position.	6. These positions help you to see the client's urinary meatus.
7. Slide a waterproof pad under the hips of the female client or slide it under the penis and on top of the thighs of the male client.	7. Prevents any urinary leakage from soiling the bed linens.
8. Attach a syringe to the balloon portal and withdraw the solution from the balloon. The entire amount of the solution should be withdrawn from the balloon. The balloon capacity is stamped on the balloon port.	8. The balloon deflates when the solution is withdrawn. If the catheter is removed without fully deflating the balloon, it will cause trauma to the urethra and the urinary meatus.

▼ *ACTION*	▼ *RATIONALE*
9. Gently withdraw the catheter. Observe for any signs of irritation around the meatus.	9. The catheter is withdrawn slowly to reduce any irritation to the urethra or meatus.
10. Use warm soapy water to cleanse the client's perineal area.	10. The area is cleansed to remove any urine that may have leaked out, to remove secretions, and to increase the client's sense of well-being.
11. Rinse and dry the person's perineal area.	11. A warm, moist environment could lead to further growth of microorganisms.
12. Remove the waterproof pad and fold down the client's gown and top linens.	12. Helps to maintain the client's privacy.
13. Empty the drainage bag and measure the amount of urinary output.	13. An accurate measurement of urinary output is obtained prior to disposing of the drainage bag.
14. Properly dispose of the drainage bag, catheter, and tubing.	14. Prevents the transmission of microorganisms.
15. Place a urine collection container in the toilet or give a urinal to the male client, and instruct the client to measure the first voided specimen after the catheter is removed.	15. Allows you to assess the characteristics and volume of the urine.
16. Remove the gloves and wash your hands.	16. Prevents the possible transmission of microorganisms.
17. If the client has not voided in several hours, assess for bladder distention. When the client voids, note the amount and color of the urine and the presence of any sediment in the urine.	17. The client may have decreased bladder function after the catheter is removed. The amount of urine will determine if the client is able to fully empty the bladder. The urine may be cloudy and contain sediment if a urinary tract infection has developed.
18. In the client's chart, record the procedure and the amount of urinary output.	18. Communicates the findings to the other members of the health care team and contributes to the legal record by documenting the care given to the client.

Example of Documentation

DATE	*TIME*	*NOTES*
10/18/93	1030	Retention catheter removed. No signs of irritation of meatus noted. 750 ml urine in bag. Client instructed to void in toilet specimen container, to save the urine, and to drink plenty of fluids.
		S. Williams, RN
10/18/93	1230	Client voided 200 ml of clear, yellow urine. No sediment noted or pain upon urination.
		S. Williams, RN

Teaching Tips

The procedure for catheter removal should be explained to the client and his or her family or caregiver. The client's family or caregiver should be taught to assess the urinary output after the catheter is removed.

Home Care Variations

The client's family or caregiver can be taught to remove the catheter in the client's home using the same procedure. The used catheter can be put into a resealable plastic bag for disposal.

SKILL 16–7   APPLYING A CONDOM CATHETER

Clinical Situations in Which You May Encounter This Skill

The condom catheter is an external drainage system for urine that is used for male clients who have urinary incontinence. It should be removed at least once every 24 hours and hygienic care should be given. The condom catheter also may be referred to as an external catheter or a Texas catheter.

Anticipated Responses

▼ The client has an adequate urinary output through the condom catheter.

Adverse Responses

▼ The client's penis is irritated from the condom catheter.
▼ The client has an erection.

Materials List

Gather these materials before beginning the skill:

▼ Prepackaged kit containing condom catheter and double-sided adhesive strip
▼ Urinary drainage bag
▼ Razor
▼ Examination gloves
▼ Basin of warm water and soap
▼ Towel and washcloth

▼ *ACTION*	▼ *RATIONALE*
1. Assess the client's penis for any signs of irritation or skin breakdown.	1. The client may need to use a retention catheter if there is a significant amount of skin breakdown. This assessment also gives you baseline data to compare with future assessments.
2. Screen the client by closing the door and the curtains around the bed.	2. Provides privacy for the client.
3. Raise the bed to a comfortable position.	3. Protects you from back strain.
4. Put on gloves.	4. Gloves should be worn to prevent the possible transmission of microorganisms when there is a chance of coming into contact with any body fluid.
5. Raise the client's gown and fold it across the client's abdomen. Pull the sheet up over the client's legs.	5. Provides minimal exposure of the client, reducing the client's embarrassment.
6. Place the client in the supine position.	6. Facilitates cleansing of the client's penis and application of the condom catheter.
7. Cleanse the client's penis with warm soapy water. Retract the foreskin on the uncircumcised male and cleanse it.	7. This area is washed to remove the microorganisms present in any drainage or feces that could enter the urinary meatus and cause a urinary tract infection.

▼ *ACTION* — — — — — — — — — | ▼ *RATIONALE* — — — — — — — —

8. Return the person's foreskin to its normal position.

8. Failure to return the foreskin can lead to swelling of the penis and complications.

9. Shave any excess hair around the base of the penis.

9. Prevents additional discomfort from the adhesive strip when the condom catheter is removed.

10. Rinse and dry the area.

10. A warm, moist environment could lead to the growth of microorganisms.

11. If provided with the condom kit, open the package containing the skin preparation wipe and apply to the shaft of the penis. If the client has an erection, wait for it to terminate before applying the catheter.

11. Helps to protect the client's skin from irritation. An erection may occur due to manipulation of the penis while cleaning the area. This is a normal reaction and will terminate in a few minutes.

12. Apply the double-sided adhesive strip to the base of the client's penis in a spiral fashion. The strip is applied 1 inch from the proximal end of the penis. *Do not* completely encircle the penis.

12. Applying the adhesive in a spiral fashion does not compromise circulation in the penis. Encircling the penis can impair circulation.

13. Place the rolled condom at the distal portion of the penis and unroll it, covering the penis and the double-sided strip of adhesive. A 1- to 2-inch space should be left between the tip of the penis and the end of the condom.

13. The condom sticks to the adhesive and remains in place. The space prevents pressure and erosion of the tip of the penis.

14. Gently press the condom to the adhesive strip.

14. Causes the condom to adhere evenly to the adhesive strip.

15. Attach the drainage bag tubing to the catheter tubing and secure the drainage bag to the side of the bed below the level of the client's bladder or to the drainage bag attached to the leg (Fig. 16–16).

15. The drainage bag is positioned below the level of the client's bladder to prevent reflux of the urine onto the penis. The urine could irritate the penis.

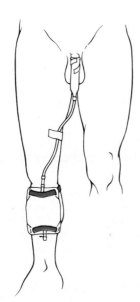

▼ **FIGURE 16–16.** Condom catheter with drainage bag attached to the client's leg.

▼ *ACTION*	▼ *RATIONALE*
16. Cover the client again.	**16.** Maintains the client's privacy and sense of well-being.
17. Dispose of the used equipment according to agency procedure.	**17.** Decreases the transmission of microorganisms.
18. Return the client's bed to the lowest position.	**18.** Reduces potential injury from falls.
19. Remove the gloves and wash your hands.	**19.** Prevents the possible transmission of microorganisms.
20. Determine that the condom and the tubing are not twisted.	**20.** If the condom or tubing is twisted, the urine cannot flow out and the condom will leak or come off.
21. Assess the client's urinary output.	**21.** It is important to determine that the output is normal.
22. Record the procedure in the client's chart.	**22.** Communicates the findings to the other members of the health care team and contributes to the legal record by documenting the care given to the client.

To give hygienic care for the condom catheter:

1. Remove the condom catheter by simultaneously unrolling the condom and the double-sided adhesive toward the distal end of the client's penis.	**1.** Both should be removed to provide good hygienic care.
2. Cleanse the penis with warm soapy water. Retract the foreskin on the uncircumcised male and cleanse. Rinse and dry the area.	**2.** Prevents skin irritation and reduces the possibility of bacterial growth.
3. Return the client's foreskin to its normal position.	**3.** Failure to return the foreskin can lead to swelling of the penis and complications.
4. Assess the client's penis for areas of redness or skin breakdown.	**4.** The condom catheter can lead to skin breakdown, which should be detected early and treated immediately.
5. Apply a new condom catheter as previously described.	

Example of Documentation

DATE	TIME	NOTES
10/18/93	1200	Voided three times in the bed. Condom catheter applied. No signs of irritation noted on penis. Purpose of condom catheter explained to Mr. B.'s family.

S. Williams, RN

Teaching Tips

The purpose and the procedure for applying a condom catheter and providing hygienic care should be explained to the client's family or caregiver. Stress that the condom should not be applied too tightly and the foreskin should be returned to its normal position if it has been retracted for cleansing. If the client has an erection during application, the client's family or caregiver should wait a little while before applying the condom catheter.

Home Care Variations

A family member or caregiver can be taught to apply a condom catheter to the client's penis and to provide hygienic care using the same skill in the client's home. The used condom catheter can be placed in a resealable bag for disposal.

SKILL 16–8 PERFORMING CONTINUOUS BLADDER IRRIGATION

Clinical Situations in Which You May Encounter This Skill

Continuous bladder irrigation is a closed irrigation system. An advantage of this type of system is the avoidance of bacterial contamination. A triple-lumen catheter is often inserted after bladder or prostate surgery for continuous bladder irrigation.

A triple-lumen catheter has three ports. An irrigation solution is connected to one port of the catheter at a set flow rate to continuously irrigate the bladder to flush out clots and mucus. The second port is used to inflate the balloon inside the bladder and the third port is connected to the urinary drainage bag (Fig. 16–17). Since fluid is constantly flowing into the bladder, the drainage bag should be emptied frequently. This procedure requires sterile technique.

Anticipated Responses

▼ Clots and mucus are flushed from the client's bladder.
▼ Irrigation fluid flows without obstruction into the client's bladder.
▼ Irrigation fluid and urine flow freely into the urinary drainage bag.

Adverse Responses

▼ The output is less than or only equal to the total amount of fluid instilled.

Materials List

Gather these materials before beginning the skill:

▼ 3,000-ml bag of irrigation solution (usually normal saline with an antibiotic added)
▼ Irrigation tubing
▼ IV pole
▼ Alcohol wipes
▼ Graduated container
▼ Triple-lumen urinary catheter with drainage bag (this is usually inserted in surgery)

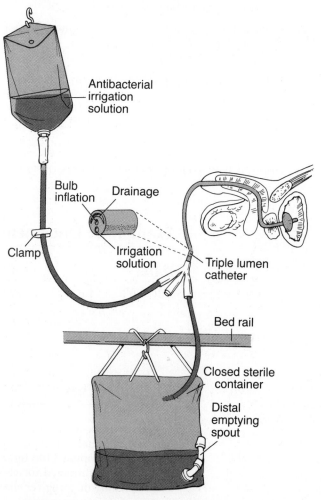

▼ FIGURE 16–17. Continuous bladder irrigation system.

▼ _ACTION_ _____   ▼ _RATIONALE_ _____

1. Check the physician's order for the type of fluid, any drugs added, and the flow rate.

2. Check the diagnosis of the medical condition and the purpose of the irrigation.

3. Screen the client by closing the door and the curtains around the bed.

4. Using sterile technique, close the clamp on the tubing and insert the irrigation tubing spike into the portal on the bag of irrigation fluid.

5. Open the clamp on the tubing and allow the fluid to flow to the end of the tubing.

6. Close the clamp.

7. Hang the bag of irrigating solution on an IV pole 3 feet above the level of the client's bladder.

8. Squeeze the drip chamber to one-half to one-third full.

9. Using sterile technique, wipe off the inflow port of the catheter and connect the irrigation tubing to the inflow port of the catheter.

10. If the urinary drainage bag has not been attached to the outflow port, one should be attached at this time.

11. Open the irrigation tubing clamp and adjust the flow rate according to the prescribed flow rate.

12. Wash your hands.

13. After approximately 15 minutes:
    a. Assess the color of the drainage in the outflow system. If the drainage is bright red, check the client's vital signs and notify the physician.
    b. Assess the client's bladder for distention.

    c. Assess for clots in the outflow tubing. If clots are present, milk or strip the tubing. To milk, place your nondominant hand on the outflow tubing proximal to the client. Use your dominant hand and use a squeezing and gently pulling motion on the tubing in a direction away from the client toward the drainage bag.

14. Record the procedure in the client's chart. Note the volume of the solution hung, the flow rate, the type of solution, and the observations regarding drainage and distention.

1. A physician's order is required. Allows correct fluid and additives to be hung.

2. Alerts you to the observations you will need to make. For example, if the irrigation is hung for a client who had urinary tract surgery, you would expect to possibly see urine that is pinkish in color and contains clots.

3. Protects the client's privacy.

4. The irrigation tubing connects the irrigation solution to the catheter.

5. Replaces the air in the tubing with irrigation fluid.

6. Prevents spilling of irrigation fluid.

7. The fluid flows by gravity into the bladder.

8. If the drip chamber is overfilled, you will not be able to see and satisfactorily count the flow rate.

9. The solution flows from the bag through the inflow port and into the bladder.

10. The irrigation fluid and urine flow out through the outflow port into the drainage bag.

11. The flow rate varies according to the type of solution used.

12. Decreases the possible transmission of microorganisms.

   a. The drainage in the outflow system should be pink, dark pink, or clear. Bright red drainage could indicate fresh bleeding or hemorrhage.
   b. If there is an obstruction to urinary outflow, the bladder becomes distended as it is filled with irrigating solution.
   c. The nondominant hand is used to stabilize the outflow tubing and keep it from being pulled out of the client. The squeezing and pulling motion by the dominant hand moves the clots toward the drainage bag.

14. Communicates the findings to the other members of the health care team and contributes to the legal record by documenting the care given to the client.

▼ ACTION	▼ RATIONALE

*To calculate urinary output:**

1. Empty the drainage bag into a graduated container.

2. Subtract the amount of solution infused over a specific time period from the total output for that same time period.

1. A graduated container is necessary to get an accurate measurement of the urine.

2. The drainage bag contains both urine and irrigating solution. By subtracting the amount of irrigating solution (inflow) from the total amount of drainage (outflow), you get the actual output.

Example of Documentation

DATE	TIME	NOTES
10/18/93	1100	Continuous bladder irrigation begun for Mr. B upon return from surgery for transurethral resection of prostate. 3,000 ml normal saline connected to inflow port and is infusing at 40 drops/minute. Urine is dark pink without clots. Urine flowing freely into drainage bag.
		S. Williams, RN

Teaching Tips

The purpose of the continuous bladder irrigation should be explained to the client and his or her family. The client should be encouraged not to lie down on the drainage tubing or let the tubing become kinked. The collection bag should stay below the level of the bladder.

Home Care Variations

This procedure usually is not performed in the client's home.

Usually calculated once per shift at end of shift, more often if client's output is low.

SKILL 16–9   CARING FOR THE CLIENT WITH A URINARY DIVERSION

Clinical Situations in Which You May Encounter This Skill

A urinary diversion may be created for a client who has a urinary tract dysfunction from disease, trauma, or congenital anomaly. There are several types of urinary diversion operations: ileal conduit, cutaneous ureterostomy, ureterosigmoidostomy, and Kock pouch (Fig. 16–18). The client with an ileal conduit or cutaneous ureterostomy should wear an external ostomy appliance (Fig. 16–19) because of continuous urine drainage and requires urinostomy care. The best time to change the appliance is prior to breakfast since there is less urinary drainage at this time.

Anticipated Responses

▼ After a demonstration of skin care and bag changes, the client is able to perform these procedures.
▼ The client's skin integrity is good with no signs of irritation or breakdown.

Adverse Responses

▼ The client refuses to look at the stoma.
▼ The client has difficulty learning or does not want to learn the procedure.
▼ The client's skin appears irritated from leakage of urine.
▼ The client's stoma appears dark.

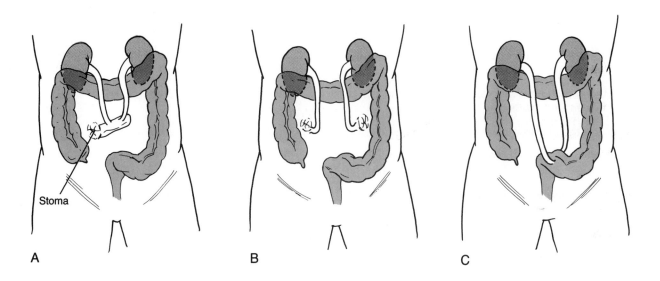

A   B   C

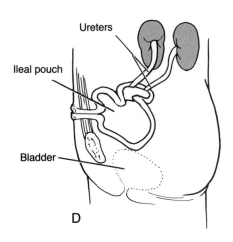

D

▼ **FIGURE 16–18.** Methods of urinary surgical diversion: ileal conduit *(A)*, cutaneous ureterostomy *(B)*, ureterosigmoidostomy *(C)*, and Kock pouch *(D)*.

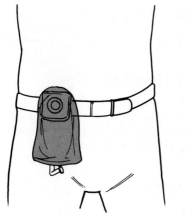

▼ **FIGURE 16–19.** Appliance for management of urinary diversion.

Materials List

Gather these materials before beginning the skill:

▼ Basin of warm soapy water
▼ Towel and washcloth
▼ Measuring guide
▼ Appliance
▼ Karaya paste
▼ Skin prep
▼ Skin barrier
▼ Scissors
▼ Waterproof tape (1 inch)
▼ 4- × 4-inch gauze pads
▼ 1,000-ml graduated container
▼ Waterproof pad × 2
▼ Plastic bag
▼ Examination gloves
▼ Graduated container

▼ *A C T I O N*

▼ *R A T I O N A L E*

1. Assess the client's readiness to learn the urostomy care.

   1. The client's ability to learn is affected by the readiness to learn.

2. Assess the client's knowledge of the procedure.

   2. You can individualize the teaching based on the client's knowledge and acceptance.

3. Screen the client by closing the door and the curtains around the bed.

   3. Protects the client's privacy.

4. Raise the bed to a comfortable working height.

   4. Protects you from back strain.

5. Place the client in either a supine or sitting position.

   5. The sitting position allows the client to observe the procedure.

6. Position the client's gown and place a waterproof pad around the edge of the gown and on the bed beside the client.

   6. The gown is positioned so that you can access the ostomy. A waterproof pad is placed to protect the client's gown.

7. Put on gloves.

   7. Gloves should be worn to prevent the possible transmission of microorganisms when there is a chance of coming into contact with any body fluid.

8. Explain each of the steps to the client.

   8. Explanations are necessary for the client to learn to do the procedure.

9. Empty the appliance and observe the color and clarity of the urine.

   9. Prevents spilling of the urine when the appliance is removed.

10. Loosen the skin barrier with a 4- × 4-inch gauze pad soaked in alcohol.

    10. The alcohol loosens the adhesive on the back of the barrier.

11. Support the client's skin and gently pull the barrier and bag diagonally away from the client.

    11. There will be less pulling and skin irritation when the appliance is removed diagonally.

12. Place the used appliance in the plastic bag and discard it.

    12. Helps to prevent the spread of microorganisms.

13. Place a rolled 4- × 4-inch gauze pad in the opening of the stoma.

    13. The rolled pad will absorb any urinary leakage from the stoma until a new ostomy appliance can be applied.

14. Wash the skin around the stoma with warm water and mild soap and wash the stoma with clear water.

    14. The area is cleansed to decrease the growth of microorganisms and to prevent skin irritation from the adhesive.

▼ *ACTION*

▼ *RATIONALE*

15. Rinse and pat the area dry.

15. The skin barrier will not stick to moist skin. Wetness causes skin excoriation and breakdown. Rubbing can irritate the skin.

16. Assess the color, moisture, and protrusion of the stoma and the condition of the surrounding skin.

16. It is easiest to fit an appliance over a protruding stoma. The stoma should be pink and moist. A dark color can indicate poor circulation and necrosis. Other problems can include hematoma, poor placement of the stoma, stenosis, and retraction. The client also may develop dermatitis or a yeast infection of the skin around the stoma.

17. Measure the stoma with the stoma measuring guide, trace the stoma size on the skin barrier, and cut out a hole.

17. The skin barrier must fit snugly around the stoma to prevent skin irritation and leakage.

18. Add one-eighth to one-sixteenth inch to the measured size and trace that size on the back of the appliance and cut out the hole.

18. The skin barrier and appliance should closely approximate the edges of the stoma. If not, the skin will be in constant contact with urine, which will lead to skin breakdown.

19. Prepare the barrier and the appliance to be applied as a unit by removing the paper from the adhesive side of the appliance and positioning it over the skin barrier.

19. It is easiest to apply the barrier and appliance as a unit.

20. Gently smooth the adhesive to remove all air bubbles.

20. A good seal is necessary to prevent leakage of urine onto the skin.

21. If the stoma borders are irregular, fill in the irregularities with karaya paste.

21. Prevents urine from undermining the skin barrier and the appliance and causing skin breakdown.

22. Remove the gauze pad from the stoma.

22. When the appliance is in place, you cannot remove the gauze.

23. To apply the unit as a whole, remove the paper from the adhesive side of the skin barrier and apply it around the stoma. Place the appliance so the bag hangs in a dependent position.

23. The adhesive is smoothed to provide a good seal.

24. Attach the dependent edge first.

24. Prevents leakage before the entire appliance is attached.

25. Smooth down the adhesive around the stoma.

25. Provides a good seal.

26. Close the outlet port at the bottom of the appliance (see Fig. 16–19).

26. Urine drains out of the port.

27. Place 1-inch waterproof tape around the outer edges in a picture-frame fashion (optional). A belt also may be used to hold the appliance in place.

27. The tape makes the appliance more secure.

28. Cover the client and remove the contaminated equipment.

28. Maintains the client's privacy and promotes his or her sense of well-being.

29. Return the client's bed to the lowest position.

29. Reduces potential injury from falls.

30. Remove the gloves and wash your hands.

30. Decreases the possible transmission of microorganisms.

31. Assess the appliance to determine that it adheres smoothly to the skin and that it is not leaking.

31. If the appliance does leak, it should be reapplied.

32. Ask the client if he or she has any questions about the procedure.

32. Questions should be answered immediately to help the client understand and retain the information.

▼ *ACTION*	▼ *RATIONALE*
33. Record the procedure. Note the appearance of the skin and the stoma. Also note the color, amount, and odor of the urine.	33. Communicates the findings to the other members of the health care team and contributes to the legal record by documenting the care given to the client.

Example of Documentation

DATE	TIME	NOTES
10/20/93	1100	Urostomy appliance changed. Stoma pink, moist, and flush with the skin. Skin intact with no redness. 200 ml of clear, yellow urine.
		S. Williams, RN

Teaching Tips

The purpose of and the procedure for caring for a urinary diversion should be explained to the client and the client's family or caregiver. Mucus secretion in the urine is a normal occurrence and the client or family should not be alarmed by it. Encourage the client to have an increased fluid intake to maintain an adequate flow of urine. The appliance should be emptied when it is approximately one-third full. The client should report any signs and symptoms of infection such as an increased temperature, pain in the abdomen or back, and nausea and vomiting. The client also should report a decrease in or absence of urine drainage.

Home Care Variations

The client and his or her family or caregiver can be taught to care for the urinary diversion using this same procedure in the client's home. The used appliance can be placed in a resealable bag for disposal.

References

Classen, D. C., et al. (1991). Daily meatal care for prevention of catheter-associated bacteriuria: Results using frequent applications of polyantibiotic cream. *Infection Control and Hospital Epidemiology*, 12 (3), 157–162.

Classen, D. C., et al. (1991). Prevention of catheter-associated bacteriuria: Clinical trial of methods to block three known pathways of infection. *American Journal of Infection Control*, 19 (3), 136–142.

Dodaro-Surrusco, D., and Zweig, N. (1994). Meeting urinary elimination needs. In V. Bolander (Ed.), *Basic nursing* (3rd ed.). Philadelphia: W. B. Saunders.

Dodds, P., and Hans, A. L. (1990). Distended urinary bladder drainage practices among hospital nurses. *Applied Nursing Research*, 3 (2), 68–69.

Ehrenkranz, N. J., and Alfonso, B. C. (1991). Failure of bland soap handwash to prevent hand transfer of patient bacteria to urethral catheters. *Infection Control and Hospital Epidemiology*, 12 (11), 654–662.

CHAPTER 17

Meeting Respiratory Needs

- -

You have the primary responsibility for monitoring the client's respiratory status. Since changes in the client's respiratory status can occur quickly, you must make frequent assessments and monitor arterial blood gases and the results of pulse oximetry. Clients with impaired oxygenation require the administration of oxygen. The physician orders the amount of oxygen and the method of delivery. You or the respiratory therapist sets up the oxygen equipment, and you monitor the effects of the oxygen therapy on the client.

If a client has difficulty breathing or maintaining a patent (open) airway, an artifical airway such as an endotracheal tube or tracheostomy tube may be inserted. You must keep the artificial airway free of respiratory secretions by suctioning. You must also supervise the administration of oxygen through the airway and provide the care necessary to prevent complications from the presence of the airway.

- -

- -

OVERVIEW OF RELATED RESEARCH

ARTERIAL BLOOD GASES

Preusser, B. A., et al. (1989). Quantifying the minimum discard sample required for accurate arterial blood gases. *Nursing Research*, 38 (5), 276–279.

There are questions about the amount of blood that should be discarded from arterial lines prior to drawing a blood sample for arterial blood gases. A study was conducted "to quantify the minimum discard sample required to remove all heparinized flush solution from an indwelling arterial catheter prior to the withdrawal of an arterial blood gas sample in order to obtain accurate pH, PCO_2, PO, and HCO_3 values." A review of related literature was presented, followed by the method for the collection of data. The results suggest that a 2-cc (2 ml) discard is required for accurate determination of all four values in situations when the heparinized arterial system deadspace volume measures 1 cc. The authors further state that these results should *not* be applied to hypoxic blood. They suggest that further studies be conducted to look at the accuracy of other laboratory values in relation to the amount of the discard sample.

ASSISTING A CLIENT WITH AN INCENTIVE SPIROMETER

Davies, B. L., Macleod, J. P., and Ogilvie, H. M. J. (1990). The efficacy of incentive spirometers in postoperative protocols for low-risk patients. *The Canadian Journal of Nursing Research*, 22 (4), 19–36.

This study compared the effectiveness of incentive spirometry to deep breathing and coughing in low-risk surgical patients with no history of respiratory problems. A third control group received the usual preoperative teaching. The researchers found no differences among the three groups in their postoperative pulmonary status.

SUCTIONING WITH AN ENDOTRACHEAL TUBE

Clark, A. P., et al. (1990). Effects of endotracheal suctioning on mixed venous oxygen saturation and heart rate in critically ill adults. *Heart and Lung*, 19, 552–557.

Mixed venous oxygen saturation measurements and recordings were collected from 189 critically ill adults before and after endotracheal tube suctioning. A closed-system method of suctioning was used for 62 patients and 127 patients were removed from the ventilator, manually hyperoxygenated and ventilated, suctioned, manually hyperoxygenated and ventilated again, and reconnected to the ventilator. No significant differences between the two groups were found in relation to baseline mixed oxygen venous saturation or heart rate. A statistically significant decrease from baseline values was found in the mixed venous oxygen saturation immediately after suctioning for the overall sample. A decrease of 4% from baseline occurred and the values returned to baseline within 3 minutes. However, for the closed-suction method group, no decrease was noted after suctioning. A statistically significant difference was also found in the heart rate values before and after suctioning. No difference was found in heart rate in relation to the method of suctioning.

Stone, K. S., et al. (1989). Effects of lung hyperinflation on mean arterial pressure and postsuctioning hypoxemia. *Heart and Lung*, 18, 377–385.

Data were collected from 8 subjects "to determine the effect of five different lung hyperinflation volumes (tidal volume, 12 cc/kg, 14 cc/kg, 16 cc/kg, and 18 cc/kg lean body weight) on mean arterial pressure and postsuctioning hypoxemia (arterial blood gasses)" (p. 377). No relationships were found between the O_2 saturation, CO_2, partial pressure of arterial carbon dioxide, mean arterial pressure, and the five different lung hyperinflation volumes.

Tyler, D. O., Clark, A. P., and Ogburn-Russell, L. (1991). Developing a standard for endotracheal tube cuff care. *Dimensions of Critical Care Nursing*, 10 (2), 54–61.

The investigators were concerned about the incidence of complications from tracheal intubation. The study consisted of a two-page survey that was mailed to critical care nurses. The survey asked questions "to identify the types and frequency of methods used by critical care nurses to prevent complications from endotracheal tubes." The survey results showed a variety of methods used by the respondents. Approximately 50% used intracuff pressure monitoring (IPM). Respiratory therapists and critical care nurses shared the cuff care, although most of the IPM was done by respiratory therapists. Some respondents did not use either minimal occlusive volume (MOV) or minimal leak technique (MLT) and approximately 50% did not measure cuff pressures. Some respondents also mentioned that no policy existed that addressed methods of cuff care. The authors suggest that the practice of appropriately using MLT or MOV in cuff care should be incorporated into standards of care for patients with cuffed endotracheal tubes.

MANAGING A CHEST TUBE

Gift, A. G., Bolgiano, C. S., and Cunningham, J. (1991). Sensations during chest tube removal. *Heart and Lung*, 20, 131–136.

Thirty-six patients were asked to indicate using a visual analog scale the sensations and the intensity of the sensations they experienced during and 15 minutes after chest tube removal. Burning was the most common sensation during removal. Patients also reported pain or hurting, pulling or yanking, or pressure during removal. Few sensations were experienced 15 minutes after removal of the chest tube.

SKILL 17–1   ASSESSING OXYGENATION STATUS WITH ARTERIAL BLOOD GASES

Clinical Situations in Which You Might Encounter This Skill

Clients who have a compromised respiratory system frequently have their ventilatory function assessed by arterial blood gas (ABG) measurements. The levels of oxygen saturation (SaO_2) and partial pressures of oxygen and carbon dioxide (PaO_2 and $PaCO_2$) are determined, as well as the acid-base balance (pH level) of the arterial blood. The effectiveness of supplemental oxygen, respiratory therapy, or ventilatory support can be evaluated by examining ABG measurements. Each institution has its own policies concerning who may draw ABG samples. Physicians, registered respiratory therapists, and registered nurses with special certification may collect arterial blood specimens for blood gas determination.

The normal ranges for ABGs are:

$$pH \quad = 7.35\text{–}7.45$$
$$PaO_2 \quad = 80\text{–}100 \text{ mmHg}$$
$$PaCO_2 = 38\text{–}42 \text{ mmHg}$$
$$SaO_2 \quad = 96\%\text{–}100\%$$
$$HCO_3 \quad = 24\text{–}30 \text{ mEq/L}$$

If the pH is less than 7.35 and the $PaCO_2$ is higher than 42 mmHg, the blood gases indicate respiratory acidosis. A pH less than 7.35 and an HCO_3 less than 24 mEq/L suggest metabolic acidosis. If the pH is greater than 7.45 and the $PaCO_2$ is less than 38 mmHg, the client may have respiratory alkalosis. A pH greater than 7.45 and an HCO_3 greater than 30 mEq/L suggest metabolic alkalosis.

Anticipated Responses

▼ The client's blood gas levels are within the normal range.

Adverse Responses

▼ The client's blood gas levels are outside the ranges listed above.

Materials List

Gather these materials before beginning the skill:

▼ Examination gloves
▼ Cup or plastic bag filled with crushed ice
▼ Blood gas kit *or*
▼ Ampule of sodium heparin (1:1,000 solution) (if syringe is not heparinized)
▼ Disposable waterproof pad
▼ 22-gauge, 1-inch needle (for most sticks)
▼ 22-gauge, 1½-inch needle (for deep femoral sticks)
▼ Alcohol prep pads
▼ Sterile 4- × 4-inch gauze pads (at least two)
▼ Adhesive tape or bandage
▼ Label

▼ *ACTION*

1. Assess the client's status, the need for ABG levels, and whether the client is taking any type of anticoagulant.

2. Determine if the client has an arterial line in place.

3. Take the client's blood pressure and temperature.

▼ *RATIONALE*

1. Validates the need for the procedure. Anticoagulants prolong the clotting time and pressure should be applied longer after the blood is drawn.

2. Blood may be drawn from the arterial line.

3. If the blood pressure is low, it may be harder to obtain the sample. If the blood pressure is high, the site may bleed longer. Temperature extremes can change CO_2 and O_2 results.

▼ *ACTION*

▼ *RATIONALE*

4. Assess the client's radial, brachial, and femoral sites for the availability of the artery; the proximity to veins, nerves, and bones; and the condition of the surrounding tissue. The radial site is usually preferred in adults.

   Test for alternative circulation to the hand before performing the arterial puncture by conducting Allen's test (Fig. 17–1):
   a. Ask the client to make a tight fist.
   b. With the pads of your middle 2 or 3 fingers, apply direct pressure over the client's ulnar and radial arteries.
   c. While pressure is being applied, ask the client to open his or her hand.
   d. Remove the pressure from the client's ulnar artery. Observe the color of the extremity distal to the pressure point.

   e. Check the client's other hand, if needed.

4. Arterial puncture should avoid other structures. Complications of arterial puncture include vasospasm and clotting; therefore, collateral circulation is desirable. The radial artery is the preferred site since the ulnar artery provides collateral circulation.
   Verifies the presence of collateral blood flow to the hand through the ulnar artery.

   d. The client's hand and fingers should flush within 15 seconds. This is considered a positive test. If the test is negative, the radial artery should *not* be used to draw the sample.

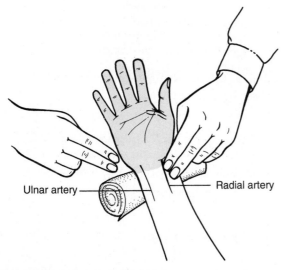

▼ FIGURE 17–1. Testing for alternative circulation to the hand with Allen's test.

5. Assess other elements that may affect the accuracy of the ABG measurement:
   a. Changes in O_2 settings within the last 20 to 30 minutes.
   b. Suctioning 20 minutes prior to drawing the ABG.
   c. The client's activities and their effects on respiration.
   d. Emotions and their effects on respiration.

5. Helps ensure accuracy of the results.

   a. The ABG results will not be accurate.

NOTE: If the syringe is heparinized, the following step may be deleted.

▼ *ACTION* ‾ ▼ *RATIONALE* ‾ ‾ ‾ ‾ ‾ ‾ ‾ ‾ ‾ ‾

6. The person collecting the specimen uses a heparinized syringe. If a preprepared heparinized syringe is not available, prepare one by:
  a. Withdrawing 0.5 ml of sodium heparin (1:1000 solution) into a syringe from an ampule or vial.
  b. While firmly holding the syringe, pull the plunger back so that the entire length of the inside of the barrel is exposed to the heparin.
  c. Push the plunger back down the barrel so that all excess heparin is expelled outside the syringe.
  d. Cover the needle and lay the syringe aside.

6. a. Prevents the specimen from clotting prior to being analyzed.

  b. Ensures that all of the specimen is prevented from clotting.

  c. Discards unneeded heparin.

  d. Prevents contamination.

7. Fill a cup with crushed ice and set it aside.

7. Ice decreases the metabolism of red blood cells, which can alter the specimen O_2 reading.

8. Place the client's bed at a comfortable working level. Lower the side rail, if appropriate.

8. Promotes proper body mechanics.

9. Put on gloves.

9. Decreases the transmission of microorganisms.

10. Provide support for the client as needed during the specimen withdrawal.

10. Provides for the client's comfort.

11. To draw an arterial sample from the client's radial artery:
  a. Place a waterproof drape under the puncture site.
  b. Hyperextend the client's wrist by placing a rolled towel beneath it.
  c. Put on gloves.
  d. Cleanse the puncture site with an alcohol wipe. Use a circular motion. In some institutions a povidone-iodine solution may also be used for cleansing.
  e. Locate the client's radial artery between your index finger and middle finger.
  f. Ask the client to remain very still as you make the puncture.
  g. Insert the needle through the client's skin at a 45- to 90-degree angle and parallel to the long axis of the client's arm (Fig. 17–2).

  a. Protects the bed linens from becoming soiled with blood.
  b. Exposes the puncture site and facilitates the arterial stick.
  c. Prevents contact with the client's blood.
  d. Reduces the transmission of skin organisms into the puncture site.

  e. Identifies the location of the puncture.

  f. Facilitates a successful stick.

  g. This is the least traumatic method of insertion.

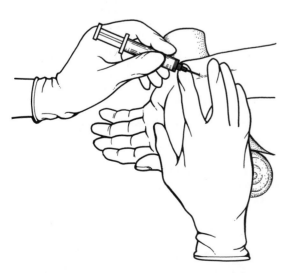

▼ **FIGURE 17–2.** Drawing a sample from the radial artery.

▼ *ACTION*   ▼ *RATIONALE*

  h. Observe for a flashback of blood in the syringe. Do not pull back on the plunger. If you missed the artery, withdraw the needle as far as possible without completely removing it, repalpate the position of the artery, and redirect the angle of the needle. Avoid repeated attempts.

  i. Collect 3 to 5 ml of arterial blood.

  j. Withdraw the needle and apply immediate pressure to the puncture site with a dry 4- × 4-inch gauze sponge for 5 minutes. If the client is taking anticoagulant medication or has high blood pressure or a bleeding disorder, pressure must be applied to the site for at least 10 minutes. A dressing may be applied at the end of the pressure time, if needed.

  h. The arterial blood pressure forces blood into the syringe when you enter the artery with the needle. Repeated attempts traumatize the tissue and may result in complications such as laceration of the artery.

  i. Sufficient blood is required to obtain accurate results.

  j. Prevents hemorrhage or hematoma formation by promoting clotting at the puncture site. A longer period of pressure helps to ensure clotting of the arterial site.

12. After you remove the syringe from the puncture site, expel air bubbles from the syringe while maintaining pressure on the puncture site.

12. Prevents false O_2 or CO_2 readings from contamination of the specimen by air.

13. Stick the needle in a rubber stopper. Rotate the syringe gently before placing it in the cup of ice.

13. Helps prevent needlestick injuries. Ice decreases the metabolism of red blood cells, which can alter the measurement of O_2. Rotation of the syringe mixes blood with anticoagulant.

14. Appropriately label the specimen and place the iced specimen in a bag before transporting it for analysis.

14. Ensures that the results are reported for the correct client. Decreases the transmission of microorganisms.

15. Remove your gloves and discard them.

15. Decreases the transmission of microorganisms.

16. Lower the bed and raise the side rails.

16. Helps to ensure the safety of the client.

17. Record information on the requisition slip (such as supplemental O_2, or the fraction of inspired oxygen [FiO_2], and the client's temperature).

17. Ensures accurate results.

18. The specimen should be transported as soon as possible.

18. Decreases sample changes from delay.

19. Inspect the puncture site at intervals.

19. Helps to ensure the integrity of the skin and adequate clotting.

20. Evaluate the ABG results.

20. Provides information for client care.

21. Record the results.

21. Communicates the findings to other members of the health care team and contributes to the legal record by documenting the care given to the client.

Example of Documentation

DATE	TIME	NOTES
11/14/93	1000	Allen's test positive. ABG drawn from L radial site and sent for analysis. Site clear, dry, and intact at 20 minutes. No hematoma or overt bleeding noted.
		R. Crawford, RN

Teaching Tips

Explain the purpose of drawing the ABGs to the client and his or her family. Explain that pressure should be applied after the puncture for at least 5 minutes and that the client should report any bleeding from the site.

Home Care Variations

ABGs are not usually drawn in the client's home.

SKILL 17–2   ASSESSING OXYGENATION STATUS WITH PULSE OXIMETRY

Clinical Situations in Which You May Encounter This Skill

Pulse oximetry is a noninvasive method of assessing a client's arterial blood oxygen saturation (SaO_2) using a pulse oximeter sensor. The sensor contains two parts. On one side of the sensor there are two light-emitting diodes (LED), one red and the other infrared. On the other side of the sensor there is a light detector called a photo detector. The LED beams light through the tissues and blood vessels and the photo detector receives the light and measures the amount of light that was absorbed by oxygenated and unoxygenated hemoglobin. Oxygenated hemoglobin tends to absorb more infrared light and unoxygenated hemoglobin absorbs more red light. By a process called spectrophotometry, SaO_2 is determined based on the amounts of each type of light that the photodetector receives.

There are several different types of sensors. Sensors are designed for use on the finger, toe, nose, ear, forehead, or around the hand or foot of the newborn. You should select the correct sensor for the measurement site you plan to use.

Before using pulse oximetry to assess the client's oxygenation status, first assess his or her hemoglobin level. Since pulse oximetry measures the percent of SaO_2, the result could appear to be normal when the hemoglobin is low since all of the available hemoglobin to carry O_2 is completely saturated.

Anticipated Responses

▼ The client's O_2 saturation is 96% to 100%.
▼ The client is able to tolerate the presence of the sensor.

Adverse Responses

▼ The client's O_2 saturation is low (<70% is life threatening).
▼ Pressure areas develop in the tissue at the site of a spring clip sensor.
▼ Skin irritation develops at the site of an adhesive sensor.

Materials List

Gather these materials before beginning the skill:

▼ Pulse oximeter with correct sensor
▼ Alcohol wipe
▼ Sheet or towel
▼ Nail polish remover (optional)

▼ *A C T I O N*   ▼ *R A T I O N A L E*

1. Select an appropriate sensor.

2. Select an appropriate site for the sensor. If you are using a finger (Fig. 17–3) or toe, assess for capillary refill and proximal pulse. If the client has poor circulation, use a forehead or nasal sensor instead.

1. The sensor should be selected based on the size of the person and the intended application site.

2. Decreased circulation alters the O_2 saturation measurement.

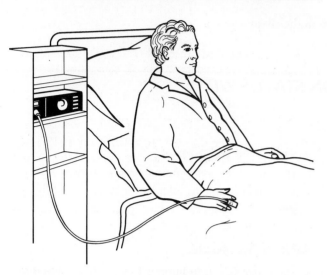

▼ **FIGURE 17–3.** Assessing oxygen status with pulse oximetry.

3. Cleanse the site with an alcohol wipe. Remove artificial nails or nail polish if present.

3. Polish and artificial fingernails alter the results.

4. Apply the sensor. Make sure the LED and photo detector are aligned on opposite sides of the selected site.

4. Proper application is necessary for accurate results.

5. Connect the sensor to the oximeter with a sensor cable. Turn on the machine. You should hear a tone and see a waveform fluctuation with each arterial pulsation.

5. The tone and waveform fluctuation indicate that the machine is detecting blood flow.

6. Adjust the alarm limits for high and low O_2 saturation levels according to the manufacturer's directions.

6. Alarms alert you to abnormal O_2 saturation levels.

7. Move the site of spring sensors every 2 hours and adhesive sensors every 4 hours.

7. Prevents skin breakdown from pressure and skin irritation from the adhesive.

8. Protect the sensor from exposure to bright light sources by covering it with a sheet or towel.

8. Light may alter the SaO_2 results.

9. Notify the physician of abnormal results.

9. Low SaO_2 levels require medical attention.

10. Record the results of the O_2 saturation measurements, the type of sensor used, the hemoglobin levels, and your assessment of the client's skin at the sensor site.

10. Communicates the findings to the other members of the health care team and contributes to the legal record by documenting the care given to the client.

Example of Documentation

DATE	TIME	NOTES
1/1/94	0800	Finger-clip pulse oximeter in place. SaO$_2$ = 98%. Hemoglobin within normal limits. No signs of redness or skin breakdown at sensor site.
		L. White, RN

Teaching Tips

Teach the client to avoid moving the extremity as much as possible since movement can be interpreted by the oximeter as an arterial pulsation and will alter the results.

Home Care Variations

SaO$_2$ can be monitored in the client's home using the same equipment and techniques. Family members should be taught to rotate the site of the sensor and assess the client's skin for irritation and breakdown.

SKILL 17–3   ADMINISTERING OXYGEN BY NASAL CANNULA, MASK, NASAL CATHETER, AND CROUPETTE, MIST TENT, OR OXYGEN TENT

Clinical Situations in Which You May Encounter This Skill

When a client's oxygen (O$_2$) saturation is below normal, O$_2$ administration is indicated. Supplemental O$_2$ is also indicated when a client's O$_2$ demand is increased, especially if the physiological supply is compromised.

In health care facilities, O$_2$ is supplied either from a portable O$_2$ tank or from a pressurized central reservoir that "pipes in" O$_2$ to the client's bedside. The flow of O$_2$ from both types of storage systems is regulated by a device called a pressure flow regulator, or flowmeter (Fig. 17–4).

O$_2$ has a drying effect as it flows over normally moist mucous membranes. This effect results in dry tissues and thick or viscous respiratory secretions that may further complicate the client's respiratory problems. To prevent this drying effect, O$_2$ is usually humidified before delivery to the client. The bubble humidifier (Fig. 17–5) is one of the most common devices used to add moisture to the O$_2$. With this

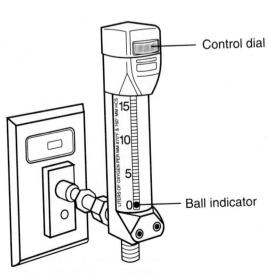

▼ FIGURE 17–4. An oxygen flowmeter.

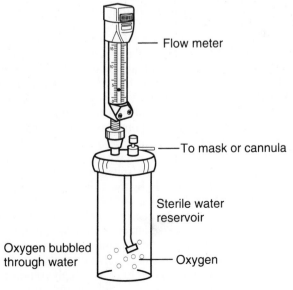

▼ FIGURE 17–5. A bubble humidifier.

device, O_2 is bubbled through water under pressure, where it picks up moisture and then is delivered to the client.

There are many devices that can be used to deliver O_2 in varying concentrations to the client. The nasal cannula (Fig. 17–6) is the most common device

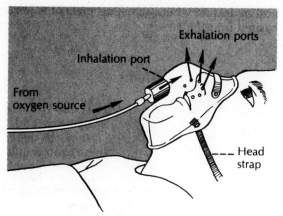

▼ **FIGURE 17–7.** A standard face mask.

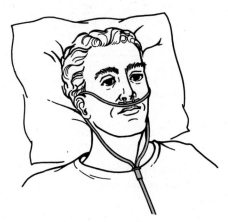

▼ **FIGURE 17–6.** A nasal cannula.

used to deliver low concentrations of O_2. The liter flow rate is usually 1 to 6 liters per minute (LPM) and delivers approximately 22 to 40% O_2. Advantages of O_2 delivery by nasal cannula include the client's comfort and ability to continue most activities such as talking and eating without disrupting the O_2 therapy. A disadvantage is that the nasal cannula can be easily dislodged by a restless patient. Nasal O_2 delivery can also be irritating to the nares.

There are several types of masks that may be used to deliver O_2. The masks are either low-flow (low-concentration) or high-flow (high-concentration) systems. All masks are designed to fit snugly over a portion of the lower face, to cover the nose and mouth, and are held in place with an elastic strap. The most common types of masks include the standard face mask, the O_2 mask with a reservoir bag (the nonrebreathing mask), the partial rebreathing mask, and the Venturi mask.

The standard face mask (Fig. 17–7) is made of clear plastic and is designed to cover both the nose and mouth. O_2 enters the mask by way of an O_2 port. The mask has small holes in the sides that allow air to be exhaled. O_2 flow should be set at 6 to 12 LPM to deliver 40 to 65% O_2. Disadvantages of the face mask include a feeling of claustrophobia and the need to remove the mask for talking and eating. The mask should be replaced with a nasal cannula during meals to prevent hypoxemia and respiratory distress. Masks should be used cautiously by the client who may vomit because of the possibility of aspiration.

The nonrebreathing mask (Fig. 17–8) is a standard mask with a reservoir bag attached. Inhaled air enters the mask from the reservoir bag and exhaled air leaves the mask by way of a one-way valve on the side of the mask. This mask is designed to deliver high volumes of O_2. The O_2 flow rate should be high enough, usually 6

to 15 LPM, to keep the reservoir bag inflated at least one-third full during inspiration. The nonrebreathing mask supplies between 60 and 90% O_2.

The partial rebreathing mask is similar to the nonrebreathing mask with the exception that there is no one-way valve for exhaled air. The partial rebreathing mask delivers slightly lower O_2 concentrations than the nonrebreathing mask.

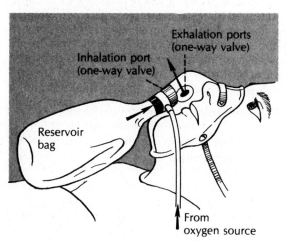

▼ **FIGURE 17–8.** A nonrebreathing mask.

The Venturi mask (Fig. 17–9) is a clear plastic mask with entrance ports that vary in size at the base of the mask. These ports are adjustable to permit delivery of specific O_2 concentrations from 24% to 50%. The O_2 flowmeter setting is determined by the required O_2 concentration. Consult the manufacturers' literature for the proper LPM of O_2 to deliver the required O_2 concentration.

The nasal catheter (Fig. 17–10) is used to administer O_2 in concentrations of up to 40% to 50% directly into the client's nasopharynx. The nasal catheter is often used when a client cannot use a nasal cannula because of mouth breathing or when a higher concentration of O_2 is needed. Disadvantages of the nasal catheter include discomfort to the nares and possible erosion of the mucous membranes of the nares. Also, improper placement of the catheter may result in air swallowing and gastric distention.

Text continued on page 514

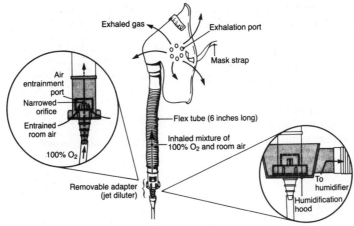

▼ FIGURE 17–9. A Venturi mask.

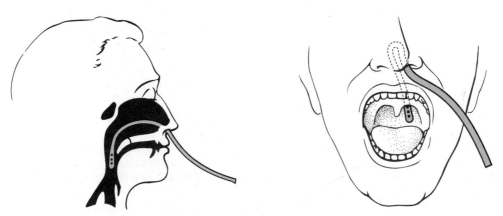

▼ FIGURE 17–10. A nasal catheter.

SAFETY CONSIDERATIONS

Safety considerations should be followed whenever O_2 is being administered, whether at the client's home or in a clinic or hospital. Although O_2 does not explode, it does support combustion. Therefore, the following guidelines should be followed to prevent injuries and fires.

1. Open flames should be avoided. A minimum of 10 feet must separate O_2 apparatus and open flames.

2. Instruct the client and his or her family that *no smoking* is allowed around O_2. No Smoking signs should be posted in conspicuous places near areas where O_2 is in use. A No Smoking sign should be placed on the client's door and over his or her bed. Cigarettes, matches, and lighters should be secured out of the client's reach or given to family members to take home while O_2 therapy is in progress.

3. Maintain proper working order of the equipment in the area, including the O_2 equipment itself. Cylinders of O_2 should be secured in upright positions. All electric equipment should be intact and should not emit sparks. (The maintenance departments of most agencies can easily check equipment.)

4. Avoid the use of synthetic fabrics that can build up static electricity.

5. Avoid the use of oils in the area. These are known to ignite spontaneously when used around O_2. Petroleum products, including petroleum jelly, should not be used around the client's face.

6. O_2 is a type of medication for your client. All guidelines that pertain to medications also apply to O_2.

Children between the ages of 1 month and 10 years who are experiencing hypoxemia may receive supplemental oxygen by way of a Croupette or mist tent. Children older than 10 years may receive supplemental oxygen via an oxygen tent. Oxygen concentrations of 21% to 60% may be delivered, along with humidification. Children and their families need education about these devices and assistance with their anxiety. A common illness that requires the use of a Croupette or mist tent is viral laryngotracheobronchitis.

Anticipated Responses

▼ The client has increased O_2 saturation levels.
▼ There is increased O_2 perfusion to the tissues of the client's body.

Adverse Responses

▼ O_2-induced hypoventilation may occur in clients with chronic lung diseases. Because of chronic hypercarbia and acidosis, rising CO_2 levels do not stimulate the respiratory center in these clients. Instead, low O_2 tension in the arterial blood is the stimulus for breathing. Administering O_2 to clients with chronic lung diseases therefore carries the risk of suppressing the respiratory drive. Do not administer more than 2 LPM of O_2 to a client with a chronic lung disease.
▼ O_2 toxicity may occur with continued administration of high O_2 concentrations. The exact mechanism for cellular damage from O_2 toxicity is not well understood. It is believed that administration of high O_2 concentrations causes a chemical reaction that results in products that cause cellular damage. Signs and symptoms include a tickling sensation in the throat, a cough, dyspnea, chest pain, fatigue, headache, anorexia, paresthesias, and alveolar collapse. Delivery of high concentrations of O_2 to neonates can also result in blindness.

▼ O_2 therapy results in dry mucous membranes and viscous respiratory secretions.

For Croupette, mist tent, or oxygen tent:
▼ The child feels cool.
▼ The inside of the tent is wet.

Materials List

Gather these materials before beginning the skill:

▼ O_2 delivery device (mask, cannula, or catheter)
▼ For a nasal catheter:
  ½-inch tape
  Examination gloves
  Sterile water-soluble lubricant
  Tongue blade
  Penlight
▼ Flowmeter with O_2 tube adapter if needed
▼ Humidification device (not for use with a Venturi mask)
▼ Sterile distilled water
▼ O_2 tubing
▼ No Smoking signs

For Croupette:
▼ Croupette or mist tent (nebulizing unit)
▼ Humidifier
▼ Sterile distilled water
▼ Ice or refrigeration unit
▼ Oxygen with flowmeter
▼ Additional clothing to fit the child
▼ Developmentally appropriate toys that will not create a fire hazard
▼ Tissues and disposal bag

For oxygen tent:
▼ Tent
▼ Oxygen tubing
▼ Oxygen with flow regulator
▼ Humidifier
▼ Sterile distilled water
▼ Tissues and disposal bag

▼ *ACTION*

1. Check the physician's order on the client's chart regarding O_2 therapy.

2. Assess the laboratory results, especially the ABG analyses.

3. Insert the flowmeter into a wall outlet for O_2 or set up the O_2 tank.

4. Connect the adapter to the humidifier bottle. (This step is optional in some settings.)

5. Screw the adapter onto the flowmeter.

6. Fill the humidification reservoir with sterile distilled water.

▼ *RATIONALE*

1. It is your responsibility to ascertain the accuracy of the physician's order prior to initiating O_2 therapy.

2. Provides data with which to compare future laboratory results.

3. Connects the flowmeter to the hospital supply of O_2. In the client's home, a tank is necessary.

4. Provides for moisture in the system.

5. Regulates the amount of O_2 that is delivered.

6. Humidification prevents the drying effects of O_2 administration. Sterile water decreases bacterial growth.

▼ *ACTION*   ▼ *RATIONALE*

7. Connect the O_2 tubing to the outlet port of the humidifier bottle.

7. Humidification prevents the drying effects of O_2 administration. Allows for O_2 in the system.

8. Connect the distal end of the O_2 tubing to the O_2 delivery device.

8. Completes the tubing system.

9. Turn on the flowmeter to 2 LPM and check to see if you feel O_2 flowing through the system.

9. Assesses the patency and operation of the equipment.

10. Position the O_2 delivery device on the client.

Administering Oxygen with a Nasal Cannula

a. Position the nasal cannula so that the two prongs are barely inside the external meatus of the client's nares. There are two types of straps that help the cannula to stay in place. One type goes around the back of the person's head and can be adjusted so the cannula is held in place comfortably. Do not allow the elastic straps to apply pressure on the client's ears. The other type loops around the person's ears and adjusts under the chin for a correct fit.

a. Allows for accurate position of the cannula and appropriate administration of O_2.

b. Instruct the client to breathe through his or her nose.

b. Provides the prescribed O_2.

Administering Oxygen with a Mask

a. Place the O_2 mask over the client's face from the nose to the chin comfortably but snugly. Secure the mask by placing an elastic strap around the back of the head. Do not allow the elastic straps to apply pressure on the client's ears.

a. A mask that is too loose allows O_2 to escape. A mask that is too tight can cause discomfort and skin irritation.

Administering Oxygen with a Nasal Catheter

a. Take the nasal catheter and holding the distal tip at the bottom of the client's earlobe measure the distance on the tube from the bottom of the earlobe to the tip of the nose (Fig. 17–11). Mark the distance on the tube with ½-inch adhesive tape or a pen.

a. Provides for proper catheter placement and delivery of O_2 at the level of the nasopharynx.

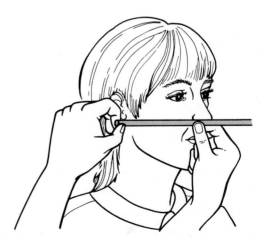

▼ **FIGURE 17–11.** Measuring the length of the nasal catheter to be inserted.

▼ *A C T I O N*   ▼ *R A T I O N A L E*

b. Put on gloves.
c. Coat the distal one-third of the catheter with the sterile water-soluble lubricant.

d. Assess the patency of the nares by occluding one side and having the client breathe through the other naris.
e. Gently place the catheter into the naris that you have determined is more open. Gently push the catheter into the naris in a back-and-down direction. Insert the catheter until the tape or pen marker reaches the entrance to the naris.
f. Lightly fasten the catheter to the client's nose with tape.
g. With a tongue blade and a penlight have the client open his or her mouth as you look at the back of his or her throat. The catheter should lie just below the nasopharynx next to the uvula (see Fig. 17–10). Adjust the catheter so that it is barely visible.
h. Securely fasten the catheter to the client's nose with tape.
i. Remove the gloves and dispose of them properly.
j. Change the catheter every 8 hours preferably to the other naris if it is patent.

11. Adjust the flowmeter to the ordered number of liters of O_2 per minute.

12. Observe the effects of O_2 on the client.
a. Assess the ABG or pulse oximetry readings.
b. Assess the client's respiratory rate for any deviations from the normal rate of 12 to 20 breaths per minute.
c. Assess for any alteration in the person's respiratory pattern.
d. Assess for any change in the person's level of consciousness.

13. Wash your hands.

14. Attach the No Smoking sign to the door of the client's room and above the bed.

15. Record the procedure.

---

b. Decreases the transmission of microorganisms.
c. Lubricates the catheter so that insertion is less traumatic. Sterile lubricant prevents contamination of the catheter and respiratory tract with microorganisms. Petroleum products are contraindicated with O_2.
d. The more patent naris is best suited for the nasal catheter.

e. Allows for the least traumatic proper placement of the catheter. Nasal turbinates are sensitive.

f. Temporarily securing the catheter prevents the catheter from slipping.
g. Ascertains the proper placement of the catheter. Coughing or gagging indicates improper placement.

h. Prevents the catheter from becoming accidentally dislodged.
i. Prevents the transmission of microorganisms.
j. Protects the client's nasal tissue from irritation and erosion.

11. O_2 is considered to be a medication and the physician orders the dosage.

12. Allows you to evaluate the effects of the treatment.

13. Decreases the transmission of microorganisms.

14. Protects the client and others from a fire hazard. Provides for a smoke-free environment.

15. Communicates the findings to the other members of the health care team and contributes to the legal record by documenting the care given to the client.

▼ *ACTION* _ _ _ _ _ _ _ _ _ _ _ _ _ _   ▼ *RATIONALE* _ _ _ _ _ _ _ _ _ _

16. Periodically observe the equipment to determine if:
    a. The humidifier is adequately filled.
    b. The O_2 flow rate is still set properly.
    c. The tubing is kinked and requires replacement.
    d. The delivery device is in place.

16. Ascertains that the equipment is working properly so that the client's care is optimized.

NOTE: Any moisture in the tubing or reservoir bag should be discarded.

Moisture can lead to bacterial growth.

Administering Oxygen with a Croupette, Mist Tent, or Oxygen Tent

1. Assess the client's respiratory status, including arterial blood gases. Assess the anxiety levels of the client and his or her family.

1. Provides information in order to plan optimum care.

2. Read the physician's orders. Especially note orders for oxygen delivery.

2. Provides for proper implementation of care.

3. Wash your hands. Put on gloves if needed. Discard them when they are no longer needed.

3. Decreases the transmission of microorganisms.

4. Assess the client's ability to clear his or her own airway of secretions.

4. Further assesses respiratory status and the client's ability to participate in care.

5. Bring the equipment to the client's bedside. While proceeding with the setup, explain the equipment and procedure to the client and his or her family.

5. Provides for efficiency. Provides teaching and decreases anxiety.

6. Place a cooling nebulizer unit or humidifying unit on the bed or crib or at the side of the bed or crib. Connect the canopy and situate it so that the complete bed or crib area is covered. Connect the unit to the oxygen source as needed. Ensure that connections are secure.

6. Maintains oxygen and humidity inside the tent.

7. Start the refrigeration unit on the Croupette. If an ice reservoir is to be used instead, stock it with ice.

7. Provides for cool air that allows for increased ease of breathing.

8. Fill the nebulizing container or humidifier unit with sterile water to the fill line. Set the oxygen flowmeter to the manufacturer's specifications, usually at least 10 L/min.

8. Provides for humidification of oxygen without overstressing the unit.

9. When a child is to be placed where the air is cooled by a refrigerator unit or ice, extra clothes should be put on the child, including socks, sweatshirt, and hat.

9. Decreases the possibility of hypothermia, which is possible due to the large body surface area in children exposed to a cool environment.

10. With the family's help, place the child in the bed or crib in a semi-Fowler's or high Fowler's position. Place a developmentally appropriate toy in with child. The toy must not be able to produce a spark, friction, or static electricity.

10. Allows for family participation and may decrease the child's anxiety. Toys help keep the child occupied in the tent. Battery-operated or electrical toys that produce sparks, friction, or static electricity can cause a fire.

▼ *ACTION*	▼ *RATIONALE*
11. Carefully tuck the top and both sides of the canopy under the mattress. Place the top sheet over the front section of the tent.	11. Keeps the oxygen and humidity inside tent.
12. Place No Smoking and Oxygen In Use signs on the client's door and over the bed. Ask the family not to smoke in the room.	12. Provides safety.
13. Organize nursing care so the tent is opened as infrequently as possible. Encourage the family to participate in care. If the child is old enough, place tissues and a disposal bag inside the tent.	13. Allows for the most effective use of the tent. Allows for disposal of contaminated tissues.
14. After the tent has been open for a time, secure the sides and flush with oxygen by raising the flow-meter rate for 30 to 60 seconds. Return to the prescribed settings.	14. Quickly restores oxygen and humidity levels.

15. Frequently evaluate the following:
a. The client's needs, as a call light cannot be placed inside the tent.
b. The client's respiratory status, including arterial blood gas results.
c. The client's comfort level, level of consciousness, and anxiety level.
d. The client's mucous membranes.
e. The water level in the nebulizing container or humidifier.
f. The moisture content inside the tent.
   i. Wipe off excess moisture on the tent sides.
   ii. Change the client's clothing and bedding as needed.
   iii. If moisture is a continuous problem, lower the humidification (if possible).
g. The oxygen level inside the tent.
h. The temperature in the Croupette should be 18 to 20° C.
i. The security of all tent sides.
	15. Provides information:
	a. Provides for client care without electrical hazard.
	
	b. Respiratory status.
	
	c. Coolness, hypoxia.
	
	d. Dryness.
	
	f. Increased moisture promotes heat loss by skin evaporation.
	
	   iii. Could increase hypothermia.

Example of Documentation

DATE	TIME	NOTES
1/12/94	1100	O_2 therapy started at 4 L/min with nasal cannula. Skin color pink. RR = 24. No accessory muscle use noted. Client states he is "breathing easier." *S. Smart, RN*

Teaching Tips

Explain the purpose of the O_2 therapy to the client and his or her family and the hazards of smoking around O_2. Explain the need for frequent oral and nasal care to prevent drying of the mucous membranes.

Home Care Variations

Many clients use supplemental O_2 systems at home, as well as portable systems that allow them to go about their activities of daily living. Good discharge planning, referral to a home respiratory therapy service, and identification of the range of home products and services available through sources such as the yellow pages of the phone book can assist clients in setting up and maintaining O_2 systems at home. Teach clients how to assess their respiratory status and how to respond in emergencies. Inform clients about their respiratory condition and how to adjust their O_2 needs to the O_2 supply to prevent further problems.

SKILL 17–4   ORAL AND NASAL CARE FOR A CLIENT WHO IS RECEIVING OXYGEN

Clinical Situations in Which You May Encounter This Skill

Clients who are receiving O_2 need special oral and nasal care, regardless of whether they are conscious or unconscious.

Anticipated Responses

▾ The client's mucous membranes remain moist and pain-free.

Adverse Responses

▾ The client's mucous membranes are uncomfortable and dry.
▾ The areas of skin around the client's nose and lips crack.

Materials List

Gather these materials before beginning the skill:

▾ Oral hygiene equipment
▾ Washcloth or gauze
▾ Towel
▾ Water-based lubricant
▾ Gloves

▾ ACTION	▾ RATIONALE
1. Assess the integrity of the client's mucous membranes.	1. Provides information for effective care.
2. Put on gloves.	2. Decreases the transmission of microorganisms.
3. If the client is receiving O_2 by mask and is unable to tolerate short periods off of O_2, then a nasal cannula should be used while you provide oral care.	3. Decreases the possibility of hypoxia.
4. Assist the client with oral hygiene, as needed (see Skill 10–1).	4. Cleanses the person's oral cavity.
5. With a moistened washcloth, cleanse around the outside and just inside the person's nares. Allow the client to gently blow his or her nose, if needed. (Briefly remove the cannula or catheter.)	5. Provides for the client's hygiene and comfort. Harsh blowing can cause irritation and bleeding of the mucous membranes.
6. With a gloved finger, gently apply a small amount of water-soluble lubricant to the client's lips and the external orifices of his or her nares.	6. Provides moisture and protection.

▼ *A C T I O N* ▼ *R A T I O N A L E*

NOTE: Petroleum products are never used around O_2.	The combination of petroleum and O_2 is a potential fire hazard.

7. Reapply the O_2 delivery device. Try to position the nasal piece or face mask and head straps a little differently than before.

7. Provides O_2. Assists in preventing pressure areas.

8. Small pieces of gauze may be placed between the cannula and the client's nose and under the head strap above the ears.

8. Assists in preventing pressure areas.

9. Remove the gloves and wash your hands.

9. Decreases the transmission of microorganisms.

10. Ascertain whether the O_2 settings are correctly set.

10. Provides the appropriate amount of O_2.

11. Evaluate the client's comfort.

11. Provides information for planning care.

12. Record the procedure and other relevant information.

12. Communicates the findings to the other members of the health care team and contributes to the legal record by documenting the care given to the client.

Example of Documentation

DATE	TIME	NOTES
9/10/93	1100	Oral and nasal care given. No areas of irritation noted. O_2 per nasal cannula continues 4 L/min.
		R. Holmes, RN

Teaching Tips

While providing oral and nasal care, explain the purpose of the O_2 and the necessity for meticulous oral and nasal hygiene.

Home Care Variations

The same procedure can be used to provide oral and nasal hygiene in the client's home.

ASSISTING THE CLIENT WITH PULMONARY PHYSIOTHERAPY

Pulmonary physiotherapy includes a group of nursing techniques that are designed to clear the respiratory tract and lungs of excessive sputum and promote optimal ventilation in clients with chronic obstructive lung diseases.

Nursing measures to clear excessive respiratory secretions include increasing the client's mobility; encouraging coughing and deep breathing; helping the client to use an incentive spirometer; and providing for postural drainage, vibropercussion, and adequate hydration.

Measures to promote optimal ventilation include teaching breathing techniques that optimize respiratory function such as pursed-lip breathing and diaphragmatic breathing.

SKILL 17–5 ASSISTING A CLIENT WITH DEEP BREATHING, COUGHING, AND BREATHING TECHNIQUES

Clinical Situations in Which You May Encounter This Skill

Chronic respiratory disorders are often characterized by excessive respiratory secretions. These secretions must be removed to prevent atelectasis and other complications such as pneumonia. In addition, whenever a client faces a period of immobility, such as after a serious illness or operation, the respiratory system is affected. Immobility leads to pooling of respiratory secretions in the gravity-dependent areas of the lungs and closure of some small airways; this causes inadequate ventilation and respiratory impairment that result in hypoventilation, hypercapnia, and hypoxemia. Deep breathing reopens these small airways, and coughing facilitates removal of respiratory secretions.

In addition to coughing and deep breathing there are two other breathing techniques that promote optimal ventilation and open airways: pursed-lip breathing and diaphragmatic breathing. These special breathing techniques are primarily used by persons with chronic obstructive pulmonary diseases to improve their respiratory status.

Anticipated Responses

▼ The client is able to breathe deeply and fully expand his or her lungs.
▼ The client is able to use breathing techniques to enhance his or her ventilation.
▼ The client is able to cough productively.
▼ The client does not develop atelectasis or pneumonia.

Adverse Responses

▼ The client experiences atelectasis or pneumonia.
▼ The client experiences hypoxemia and hypercapnia.

Materials List

Gather these materials before beginning the skill:

▼ Facial tissues
▼ Emesis basin
▼ Stethoscope
▼ Pillows for splinting the client's chest and abdomen

▼ *ACTION*

Teaching Deep Breathing

1. Explain the importance of deep breathing to the client.

2. Help the client to sit at the side of the bed or place the bed in a high-Fowler's position.

3. Instruct the client to slowly breathe in as deeply as possible. Place your palms on the client's rib cage to assess for full chest expansion. You should see the rib cage rising with each breath (Fig. 17–12).

▼ *RATIONALE*

1. Elicits the client's cooperation.

2. An upright posture allows maximal lung expansion.

3. Produces maximum lung expansion and opens the airways.

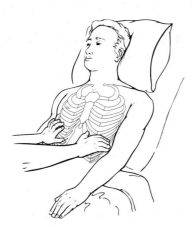

▼ **FIGURE 17–12.** Assisting a client with deep breathing.

▼ *ACTION*   ▼ *RATIONALE*

4. Instruct the client to exhale slowly.

5. Repeat Steps 3 and 4 10 to 20 times. Observe for dizziness, shortness of breath, or other respiratory problems.

Helping the Client to Cough

1. Explain to the client the importance of coughing effectively.

2. Don a mask, goggles, gloves, and gown if indicated.

3. Help the client to cough.

    a. Instruct the client to take two or three deep breaths. Follow the procedure for deep breathing.

    b. As the client takes the next breath, instruct him or her to lean forward, hold his or her breath for a second, and contract his or her abdominal muscles.

    c. Instruct the client to cough forcefully, and expel secretions into a tissue or basin as you splint his or her thoracic and abdominal area.

    d. Splint the client's abdomen and chest while he or she coughs by pressing on his or her lower chest wall and abdomen with your hands, a pillow, or a folded towel during expiration (Fig. 17–13).

4. Produces the maximum expiration.

5. May indicate hyperventilation.

1. Elicits cooperation.

2. Respiratory disorders such as tuberculosis are transmitted by droplet nuclei during coughing.

3. Promotes maximal inspiration. Deep inspiration increases lung volume and opens the airways to allow air to get behind mucus and propel it forward.
    a. Promotes maximal inspiration. Deep inspiration increases lung volume and opens the airways to allow air to get behind mucus and propel it forward.
    b. Uses the force of air behind the mucus and muscle contraction to cough more forcefully.

    c. Clears secretions from the person's airway.

    d. Thoracic and abdominal splinting limits pain during coughing and promotes more forceful contraction of expiratory muscles.

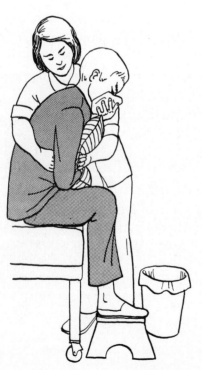

▼ **FIGURE 17–13.** Helping a client to cough.

▼ *ACTION*	▼ *RATIONALE*
e. Repeat the previous steps as necessary.	e. It may take several efforts to clear the person's airways of secretions.
f. Auscultate the client's lungs to assess for adequate removal of secretions.	f. Determines the effectiveness of the treatment.
4. Dispose of the tissues and clean the basin.	**4.** Decreases the transmission of microorganisms.
5. Offer mouth care to the client.	**5.** Promotes the client's comfort.
6. Return the patient to a position of comfort.	**6.** Coughing is tiring; allow rest time.
7. Remove any protective equipment and wash your hands.	**7.** Decreases the transmission of microorganisms.
8. Encourage the client to drink fluids if they are not contraindicated.	**8.** Hydration decreases the viscosity of pulmonary secretions and makes them easier to remove by coughing.

Teaching Pursed-Lip Breathing

1. Explain the rationale for using the pursed-lip breathing technique to the client.	**1.** This technique facilitates maximal expiration for clients with obstructive lung disease.
2. Instruct the client to inhale through his or her nose and then to purse the lips as if to kiss someone. The client should exhale slowly through the pursed lips (Fig. 17–14).	**2.** Allows better expiration by increasing airway pressure that keeps air passages open during exhalation.

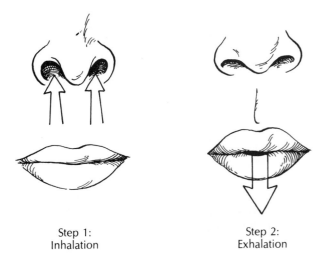

Step 1:
Inhalation

Step 2:
Exhalation

▼ **FIGURE 17–14.** Pursed-lip breathing.

Teaching Diaphragmatic Breathing

1. Help the client to assume a position of comfort.	
2. Have the client place one hand on his or her upper abdomen and one hand on his or her upper chest.	**2.** Enables the client to monitor the movement of his or her diaphragm and enables the client to monitor the use of the accessory muscles.

▼ *ACTION*   ▼ *RATIONALE*

3. As the client exhales, instruct him or her to consciously pull upward with the abdominal muscles (Fig. 17–15). The client should not use the accessory muscles in the chest.

3. Moves the diaphragm upward and results in more complete exhalation.

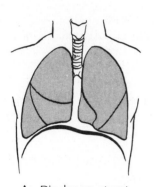
A Diaphragm at rest

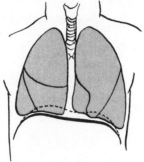
B Inhalation

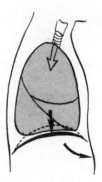
C Inhalation

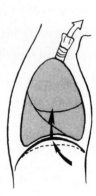
D Exhalation

▼ **FIGURE 17–15.** Diaphragmatic breathing.

4. During inhalation, instruct the client to consciously pull his or her diaphragm down (see Fig. 17–15).

4. Assists in increasing the negative pressure in the person's thoracic cavity and results in an increased volume of air inhaled.

5. Observe the client for dizziness, shortness of breath, or other respiratory symptoms.

5. May indicate hyperventilation.

Example of Documentation

DATE	TIME	NOTES
1/5/94	0900	Pursed-lip breathing and diaphragmatic breathing exercises discussed and demonstrated. Client was able to return the demonstration. *M. Jones, RN*
1/20/94	1000	Assisted client with deep breathing and coughing. Moderate amount of yellowish green sputum produced. Specimen obtained for culture and sensitivity testing and sent to lab. *C. Lammon, RN*

Teaching Tips

Be sure the client understands the importance of and rationale for deep breathing, coughing, and breathing exercises. Use a demonstration–return demonstration style of teaching to ensure that learning has taken place.

Home Care Variations

Coughing, deep breathing, and breathing exercises may be carried out in the client's home as described in this skill.

SKILL 17–6   ASSISTING A CLIENT WITH AN INCENTIVE SPIROMETER

Clinical Situations in Which You May Encounter This Skill

Incentive devices encourage the client to sustain a maximum inspiration. They are used to encourage voluntary deep breathing for postoperative clients, chest trauma victims, and clients with respiratory disorders such as atelectasis. Incentive spirometers stimulate coughing, open airways, and reduce atelectasis.

There are two basic types of incentive spirometers that provide visual feedback to clients to enhance their voluntary deep breathing:

1. Volume-oriented instruments generally have a bellows that may be raised to a preset volume by an inhaled breath. They may have a light that illuminates when the preset volume is reached instead of a bellows.
2. Flow-oriented instruments have colored balls that move as the client inhales a breath. The balls are elevated as long as the client maintains that inhaled breath.

Anticipated Responses

▼ The client's inspiratory lung expansion is at one-half to one-third of his or her preoperative inspiratory capacity.
▼ The client's lung sounds are bilaterally clear and equal upon auscultation.
▼ The client has no symptoms of atelectasis.
▼ The client's PaO$_2$ remains at normal levels.

Adverse Responses

▼ The client's inspiratory lung expansion is below one-third of his or her preoperative inspiratory capacity.
▼ A worsening or development of respiratory disorders including adventitious breath sounds, atelectasis, or pneumonia occurs.
▼ The client becomes dizzy from hyperventilation.
▼ The client's PaO$_2$ levels are below normal.

Materials List

Gather these materials before beginning the skill:

▼ Incentive spirometer
▼ Pillow

▼ ACTION

1. Review the client's respiratory status, including ABG results if appropriate.

2. Obtain a preoperative normal inspiratory volume.

3. Review the client's history to ascertain any respiratory disorders or other information, such as a history of smoking, which may affect the client's respiratory status.

4. Provide the client with oral care and insert dentures if possible.

5. Assess the client's comfort level and provide medication if appropriate.

6. Raise the bed to a comfortable working level. If you are helping the client to get out of bed, lower the bed to the lowest level.

7. Help the client to assume a semi-Fowler's or a high-Fowler's position in the bed or a chair.

▼ RATIONALE

1. Provides information for optimum care and comparison of later results.

2. Allows for appropriate goal settings for the client.

3. Provides information for an optimum plan of care and identifies potential problems.

4. Allows for a better lip seal around the mouthpiece.

5. A decreased pain level allows the client to participate in the procedure more comfortably.

6. Decreases the potential of back injury. Provides for the client's safety.

7. Allows for the greatest lung expansion.

▼ *ACTION*   ▼ *RATIONALE*

8. After he or she has exhaled to a point of comfort, direct the client to place his or her lips over the mouthpiece so that the complete mouthpiece is covered and an adequate seal is made.

8. Allows for an intact system for an effective use of the incentive spirometer.

9. Direct the client to inhale through his or her nose slowly, steadily, and continuously and at the same time to maintain a lip seal over the mouthpiece. When the client has inhaled to his or her maximum inhalation, direct him or her to hold the breath for at least 3 seconds and then exhale slowly and steadily. For a flow spirometer, tell the client to watch the ball or gauge rise to the desired level (Fig. 17–16). For a volume spirometer, tell the client to watch the gauge rise to the preset limit. A pillow may be used over the incisional area if needed.

9. Allows for optimum lung and alveolar expansion. Helps to prevent collapse of the alveoli. Ensures adequate depth of inspiration. Provides comfort.

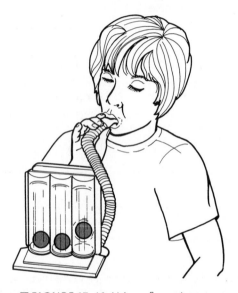

▼ **FIGURE 17–16.** Using a flow spirometer.

10. Direct the client to take 2 to 4 normal breaths and then repeat the procedure the prescribed number of times (usually 10–20 times an hour). Remind the client to report any dizziness, shortness of breath, or other problems. This procedure is repeated every hour while the client is awake.

10. Helps prevent fatigue and hyperventilation. May indicate hyperventilation or other problems. Helps to maintain adequate lung expansion.

11. Help the client to assume a position of comfort. Return the bed to its lowest position and raise the side rails, if appropriate.

11. Provides for the client's comfort and safety.

12. Evaluate the client's respiratory status, including sputum production.

12. Provides information for an optimal plan of care. Provides information on the effectiveness of the procedure.

13. Remove the mouthpiece and rinse it with cold water. Store the unit at the client's bedside.

13. Removes sputum and reduces the presence of microorganisms.

14. Record the procedure.

14. Communicates the findings to the other members of the health care team and contributes to the legal record by documenting the care given to the client.

Example of Documentation

DATE	TIME	NOTES
12/17/93	1300	Incentive spirometer used times 10. Preset volume attained. RR = 24. Lungs bilaterally clear and equal on auscultation. Nonproductive cough noted. Client states he is comfortable, but "somewhat tired." Client positioned on L side for rest period.

J. Markham, RN

Teaching Tips

Explain the procedure and the purpose of the procedure to the client or his or her family. Allow time for the client to perform a return demonstration.

Home Care Variations

With more same-day operations being performed, clients may be sent home with an incentive spirometer. Those clients with respiratory disorders and histories of smoking are more likely than others to have this procedure ordered. You should make sure the client knows how to use the equipment and have the client demonstrate the skill prior to discharge, if possible. The client should also be told what problems he or she needs to report to the health care provider, such as increased production of discolored sputum.

SKILL 17–7 USING A HUMIDIFIER

Clinical Situations in Which You May Encounter This Skill

A humidifier provides increased moisture in the air for clients who have respiratory conditions such as pneumonia, bronchitis, croup, and influenza. The moisture helps to loosen secretions and prevents drying of the respiratory tract.

Anticipated Responses

▼ The air in the client's area has a higher moisture content and facilitates the respiratory efforts of the client.
▼ The client is able to expectorate secretions more easily and the secretions are thinner.

Adverse Responses

▼ The client is unable to expectorate secretions.
▼ The client's respiratory secretions are thick and tenacious.
▼ The client develops respiratory problems from an unclean humidifier.

Materials List

Gather these materials before beginning the skill:

▼ Humidifier
▼ Distilled water
▼ Table
▼ Towel

▼ *ACTION*   ▼ *RATIONALE*

1. Review the physician's order, the diagnosis of the client's condition, and the reason for the humidifier.

1. Assists in planning care.

2. Determine if the humidifier is clean. If not, clean it according to the manufacturer's directions.

2. Prevents the growth of microorganisms.

NOTE: Make sure the humidifier is disconnected from the power source.

Prevents electric shock. Water is an excellent conductor of electricity.

---

3. Prior to using the equipment, ascertain that it is properly grounded.

3. Provides for safety.

4. The manufacturer usually includes specific directions for the filling and operation of the equipment. Generally, the following steps are included:
   a. Rinse the base of the humidifier.
   b. Fill to the "fill" mark on the base with distilled water.

   c. Reassemble the humidifier.
   d. Place a table in the client's room where the humidifier will provide the moisture needed without being a mechanical safety hazard.
   e. Place a towel on the table.
   f. Place the humidifier on top of the towel on the table.
   g. Plug the unit into the appropriately grounded electric outlet.
   h. Turn the humidifier on and watch for water vapor to appear. When it does, adjust the humidifier to the desired mist level (Fig. 17–17). If no vapor appears, check the manufacturer's directions.

4. Each piece of equipment should be operated according to the manufacturer's directions for the safest, most efficient use.
   a. Rinses out impurities.
   b. Overfilling can lead to splattering of the liquid or damage to the motor. Underfilling causes the humidifier to run out in a short period of time.

   d. Humidity should be increased in the client's vicinity. Tripping over cords leads to falls.

   e. Helps collect excess condensation.
   f. To work properly, the humidifier should be on a flat surface.
   g. Prevents electric hazards.

   h. Water vapor shows that the humidifier is operating properly.

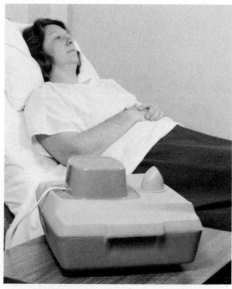

▼ **FIGURE 17–17.** Using a humidifier.

▼ *ACTION*	▼ *RATIONALE*
5. Wash your hands.	5. Decreases the transmission of microorganisms.
6. Record the procedure.	6. Communicates the findings to the other members of the health care team and contributes to the legal record by documenting the care given to the client.
7. Periodically check the humidifier to ascertain the need for refilling.	7. Water should be replaced for the humidifier to do its job.
8. Clean the humidifier every 24 hours according to the manufacturer's directions.	8. Prevents the growth of microorganisms and infection of the respiratory tract.

Example of Documentation

DATE	TIME	NOTES
10/24/93	0930	Humidifier set up in client's room. Fine mist flows easily from vented areas.
		S. Williams, RN

Teaching Tips

Explain the purpose of the humidifier to the client or the client's family. Explain that the client should stay in the room so that the humidifier can have the proper effect. Instruct the client to notify you if the bed linen becomes moist so that it can be changed.

Home Care Variations

Clients are often asked to set up humidifiers at home. Make them aware of the safety hazards of this equipment. They must also know to keep the equipment clean or it can grow microorganisms that may be harmful.

SKILL 17–8 PROVIDING CHEST PHYSIOTHERAPY

Clinical Situations in Which You May Encounter This Skill

Clients who are experiencing secretion retention and impaired oxygenation, such as in pneumonia, chronic obstructive pulmonary disease, or cystic fibrosis, may need assistance to loosen and expectorate secretions. Chest physiotherapy involves three techniques: postural drainage, chest percussion, and vibration. The optimal time to perform these techniques is before the client's meals and bedtime.

Postural drainage involves placing the client in various and specific positions to facilitate drainage of mucus and secretions from the lung fields. Gravity is used to promote drainage of the secretions. Percussion is done by cupping each of your hands to make wide "half moons" with your fingers held firmly together. Rhythmically alternate your hands with a clapping sound over the client's chest. Encourage the client to cough up and expectorate the secretions. Vibration involves placing the hands in a flat position over the chest wall and vibrating the hands.

Anticipated Responses

▼ Pooling of secretions is prevented.
▼ Promotion of tracheobronchial drainage and improvement in ventilation occurs.

Adverse Responses

▼ Secretions pool, especially in gravity-dependent areas of the person's lungs.
▼ The client experiences impaired oxygenation.

Materials List

Gather these materials before beginning the skill:

▼ Pillows
▼ Gown or other nonirritating cloth
▼ Adjustable bed
▼ Tissues
▼ Emesis basin
▼ Mouthwash, toothbrush, toothpaste, cup of water for oral hygiene
▼ Masks, goggles, gown, gloves if indicated

▼ ACTION	▼ RATIONALE
1. Auscultate for the client's breath sounds.	1. Provides baseline information.
2. Assess the client's respiratory pattern and quality of secretions.	2. Provides baseline information.
3. Assess the client's heart rate and rhythm pattern.	3. Provides baseline information.
4. Review the client's history and physical condition for hypertension, congestive heart failure, pulmonary edema, increased intracranial pressure, abdominal complications, and lung segments that require treatment.	4. Some positions are contraindicated with certain physical conditions.
5. Determine when the client last ate and allow the client to urinate.	5. Increases the client's comfort. A time interval of more than 1 hour since the last meal is best to prevent vomiting.
6. Instruct the client to tell you if he or she experiences nausea, chest pain, or increased dyspnea.	6. Indicates that the procedure should be stopped.
7. Administer any medications that will help to liquefy secretions.	7. Increases the effectiveness of the chest physiotherapy.
8. Don a mask, goggles, gown, and gloves if indicated.	8. Some respiratory disorders are transmitted by droplet and are accompanied by productive coughing.
9. Begin chest physiotherapy.	

Assisting with Postural Drainage

a. Loosen the client's clothing and provide tissues and a sputum collection device.	a. Allows for unrestricted movement and proper disposal of microorganisms.
b. Place the client in the position best suited for proper lung segment drainage (Figs. 17–18 and 17–19). Pillows may be used to maintain the client's position. Leave the side rails of the bed up, if this does not interfere with correct body mechanics.	b. Drainage of lung segments is aided by gravity. Provides comfort and safety.

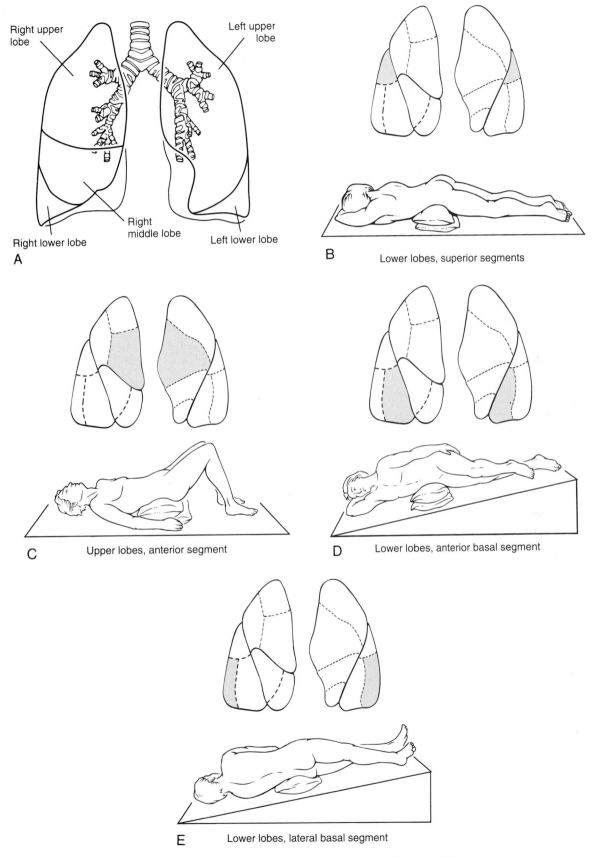

A

B   Lower lobes, superior segments

C   Upper lobes, anterior segment

D   Lower lobes, anterior basal segment

E   Lower lobes, lateral basal segment

▼ **FIGURE 17–18.** Positions for proper lung segment drainage (adult).

▼ *ACTION* _____ ▼ *RATIONALE* _____

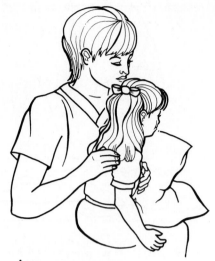

A Posterior segments

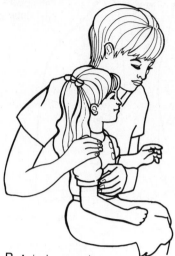

B Apical segments

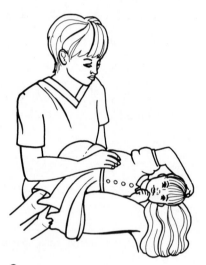

C Lateral and basal segments

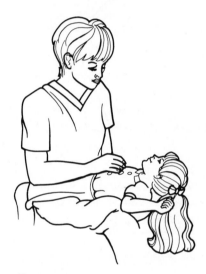

D Anterior segments

▼ **FIGURE 17–19.** Positions for proper lung segment drainage (child).

c. Cover any exposed area with a gown.

d. Have the client maintain this position for 5 minutes. Gradually increase the duration in this position to 15 minutes.

e. Encourage the client to cough and expectorate secretions.

Performing Percussion

a. Stand on the opposite side of the client's chest area to be percussed.

b. Cup each of your hands to make wide "half moons" with your fingers held firmly together.

c. Rhythmically alternate your hands with a clapping sound over the covered chest area. This technique is best done by allowing your wrists to control the hand motion.

c. Provides comfort to the client and lessens skin irritation.

d. Allows for adequate lung drainage and allows the client to gradually increase his or her tolerance.

e. Promotes respiratory hygiene.

a. Provides for your comfort and correct body mechanics.

b. Air that is trapped beneath your hands provides comfort to the client.

c. Aids the loosening of secretions in the client's lungs.

▼ _ A C T I O N_

▼ _ R A T I O N A L E_

d. Percuss the area for approximately 3 minutes.

e. Encourage the client to cough and expectorate secretions.

d. Allows for effective loosening of secretions.

e. Provides for removal of loosened secretions.

Performing Vibration

a. Instruct the client to take deep slow breaths in through his or her nose and out through his or her mouth with the lips pursed during the vibration process.

b. Keep your hands flat and place them over the client's chest area to be vibrated.

c. Ask the client to take a breath and as the client exhales vibrate your hands gently over the chest area.

a. Lengthens the expiratory phase.

b. Allows for the most contact.

c. Enhances the removal of secretions from the client's lungs.

NOTE: Use vibration only during the expiratory phase.   Vibration performed during inspiration may cause unwanted effects.

---

d. Encourage the client to cough and expectorate secretions.

10. Reassess the client's status after completion of postural drainage, percussion, and vibration of each lung segment.

11. Repeat the chest physiotherapy technique for each lung segment.

12. Slowly return the bed to its normal position.

13. Slowly help the client to assume a position of comfort.

14. Provide oral hygiene and wash the client's hands.

15. Lower the bed to the lowest level and raise the side rails.

16. Remove protective equipment if used and wash your hands.

17. Evaluate the client's respiratory pattern and the quality of secretions.

18. Evaluate the client's heart rate and rhythm pattern.

19. Record the procedure. Note the type and amount of secretions removed and the client's respiratory status.

d. Promotes respiratory hygiene.

10. Provides data regarding the effectiveness of the procedure and the client's tolerance.

12. Promotes the client's comfort and safety.

13. The client may be tired and a comfortable position facilitates rest.

14. Provides comfort and removes microorganisms.

15. Provides safety.

16. Decreases the transmission of microorganisms.

17. Provides information for optimal planning of care.

18. Provides information for planning further care.

19. Communicates the findings to the other members of the health care team and contributes to the legal record by documenting the care given to the client.

Example of Documentation

DATE	TIME	NOTES
3/24/94	1000	Assisted with chest physiotherapy of posterior right upper lobe. Client tolerated procedure well. Expectorated 10 to 20 ml thick, yellow secretions. RR = 24. Diminished breath sounds bilaterally in right upper lung fields. HR = 90. Monitor shows normal sinus rhythm.
		L. Long, RN

Teaching Tips

Students should practice hand positions, percussion, and vibration on their thighs and then on each other. It takes practice to perfect this skill.

Home Care Variations

Clients may be asked to perform this procedure or parts of it at home. Therefore, include instructions as part of the client's discharge plan.

MAINTAINING A PATENT AIRWAY

An open airway, or patent airway, provides the body with the means to obtain oxygen and to rid itself of carbon dioxide. Maintaining an open airway is crucial since brain death results within 4 to 6 minutes after an airway is completely obstructed or blocked. The airway can be occluded by a foreign body, respiratory secretions, or a neuromuscular impairment such as a bronchospasm. Refer to Skill 3–3 regarding clearing the airway of a foreign-body obstruction. If the airway occlusion is from respiratory secretions or a neuromuscular impairment, an artificial airway should be inserted to maintain the open airway. There are four types of commonly used artificial airways:

1. The oral airway, or oropharyngeal airway (Fig. 17–20), is a hard plastic curved device that fits over the tongue and prevents it from occluding the posterior pharynx.
2. The nasal airway, or nasal trumpet (Fig. 17–21), is a flexible airway inserted into the nasal passageway to facilitate nasotracheal suctioning.

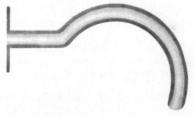

▼ **FIGURE 17–20.** An oral, or oropharyngeal, airway.

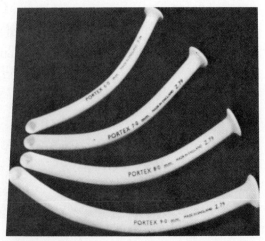

▼ **FIGURE 17–21.** Nasal airways, or nasal trumpets.

3. The endotracheal tube (Fig. 17–22) is a plastic tube that is inserted orally or nasally into the trachea. The tube may or may not have an inflatable cuff at its distal end. A cuffed tube is inflated by using a syringe to inject air through the air valve. The cuff serves three purposes. It helps to hold the endotracheal tube in proper position, it seals the trachea so that air cannot leak around the endotracheal tube, and it prevents upper airway secretions from draining down into the lungs. The cuff is deflated at intervals to prevent tracheal necrosis.

4. The tracheostomy tube (Fig. 17–23) is a plastic or metal tube that is inserted surgically into the trachea through the neck. The tracheostomy tube can be cuffed or uncuffed and may or may not include a removable inner cannula. The major purpose of an inflated cuff is to separate the upper and lower airways. An inflated cuff prevents air leakage around the cuff and prevents upper airway secretions from draining into the lungs.

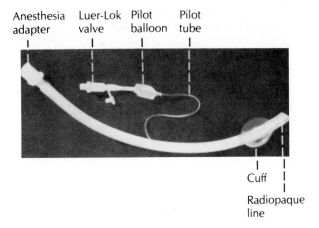

▼ **FIGURE 17–22.** An endotracheal tube.

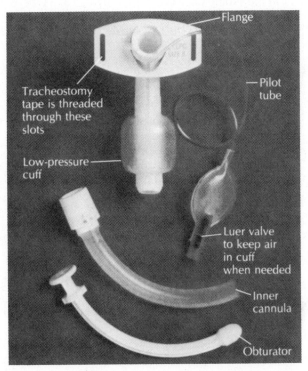

▼ **FIGURE 17–23.** A tracheostomy tube.

SKILL 17–9   INSERTING AN ORAL AIRWAY

Clinical Situations in Which You May Encounter This Skill

Clients who are semiconscious or unconscious or recovering from anesthesia may have an oral airway inserted to maintain an open airway. Clients who are intubated with an endotracheal tube or oral gastric tube may need an oral airway to facilitate suctioning or prevent biting of the other tubes.

The airway is a curved piece of plastic that is inserted through the mouth and the distal end is positioned in the area of the posterior pharynx and base of the tongue. The airway may be changed daily to promote oral hygiene.

Anticipated Responses

▼ The client's airway remains open with his or her tongue in place.

Adverse Responses

▼ Irritation and ulceration of the mucous membranes occur.
▼ The gag reflex may be initiated, especially if the airway is misplaced.

Materials List

Gather these materials before beginning the skill:

▼ Oral airway (sizes 4–10 are used for adults and sizes 000, 00, 0, and 1–3 are used for children) (The oral airway should be sterile for first insertion and clean thereafter.)
▼ Towel
▼ Examination gloves
▼ 1/2- to 1-inch tape
▼ Tissues
▼ Suction equipment

▼ ACTION

1. Assess the need for the airway and its size.

2. Put on gloves.

3. Place the client in the supine position and tilt (hyperextend) his or her head backward. A rolled towel under the neck facilitates this position. A semi-Fowler's position may be used.

4. Ask the client to open his or her mouth. If the client is unable to open his or her mouth, gently open it.

▼ RATIONALE

1. An oral airway that is too large can block the client's airway, and an oral airway that is too small will not keep the tongue properly positioned.

2. Decreases the transmission of microorganisms.

3. Opens the client's airway and allows for proper placement of the oral airway. The supine position may cause respiratory distress.

4. Facilitates insertion of the airway.

▼ _A C T I O N_ _____ ▼ _R A T I O N A L E_ _____

5. With the oral airway in a horizontal position, gently insert it until it reaches the posterior portion of the oropharynx and gently rotate the airway until it is flat against the person's tongue (Fig. 17–24).

5. Allows for proper placement of the oral airway and assists in holding the tongue in a forward position.

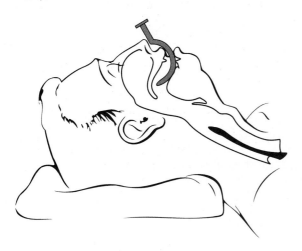

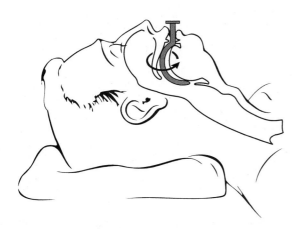

▼ **FIGURE 17–24.** Inserting and rotating an oral airway.

6. Check for proper placement of the oral airway.

6. Improper placement can stimulate the gag reflex and could hamper the client's respiration.

7. Secure the airway well with tape.

7. The airway may become displaced and lead to respiratory distress.

8. Suction the client's oral cavity if needed.

8. Helps to maintain a patent airway.

9. Wipe the client's face.

9. Removes any secretions and promotes comfort.

10. Remove the gloves and wash your hands.

10. Decreases the transmission of microorganisms.

11. Assess the client's respiratory status. Check for gagging.

11. An improperly sized or placed airway may cause gagging or airway obstruction.

▼ *ACTION*	▼ *RATIONALE*
12. Record the procedure and other relevant information.	**12.** Communicates the information to the other members of the health care team and contributes to the legal record by documenting the care given to the client.

> **NOTE:** Remember to change the client's position frequently to decrease pooling of secretions.

Example of Documentation

DATE	TIME	NOTES
10/21/93	0800	No. 5 oral airway inserted. RR = 22, with ease and no accessory muscle use or gagging noted. Client suctioned with moderate amount clear secretions obtained.
		H. Noles, RN

Teaching Tips

Explain the purpose of the airway to the client or the client's family.

Home Care Variations

The client's family can be taught to insert an oral airway using this same procedure.

SKILL 17–10   SUCTIONING THE OROPHARYNGEAL CAVITY

Clinical Situations in Which You May Encounter This Skill

Oral suctioning is useful for clients who have had oral or maxillofacial trauma or surgery. This procedure is also used for clients who have dysphagia from conditions such as cerebrovascular accidents. It is especially useful when the secretions are thick or abundant. The Yankauer suction tip, or tonsillar tip (Fig. 17–25), is only used to suction oral or pharyngeal secretions or those secretions external to the nares. Clients frequently are taught how to use this type of suctioning on their own.

Anticipated Responses

▼ The client has a clear, patent oral or pharyngeal airway.

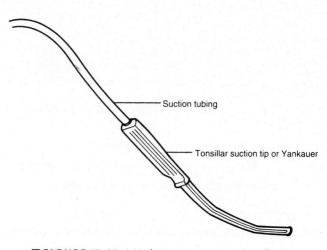

Suction tubing

Tonsillar suction tip or Yankauer

▼ **FIGURE 17–25.** A Yankauer suction tip, or tonsillar tip.

Adverse Responses

▼ The client has an airway with thick, abundant amounts of mucus.

Materials List

Gather these materials before beginning the skill:

▼ Tonsillar-tip suction device
▼ Disposable cup
▼ Water
▼ Towel
▼ Washcloth
▼ Suction setup including:
    Collection bottle
    Connecting tubing
▼ Gloves
▼ Mask
▼ Gown
▼ Goggles

▼ ACTION	▼ RATIONALE
1. Assess the client's respiratory status.	1. Provides baseline data with which to make future comparisons.
2. Review the client's chart to assess the position of his or her sutures or trauma.	2. Prevents further damage to the tissue from suctioning.
3. Observe the client's oral or pharyngeal cavity.	3. Allows for direct assessment of the area to prevent further damage.
4. Place a cup in an easily accessible area and fill it two-thirds full with water.	4. Water is used to clear secretions from the suction catheter.
5. Put on gloves and a mask, goggles, and gown if needed.	5. Decreases the transmission of microorganisms.
6. Place the bed at a comfortable working level and lower the side rail.	6. Decreases the strain on your back.
7. Help the client to assume a semi-Fowler's position or help the client to assume a position that allows for easy access to his or her oral cavity.	7. Promotes visibility of the oral cavity and easy access for suctioning.
8. Place a towel across the client's chest.	8. Protects the client's clothes.
9. Attach the connecting tubing to the suction unit and the oral suction catheter to the other end of the connecting tubing.	9. The connecting tubing links the suction device to the suction catheter.
10. Turn on the suction device at the wall or portable unit.	10. Provides suction.

NOTE: Keep the suction at low negative pressure. See the suction unit manual for the appropriate negative pressure setting according to the client's age. | Reduces tissue trauma. A higher pressure may cause damage to the client's oral mucosa.

▼ _ACTION_ _ _ _ _ _ _ _ _ _ _ _ _ _ _ _ _ _ _ ▼ _RATIONALE_ _ _ _ _ _ _ _ _ _ _ _

11. Determine the suction capability by suctioning a small amount of water into the system from the cup. Refill the cup if needed.	11. Ascertains the proper functioning of the unit.
12. Remove the oxygen mask if the client is using one.	12. Provides access to the client's oral cavity.

> **NOTE:** A nasal cannula may be left in place.

13. Gently insert the tip of the suction into the client's mouth along the lower gum line to the back of the oral cavity.	13. Causes the least gagging and trauma.

> **NOTE:** Do not apply suction at this time. Stop progression of the suction device and withdraw it slightly if the client starts to gag.

14. Apply suction and remove secretions by encircling the oral cavity with suction. The client may be encouraged to cough. (You may wear a mask and gown.)	14. Provides for efficient removal of secretions. Decreases the transmission of microorganisms.
15. Remove the suction device from the client's mouth and replace the client's oxygen.	15. Reduces hypoxia.
16. Rinse the oral suction device by suctioning water from the cup.	16. Removes secretions that can impede suction flow.
17. Reassess the client's respiratory status and need for further suctioning.	17. Determines the effectiveness of the suctioning.
18. Resuction, using the above steps, if needed. Remember to replace the oxygen after suctioning.	18. Provides for adequate removal of secretions.
19. After suctioning is completed, turn off the suction unit. Place the cleaned oral suction tip in its package and place it in an appropriate storage area. (The suction device may be cleaned with a solution of hydrogen peroxide and water. Rinse it well and dry it.) Fold the connecting tubing around the suction unit so that it is confined and cannot reach the floor.	19. An oral suction tip may be reused and should be cleaned before it is stored. Provides for removal of secretions and microorganisms. Decreases the transmission of microorganisms.
20. Wipe the client's face with a damp washcloth and dry it.	20. Removes secretions. Provides comfort.
21. Discard the water and cup.	21. Decreases the transmission of microorganisms.
22. Remove and discard your gloves. Remove your mask and gloves, and wash your hands.	22. Decreases the transmission of microorganisms.
23. Raise the side rails and lower the bed.	23. Provides safety.

▼ *ACTION*

24. Evaluate the client's oral cavity.

25. Record the procedure. Note the type and amount of secretions removed.

▼ *RATIONALE*

24. Assists in planning further care.

25. Communicates the findings to the other members of the health care team and contributes to the legal record by documenting the care given to the client.

Example of Documentation

DATE	TIME	NOTES
12/15/93	0800	Oral cavity suctioned with oral suction. Moderate amount thick slightly blood-tinged secretions obtained. O_2 at 4 L/min nasal cannula. RR = 22. Skin color pink. No accessory muscle use noted. No fresh bleeding noted at suture line.
		L. Smith, RN

Teaching Tips

Explain the purpose of and the procedure for suctioning to the client or the client's family.

Home Care Variations

Teach clients who will be using oral suction at home how to care for the equipment and how to assess their respiratory status and oral cavity.

SKILL 17–11 SUCTIONING AN INFANT WITH A BULB SYRINGE

Clinical Situations in Which You May Encounter This Skill

Newborns who have mucus or amniotic fluid in the upper airway are often suctioned with a bulb syringe. Newborns are nose breathers and their noses should be cleared to allow them to breathe comfortably. Infants and toddlers who have not learned to blow their noses may need to have the upper airway cleared of mucus from respiratory conditions such as colds or allergies. The bulb syringe exerts a gentle controlled pressure that easily clears the upper airway.

Anticipated Responses

▼ The infant's upper airway sounds clear of mucus and amniotic fluid.
▼ The infant does not demonstrate signs and symptoms of upper respiratory distress such as increased respiratory rate, use of accessory muscles, nasal flaring, gasping, and restlessness.

Adverse Responses

▼ The infant's airway does not sound clear of mucus or amniotic fluid.
▼ The infant demonstrates signs and symptoms of upper respiratory distress. If the infant's upper airway is clear but there are still signs of respiratory distress, then other possibilities should be assessed, such as lower respiratory distress or neurologic dysfunction.

Materials List

Gather these materials before beginning the skill:

▼ Bulb syringe
▼ Tissues
▼ Soft cloths (such as those used for burping)
▼ Soft receiving blanket or larger infant's blanket
▼ Examination gloves

▼ _A C T I O N_   ▼ _R A T I O N A L E_

ACTION	RATIONALE
1. Assess the child for signs and symptoms of upper respiratory distress and the need for suctioning.	1. Provides baseline data with which to compare future assessments.
2. Place the materials where they are easily accessible.	2. Provides for an efficient procedure.
3. Put on gloves.	3. Decreases the transmission of microorganisms.
4. Firmly yet gently position the infant in one of the following positions:	4. Provides for effective restraint of the infant to allow for better management of the procedure.
a. Position one:	
i. Place the infant horizontally across your upper body. Let the infant's head rest on your nondominant arm.	i. Provides gentle restraint of the baby while providing you with a free dominant hand for suctioning.
ii. Place the infant's arm that is nearest to your body comfortably around your back.	
iii. Use your arm on which the infant's head is resting to block the infant's arm from returning to your front.	
iv. With your hand from the arm that is holding the baby, grasp the baby's free arm.	
b. Position two:	
i. Place a receiving blanket or towel horizontally on a flat surface.	i. Provides gentle restraint of the baby while providing you with a free dominant hand for suctioning.
ii. Lay the infant on the covering so that the lengthwise top of the covering is at the height of the infant's shoulders.	
iii. Place the infant's arms straight alongside his or her body.	
iv. Wrap one side of the covering across the anterior of the infant's body and arms and tuck it under his or her back on the opposite side.	
v. Bring the opposite side of the covering across the infant's body and tuck the covering under his or her back on the first side.	
vi. Pick up the infant and place him or her in your nondominant arm.	
c. Position three (usually used with a large infant or toddler):	
i. Position the child in a supine position with his or her head slightly raised and his or her arms straight along the sides.	i. Provides gentle restraint of the child while providing you with a free dominant hand for suctioning.
ii. Face toward the child's head. Sit next to the child with your dominant hand closest to him or her.	
iii. Lightly lay your upper body over the child's chest and arms. Leave your arms and hands free to hold the child's head still while you suction.	iii. Your body also provides more restraint that is needed with a bigger and stronger child.
5. Place a cloth across the child's chest. Place tissues beside the child.	5. Decreases the transfer of microorganisms to the client's clothes. Tissues provide a place to discharge mucus.

▼ *A C T I O N* _____ ▼ *R A T I O N A L E* _____

6. Hold a bulb syringe in your dominant hand and compress the bulb until it is fairly flat and air has been removed from the bulb.

6. Prepares the bulb for suction. Prevents mucus from being pushed further into the child's respiratory tract.

7. Gently insert the tip of the syringe into one naris or the child's mouth.

7. Allows for suction of the upper airway.

8. After the tip is inserted, gradually release the pressure on the bulb (Fig. 17–26).

8. Allows for steady low-pressure suction.

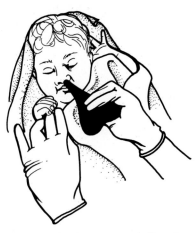

▼ **F I G U R E 17–26.** Using a bulb syringe.

NOTE: Do not allow the tip of the bulb to press against the child's mucosa.

Prevents damage to the child's mucosa from suction.

9. Following the release of all pressure, remove the syringe and discharge the suctioned secretions onto the tissues beside the child by quickly squeezing and releasing the bulb.

9. Removes mucus and fluid from the syringe. Allows for visibility of the secretions. Prepares the syringe for further use.

10. Reassess the child's respiratory status and repeat the procedure if needed. Allow the child to take several breaths between suctionings. Stop the suctioning if the child's status worsens.

10. Provides information for optimal care. Provides for reoxygenation. Indicates the need for further assessment.

11. After suctioning is completed, wipe the child's face with a damp cloth.

11. Removes secretions from the facial area.

12. Unrestrain the child and provide comfort.

12. Calms the child and assists his or her respiratory effort.

13. Place the child in a comfortable position that allows for ease of respiration.

13. Promotes adequate breathing.

14. Discard the tissues and clean the other materials for future use. Store the bulb syringe as required by your agency policy. Discard washables in an appropriate area.

14. Decreases the transfer of microorganisms. Allows for more efficient care.

15. Remove the gloves and wash your hands.

15. Decreases the transmission of microorganisms.

▼ ACTION	▼ RATIONALE
16. Evaluate the child's respiratory status.	**16.** Determines the effectiveness of the procedure. Provides information needed to plan for optimal care.
17. Record the results.	**17.** Communicates the findings to the other members of the health care team and contributes to the legal record by documenting the care given to the client.

Example of Documentation

DATE	TIME	NOTES
12/15/93	1100	Child suctioned with bulb syringe. Moderate amount of clear mucus obtained. Child calmed easily after suctioning procedure. RR = 42. No nasal flaring or accessory muscle used noted. Skin color pink.
		G. Garrity, RN

Teaching Tips

Many infants and young children have problems with mucus in the upper airway, such as with upper respiratory infections. Teach parents how to appropriately suction their children's airways until the children are able to blow their noses or otherwise learn to clear the airway. Caution parents that the nose is very sensitive and care should be taken during the suctioning procedure so as not to cause injury to the delicate tissue.

Home Care Variations

Encourage parents to learn to use a bulb syringe. It can be used in the child's home according to the above procedure.

SKILL 17–12   TRACHEOBRONCHIAL SUCTIONING VIA THE NASOTRACHEAL, ENDOTRACHEAL, AND TRACHEOSTOMY ROUTES

Clinical Situations in Which You May Encounter This Skill

When respiratory secretions accumulate in the tracheobronchial airway, they must be removed to maintain a patent airway. Suctioning the airway is a sterile procedure. Suctioning temporarily deprives the individual of oxygen and it can alter arterial blood gas (ABG) results. Thus, it is best to wait at least 30 minutes after suctioning before ABGs are drawn.

Anticipated Responses

▼ The client's airway is open and not blocked by secretions.
▼ Adequate oxygenation, as determined by ABGs, is maintained.
▼ Contamination of the client's respiratory tract does not occur.
▼ The skin and oral mucosa around the client's endotracheal tube or tracheostomy are clear and intact.
▼ There is no tracheal damage from the suction catheter, endotracheal or tracheostomy tube, or cuff.

Adverse Responses

▼ The client's airway has secretions that cause airway obstruction.
▼ The client's oxygenation is compromised.
▼ Cardiac dysrhythmias occur.
▼ Trauma to the client's tracheal or bronchial membranes occurs.
▼ Respiratory infections occur.
▼ Skin and oral mucosa irritation and breakdown around the artificial airway occur.
▼ Tracheal damage, such as necrosis, occurs.

Materials List

Gather these materials before beginning the skill:

▼ (A sterile suctioning kit may contain many of the items listed below.)
▼ Appropriate-sized sterile suction catheter (the catheter diameter should not exceed one-half the diameter of the airway):

Age	Catheter size
Newborn–18 mo	6–8 French
18–24 mo	8–10 French
2–4 yr	10–12 French
4–7 yr	12 French
7–10 yr	12–14 French
Adult	12–16 French (14 French is standard)

▼ Nasal trumpet for nasotracheal suctioning
▼ Sterile bowl or container
▼ Sterile normal saline
▼ Towel
▼ Resuscitation bag with mask and adapter for fitting to an endotracheal or tracheostomy tube
▼ Oxygen administration equipment (flowmeter, tubing, mask, or cannula)
▼ Wall suction or portable suction setup (vacuum gauge, collection container, and tubing)
▼ Sterile gloves, mask, goggles, gown
▼ Examination gloves for oral hygiene
▼ Toothbrush, toothpaste, mouthwash, emesis basin, and cup of water for oral hygiene

▼ ACTION

1. Assess the client's respiratory status and need for suctioning.

2. Place the materials on the bedside table within reach.

3. Raise the bed to a comfortable working level and lower the side rail.

4. Help the client assume a semi-Fowler's position.

5. Attach the connecting tubing to the suction apparatus, place the end of the tubing where it is accessible, and turn on the suction.

6. Place a towel across the client's chest.

7. Insert a nasal airway if nasotracheal suctioning is to be done.

8. Wash your hands.

9. Aseptically open the suction kit or equipment.
   a. Place a sterile bowl or container on top of the overbed table without touching the inside of the bowl.

▼ RATIONALE

1. Provides baseline data to compare with future assessments and helps to determine the effectiveness of the suctioning.

2. Increases efficiency. Decreases the possibility of contamination.

3. Protects your back.

4. A sitting position facilitates coughing and suctioning.

5. Connecting tubing links the suction device to the suction catheter.

6. Protects the client's clothing.

7. Reduces trauma to the client's nasal membranes.

8. Reduces the transmission of microorganisms.

   a. The inside of the bowl or container is considered to be sterile and your hands are contaminated.

▼ *A C T I O N*   ▼ *R A T I O N A L E*

b. Pour approximately 100 ml of sterile saline into the bowl.

c. If it is separate, open the package containing the suction catheter. Use sterile technique.

d. Put on a gown, mask, and goggles if needed. Put on sterile gloves.

> **NOTE:** Your dominant hand must remain sterile.

e. Hold the connecting tubing with your non-dominant hand and attach the sterile suction catheter with your sterile dominant hand (Fig. 17–27).

b. The saline is used to lubricate the suction catheter and clear secretions from the catheter.

c. Sterile technique is used to decrease contamination of the respiratory tract with microorganisms.

d. Aerosolization of microorganisms may occur. Decreases the spread of microorganisms. The dominant hand is used to manipulate the sterile equipment.

e. The nondominant hand is used to manipulate nonsterile equipment such as the connecting tubing. The suction catheter is sterile.

▼ **FIGURE 17–27.** Attaching a suction catheter.

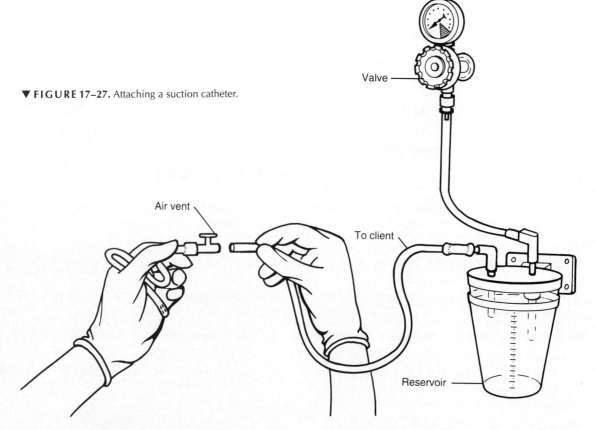

f. Suction a small amount of saline through the tubing. Control the suction by using the thumb of your dominant hand while holding the catheter in the same hand.

g. Holding the tip of the sterile catheter between your index finger and the thumb of your dominant hand, wrap the rest of the sterile catheter around your dominant hand.

10. Ask the client to take several deep breaths or hyperinflate or oxygenate the client by using the resuscitation bag or sigh device on the ventilator with your nondominant hand.

f. Checks for proper functioning of the suction apparatus and catheter.

g. Decreases the potential contamination of the catheter.

10. Decreases the potential for hypoxia during suctioning.

▼ *ACTION*	▼ *RATIONALE*

11. Use your sterile hand to insert the catheter.

11. Sterile technique prevents contamination of the respiratory tract with microorganisms.

12. Begin suctioning.

Suctioning via the Nasotracheal Route

a. Insert and advance the catheter through the client's nasal airway as the client inhales (Fig. 17–28). Do not apply suction while you insert the catheter.

a. The nasal airway reduces trauma to the nasal mucosa. Inhalation moves the epiglottis out of the way of the trachea. Suctioning while inserting the catheter causes trauma and hypoxia.

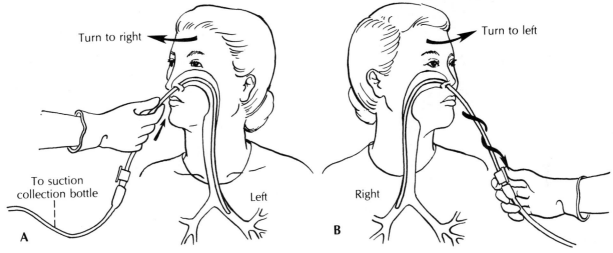

▼ **FIGURE 17–28.** Inserting a catheter for nasotracheal suctioning.

b. Advance the catheter until resistance is met, cough is stimulated, or secretions are located. Apply an intermittent vacuum as you rotate and withdraw the catheter. (Do not suction longer than 10–15 sec.)

b. Removes secretions. Prolonged suctioning results in hypoxia.

Suctioning via the Endotracheal Route

a. Using your sterile dominant hand gently and quickly insert the catheter during inspiration into the client's endotracheal tube until an obstruction is met, cough is stimulated, or secretions are located. Pull back slightly.

a. Reduces trauma to the mucosa.

NOTE: *Do not* apply suction during insertion of the catheter.

Suction can increase hypoxia.

▼ *ACTION*

▼ *RATIONALE*

b. Apply intermittent suction and rotate the catheter while you remove the catheter from the endotracheal tube (Fig. 17–29). Ask the client to cough if he or she is able.

b. Removes secretions. Rotating the catheter removes secretions from all sides of the tube.

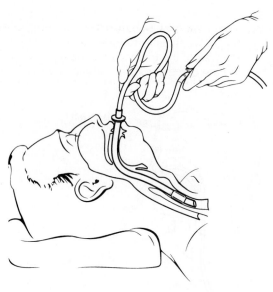

▼ **FIGURE 17–29.** Suctioning an endotracheal tube.

NOTE: *Do not* leave the catheter inserted longer than 10 to 15 seconds.

Longer insertion increases hypoxia.

---

c. Give the client oxygen or ask him or her to take deep breaths or hyperventilate with the resuscitation bag for five breaths.
d. Suction saline through the catheter.
e. Repeat steps a through d if needed.

c. Suctioning decreases oxygenation.

d. Rinses and removes debris from the tubing.
e. Provides for removal of secretions.

NOTE: Wait 1 full minute between suctionings. Assess the client's respiratory and cardiac status between suctionings.

Allows time for reoxygenation. Suctioning can stimulate cardiac dysrhythmias and respiratory distress.

Use a fresh suction catheter, glove, cup, and saline for each time tracheal suctioning is done.
f. Replace the ventilator, oxygen, or humidification device.

Prevents infection of the tracheobronchial airway.

f. Promotes breathing or adequate oxygenation, or both.

▼ *A C T I O N*   ▼ *R A T I O N A L E*

Suctioning via the Tracheostomy Route

a. Gently but quickly insert the catheter into the tracheostomy until an obstruction is met. Pull back slightly.

a. Helps to encourage the cough reflex. Decreases trauma to the wall of the mucosa.

NOTE: *Do not* apply suction while inserting the catheter.

Suction can increase hypoxia.

---

b. Apply intermittent suction and rotate the catheter while removing the catheter from the tracheostomy (Fig. 17–30). Ask the client to cough if he or she is able.

b. Decreases trauma to the wall of the mucosa and removes secretions.

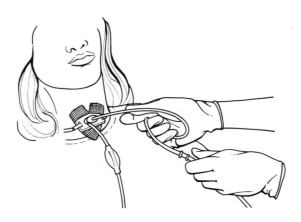

▼ **FIGURE 17–30.** Suctioning a tracheostomy.

NOTE: *Do not* leave the catheter inserted for longer than 10 15 seconds.

Longer insertion can increase hypoxia.

---

c. Give the client oxygen and ask him or her to take deep breaths or give five breaths with the resuscitation bag.

c. Helps to reoxygenate the client.

NOTE: A second person is needed to use the resuscitation bag because your hand with the catheter must remain sterile.

▼ *ACTION*   ▼ *RATIONALE*

   d. Rinse the suction catheter with saline.

   e. Repeat steps a through d if needed.

   d. Removes debris from the catheter.

NOTE: Wait 1 full minute between suctionings.

Allows time for reoxygenation.

---

   f. Assess the client's respiratory and cardiac status between suctionings.

   g. If tracheostomy care or cleaning is to be done, see Skill 17–13.

   h. Replace the oxygen or humidification device.

   f. Provides data with which to determine if continued suctioning is necessary.

   h. Allows for the prescribed oxygenation.

13. After the tracheobronchial airway has been cleared of secretions, suction the client's oral and nasal cavities if needed.

13. Removes secretions from the upper airways.

NOTE: Once the catheter has been used to suction these areas, it may not be used to suction the endotracheal tube again. A new sterile catheter must be obtained.

The upper airway is contaminated.

---

14. Remove the catheter from the connecting tubing, wrap the catheter around your gloved hand, and pull the glove off your hand over the catheter. Discard it into an appropriate container.

14. Decreases the transmission of microorganisms.

15. Using your other gloved hand discard the saline bowl, towel, and other articles. Disinfect the goggles. Remove the glove and discard it.

15. Decreases the transmission of microorganisms.

16. Put on examination gloves and provide the client with oral hygiene. Change the tape or ties holding the tube in place if needed.

16. Provides comfort and hygiene.

NOTE: The endotracheal or tracheostomy tube cuff must be inflated during oral hygiene.

Helps to prevent aspiration.

---

17. Reposition the client, put up the side rails, and lower the bed.

17. Provides comfort and safety.

18. Evaluate the client's cardiac and respiratory status.

18. Suctioning can stimulate cardiac dysrhythmias. The lungs should sound clearer on auscultation and there should be no signs of respiratory distress.

▼ *ACTION*

▼ *RATIONALE*

19. Record the procedure. Note the type and amount of secretions removed and the client's respiratory status.

19. Communicates the findings to the other members of the health care team and contributes to the legal record by documenting the care given to the client.

Example of Documentation

DATE	TIME	NOTES
1/21/94	1000	Endotracheal tube suctioned. Moderate amount clear secretions obtained. HR = 88, regular; RR = 24 with ease. Skin color pink. Client resting.
		M. Naylor, RN

Teaching Tips

Explain the purpose of and the procedure for suctioning to the client and the client's family. Encourage all family members with respiratory infections not to visit the client or to wear a mask if they must visit.

Home Care Variations

A portable suction unit can be used in the client's home. The client and his or her family should be encouraged to use sterile technique at all times and their technique should be periodically assessed.

SKILL 17–13   CARING FOR A CLIENT WITH A TRACHEOSTOMY

Clinical Situations in Which You May Encounter This Skill

A tracheostomy provides an artificial airway for clients who require either a temporary or permanent opening through which oxygenation may be maintained. You should cleanse and dress the tracheostomy stoma as well as clean the inner cannula if the tracheostomy tube has one. Cuffed tracheostomy tubes require deflation of the cuff periodically to prevent tracheal necrosis.

Anticipated Responses

▼ The client's airway is open and not blocked by secretions.
▼ Adequate oxygenation, as determined by arterial blood gases (ABGs), is maintained.

▼ Respiratory infections improve or do not occur after the tube is inserted.
▼ The skin site around the tracheostomy is free of infection and is intact.
▼ There is no tracheal damage from the tube and cuff (if one is present).

Adverse Responses

▼ The client's airway and tracheostomy have secretions that cause airway obstruction.
▼ Respiratory infections occur.
▼ Skin irritation and breakdown occur around the tracheostomy.
▼ Tracheal damage such as necrosis occurs.

Materials List

Gather these materials before beginning the skill:

▼ Suction equipment (see Skill 17–12)
▼ Suction setup (either wall or portable)
▼ Sterile gloves (2 pairs), mask, goggles, and gown
▼ Sterile drape or disposable sterile field
▼ To cleanse the tracheostomy:
Hydrogen peroxide
Normal saline
Cleansing brush
Sterile cotton-tipped swabs (two pkgs.)
Sterile bowl
Tracheostomy necktie
Scissors
4- × 4-inch non-cotton gauze pads (three pkgs. if single or two pkgs. if double)

Tracheostomy bib (or dressing made from non-cotton gauze 4- × 4-inch strips)
Sterile gloves (2 pairs)
Disposable inner cannula (if required by the tracheostomy)
(If a disposable inner cannula is to be used, a sterile bowl with hydrogen peroxide and the cleansing brush are not needed.)
▼ To deflate and inflate the cuff:
Oropharyngeal suction equipment
Sterile gloves, mask, goggles, and gown
5- to 10-ml syringe
Resuscitation bag
Stethoscope
Rubber-shod hemostat
Manometer to measure cuff pressure

▼ ACTION

1. Assess the client's respiratory status including the need for suctioning and tracheostomy cleansing.

2. Place the materials on a bedside table within reach.

3. Raise the bed to a comfortable working level and lower the side rail on the working side.

4. Help the client to assume a semi-Fowler's position. A side-lying position may be best if the client is unconscious.

5. Attach the connecting tubing to the suction apparatus, place the end of the tubing where it is accessible, and turn on the suction.

6. Place a towel across the client's chest.

7. Open the suction kit or equipment. Also open the materials needed for tracheostomy cleansing at this time.
   a. Place the drape down first and set up the suction equipment (see Skill 17–12).
   b. Set a second sterile bowl near but out of the way of the first bowl. Do not touch the inside of the bowl.

> **NOTE:** The second bowl of hydrogen peroxide and a cleansing brush are not needed if you are replacing the inner cannula with a sterile disposable one.

   c. Pour approximately 50 ml of sterile hydrogen peroxide into the second bowl. Do not drip it on the drape.

▼ RATIONALE

1. Provides baseline data with which to compare future assessments and helps to determine the effectiveness of the suctioning.

2. Increases efficiency. Decreases the possibility of contamination.

3. Protects your back.

4. A sitting position facilitates coughing and suctioning. A side-lying position helps to prevent choking and aspiration.

5. Connecting tubing links the suction device to the suction catheter.

6. Protects the client's clothing.

   a. Use of a sterile field decreases the possibility of contamination.
   b. The first bowl is used for suctioning and is contained in the suctioning kit. The second bowl is used for cleaning the inner cannula.

   c. The hydrogen peroxide is used to clean the inner cannula. The sterile field is considered contaminated if any fluid drips on it.

▼ *ACTION*   ▼ *RATIONALE*

d. Open the sterile brush and place it next to the bowl with hydrogen peroxide.

e. Open packages of three 4- × 4-inch gauze pads. Maintain sterility of the gauze. Pour hydrogen peroxide on one gauze pad and saline on the second. Leave the third open and dry.

f. Open the cotton-tipped swabs. Pour hydrogen peroxide on one set and saline on the other. Set the bottles of saline and hydrogen peroxide aside with their caps off.

g. If you are using a disposable inner cannula, open the package so that the cannula may be easily removed. Maintain the sterility of the inner cannula.

h. Determine the needed length of the tracheostomy necktie by doubling the circumference of the neck plus 2 inches and cutting the tie to that length.

8. Follow the suctioning procedure (see Skill 17–12). Be sure to wear protective clothing and sterile gloves.

9. Remove the tracheostomy bib from around the tracheostomy tube and discard it.

10. Discard the soiled gloves and put on new sterile gloves. Your dominant hand should remain sterile throughout the remainder of the procedure.

11. Clean the inner cannula.

Replacing a Disposable Inner Cannula

a. Unlock and carefully remove the inner cannula with your nondominant hand.

b. Suction the client again with sterile technique, if needed.

c. Remove the fresh sterile inner cannula from the package and pour a small amount of sterile saline over the new cannula.

d. Allow the excess saline to drip off the inner cannula.

e. Carefully insert the inner cannula into the outer cannula and lock it into place.

f. Reattach the oxygen source.

---

d. The brush is used to clean the inner cannula.

e. One gauze pad is used to cleanse the skin around the tracheostomy. The second is used to remove the debris loosened by the hydrogen peroxide, and the third is used to dry the skin.

f. The swabs are used to cleanse around the tracheostomy.

g. The sterile inner cannula should be ready to insert after you cleanse the skin.

h. The tie should hold the tracheostomy in place without constricting circulation.

8. Clears the airway for more efficient cleansing of the tracheostomy. Suctioning is a sterile procedure. Protective clothing prevents contact with body fluids.

9. The skin should be cleansed to prevent skin breakdown.

10. Decreases the transmission of microorganisms.

a. The inner cannula must be removed and changed to decrease the transmission of microorganisms and to enhance breathing.

b. Removing the inner cannula may stimulate coughing and the client may need suctioning.

c. Lubricates the cannula for easier insertion.

d. Saline dripped into the tracheostomy causes the client to cough.

e. Prevents the inner cannula from accidentally coming out and disrupting the integrity of the tracheostomy.

f. Provides oxygenation.

▼ *ACTION* _ _ _ _ _ _ _ _ _ _ _ _ _ _ _ ▼ *RATIONALE* _ _ _ _ _ _ _ _ _ _ _ _

Cleaning a Nondisposable Inner Cannula

a. Remove the inner cannula with your nondominant hand and place it in a bowl with hydrogen peroxide.

a. Removes mucus and microorganisms from inner cannula.

NOTE: Attempt to keep the oxygen source as close as possible to the outer cannula. If the client is unable to breathe without mechanical assistance, a second nurse or respiratory therapist should maintain respirations with a mechanical resuscitation device.

Provides for adequate oxygenation.

---

b. Pick up the brush with your dominant hand and the inner cannula with your nondominant hand and clean the inner cannula with the brush.

b. Removes stubborn mucus and crusted secretions.

c. Hold the cannula above the peroxide bowl with your dominant hand and pour the saline over the cannula until it is well rinsed.

c. Removes hydrogen peroxide and other residue.

d. Allow the excess saline to drip off the inner cannula.

d. Saline dripped into the tracheostomy causes the client to cough.

e. Reinsert the inner cannula into the outer cannula and lock it in place (Fig. 17–31).

e. Prevents the inner cannula from accidentally coming out and disrupting the integrity of the tracheostomy.

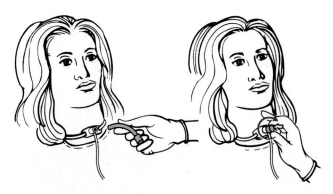

▼ **FIGURE 17–31.** Reinserting an inner cannula to an outer cannula and locking it in place.

f. Reattach the oxygen source.

f. Provides oxygenation.

NOTE: Cleaning the cannula should be done as quickly as possible.

Decreases possible hypoxia.

▼ *A C T I O N* _____ ▼ *R A T I O N A L E* _____

12. Use the hydrogen peroxide–saturated 4- × 4-inch piece of gauze and swabs to cleanse the outer surfaces of the outer cannula and the skin areas around it. Remember to cleanse the skin area directly adjacent to the cannula. Cleanse from the stoma out (Fig. 17–32).

12. Removes mucus and microorganisms.

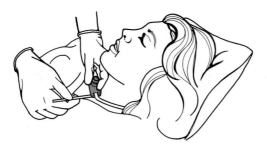

▼ **FIGURE 17–32.** Cleansing around a tracheostomy.

13. Rinse the same areas with the saline-saturated 4- × 4-inch gauze and swabs.

13. Removes hydrogen peroxide, which can be irritating to tissues.

14. Gently dry the same areas with the dry 4- × 4-inch piece of gauze.

14. Decreases moisture that may enhance microorganism growth. Protects skin integrity.

15. Obtain the precut necktie.

16. To change the necktie:
   a. Leave the present necktie in place.
   b. Thread the clean tie through one side of the faceplate.
   c. Bring both free ends around the back of the client's neck to the other side of the faceplate.
   d. Thread one free end through the other side of the faceplate and tie it firmly but not tightly.
   e. Cut the old necktie so that it can be removed and discarded.

   a. Prevents the tracheostomy from slipping out.

   d. A clean tracheostomy bib should be placed under the faceplate.

> **NOTE:** This process can be done by having a second person hold the tracheostomy tube in place while the original necktie is removed and a clean one is applied.

▼ *ACTION* | ▼ *RATIONALE*

17. Place a clean tracheostomy bib or dressing in place around the outer cannula under the ties and faceplate (Fig. 17–33). Check to make sure the necktie is not too tight but the tracheostomy tube is safely held in place.

17. Allows for collection of mucus from the tracheostomy. Protects skin integrity.

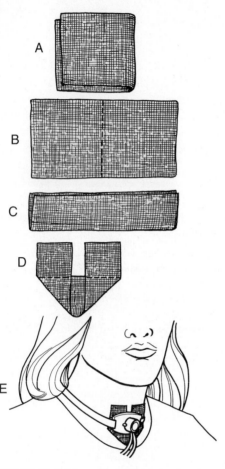

▼ **FIGURE 17–33.** Folding and applying a tracheostomy dressing.

18. Suction the client if needed.

18. Provides for a clear airway.

19. Replace the oxygen or humidification device, if not already done.

19. Allows for prescribed oxygenation.

20. Provide oral care.

20. Decreases the growth of microorganisms in the client's mouth.

21. Using your gloved hands discard the bowls and other articles.

21. Decreases the transmission of microorganisms.

22. Remove the gloves and dispose of them properly.

22. Decreases the transmission of microorganisms.

▾ *A C T I O N* _____ ▾ *R A T I O N A L E* _____

> **NOTE:** The following procedure can also be used to deflate and inflate an endotracheal tube cuff.

23. To deflate and inflate the tracheostomy tube cuff:
   a. Put on gloves.
   b. Suction the client's oropharyngeal airway.

   c. If a clamp is present on the cuff inflation tube, release it. Attach the syring to the inflation tube.
   d. Ask the client to inhale or give a breath with the resuscitation bag as you slowly withdraw the amount of air from the cuff as recommended by the manufacturer (usually 5 cc).
   e. Observe for respiratory difficulties.

24. To inflate the cuff using the minimal occlusive volume (MOV) and minimal leak technique (MLT):
   a. Place the stethoscope on the client's neck.

   b. While listening with the stethoscope, inflate the cuff with a syringe (Fig. 17–34). Use the smallest amount of air needed to obtain a seal (usually 2–5 ml).

a. Decreases transmission of microorganisms.
b. Prevents secretions from draining down into the lower respiratory tract when the cuff is deflated.
c. Prepares for releasing air from the cuff.

d. Creates pressure in the airway that forces secretion upward.

e. If difficulties are seen immediately reinflate the cuff.

a. The stethoscope is used to auscultate for the presence of an air leak around the cuff.
b. Using MOV prevents overinflation of the cuff that results in pressure on the tracheal membranes and necrosis.

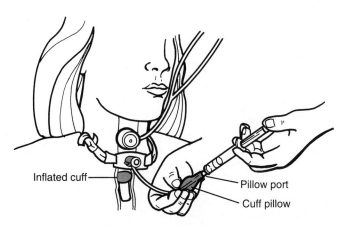

Inflated cuff

Pillow port
Cuff pillow

▾ **FIGURE 17–34.** Inflating a tracheostomy tube cuff with a syringe.

   c. Aspirate a small amount of air (0.1–3 ml) until a very slight air leak is auscultated.
   d. Note the total amount of air inserted in the cuff. Then clamp the tube with the rubber-shod hemostat if necessary and remove the syringe.
   e. Measure the cuff pressure with a manometer.

c. MLT ensures that excessive pressure on the tracheal mucosa is avoided.
d. Holds air in the cuff.

e. Assesses the amount of pressure on the tracheal mucosa.

▼ *ACTION*	▼ *RATIONALE*
f. Document the time of the cuff deflation, the amount of air reinserted into the cuff, how the client tolerated the procedure, and the measurement of cuff pressure.	f. Communicates the findings to the other members of the health care team and contributes to the legal record by documenting the care given to the client.
25. Reposition the client, put up the side rails, and lower the bed.	**25.** Provides comfort and safety.
26. Remove gloves and wash your hands. Put away the articles.	**26.** Decreases transmission of microorganisms. Provides for an uncluttered area.
27. Evaluate the client's cardiac and respiratory status.	**27.** Cleaning and suctioning the tracheostomy may alter the client's cardiac or respiratory status.
28. Determine if more suctioning or tracheostomy care equipment are needed and order them. Have at least one suctioning kit accessible.	**28.** Provides for an efficient and prompt procedure next time.
29. Record the procedure. Note the type and amount of secretions removed and the client's respiratory and cardiac status.	**29.** Communicates the findings to the other members of the health care team and contributes to the legal record by documenting the care given to the client.

Example of Documentation

DATE	*TIME*	*NOTES*
1/10/93	1000	Tracheostomy care given. Stoma area slightly reddened, without drainage. Moderate amount of clear mucus obtained when suctioning. HP = 88, RR = 24, with ease. Skin color pink. Client resting.
		L. Marson, RN

Teaching Tips

Explain the purpose of and the procedure for the tracheostomy cleaning to the client and the client's family. Encourage all family members with respiratory infections to not visit the client or to wear a mask if they must visit.

Home Care Variations

Clients are sent home with tracheostomy tubes that require suctioning and care. Teach the client the proper procedure for suctioning and cleaning. Stress the necessity of keeping all equipment clean and suctioning catheters sterile.

SKILL 17–14   PROVIDING ENDOTRACHEAL TUBE CARE

Clinical Situations in Which You May Encounter This Skill

An endotracheal tube provides an artificial airway for clients who require temporary assistance with oxygenation. If long-term oxygenation assistance is needed, a tracheostomy is performed. Clients with certain neuromuscular diseases, respiratory conditions, and other situations that cause an interference in the normal airway flow may require an endotracheal tube. Endotracheal tubes are cuffed in order to maintain proper placement and to prevent the tube from coming out or slipping down into one of the bronchi, which would prevent air exchange in one lung.

Anticipated Responses

▼ The client's airway is clear.
▼ Adequate oxygenation, as determined by arterial blood glases, is maintained.
▼ Respiratory infections do not occur or improve after the tube is inserted.
▼ The skin and oral mucosa around the endotracheal tube are clear and intact.
▼ There is no tracheal damage from the tube or cuff.

Adverse Responses

▼ The airway or endotracheal tube has secretions that cause airway obstruction.
▼ Oxygenation is compromised.
▼ Respiratory infections are present.
▼ Skin and oral mucosal irritation and breakdown around the endotracheal tube occur.
▼ Tracheal damage such as necrosis may occur.
▼ The endotracheal tube and oral cavity are dirty.

Materials List

Gather these materials before beginning the skill:

> **NOTE:** A sterile suctioning kit may have all the items listed.

Suctioning
▼ Clean area (overbed table is best)
▼ Suction catheter (use appropriate size)

Age	Catheter Size
Newborn–18 mo	6–8 French (Fr.)
18–24 mo	8–10 Fr.
2–4 yr	10–12 Fr.
4–7 yr	12 Fr.
7–10 yr	12–14 Fr.
Adults	12–16 Fr. (14 Fr. is standard)

▼ Water-soluble lubricant
▼ Sterile bowl
▼ Sterile normal saline
▼ Towel
▼ Waterproof drape (inside should be sterile, if possible)
▼ Suction (either wall or portable)
▼ Connecting tubing
▼ Gloves (one must be sterile)
▼ Ambu bag with oxygen connector

Cleaning the endotracheal tube
▼ Adhesive tape or waterproof tape (1–1.5 inches in diameter)
▼ Twill tape (at least 2 feet long)
▼ Scissors
▼ Nonsterile gloves
▼ Adhesive remover (if adhesive tape is used)
▼ Clean bowl
▼ Hydrogen peroxide
▼ Oral airway cleaning brush
▼ Oral hygiene swabs
▼ Washcloths (2: one to wash and one to rinse)
▼ Towels (2)
▼ Bath basin with warm water
▼ Oral hygiene equipment
▼ Tincture of benzoin and applicator

▼ ACTION

1. Assess the client's respiratory status including the need for suctioning and endotracheal tube care.

2. Place materials on the client's bedside table within reach.

3. Raise the bed to a comfortable working level. Lower the side rail on the working side(s).

▼ RATIONALE

1. Gathers data for optimal care.

2. Increases efficiency. Decreases the possibility of contamination.

3. Protects your back.

▼ *ACTION*   ▼ *RATIONALE*

4. Help the client to assume a semi-Fowler's or supine position. Side-lying may be needed if the client is unconscious.

4. Increases efficiency. Side-lying decreases the possibility of aspiration.

5. If needed, attach connecting tubing to the suction apparatus. Place the end of the tubing where it is accessible. Turn on the suction.

5. Increases efficiency. Provides suction when needed.

6. Place a towel across the client's chest.

6. Protects the client's clothing.

7. When opening the suction kit or equipment, also open materials needed for endotracheal tube cleaning.

7. Increases efficiency.

   a. Place the drape down first and set up the suction equipment. (See Skill 17–12 for setup of suctioning equipment.)

   a. Decreases the possibility of contamination.

   b. Open and place the oral hygiene items, including the washcloths, towel, and bath basin, on a separate towel.

   b–f. Increases efficiency.

   c. Set the second bowl near the oral hygiene materials.

   d. Pour approximately 50 ml of sterile hydrogen peroxide into the bowl.

   e. Open the oral airway cleaning brush and place it next to the bowl with the hydrogen peroxide.

   f. Place the opened adhesive remover swabs beside the oral hygiene items (if you are using adhesive tape).

   g. Prepare the tape for securing the tube. Use one of the two following methods:
      i. Using adhesive tape:

      • Cut one strip of adhesive tape as long as the circumference of the client's head plus 6 to 8 inches with the client's nose as the starting point.

      • Prevents the tape from sticking to the client's hair.

      • Cut a second strip of adhesive tape long enough to cover the adhesive side of the center of the first strip from in front of one ear around the back of the head to the front of the other ear.

      • Prevents unnecessary skin irritation.

      • Attach the adhesive tapes to each other.

      • Prepare the tincture of benzoin.
      ii. Using twill tape:

      • Cut a 2-foot piece of twill tape and double it over.

   h. Place the tape near the other nonsterile equipment.

   h. Separates sterile and nonsterile equipment.

   i. Ensure that all needed equipment is in place.

   i. Increases efficiency.

8. Follow the suctioning procedure. (See Skill 17–13.)

8. Clears the client's airway for a more efficient cleaning of the endotracheal tube.

▼ *ACTION*

▼ *RATIONALE*

9. While the client is reoxygenating, again ascertain that all equipment needed is present. Have suctioning equipment set up for oral suctioning. (A Yankuer may also be used.)

   Have a sterile suction catheter readily available. Leave the client connected to the mechanical ventilation, unless contraindicated. The client may be ambued, if needed.

9. Increases efficiency.

   Provides for sterile suctioning of the endotracheal tube, if needed. Provides for oxygenation.

10. Obtain assistance from another health professional.

10. Assists in maintaining tube placement.

11. Ask a gloved assistant to hold the endotracheal tube firmly in place at the client's lip line.

11. Helps maintain tube placement and client comfort.

12. Carefully remove all tape from around the tube and the client's skin. Adhesive remover may be used to completely remove all adhesive tape. Discard the tape.

12. Allows for skin and oral hygiene. Tape may cause skin irritation.

13. If an oral airway or a bite-block is in place, remove it and place it in a bowl of hydrogen peroxide.

13. Allows for access to the oral cavity while the airway is soaking.

14. Perform oral hygiene. If the client has a nasotracheal tube, complete oral hygiene and clean around the nasotracheal tube. If the client has an orotracheal tube:
    a. Perform oral care on the side of the oral cavity that is unencumbered by the tube.
    b. Note the centimeter mark of the tube in reference to the client's lips.
    c. With an assistant's help, grasp the tube at this mark and carefully move the tube to the other side of the client's mouth.
    d. Ascertain that the reference mark remains the same.
    e. Use oral suction as needed.

14. Provides for comfort. Decreases oral bacteria and the possibility of infection to the client's teeth and gums.

    b–d. Helps maintain tube placement.

    e. Removes excess secretions.

15. Wash the client's face and neck area with a soapy washcloth, rinse with a wet washcloth, and dry the area with a towel. A facial shave for male clients may be done at this time.

15. Provides comfort and hygiene.

16. Use Step 17 or 18 to secure the endotracheal tube.

17. To secure the endotracheal tube with adhesive tape:
    a. Using a prepared tincture of benzoin swab, lightly brush the facial areas that will be covered with tape.
    b. Allow the area to dry.

    c. While the tincture of benzoin is drying and prior to securing the endotracheal tube, auscultate the lung fields.
    d. Slide the prepared adhesive tape under the client's neck with the sticky side up and the covered area stretching from ear to ear.
    e. Adhere one side of the adhesive tape from the client's ear to the endotracheal tube, then tear that leftover portion of the tape into two sections.

    a. Increases adhesive tape adherence with decreased skin irritation.

    b. The skin must be dry for the procedure to work properly.
    c. Helps ascertain that the endotracheal tube is in place and has not slipped into one of the bronchi.
    d. Maintains appropriate placement of the endotracheal tube for adequate oxygenation.

    e–l. Allows for the most secure grasp of the tube.

▼ *ACTION*   ▼ *RATIONALE*

f. Wrap the top portion of the torn tape around the endotracheal tube from top to bottom.

g. Adhere the bottom portion of the tape along the client's skin next to the tube. Cut off the leftover tape.

h. Pull the other side of the adhesive tape so there is no excess.

i. Adhere this side of adhesive tape from the client's ear to the endotracheal tube.

j. Again tear that leftover portion of tape into two sections.

k. Wrap the bottom portion of the torn tape around the endotracheal tube from bottom to top.

l. Adhere the top portion of the tape along the client's skin next to the tube. Again cut off unneeded tape.

18. To secure the endotracheal tube with twill tape:
    a. Use doubled-over 2-foot twill tape.
    b. Tie the tape around the tube. Bring the ends through this loop below the mark of where the endotracheal tube leaves the client's mouth or nares.
    c. Pull the tape ends in opposite directions to reach around and behind the client's neck.
    d. Gently but firmly pull the tape snug against the neck skin. (If needed, tincture of benzoin may be applied on the skin under the tape. See step 17a.)
    e. Tie a secure knot at the side of the client's neck.

18. a–e. Allows for the most secure grasp of the tube.

e. Do not make the knot tight. A tight knot can obstruct venous flow.

19. Reconnect the client to mechanical ventilation if not already done.

19. Maintains ventilation of client.

20. Using a brush, clean the oral airway or bite-block and rinse it well with water. Remove excess water.

20. Removes secretions and microorganisms.

21. Gently and correctly reinsert the oral airway or bite-block. (See Skill 17–9.)

21. Provides for proper placement without trauma. Prevents occlusion of the orotracheal tube.

22. Reposition the client. Raise the side rails and lower the bed.

22. Provides comfort and safety.

23. With gloved hands, discard the bowls and other articles. Remove the gloves and discard them.

23. Decreases the transmission of microorganisms.

24. Wash your hands. Recap and put away articles.

24. Provides for an uncluttered area.

25. Evaluate the client's cardiac and respiratory status.

25. Provides information for planning care.

26. Evaluate the client's comfort.

26. See above.

27. Determine whether more suctioning or tracheostomy care equipment are needed and order them. Have at least one suctioning kit accessible for use.

27. Provides for an efficient and prompt procedure next time.

Example of Documentation

DATE	TIME	NOTES
1/10/94	1000	Endotracheal tube care provided. Oral area pink, moist, without obvious irritation. Moderate amount of clear mucus obtained when suctioning. HR = 88, RR = 24, with ease. Skin color pink. Client resting.
		L. Marson, RN

SKILL 17–15   MANAGING A CHEST TUBE

Clinical Situations in Which You May Encounter This Skill

Chest tubes are inserted into the client's thoracic cavity to remove abnormal accumulations of air or fluids such as blood from the pleural space. These accumulations result from conditions such as trauma, chronic respiratory diseases, or thoracic surgery. The presence of air in the pleural space is called a pneumothorax, the presence of serous fluid is called a pleural effusion, and the presence of blood is called a hemothorax.

These conditions disrupt the negative intrapleural pressure of the pleural space and result in a collapsed lung and compromised ventilation. To restore the negative pressure, a chest tube is inserted into the pleural space and attached to a water-sealed drainage system. The purpose of the water seal is to prevent air from reentering the pleural space as the accumulation

of air and fluid is draining from it. There are four types of drainage systems that may be used with the chest tube:

1. The single-bottle system (Fig. 17–35) uses gravity alone to encourage drainage of air or fluid from the pleural space. There is an air vent to prevent a buildup of air and pressure in the system. The single-bottle system is primarily used for resolving a pneumothorax.
2. The two-bottle system (Fig. 17–36) adds a second bottle that allows for drainage of fluid as well as air from the pleural space. The two-bottle system is used to resolve a hemothorax (blood), hemopneumothorax (blood and air), and pleural effusion (serous fluid). The first bottle is for collection of fluid and air and the second bottle provides the water seal.
3. The three-bottle system (Fig. 17–37) includes a third bottle that allows connection to a suction control device. This system may be used for any of the above-named conditions. The purposes of the first and second bottles are the same as in the two-bottle system.
4. Disposable commercial systems (Pleur-evac, Thoraclex, Argyle) (Fig. 17–38) work either as a two-bottle system when there is no suction or a three-bottle system when suction is provided. Some of these

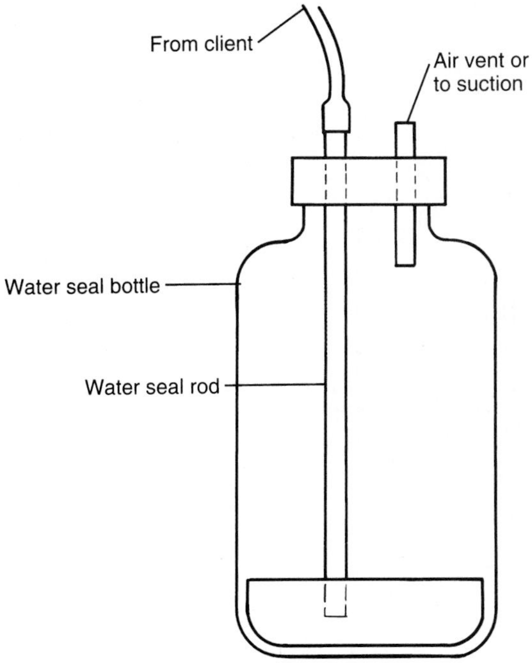

▼ **FIGURE 17–35.** A single-bottle drainage system.

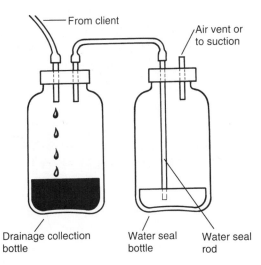

▼ **FIGURE 17–36.** A two-bottle drainage system.

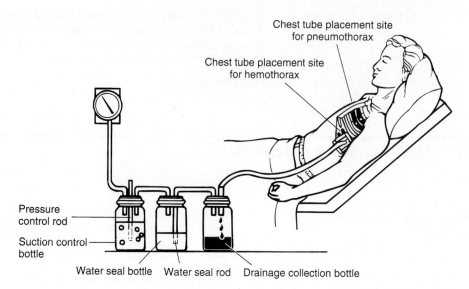

Chest tube placement site
for pneumothorax

Chest tube placement site
for hemothorax

Pressure
control rod

Suction control
bottle

Water seal bottle   Water seal rod   Drainage collection bottle

▼ FIGURE 17–37. A three-bottle drainage system.

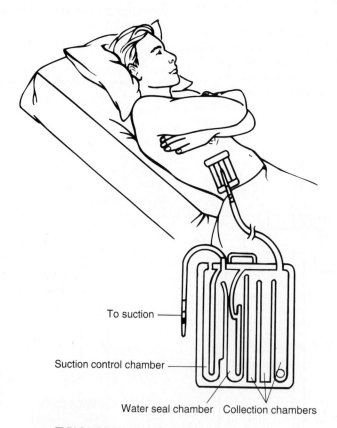

To suction

Suction control chamber

Water seal chamber   Collection chambers

▼ FIGURE 17–38. A disposable drainage system.

devices require that sterile water be added to the chambers and others require no additions of sterile water to maintain a closed system. Follow the manufacturer's directions when setting up these systems.

Anticipated Responses

▼ Removal of air, fluid, or blood from the pleural space occurs along with restoration of negative pressure.
▼ Auscultated breath sounds improve and the client begins to subjectively "feel better."
▼ Arterial blood gas (ABG) readings are more normal.

Adverse Responses

▼ Removal of air, fluid, or blood from the pleural space is obstructed, possibly by a malfunction in the closed drainage system.
▼ The negative pressure is not restored, possibly because of air leaks.
▼ Auscultated breath sounds do not improve and may deteriorate.
▼ The client complains of continued or increased shortness of breath.
▼ ABG readings remain unchanged or deteriorate.
▼ A tension pneumothorax develops.

Materials List

Gather these materials before beginning the skill:

▼ Razor, soap, water, towel, and examination gloves to prep the insertion site

▼ Chest-tube insertion tray:
4- × 4-inch gauze pads
Antiseptic solution
Sterile gloves
Lidocaine 1% without epinephrine
Scalpel handle with blades
Non–Luer-Lok syringes (10 and 30 ml) (several)
Sutures
Clamps
Forceps
Scissors
Sterile five-in-one barrel connector (at least two)
Sterile "Y" connecter if there is more than one chest tube
Sterile dressing materials including adhesive-backed elastic dressing and petrolatum gauze dressing
▼ Chest tubes of various sizes with obturators (at times included in chest-tube insertion tray)
▼ Drainage system (one-, two-, or three-bottle, or disposable)
▼ Sterile water or saline
▼ 60-ml sterile Asepto syringe
▼ Suction source (wall or Emerson)
▼ Drainage tubing
▼ Adhesive tape (0.5–1 inch)
▼ Rubber-shod Kelly clamps (two for each chest tube)
▼ Surgical prep tray if shaving is required
▼ Lotion or alcohol wipes if "milking or stripping" is required

▼ ACTION

Assisting with Insertion of a Chest Tube

1. Assess the client's respiratory and cardiac status.

2. Set up a sterile field and chest tube insertion tray.

3. Prepare the drainage system. Note whether or not a one-, two-, or three-bottle system or a disposable system is to be used.

Using a One-Bottle System Setup

a. Obtain one sterile vented water-seal chest tube bottle.
b. Remove the cover from the vent.

c. While maintaining the sterility of the system, place enough sterile water or saline in the bottle so that the longer tube is covered by 1 inch (2 cm) of fluid.

▼ RATIONALE

1. Provides baseline data with which to compare future assessments.

2. Sterile technique is used to decrease the transmission of microorganisms.

3. Allows for prompt connection of the chest tubes to drainage system. Allows for proper implementation of the physician's order.

a. This type of bottle is generally used for resolution of a pneumothorax.
b. Allows for release of excess air from the system.
c. Prevents air from entering back into the intrapleural space.

▼ *A C T I O N*   ▼ *R A T I O N A L E*

    d. Assess the system's integrity for airtightness, sterility, an open air vent, and appropriately submerged longer tube.

    d. Prevents air leaks.

Using a Two-Bottle System Setup

    a. Obtain and set up a water-seal bottle (bottle No. 2) as described above.

    b. Obtain a sterile drainage collection bottle (bottle No. 1) and a connecter rod.

    c. Using sterile technique, attach the connecter rod from the vent opening of the drainage collection bottle (bottle No. 1) to the submerged longer tube of bottle No. 2.

    d. The second shorter (nonsubmerged) tube on bottle No. 2 remains open to the atmosphere.

    e. The second tube on bottle No. 1 is connected to the client.

    f. Assess the system's integrity for airtightness, sterility, an open air vent, an appropriately submerged longer tube, and other relevant connections.

    a. Prevents air from entering back into the intrapleural space. Allows excess air to escape from the system.

    b. Provides for separate collection of fluid.

    c. Allows for excess air to flow from bottle No. 1 to bottle No. 2 and escape from the system. Prevents air from flowing back into the intrapleural space.

    d. Allows excess air to escape from the system.

    e. Completes the system.

    f. Decreases the possibility of air leaks.

Using a Three-Bottle System Setup

    a. Obtain and set up a water-seal bottle (bottle No. 2) and a sterile drainage collection bottle (bottle No. 1) as described above under the two-bottle system setup.

    b. Obtain a suction control bottle (bottle No. 3) and a second connecter rod.

    c. While maintaining the sterility of the system, place enough sterile water or saline in bottle No. 3 so that the longer tube is covered by 1 inch (2 cm) of fluid. The opposite end of this tube should remain vented to the air.

    d. Using sterile procedure, attach the second connecter rod from the vent opening (short tube) of the water-seal bottle (bottle No. 2) to one of the two short tubes of bottle No. 3.

    e. Connect the second short tube on bottle No. 3 to the suction source.

    f. The second tube on bottle No. 1 is connected to the client.

    g. Assess the system's integrity for airtightness, sterility, an open air vent, an appropriately submerged longer tube, and other relevant connections.

    a. Prevents air from flowing back into the system. Allows excess air to escape from the system.

    b. Allows for suction while maintaining the integrity of the system.

    c. Prevents air from flowing back into the intrapleural space while allowing excess air to escape.

    d. Allows for suction to be attached to the system.

    e. Allows for the suction source to be attached to the system.

    f. Completes the system.

    g. Prevents the possibility of air leaks.

Using a Disposable System

    a. Follow the manufacturer's directions.

4. Place a strip of adhesive tape vertically on the collection bottle next to the calibrated numbers.

4. Allows for accurate assessment of the amount of fluid collected in the chest tube drainage system.

5. Place the client in a Fowler's or semi-Fowler's position.

5. Allows for optimal evacuation of fluid or air.

6. Put on examination gloves.

6. Decreases the transmission of microorganisms.

▼ *A C T I O N* _____   ▼ *R A T I O N A L E* _____

7. Shave the chest tube insertion site, if needed. Discard used supplies and gloves.

7. Hair harbors microorganisms. Hair removal promotes easier application and removal of tape.

8. Assist the physician, as needed, during the insertion procedure. Wear sterile gloves to protect you from contact with body fluids.

| **NOTE:** Monitor the client's respiratory, cardiac, and psychologic status during the procedure. | Chest tube insertion can compromise the client's respiratory and cardiac status. |

---

9. Connect the distal end of the chest tubes to the functional drainage system.

9. Establishes a closed drainage system.

10. If there are two chest tubes, connect both to the drainage system via a "Y" connecter.

10. Allows for adequate drainage of two sites with one drainage system.

11. Ascertain that all connections and stoppers are firmly attached.

11. Prevents air from entering the intrapleural space.

12. Secure all connections with adhesive tape.

12. Prevents disconnection and entrance of air.

13. Remove your gloves and discard them appropriately. Wash your hands.

13. Decreases transmission of microorganisms.

14. If the client can tolerate it position him or her in a semi-Fowler's to high-Fowler's positon.

14. Assists in evacuation of air and fluid.

15. Evaluate the client's respiratory and cardiac status.

15. Provides information for further care.

16. Periodically evaluate the client for development of a tension pneumothorax. If this does develop, examine the chest tubes for occlusion (see Step 19). Notify the physician.

16. Occluded chest tubes can lead to a build-up of air in the intrapleural space and cause a shift of tissues. This is a medical emergency.

17. Examine and record the chest tube drainage on the collection bottle or chamber as ordered (*Do not* empty the bottle):
   a. Every hour for new postoperative clients.
   b. Every hour for clients with a large amount of drainage.
   c. Every 8 hours for all clients with chest tubes.

17. Provides continuing information about the quantity and quality of the drainage.

NOTE: The time of the examination and the date on the collection bottle or chamber. Also evaluate the color of the drainage and if there is bubbling in the collection bottle or chamber.

Monitoring the Client with a Chest Tube

18. Ensure that the necessary equipment is at the client's bedside in case of emergency:
   a. Two rubber-shod Kelly clamps.

   a. Used to clamp the chest tube if a leak develops in the tubing.

▼ _ACTION_   ▼ _RATIONALE_

b. Sterile petrolatum gauze dressing.

c. Extra drainage system.

19. Periodically evaluate that:

a. Connections remain firmly attached and secure.
b. The drainage system remains below the chest-tube insertion site.
c. Tubing is not twisted and lies in a fairly straight line from the insertion site to the drainage system.
d. Sterile water or saline levels in the water-seal bottle or chamber are at the proper mark.
e. If suction is ordered, the proper level is set. The suction should be adjusted so that gentle, continuous bubbling is seen in the suction bottle or chamber. (If an Emerson pump is used for suction, the chest-tube system is connected to the Emerson and the front dial is set to the prescribed suction amount.)
f. Chest drainage does not collect in the tubing.
   i. If sluggish drainage or clots are present, "milking or stripping" tubes may be required.

b. Used to form an occlusive seal if the chest tube is accidentally dislodged.
c. Used in case of breakage or malfunction.

19. Provides for the safety, integrity, efficiency, and effectiveness of the system.
a. Reduces air leaks. Allows for the prescribed suction.
b. Allows for drainage flow away from the client's body.
c. Allows for efficient flow and the prescribed suction pressure.

d. Allows for a proper water seal to reduce air leaks and maintain adequate negative pressure.
e. The fluid level in the suction bottle or chamber determines the amount of suction. Allows for the prescribed suction without excessive evaporation of fluid in the suction bottle or chamber.

f. Provides for efficient flow.
   i. Encourages drainage. Prevents blockage of the flow

NOTE: A physician's order is needed. Check the hospital policy about this procedure since "milking or stripping" is controversial.

Since an increase in suction occurs during "milking," controversy centers on the possibility of tissue damage.

• Occlude the tube close to the client's chest with your nondominant hand.

NOTE: Never block the tubing for more than 1 minute.

A tension pneumothorax may occur.

• Using your dominant hand occlude the tube directly below your opposite hand.

• Using a controlled, continuous motion, slide your dominant hand along the tubing away from the client toward the drainage system.

• Breaks up clots and increases suction in the tube to improve flow.

• Moves the drainage toward the drainage system and away from the client's chest.

NOTE: Lotion or alcohol wipes may be used along the tubing.

Decreases friction along the tubing and facilitates the procedure.

▼ *A C T I O N* _____ | ▼ *R A T I O N A L E* _____

- Repeat the previous three steps. Move along the chest tubing until the drainage system is reached.

  ○ Moves the drainage toward the drainage system and away from the client's chest.

- If "milking" is ordered and there is hospital policy approval for this procedure, "milk" the chest tubes every 4 to 8 hours if the chest drainage is serous and every 30 to 60 minutes if the drainage is bloody or contains clots.

  ○ Provides for optimal flow.

g. Air leaks are not present.
   i. Continuous bubbling in the water-seal bottle or chamber indicates an air leak.

   i. Intermittent bubbling or a rise and fall of fluid in the longer tube associated with respiration is normal. These indicators should stop when negative pressure within the intrapleural space is restored and the lung reexpands.

- To determine the location of an air leak, use rubber-shod Kelly clamps to occlude the chest tube close to the client's chest for a few seconds while observing the water-seal bottle. If bubbling continues, the leak is most likely in the drainage system. If bubbling stops, the leak is most likely with the chest-tube insertion site. (Do not clamp the tube longer than 1 minute.)

  ○ Placing a clamp between the system and the origin of the air leak stops the bubbling.

  Tension pneumothorax can occur.

- To correct a leak in the drainage system, reevaluate the integrity of all connections and stoppers. Retape the connection sites. If you are unable to correct the problem, replace the drainage system.

  ○ Air entering through loose connections is the most common cause of air leaks.

- If the leak is at the chest-tube insertion site, reinforce the occlusive chest dressing. If the leak continues, notify the physician and assess the client's condition.

  ○ The leak may occur from one of the openings on the chest tube that has slipped out of the client's chest. Physicians should correct this problem. Allows for optimal care.

h. The drainage bottle or chamber is not full.
   i. When the drainage bottle or chamber becomes full, set up a new drainage system and ascertain its integrity.
   ii. Put on gloves.

   i. Proper suction and drainage cannot occur. Allows for proper functioning of the system.
   ii. Decreases the transmission of microorganisms.
   iii. Prevents air from entering the system.

   iii. Using rubber-shod Kelly clamps occlude the chest tube close to the client's chest just long enough to disconnect the chest tube from the drainage system and reconnect the chest tube to the new drainage system. Maintain the sterility of the system during the transfer.

NOTE: Do not leave the chest tube clamped for more than 1 minute.

A tension pneumothorax may occur.

▼ _ACTION_	▼ _RATIONALE_
iv. Ascertain whether all connections and stoppers are firmly attached.	iv. Prevents air from entering the intrapleural space.
v. Secure all connections with adhesive tape.	v. Prevents air from entering the intrapleural space.
vi. Assess the client's status.	vi. Provides information for optimal care.
vii. Dispose of the used drainage system in the proper area.	vii. Decreases the transmission of microorganisms.
viii. Remove the gloves and discard them appropriately.	viii. Decreases the transmission of microorganisms.
20. Record the procedure.	**20.** Communicates the findings to the other members of the health care team and contributes to the legal record by documenting the care given to the client.

Example of Documentation

DATE	TIME	NOTES
6/25/93	1200	Right-sided chest tube connected to 20 cm suction. 50 ml light red drainage measured in collection chamber since 0800. No bubbling seen in water-seal chamber. Client quietly resting in semi-Fowler's position. Skin color pink. No complaints. RR = 26 without accessory muscle use. Lung sounds bilaterally clear and equal anteriorly and posteriorly.
		S. Kelly, RN

Teaching Tips

Explain the purpose of the chest tubes and the procedure for insertion to the client and his or her family. Encourage the client to cough, deep breathe, and change positions periodically.

Home Care Variations

Chest tubes are not used in the client's home.

References

Clark, A. P., et al. Effects of endotracheal suctioning on mixed venous oxygenation saturation and heart rate in critically ill adults. _Heart and Lung,_ 19, 552–557.

Davies, B. L., MacLeod, J. P., and Ogilvie, H. M. J. (1990). The efficacy of incentive spirometers in postoperative protocols for low-risk patients. _The Canadian Journal of Nursing Research,_ 22 (4), 19–36.

Gift, A. G., Bolgiano, C. S., and Cunningham, J. (1991). Sensations during chest tube removal. _Heart and Lung,_ 20, 131–136.

Kersten, L., and Cronin, S. N. (1994). Meeting respiration needs. In V. Bolander (Ed.). _Basic Nursing_ (3rd ed.). Philadelphia: W. B. Saunders.

Preusser, B. A., et al. (1989). Quantifying the minimum discharge sample required for accurate arterial blood gases. _Nursing Research,_ 38 (5), 276–279.

Stone, K. S., et al. (1989). Effects of lung hyperinflation on mean arterial pressure and postsuctioning hypoxemia. _Heart and Lung,_ 18, 377–385.

Tyler, D. O., Clark, A. P., and Ogburn-Russell, L. (1991). Developing a standard for endotracheal tube cuff care. _Dimensions of Critical Care Nursing,_ 10 (2), 54–61.

CHAPTER 18

Administering Medications

- -

One of the most important responsibilities nurses hold is medication administration. In order to administer medications safely and correctly, you must possess the manual dexterity and skill to manipulate equipment such as needles and syringes. You also must have knowledge of sterile technique, the pharmacology of the medication to be given, techniques of safe medication administration, the legal implications of medication administration, and an understanding of how to apply the nursing process to the client who is receiving medications.

Preventing medication errors is of utmost importance when caring for clients who are receiving medications. You should adhere to the "five rights of medication administration" when preparing and administering medications. The five rights are: right drug, right dose, right route, right time, and right person. You may administer medications by the topical, oral, or parenteral routes.

- -

- -

OVERVIEW OF RELATED RESEARCH

deSilva, M. I., et al. (1986). **Multidosage medication vials: A study of sterility, use patterns, and cost-effectiveness.** *American Journal of Infection Control,* 14 (3), 135–138.

Frequently used medications are often supplied in multidose injectable vials (MDVs) as a cost containment measure. The sterility, use patterns, and cost-effectiveness of 839 MDVs were studied. Following existing hospital guidelines, no vials had bacterial contamination, and the cost incurred by the pharmacy for medication wastage with an automatic expiration date of 7 or 14 days was $437. The second phase of the study instituted new guidelines with the significant difference of an automatic expiration date extended to either 3 months or the manufacturer's recommended date. A total of 1,070 MDVs were processed with no bacterial contamination and a cost savings from $437 to $46.

Kasmer, R. J., et al. (1986). **Sterility of preloaded insulin syringes.** *American Journal of Infection Control,* 14 (4), 180–183.

Maintaining sterility of preloaded syringes of insulin for use by elderly or blind patients is a concern to nurses. A total of 1,536 preloaded syringes of insulin were evaluated to determine their sterility after storage at room and refrigeration temperatures for up to 28 days. Seven of the 1,536 syringes were found to be contaminated after 7, 14, and 21 days of storage. Although the potential for contamination with bacteria exists, this study confirms that preloaded insulin syringes can be maintained for a prolonged period of time in an aseptic state after careful preparation and storage.

TOPICAL MEDICATIONS

Topical medications are applied directly to the skin or mucous membranes. These agents may be used for their local effect or to produce systemic effects from percutaneous absorption. Topical medications include drugs applied to the skin (such as lotions, creams, and ointments); optic medications (administered into the eye); otic medications (administered into the ear); pulmonary medications (administered by inhalation); nasal medications (instilled into the nose); rectal medications (inserted into the rectum); and vaginal medications (inserted into the vagina).

SKILL 18–1   APPLYING MEDICATIONS TO THE SKIN

Clinical Situations in Which You May Encounter This Skill

Medications can be applied to the skin to relieve itching, to prevent or treat local infections, to cause vasodilation, or to moisten the skin.

Materials List

Gather these materials before beginning the skill:

▼ Correct medication
▼ Correct applicator (tongue blade, sterile gauze pad, cotton ball)
▼ Sterile gloves (2 pairs)
▼ Basin with warm water
▼ Mild soap
▼ Washcloth and towel
▼ Examination gloves
▼ Gauze dressing
▼ Plastic wrap (for anti-anginal ointment only)
▼ Tape
▼ Disposable waterproof pad
▼ Tray
▼ Chart

▼ ACTION	▼ RATIONALE
1. Obtain a physician's order.	**1.** The physician is licensed to prescribe medications. You are licensed to administer medications.
2. Verify the correctness of the order and check the client's chart for drug allergies.	**2.** You are responsible for all medications administered to the client. A drug allergy is a contraindication to administration of the medication.

▼ *ACTION* _ _ _ _ _ _ _ _ _ _ _ _ _ _ _ _ _ _ _

▼ *RATIONALE* _ _ _ _ _ _ _ _ _ _ _ _ _ _ _

3. Wash your hands.

3. Handwashing is the single most effective measure to decrease the transmission of microorganisms from one person to another.

4. Concentrate alone.

4. Prevents medication errors from inattention.

5. Select the correct medication and read the label. (This is the first of three times that the label should be read.)

5. The label is read three times to prevent medication errors.

6. Check the expiration date.

6. Expired medications may not give the needed effect.

7. Read the medication label for a second time and place the drug on the tray with the other equipment.

7. The label is read three times to prevent medication errors.

8. Carry the medication and equipment to the client and introduce yourself.

8. Identifies the caregiver and his or her credentials. Helps to establish rapport with the client.

9. Ask the client if he or she has any drug allergies.

9. You should assess the client's chart and medication records for drug allergies. Asking the client about drug allergies serves as a final safety check.

10. Verify the client's identity by checking his or her arm band and bed tag and asking the client to state his or her name.

10. Prevents you from administering medications to the wrong client.

11. Verify the drug by reading the label for the third time.

11. The label is read three times to prevent medication errors.

12. Position the client comfortably and expose the area to be treated. Keep all unaffected areas draped.

12. Facilitates treatment and provides for the client's dignity and modesty.

13. Put on gloves.

13. Protects your hands from contact with bodily secretions and contact with the medication.

14. Pad the bed if necessary.

14. Prevents soiling of the bed linens.

15. Cleanse the area to be treated with warm water and mild soap. If the area is very irritated, use warm water only.

15. Removes exudate and drainage.

16. Pat the area dry unless moisture retention is desired (as is the case with some creams, ointments, and lotions).

16. Prevents further irritation.

17. Assess the condition of the client's skin. Note the color, temperature, circulation, texture, drainage, and any changes from the previous observation.

17. Evaluates the client's progress and identifies signs of complications such as infection or poor circulation.

18. Change your gloves if necessary.

18. If your gloves are soiled by secretions, put on new gloves before administering the medication to prevent contamination of the area.

19. Administer the medication.

Administering an Aerosol Spray

   a. Shake the container well.
   b. Follow the manufacturer's directions regarding the distance to hold the spray from the affected area.
   c. Spray the medication evenly over the affected area. Be sure to direct the spray away from the client's face.

   a. Mixes the medication.
   b. Provides the best coverage.

   c. Aerosol propellants can be irritating to the eyes and lungs.

▼ *A C T I O N*   ▼ *R A T I O N A L E*

Administering Creams, Gels, Pastes, Ointments, and Oil-based Lotions

a. Place 1 to 2 teaspoons of medication in the palm of your gloved hands or use a tongue blade.

b. Apply the medication smoothly and evenly over the surface of the area to be treated. Follow the direction of the person's hair growth.

Administering Nitroglycerine Paste or Ointment

a. Squeeze out the ordered number of inches of medication onto a paper measuring guide (Fig. 18–1).

a. This amount generally covers the area.

b. Facilitates even application of the medication to the area to be treated.

a. Use of a paper guide facilitates accurate measurement.

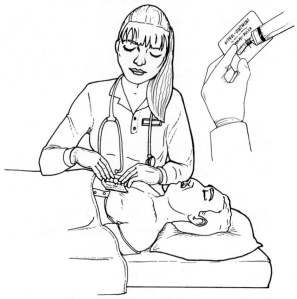

▼ **FIGURE 18–1.** Squeezing medication onto a paper measuring guide.

b. Remove the old medication patch from the client's skin and cleanse the area.

c. Place the ointment and paper on the client's skin. Avoid hairy areas. *Do not* touch the ointment.

d. Cover the ointment and paper with plastic wrap and tape the paper in place.

b. Promotes the client's comfort.

c. Promotes the best absorption. The ointment is absorbed through your skin and may cause systemic results.

d. Maintains skin contact with the drug and prevents soiling of clothing.

Applying a Transdermal Patch

a. Follow the manufacturer's directions regarding removal of the patch backing.

b. Apply the patch to a smooth skin area that is free of lesions or excess hair.

c. Remove the old patch if there is one.

a. Most medication discs have a plastic, foil, or paper backing that must be removed before application.

b. Lesions or hair may prevent the proper adhesion of the patch.

c. Promotes the client's comfort.

▼ *A C T I O N*	▼ *R A T I O N A L E*

Applying Suspension-based Lotions

a. Shake the medication well.
b. Moisten a gauze pad or cotton ball with lotion and gently pat it onto the area to be treated.

a. Evenly suspends medication in the solution.
b. After the water evaporates, a thin film of powdered medication remains on the skin.

Applying Powders

a. Be sure the area to be treated is completely dry.
b. Lightly dust the area with powder.

a. Prevents caking of the powder.

b. A thin layer of powder prevents crusting and irritation.

Applying Liniments

a. Pour 1 to 2 teaspoons of medication into your hands.
b. Apply the medication to the client's skin with long firm smooth strokes.

b. Liniments should be rubbed into the skin.

20. Cover the affected area with a dressing if indicated.

20. Keeps the medication in contact with the client's skin and prevents soiling of his or her clothing.

21. Help the client to dress and return to a position of comfort.

21. Promotes the client's comfort.

22. Dispose of soiled supplies in a proper container.

22. Decreases the transmission of microorganisms.

23. Wash your hands.

23. Decreases the transmission of microorganisms.

24. Return to the client at the appropriate time to assess the effects of the medication.

24. You are responsible for monitoring for the desired effect, potential side effects, and allergic reactions to the medication.

25. Chart the medication given; the time, dose, and route of medication; the appearance of the client's skin; his or her response to the drug; and any other related information.

25. Communicates to the other members of the health care team and contributes to the legal record by documenting the care given to the client.

Example of Documentation

DATE	TIME	NOTES
1/1/93	0900	Nystatin applied to diaper rash. Skin is red with papules noted.
		H. White, RN

Teaching Tips

The client should know the name of the medication, its purpose, and any possible side effects. Be sure the client understands the correct method of applying skin preparations to obtain the maximum effect of the drug.

Home Care Variations

Topical medications can be applied in the client's home using the same procedure.

SKILL 18–2   ADMINISTERING OPTIC MEDICATIONS

Clinical Situations in Which You May Encounter This Skill

Optic medications are frequently administered to treat infections, relieve inflammation, treat eye disorders such as glaucoma, and diagnose foreign bodies and corneal abrasions. Absorption of medications through the tear ducts can lead to systemic effects such as alterations in blood pressure and heart rate.

Anticipated Responses

▼ The medication produces the desired local effect.
▼ No side effects such as eye irritation or burning are noted.

Adverse Responses

▼ The medication produces a systemic response.

Materials List

Gather these materials before beginning the skill:

▼ Correct medication
▼ Tissue
▼ Wash basin with warm water
▼ Washcloth
▼ Sterile gloves (2 pairs)
▼ Medication tray
▼ Chart
▼ Eye patch (optional)
▼ Tape (optional)

▼ ACTION

1. Obtain a physician's order.

2. Verify the correctness of the order and check the client's chart for drug allergies.

3. Wash your hands.

4. Concentrate alone.

5. Select the correct medication and read the label. (This is the first of three times that the label should be read.)

6. Check the expiration date.

7. Gather the equipment needed to administer the drug and place it on the medication tray.

8. Read the label of the medication for the second time and place the drug on the tray.

9. Carry the medication and equipment to the client. Introduce yourself.

10. Ask the client if he or she has any drug allergies.

11. Verify the client's identity by checking his or her arm band and bed tag and asking the client to state his or her name.

12. Verify the drug by reading the label for the third time.

13. Position the client in the supine position or sitting in a chair with his or her neck hyperextended.

▼ RATIONALE

1. The physician is licensed to prescribe medications. You are licensed to administer medications.

2. You are responsible for all medications administered to the client. A drug allergy is a contraindication to administration of the medication.

3. Handwashing is the single most effective measure to decrease the transmission of microorganisms from one person to another.

4. Prevents medication errors from inattention.

5. The label is read three times to prevent medication errors.

6. Expired medications may not give the needed effect.

7. All needed equipment is available.

8. The label is read three times to prevent medication errors.

9. Identifies the caregiver and his or her credentials. Helps to establish rapport with the client.

10. You should assess the client's chart and medication records for drug allergies. Asking the client about drug allergies serves as a final safety check.

11. Prevents you from administering medications to the wrong client.

12. The label is read three times to prevent medication errors.

13. Prevents the eye medication from flowing out of the person's eye.

▼ *ACTION*	▼ *RATIONALE*
14. Put on sterile gloves.	**14.** Prevents contamination of the client's eye. Gloves should be worn whenever there is a chance of contact with bodily secretions.
15. If exudate is seen on the client's eyelids or lashes, gently cleanse the area with warm water. Wipe from the inner to outer canthus. You may need to soak the area by applying a warm moist washcloth over the eye for a few minutes.	**15.** Removing secretions provides hygienic care and removes the medium for further bacterial growth.
16. Assess the external structures of the eye for redness, drainage, crusting, or lesions.	**16.** These are signs of infection and should be recorded in the client's chart.
17. Change your gloves if needed.	**17.** If your gloves are soiled by the person's eye secretions, new sterile gloves are needed before administering the medication in order to prevent contamination.
18. Give the client a tissue to hold just below the lower eyelid.	**18.** The tissue catches any medication that inadvertently flows down the client's face.
19. With your nondominant hand, rest your index finger on the bony rim of the client's upper eye orbit. Rest your thumb on the lower bony rim of the client's eye orbit.	**19.** Stabilizes the eye area.
20. Spread your thumb and index finger to open the client's eye and create a lower pocket or conjunctival sac.	**20.** The medication is instilled into this pocket or sac.
21. Ask the client to look up and to try not to blink.	**21.** Blinking discharges some of the medication from the eye.
22. Administer the medication.	

Instilling Eye Drops

a. Hold the eye dropper in your dominant hand ½ inch above the client's conjunctival sac. Rest your dominant hand on client's forehead.	a. Prevents eye injury and dropper contamination.
b. Instill the prescribed number of drops into the sac (Fig. 18–2).	b. Ensures an accurate dosage.

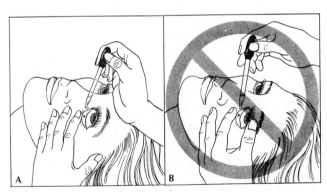

▼ **FIGURE 18–2.** Correct *(A)* and incorrect *(B)* ways to instill eye drops.

c. When administering drugs that may cause a systemic effect, apply gentle pressure to the nasolacrimal duct for 1 minute after instilling the medication.	c. Prevents the medication from flowing down the tear duct and being absorbed through the mucous membranes.

▼ *ACTION* ‾ ‾ ‾ ‾ ‾ ‾ ‾ ‾ ‾ ‾ ‾ ‾ ‾ ‾ ‾ ‾ ▼ *RATIONALE* ‾ ‾ ‾ ‾ ‾ ‾ ‾ ‾ ‾ ‾

d. Allow the client to gently close his or her eye.

e. Use a tissue to catch any stray drops of medication.

d. Squeezing the eye shut expels the medication.

e. Provides for the client's comfort.

Administering Eye Ointment

a. Apply a thin line of eye ointment from the client's inner canthus to the outer canthus along the lower eyelid inside the conjunctival sac (Fig. 18–3).

a. Spreads the medication evenly over the eye.

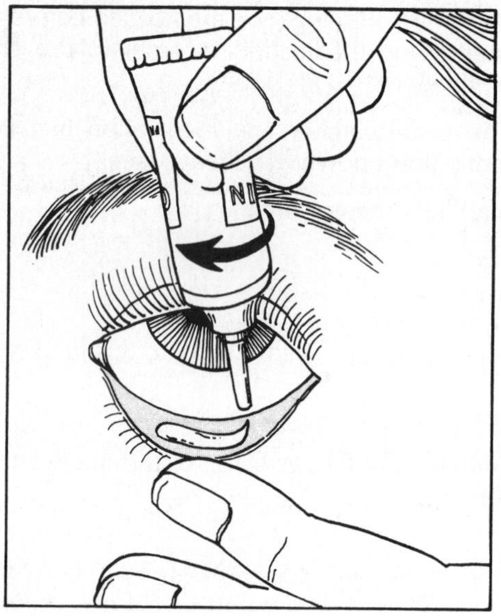

▼ **FIGURE 18–3.** Administering eye ointment.

b. Ask the client to gently close his or her eye and move the eyeball around in the socket.

c. Gently wipe away the excess medication with a tissue from the inner canthus to the outer canthus.

b. Aids in melting and spreading the medication over the eye.

c. Provides for the client's comfort. The direction of the wipe reduces the risk of infection.

23. Apply an eye patch if indicated.

23. Maintains eye closure.

24. Dispose of soiled supplies in a proper container.

24. Decreases the transmission of microorganisms.

25. Remove gloves and wash your hands.

25. Decreases the transmission of microorganisms.

26. Return to the client at the appropriate time to assess the effects of the medication.

26. You are responsible for monitoring for the desired effect, potential side effects, and allergic reactions to the medication.

27. Chart the medication given; the time, dose, and route of medication; the appearance of the client's eye; his or her response to the drug; and any other related information.

27. Communicates to the other members of the health care team and contributes to the legal record by documenting the care given to the client.

Example of Documentation

DATE	TIME	NOTES
1/1/93	0945	Betaxolol hydrochloride 1 gt OD administered now.
		H. White, RN

Teaching Tips

The client should know the name of the medication he or she is receiving, as well as its purpose and possible side effects. If the client is to use the medication at home, the technique for administration should be demonstrated and time should be provided for the client to do a return demonstration.

Home Care Variations

Eye medications can be administered in the client's home using the same procedure.

SKILL 18–3　ADMINISTERING OTIC MEDICATIONS

Clinical Situations in Which You May Encounter This Skill

Otic medications are usually administered to treat infection, relieve pain, or soften and remove impacted cerumen (wax).

Adverse Responses

▼ There is no improvement in the client's hearing acuity.
▼ Redness, drainage, or swelling of the ear canal are present.
▼ The client complains of pain in the ear.

Anticipated Responses

▼ If ear drops were used for impacted cerumen, the client's hearing is improved.
▼ If ear drops were used to combat infection, the client's ear canal has no signs of inflammation, drainage, or swelling.
▼ If ear drops were used to relieve pain, the client voices no complaints of pain.

Materials List

Gather these materials before beginning the skill:

▼ Correct medication
▼ Cotton ball
▼ Cotton-tipped applicator
▼ Medication tray
▼ Examination gloves
▼ Chart

▼ ACTION

1. Obtain a physician's order.

2. Verify the correctness of the order and check the client's chart for drug allergies.

3. Wash your hands.

4. Concentrate alone.

▼ RATIONALE

1. The physician is licensed to prescribe medications. You are licensed to administer medications.

2. You are responsible for all medications administered to the client. A drug allergy is a contraindication to administration of the medication.

3. Handwashing is the single most effective measure to decrease the transmission of microorganisms from one person to another.

4. Prevents medication errors from inattention.

▼ ACTION	▼ RATIONALE
5. Select the correct medication and read the label. (This is the first of three times that the label should be read.)	**5.** The label is read three times to prevent medication errors.
6. Check the expiration date.	**6.** Expired medications may not give the needed effect.
7. Gather the equipment needed to administer the drug and place it on the medication tray.	**7.** Increases your organization and efficiency.
8. Read the label of the medication for the second time and place the drug on the tray.	**8.** The label is read three times to prevent medication errors.
9. Carry the medication and equipment to the client and introduce yourself.	**9.** Identifies the caregiver and his or her credentials. Helps to establish rapport with the client.
10. Ask the client if he or she has any drug allergies.	**10.** You should assess the client's chart and medication records for drug allergies. Asking the client about drug allergies serves as a final safety check.
11. Verify the client's identity by checking his or her arm band and bed tag and asking the client to state his or her name.	**11.** Prevents you from administering medications to the wrong client.
12. Verify the drug by reading the label for the third time.	**12.** The label is read three times to prevent medication errors.
13. Position the client in the side-lying position with the affected ear facing upward.	**13.** Facilitates the flow of the medication down the ear canal by gravity.
14. Put on gloves.	**14.** Gloves should be worn whenever there is potential contact with body secretions to reduce the transmission of human immunodeficiency virus and other microorganisms.
15. Assess the client's external ear for drainage, inflammation, and pain.	**15.** These are signs of infection.
16. If drainage or cerumen are seen in the outer ear, gently cleanse the area with a cotton-tipped applicator. *Do not* push the applicator down into the ear canal.	**16.** Removing secretions provides hygienic care and removes the medium for further bacterial growth.
17. Grasp the person's external ear and pull to straighten the ear canal.	**17.** For adults, pull the ear up and back (Fig. 18–4). For children, pull the ear down, back, and out (Fig. 18–5).
18. Hold the medicine dropper one-half inch above the ear and rest your hand on the client's head. Instill the prescribed number of drops into the ear canal. *Do not* touch the dropper to the ear or another object.	**18.** The tip of the dropper should remain sterile. Touching the dropper to the ear or other objects contaminates it.
19. Instruct the client to continue to lie on his or her side for 2 to 3 minutes.	**19.** Facilitates the flow of the ear drops down the ear canal.
20. Apply gentle pressure on the tragus of the client's ear with your finger.	**20.** Facilitates the flow of the ear drops down the ear canal.
21. Place an ear plug or a portion of a cotton ball into the client's external ear canal if ordered by the physician. Remove the cotton after 15 to 30 minutes.	**21.** Prevents the medication from flowing out of the ear canal.
22. Help client to assume a position of comfort.	**22.** Promotes the client's comfort.

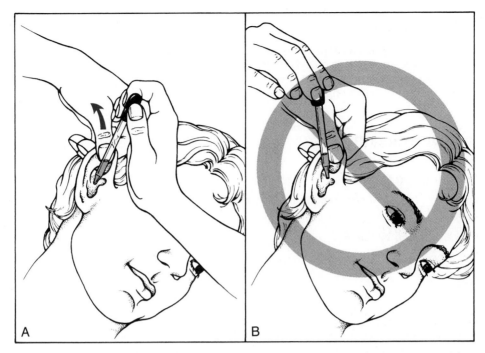

▼ **FIGURE 18–4.** Correct *(A)* and incorrect *(B)* ways to administer an otic medication to an adult.

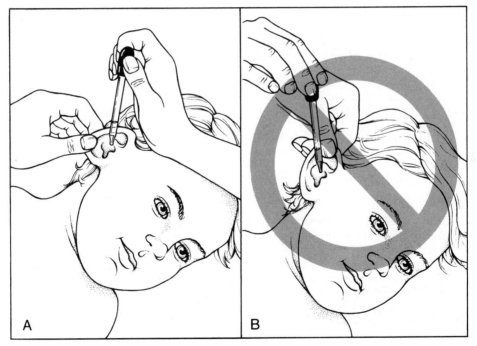

▼ **FIGURE 18–5.** Correct *(A)* and incorrect *(B)* ways to administer an otic medication to a child.

▼ *ACTION*	▼ *RATIONALE*
23. Dispose of the soiled supplies in a proper container.	**23.** Decreases the transmission of microorganisms.
24. Wash your hands.	**24.** Decreases the transmission of microorganisms.
25. Return to the client at the appropriate time to assess the effects of the medication.	**25.** You are responsible for monitoring for the desired effect, potential side effects, and allergic reactions to the medication.

▼ *ACTION*	▼ *RATIONALE*
26. Record the medication given; the time, dose, and route of medication; the appearance of the client's ear; his or her response to the drug; and any other related information in the client's chart.	**26.** Communicates to the other members of the health care team and contributes to the legal record by documenting the care given to the client.

Example of Documentation

DATE	TIME	NOTES
1/1/93	1000	2 gtt Auralgan administered to left ear canal for c/o ear pain
		H. White, RN

Teaching Tips

Teach the client never to insert objects into the ear canal when cleansing or medicating the ear. The client or his or her family member should be taught the purpose of the medication, the expected response from the medication, and the procedure for administration of the medication.

Home Care Variations

Ear drops can be administered in the client's home using the same technique.

SKILL 18–4 ADMINISTERING INHALED MEDICATIONS WITH A METERED-DOSE INHALER

Clinical Situations in Which You May Encounter This Skill

Medications may be inhaled into the respiratory tract to provide rapid absorption of the drugs for relief of symptoms of bronchospasm such as wheezing or asthma. Common medications delivered through the respiratory tract include bronchodilators, mucolytic agents, antibiotics, and steroids. In addition, medications may be inhaled to block local allergic reactions to antigens. The medications may be administered with a hand-held inhaler and dispersed through an aerosol spray, mist, or fine powder. The bronchioles provide a large surface area for absorption of the medications. The alveolar area provides a capillary network to rapidly absorb the medications.

The inhaled medications produce a local effect on the bronchioles. Dilatation of the bronchioles relieves symptoms of bronchospasm by opening narrowed bronchioles. Mucolytic agents and inhaled sterile saline help liquefy thick secretions.

Because all medications that are inhaled pass rapidly into the systemic circulation, the client should be monitored for side effects. For example, inhaled isoproterenol hydrochloride dilates the bronchioles, but it also may cause cardiac dysrhythmias.

The metered-dose form of delivering inhaled medications provides a specified amount of medication with each depression of the canister. The client must depress the canister and inhale at the same time. Clients who have chronic, debilitating disease or clients who are elderly may have a difficult time with this coordinated effort. As a result, much of the medication only sprays the nasopharynx and does not enter the lower respiratory tract. Newer methods attach the medication onto a barrel device that allows better inhalation and absorption of the medication (Fig. 18–6).

Anticipated Responses

▼ The client experiences relief from the bronchospasm and his or her breathing is easier.
▼ No wheezes are heard on auscultation.
▼ Secretions are liquefied.

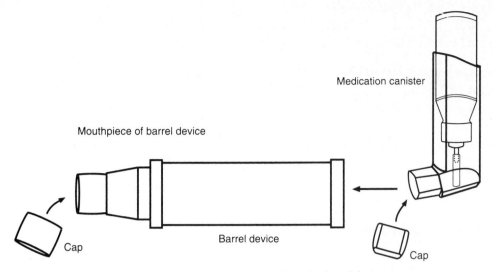

▼ **FIGURE 18–6.** Metered-dose inhaler with a barrel device.

Adverse Responses

▼ The client continues to experience bronchospasm with difficulty breathing.
▼ The client experiences anxiety from lack of oxygen.
▼ Wheezes are still heard on auscultation.
▼ Secretions remain thick and tenacious.

Materials List

Gather these materials before beginning the skill:

▼ Metered dose of medication, or
▼ Medication and inhalation device

▼ *ACTION*

1. Assess the client's ability to hold and manipulate the inhalation device.

2. Instruct the client to:
   a. Place the mouthpiece into his or her mouth.

   b. Exhale deeply through his or her nose.
   c. Inhale deeply through his or her mouth and depress the inhalation device so that the medication is inhaled (Fig. 18–7).

▼ *RATIONALE*

1. Inhaled medications should be administered by the client.

   a. The client inhales the medication through the mouthpiece.
   b. Removes air from the respiratory tract.
   c. The medication passes through to the lower respiratory tract, rather than only spraying the posterior nasopharynx.

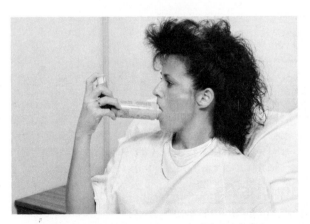

▼ **FIGURE 18–7.** Using a metered-dose inhaler.

▼ _ACTION_	▼ _RATIONALE_
d. Hold his or her breath for several seconds.	d. Allows the medication to remain on the bronchioles and be absorbed.
e. Slowly exhale through pursed lips.	e. Keeps small bronchioles open during exhalation.
3. Assess the client's ability to administer the inhaled medication.	3. Further education is required for the client who is unable to administer the medication correctly.
4. Assess the client's breathing for audible wheezing.	4. Breathing and wheezing should be improved.
5. Assess the client's pulse for evidence of cardiac dysrhythmias.	5. Some medications such as the bronchodilators can cause cardiac dysrhythmias.

Example of Documentation

DATE	TIME	NOTES
1/15/93	0900	Client complaining of shortness of breath and wheezing. Bilateral wheezes heard, R = 26, P = 90. Merered dose inhaler as prescribed by physician.
		S. Williams, RN
	0920	No further complaints of shortness of breath. No wheezes heard. R = 22, P = 90.
		S. Williams, RN

Teaching Tips

Assess the client's ability and readiness to learn the skill. When teaching the client to use a metered-dose nebulizer, ensure that the client is free of pain, fatigue, and acute shortness of breath. Readiness to learn is critical if the client is to accept responsibility for correctly administering the medication and maintaining the scheduled dose.

Tell the client to use the inhaled medication only as directed and no more frequently. Clients should be taught to monitor for side effects of the medication. Ensure that the client knows the skill by observing his or her demonstration of the procedure.

Home Care Variations

Inhaled medications are often used in the client's home. The client should understand the correct procedure and the symptoms of reactions to be reported.

SKILL 18–5   ADMINISTERING NASAL INSTILLATIONS

Clinical Situations in Which You May Encounter This Skill

Nasal instillations may be administered via drops or sprays. Nose drops may be prescribed to achieve a local effect on the nasal mucosa or the sinuses, and nasal sprays may be used to achieve a local effect on the nasal mucosa or for a systemic effect. The instillation of nose drops and sprays is usually treated as a clean procedure unless the client has just had sinus or facial surgery.

The client's position for the instillation of nose drops varies slightly, depending on the area or nasal sinus to be treated. If the medication is intended for a eustachian tube, the client assumes an upright position or a supine position with his or her head maintained in the midline. In this position, the medication passes over the nasopharynx to the eustachian tube.

Nose drops also may be used to medicate sinuses. The four groups of sinuses are: frontal, ethmoid, sphenoid, and maxillary. If the ethmoid or the sphenoid sinus is to be medicated, position the client in the Proetz position (supine with his or her head over the edge of the bed or a pillow under the shoulders with his or her head leaning backward) (Fig. 18–8). If the client lies supine with his or her head leaning back over the side of the bed, support the client's head with your hand to avoid muscle strain on the client's neck. If the person is an infant, position him or her using a football hold and allow the neck to slightly hyperextend. A small child who is not cooperative may need to be restrained. If the maxillary or frontal sinuses are to be treated, the client should assume the Parkinson position (supine with the head turned to the affected side to be treated) (Fig. 18–9).

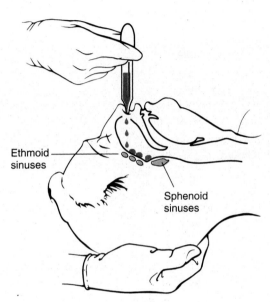

Ethmoid sinuses

Sphenoid sinuses

▼ **FIGURE 18–8.** The Proetz position.

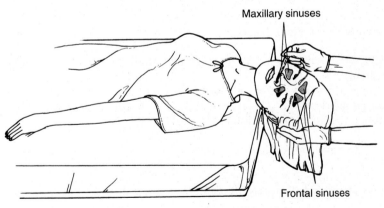

Maxillary sinuses

Frontal sinuses

▼ **FIGURE 18–9.** The Parkinson position.

Anticipated Responses

▼ The client is free of nasal congestion, discharge, and odor.
▼ The client's nasal mucosa is pink and moist.
▼ The client breathes freely through his or her nose.
▼ The client is free of pain or discomfort in the sinus areas after instillation of the medication.

Adverse Responses

▼ The client continues to complain of nasal congestion and discharge.

▼ An odor remains from the discharge.
▼ The client's nasal mucosa is red, dry, and encrusted.
▼ The client continues to have pain or discomfort in the sinus area.

Materials List

Gather these materials before beginning the skill:

▼ Nasal spray or drops
▼ Dropper
▼ Clean tissue

▼ *ACTION*	▼ *RATIONALE*
1. Ask the client if he or she has ever had the procedure before.	1. If the client is not familiar with the procedure, you can give simple explanations to relieve his or her anxiety and dispel any fears.
2. Tell the client about sensations to expect (a stinging, burning, or choking sensation as the solution drips into the throat).	2. Reduces fear and apprehension.
3. Assess the client for: a. Obstruction of breathing through the nose by asking the client to close one nostril at a time and gently exhale. b. Pain or discomfort. c. Discharge, redness, or encrustations of the nares. A nasal speculum may be used to inspect the nasal mucosa.	a. Verifies that nasal passages are patent. b. Infected sinuses are often painful or the person may have a feeling of fullness in the sinus area. c. The nares should be free of discharge, redness, and encrustations. The mucosa should be pink, moist, and free of odor.
4. Determine the purpose of the nasal instillation.	4. Determines the client's position during the instillation.

Instilling Drops

5. a. Ask the client to gently blow his or her nose. b. Inspect the discharge on the tissue for color, odor, and consistency. c. Help the client to assume the correct position for the instillation of the drops. d. Draw up the correct dosage of medication in the dropper. e. Ask the client to breathe through his or her mouth. f. Hold the dropper just above the person's nares and direct the tip toward the midline of the ethmoid bone without touching the dropper to the nares or the nasal mucosa. g. Instill the drops and ask the client to remain in the position for 5 minutes.	5. a. Clears the nasal passages and aids absorption of the medication. b. Enables you to provide objective documentation. c. The position varies depending on the sinus to be medicated. e. Reduces the chance of aspiration of the solution. f. If the medication is directed toward the posterior wall, little absorption will occur and the solution will flow immediately to the posterior nasal pharynx. Touching the dropper contaminates the dropper and may damage the nasal mucosa. g. Facilitates absorption of the medication.

Instilling Sprays

6. a. Ask the client to exhale and then close one nostril.	6. a. Closing one nostril facilitates instillation of the spray in the other nostril.

▼ *ACTION*   ▼ *RATIONALE*

   b. Ask the client to inhale while you instill the spray into the first nostril.

   b. Instilling the spray as the person inhales helps to distribute the spray.

   c. Offer the client a clean tissue to blot his or her nose. Caution the client not to blow his or her nose.

   c. Excess spray may be botted, but blowing the nose expels the solution.

   d. Help the client to assume a position of comfort.

   d. Facilitates the client's sense of well-being.

   e. Remove the soiled supplies and dispose of them according to agency guidelines.

   e. Proper disposal decreases the transmission of microorganisms.

7. Assess the client in 15 to 30 minutes for his or her response to the medication.

7. Evaluates the effectiveness of the medication.

8. Record the procedure and the client's response.

8. Communicates the findings to the other members of the health care team and contributes to the legal record by documenting the care given to the client.

Example of Documentation

DATE	TIME	NOTES
1/15/93	1000	Complaining of fullness and pressure in right supraorbital region. Positioned with head lowered and turned to right. Nasal spray instilled.
		S. Williams, RN
	1030	States that pressure and fullness are less.
		S. Williams, RN

Teaching Tips

Teach the client to instill his or her own nose drops and nasal sprays. Have the client demonstrate the skill for you. Caution clients who have a history of hypertension or cardiovascular disease not to instill nasal medications that contain vasoconstrictors. Elevated blood pressure may result if the vasoconstrictor is absorbed systemically. In addition, caution clients never to instill an oily substance into the nasal cavity. If a substance is not water-soluble and it inadvertently passes into the respiratory tract, aspiration pneumonia may result.

Caution clients not to use "over-the-counter" nose sprays for longer than 4 to 5 days. Rebound vasodilation may result if the spray or drops contain sympathomimetic drugs, and the nasal congestion symptoms may worsen.

Home Care Variations

For simple nasal congestion or for nasal drops or sprays for children, saline drops may be made in the client's home by dissovling 1 teaspoon of salt in 1 pint of warm water. To avoid bacterial growth in the saline solution, it should be discarded after 24 hours and remade if continued use is indicated.

SKILL 18–6   ADMINISTERING RECTAL MEDICATIONS

Clinical Situations in Which You May Encounter This Skill

Medications administered through the rectal route are most commonly in the form of suppositories. Absorption of medications through the rectal mucosa is not as reliable as through the oral or parenteral route. However, it does serve as an alternate route for administering medications for systemic effect when the oral or parenteral route is contraindicated.

Rectal suppositories exert local effects (defecation or symptomatic relief from painful hemorrhoids) from the medication and provide a route for administering medications when the oral route is not desirable (when the client has nausea and vomiting). The rectal route is not used if the client has had rectal surgery or is experiencing rectal bleeding.

Absorption of the medication is dependent on contact of the medication with the rectal mucosa. Therefore, it may be necessary to administer an enema before inserting a suppository.

Anticipated Responses

▼ The suppository is inserted without difficulty 4 inches into the adult client's rectum (2 inches for a child).
▼ The client retains the suppository until the medication is absorbed and the desired effect has occurred.

Adverse Responses

▼ The client has stool in the rectum and the suppository cannot be placed along the rectal mucosa.
▼ The client cannot retain the suppository and expels it before absorption and the needed effects can take place.

Materials List

Gather these materials before beginning the skill:

▼ Suppository
▼ Examination gloves
▼ Water-soluble lubricant
▼ Paper towel

▼ ACTION

1. Ask the client if he or she has ever had a suppository administered before.

2. Ask the client when he or she last had a bowel movement.

3. Close the client's door and draw the curtains around the bed.

4. Help the client to assume a left lateral position with the right leg sharply flexed. (The supine position could be used with the client's legs flexed if the side-lying position is uncomfortable or contraindicated).

5. Stand behind the client so that you face the client's back.

6. Remove the suppository from the wrapper and leave it on the wrapper.

7. Place a sufficient amount of water-soluble lubricant on a paper towel to lubricate the suppository and your index finger.

8. Don examination gloves.

9. Separate the client's buttocks.

▼ RATIONALE

1. Allows you to explain what the client can expect (rectal pressure and the feeling of needing to defecate) and the need to retain the suppository after insertion. These simple explanations can reduce fear and apprehension.

2. Helps you to determine if a small enema is needed. If the effect of the suppository is to be systemic, the rectum should be free of feces.

3. Provides privacy and protects the client's modesty.

4. The left lateral position allows the sigmoid colon to be low and decreases the chance that feces will expel the suppository.

5. Allows you to insert the suppository easily.

6. Prevents contamination of the suppository.

7. Lubrication of the suppository and your finger eases insertion and decreases discomfort and friction against the person's rectal mucosa.

8. Decreases the transmission of microorganisms to and from the client.

9. Allows you to see the client's anus.

▼ _A C T I O N_ _____   ▼ _R A T I O N A L E_ _____

10. Inspect the anal area for hemorrhoids or bleeding.

10. Internal rectal bleeding is a contraindication to the administration of a rectal suppository. Very careful insertion is necessary if the person has hemorrhoids.

11. Lubricate the suppository and your index finger.

11. Facilitates insertion.

12. Ask the client to open and breathe through his or her mouth.

12. Helps to relax the anal sphincter.

13. Tell the client that you are going to insert the suppository.

13. Lets the client know what to expect.

14. Gently insert the suppository (4 inches for an adult and 2 inches for a child) against the rectal mucosa (Fig. 18–10).

14. The suppository must be against the mucosa for absorption to occur.

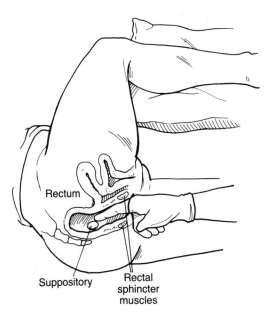

Rectum

Suppository   Rectal sphincter muscles

▼ **FIGURE 18–10.** Inserting a rectal suppository.

15. Gently compress the client's buttocks together.

15. Prevents the client from prematurely expelling the suppository.

16. Ask the client to retain the suppository for a specified amount of time.

16. The amount of time for retention of a suppository depends on the needed effect.

17. Assist the client to a position of comfort.

17. Promotes the person's sense of well-being.

18. Place the client's call bell within easy reach.

18. The client will be able to call for assistance as needed.

19. Evaluate the client for the expected results of the medication administered.

19. The results of the suppository should be documented in the client's chart.

20. Document the procedure and results in the client's chart.

20. Communicates to the other members of the health care team and contributes to the legal record by documenting the care given to the client.

Example of Documentation

DATE	TIME	NOTES
4/10/93	0900	Client complaining of nausea. Trimethobenzamide suppository, 200 mg, administered. Side rails raised.
		S. Williams, RN
	1000	Nausea relieved. Client drowsy.
		S. Williams, RN

Teaching Tips

If the client prefers to insert the suppository unassisted, ensure that the client knows the correct procedure. Provide the client with an examination glove or finger cot and stress good handwashing. If the suppository is to be administered for constipation, teach the client about potential dependency on laxatives.

Home Care Variations

The same procedure can be used in the home.

SKILL 18–7   ADMINISTERING VAGINAL MEDICATIONS

Clinical Situations in Which You May Encounter This Skill

Vaginal medications in the form of suppositories, foams, jellies, creams, or douches (irrigations) may be prescribed by the physician to deliver medication to the vagina or cervix. Because vaginal medications are often ordered to treat an infection or irritation, you should use good handwashing techniques and wear examination gloves.

Vaginal irrigations are used to therapeutically cleanse or disinfect the vagina, to soothe inflamed tissue, and to treat minor bleeding. Vaginal irrigations are administered at 43.3° centigrade (C) or 110° Fahrenheit (F) unless otherwise ordered. The bag containing the irrigant is hung no more than 2 ft above the client's hips. To achieve therapeutic effects, the vaginal irrigation should not be administered hastily, but should take from 20 to 30 minutes.

Vaginal suppositories are packaged individually in foil wrappers. The suppositories are stored in the refrigerator until they are ready for use to avoid melting. After the suppository is removed from the foil and inserted into the vagina, the client's body temperature causes it to melt. The suppository is inserted with an applicator or a gloved hand.

Often the client prefers to administer the suppository or vaginal irrigant herself. The client should be taught the safe and effective method for the procedure and should have privacy provided. She may want to wear a perineal pad to collect the drainage from the melting suppository or foam. Additionally, because vaginal medications are often prescribed to treat an infection, the client may have a foul discharge. Encourage good hygiene and frequent perineal care.

Anticipated Responses

▼ The vaginal infection, irritation, or pruritus that required the vaginal irrigation or suppository is cured.
▼ The client's vaginal tissues are smooth, pink, and without discharge or the discharge from the vagina is the color of the medication inserted.
▼ The woman does not have a recurrence of the condition.

Adverse Responses

▼ The discharge from the client's vagina remains foul-smelling.
▼ The client's vaginal walls are red and irritated, and patches of white curdlike discharge remain on the sides of the vaginal walls.
▼ The client continues to complain of itching or discomfort.

Materials List

Gather these materials before beginning the skill:

▼ For creams, suppositories, or foams:
Vaginal medication
Applicator (optional)
Examination gloves
Water-soluble lubricating jelly
Perineal pad
Toilet tissue
Paper towel

▼ For a vaginal irrigation:
Douche bag with nozzle attached
Solution for irrigation (105–110° F)
Bedpan (optional)
IV pole

▼ *ACTION*

1. Ask the client if she has ever had the procedure before.

2. Check the physician's order for the name of the drug to be given and the time of administration.

3. Have the client void.

4. Wash your hands.

5. Arrange the supplies near the client's bed.

6. Close the door and pull the curtain around the client's bed.

7. Help the client to assume a dorsal-recumbent position.

8. Drape the client's abdomen and lower extremities.

9. Adjust the lighting so that the client's vaginal orifice is illuminated adequately.

10. Don examination gloves.

11. Administer the medication.

Inserting a Suppository

   a. Remove the suppository from the foil. Place the suppository in an applicator (optional).
   b. Apply a water-soluble lubricant to the suppository.
   c. With your nondominant hand, gently retract the woman's labia.
   d. Using your dominant hand, insert the tapered end of the suppository with your index finger or the applicator along the posterior wall of the woman's vagina (about 3–4 inches) (Fig. 18–11).
   e. After inserting the suppository, wipe the client's perineal area and labia from front to back with toilet tissue.
   f. Apply a perineal pad.
   g. Remove your gloves inside out and discard them into a waste receptacle.

▼ *RATIONALE*

1. Allows you to clarify any questions and to explain exactly what the client should expect.

2. Allows you to correctly monitor the client's response to the medication given.

3. Promotes the client's comfort during the procedure.

4. Decreases the transmission of microorganisms.

5. All needed equipment is available.

6. Provides for privacy.

7. Promotes visibility and access to the client's vaginal orifice. Allows the medication to remain in the vaginal area.

8. Provides for privacy and protects the client's modesty.

9. Proper insertion requires that you adequately see the perineal area.

10. Decreases the transmission of microorganisms from and to the client.

   a. The foil is discarded. An applicator or gloved finger may be used to insert the medication.
   b. Promotes ease of insertion and reduces discomfort for the client.
   c. Exposes the person's vaginal orifice.

   d. Complete insertion of the suppository is necessary for the medication to dissolve and cover the entire vagina.

   e. Removes excess lubricant and promotes the client's comfort.

   f. Absorbs excess drainage.
   g. Microorganisms remain inside the gloves.

▼ *ACTION* _ ▼ *RATIONALE* _ _ _ _ _ _ _ _ _ _ _ _ _

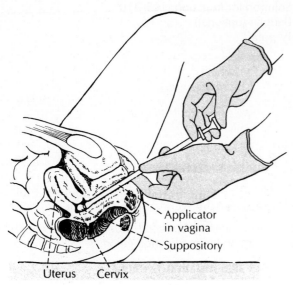

▼ **FIGURE 18–11.** Inserting a vaginal suppository.

h. Instruct the client to remain on her back for at least 10 minutes.

h. Prevents the medication from running out.

Inserting Foam, Jelly, or Cream

a. Fill the applicator with medication.

b. With your nondominant hand, gently retract the client's labia.

c. Insert the applicator plunger 2 to 3 inches into the client's vagina toward the client's sacral area.

d. Push the plunger to expel the medication.

e. Withdraw the applicator and place it on a paper towel.

f. Wipe the client's perineal area and labia from front to back with toilet tissue.

g. Follow Steps f–h under "Inserting a Suppository" above.

h. Wash the applicator with soap and warm water, dry it thoroughly, and store it for future use.

a. The applicator is used to administer the medicine.

b. Exposes the vaginal orifice.

c. Promotes ease of insertion.

d. The plunger pushes the medicine into the vagina.

e. The applicator will soil the bed or other objects.

f. Promotes comfort and removes the medication from the client's labia and perineal area.

h. Removes microorganisms and prevents contamination of the client with microorganisms.

Administering a Vaginal Irrigation (Douche)

a. Warm the solution to 105 to 110° F or until it is comfortable to your wrist.

b. Assist the client in the semirecumbent position on a bedpan. (The client also could be positioned in a clean tub or could be seated on the toilet. If the client has the vaginal irrigation while she is in the sitting position on the toilet, her labia should be held together to permit the solution to fill the entire vaginal vault.)

a. A solution that is too hot could burn the woman's vagina. A solution that is too cool could cause discomfort.

b. Facilitates infusion of the irrigant into the entire vaginal vault.

▼ _ A C T I O N _ _ _ _ _ _ _ _ _ _ _ _ _ _ _ _ _ ▼ _ R A T I O N A L E _ _ _ _ _ _ _ _ _ _ _ _

c. Allow some of the irrigant to flow out of the nozzle or lubricate the tip with a water-soluble lubricant.

c. Lubricates the tip of the applicator for easier insertion.

d. Hang the container on an IV pole no more than 2 feet above the client's hips.

d. Greater heights increase the pressure of the flow and may cause a fluid or air embolus that could result in death.

e. Insert the nozzle about 3 inches into the woman's vagina by directing the nozzle upward and back toward the sacrum.

e. This position reduces discomfort associated with insertion of the nozzle.

f. Release the clamp and allow the solution to flow into the client's vagina.
   i. Rotate the nozzle so the fluid flows around the entire mucosa.

   i. Rotating the nozzle reduces the chance of introducing fluid through the cervix into the uterus.

   ii. If the vaginal irrigation is done while the woman is on the toilet or if the purpose of the vaginal irrigation is to expose the vaginal walls to medication or moist heat, hold the woman's labia together.

   ii. Fills the vaginal vault.

   iii. Release the labia.

   iii. Allows the fluid to exit rapidly and flush out debris.

   iv. Continue filling and expelling the fluid until the solution is finished.

g. Have the client sit up and lean forward after the vaginal irrigation is completed.

g. Aids in emptying the vagina.

h. Wash the equipment used and store it in a well-ventilated place.

h. Properly cleaning equipment prevents the possible spread of infection.

i. Remove gloves and wash your hands.

i. Decreases the transmission of microorganisms.

12. Inspect the client's outer perineal area for signs of irritation or unexpected discharge.

12. Helps determine if the medication effectively reduced the client's symptoms.

13. Ask the client about pruritus, burning, or discomfort.

13. Determines whether symptoms have been relieved.

14. Record the procedure. Note the color, odor, and consistency of the discharge and the client's response to the procedure.

14. Communicates to the other members of the health care team and contributes to the legal record by documenting the care given to the client.

Example of Documentation

DATE	TIME	NOTES
4/1/93	0900	Vaginal irrigation with 1,000 ml of warm saline. Client appears relaxed and comfortable. No foul-smelling discharge noted.
		S. Williams, RN

Teaching Tips

The client should be taught the correct procedure for administering vaginal medications. Tell the client that if the suppository fails to dissolve, the expiration date should be checked because a new supply may be needed. Ensure that the client knows how to properly clean and store the equipment. She should be told to report any continued symptoms to her health care provider. Discuss simple asepsis with the client to ensure that she knows how bacteria may be transferred from the hands to other areas of the body. Teach the client to wipe her perineal area from front to back.

Home Care Variations

If the client is to perform a vaginal irrigation at home, be sure she has a clean bathtub or toilet. Ensure that the client properly washes and stores all supplies.

If the client has suppositories, they should be stored in the refrigerator. Rectal suppositories should be clearly labeled to prevent them from being used in the vagina. Vaginal suppositories are larger and more oval in shape.

ORAL MEDICATIONS

Any medication administered by mouth is considered to be an oral drug. Oral medications include drugs that are absorbed in the mouth such as sublingual drugs and those placed directly into the stomach or intestine for absorption by way of a nasogastric tube. Oral medications include solid tablets and capsules, liquid elixirs and syrups, and powders.

SKILL 18–8   ADMINISTERING ORAL MEDICATIONS

Clinical Situations in Which You May Encounter This Skill

You may administer oral medications to clients in hospitals, outpatient clinics, and the home. The physician's order and the characteristics of the medication determine the route of drug administration.

If the client is unable to swallow the medication, it can be crushed (if it is not enteric-coated) and mixed with soft foods such as applesauce. If available, the medication can be exchanged for a liquid form.

Medications may produce adverse effects or reactions that should be reported immediately to the physician. Diphenhydramine or epinephrine may be ordered to treat allergic responses.

Anticipated Responses

▼ The client is able to swallow the medication.
▼ The medication produces the expected effect without extreme side effects or allergic reactions.

Adverse Responses

▼ The client is unable to swallow the medication.

Materials List

Gather these materials before beginning the skill:

▼ Souffle cup
▼ Correct medication
▼ Chart
▼ Cup of water
▼ Medication tray
▼ Liquid medication cup
▼ Optional: Mortar and pestle
              Dropper
              Spoon
              Syringe

▼ ACTION	▼ RATIONALE
1. Obtain a physician's order.	1. The physician is licensed to prescribe medications. You are licensed to administer medications.
2. Verify the correctness of the order and check for drug allergies.	2. You are responsible for all medications administered to the client. A drug allergy is a contraindication to administration of the medication.
3. Wash your hands.	3. Handwashing is the single most effective measure to decrease the transmission of microorganisms from person to person.
4. Concentrate alone.	4. Prevents medication errors from inattention.
5. Select the correct medication and read the label. (This is the first of three times that the label should be read.)	5. The label is read three times to prevent medication errors.

▼ *ACTION* ------ -- -- -- -- -- -- | ▼ *RATIONALE* -- -- -- -- -- -- --

6. Check the expiration date.

6. Expired medications may not give the needed effect.

7. Select the appropriate container with which to administer the medication to the client.

7. A paper souffle cup is used for tablets and capsules. A plastic medication cup is used for liquids.

8. Read the label again.

8. The label is read three times to prevent medication errors.

9. Remove the cap from the medication container or open the unit dose package.

9. Facilitates medication administration.

10. Prepare the medication.

Administering Tablets or Capsules

a. Pour the correct number of capsules or tablets into the cap (Fig. 18–12).

a. You should not touch the medication as you prepare it.

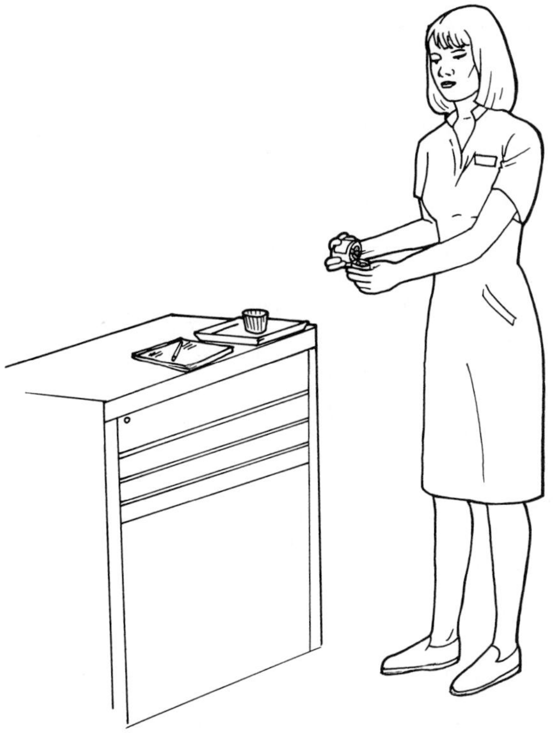

▼ **FIGURE 18–12.** Pouring tablets into a cap.

b. Pour the tablets or capsules from the bottle cap into the souffle cup and place the cap or cup on the medication tray.

c. If the client has difficulty swallowing pills, crush them with a mortar and pestle, dissolve them in liquid, or mix them with a small amount of food such as applesauce. Administer the medication in a medicine cup, syringe, dropper, or spoon.

c. Many medications can be administered in this way; however, syringes, spoons, and droppers are especially useful when administering medications to young children.

▼ *A C T I O N*   ▼ *R A T I O N A L E*

NOTE: *Do not* crush enteric-coated medications.   Releases the medication in the stomach, where it may be destroyed by gastric acid or may irritate the gastric mucosa.

Administering Liquid Medications

a. Place a liquid medication cup on a level surface.

b. While holding the label of the bottle in your palm, pour the liquid medication into the cup (Fig. 18–13).

c. Measure the correct volume of medication at the meniscus (Fig. 18–14).

a. Facilitates accurate measurement.

b. Prevents the medication from dripping down the label and rendering it illegible.

c. This technique is the most accurate way to measure liquids.

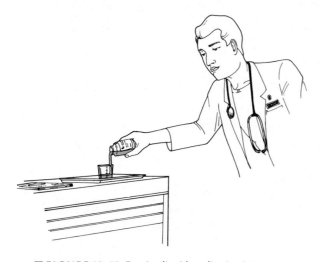

▼ **FIGURE 18–13.** Pouring liquid medication into a cup.

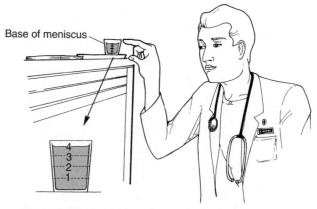

▼ **FIGURE 18–14.** Measuring medication at the meniscus.

11. Read the label of the medication container for the third time before returning it to the shelf or discarding it.

11. The label is read three times to prevent medication errors.

12. Carry the medication to the client, introduce yourself, and explain your presence.

12. Identifies the caregiver and his or her credentials.

13. Ask the client if he or she has any drug allergies.

13. You should assess the client's chart and medication records for drug allergies. Asking the client about his or her allergies serves as a final safety check.

14. Verify the client's identity by checking his or her arm band and bed tag and by asking the client to state his or her name.

14. Prevents you from administering medications to the wrong client.

15. Help the client to assume an upright position unless this position is contraindicated by the client's health status. Turn to side if not able to sit up.

15. Helps the client to swallow medications.

16. Give the client the medication cup and a glass of water to help him or her swallow. Tell the client what the medication is and its purpose.

16. Water aids in swallowing, removes unpleasant tastes from the mouth, and hastens the dissolution and disintegration of oral medications in the stomach. The client should be aware of the name of the medication and its purpose.

▼ *ACTION*   ▼ *RATIONALE*

17. Remain with the client until the medication is swallowed.

18. Return the equipment to the medication room.

19. Wash your hands.

20. Return to the client's room at the appropriate time to assess the effects of the medication.

21. Chart the medication given; the time, dose, and route of medication; the client's response to the drug; and any other related information.

17. Ensures that the client receives the medication and does not have any difficulty swallowing.

18. Nondisposable equipment can be used again.

19. Decreases the transmission of microorganisms.

20. You are responsible for monitoring for the expected effect, potential side effects, and allergic reactions to the medication.

21. Communicates to the other members of the health care team and contributes to the legal record by documenting the care given to the client.

Example of Documentation

DATE	TIME	NOTES
1/1/93	0900	Acetaminophen ii tabs given PO for complaints of abdominal surgical site.
		H. White, RN
	0930	Client states abdominal pain is relieved. BP = 122/80, R = 14/min.
		H. White, RN

Teaching Tips

You should teach the client the name of the medication, its purpose, possible side effects, and any special administration techniques.

Home Care Variations

Many clients, particularly elderly clients, take many medications and may have difficulty correctly administering them. Self-administration problems include difficulty reading the print on the labels and difficulty remembering to take the drugs at the appropriate time. You may find it necessary to prepare a week's supply of medications for the client by placing each day's medication in a resealable bag labelled in large print. Medication charts also may be used to facilitate accurate medication administration.

SKILL 18–9 ADMINISTERING MEDICATIONS THROUGH A NASOGASTRIC TUBE

Clinical Situations in Which You May Encounter This Skill

Oral medications can be administered through a gastric tube when the client is unable to swallow or when there is a gastric tube already in place.

Anticipated Responses

▼ Medication flows through the tube without difficulty.

Adverse Responses

▼ Medication flows sluggishly through the tube.

Materials List

Gather these materials before beginning the skill:

▼ 60-ml catheter-tipped syringe
▼ Glass of water
▼ Mortar and pestle or other pill-crushing device
▼ Disposable waterproof pad
▼ Stethoscope
▼ Plastic medication cup
▼ Clamp for nasogastric tube
▼ Examination gloves

▼ *ACTION*	▼ *RATIONALE*
1. Obtain a physician's order.	1. The physician is licensed to prescribe medications. You are licensed to administer medications.
2. Verify the correctness of the order and check for drug allergies.	2. You are responsible for all medications administered to the client. A drug allergy is a contraindication to administration of the medication.
3. Wash your hands.	3. Handwashing is the single most effective measure to decrease the transmission of microorganisms from person to person.
4. Concentrate alone.	4. Prevents medication errors from inattention.
5. Select the correct medication and read the label three times. (This is the first of three times that the label should be read.)	5. The label is read three times to prevent medication errors.
6. Check the expiration date.	6. Expired medications may not give the needed effect.
7. Select the appropriate container with which to administer the drug to the client.	7. A plastic cup is needed since the medication must be dissolved in a liquid to pass through the gastric tube.
8. Read the label again.	8. The label is read three times to prevent medication errors.
9. Remove the cap from the medication container or open the unit dose package.	9. Facilitates medication administration.
10. Pour the correct number of tablets into a clean mortar.	10. A mortar and pestle are used to crush tablets. To avoid contaminating the medication with previously crushed drugs, thoroughly wash the mortar and pestle.
11. Read the label of the medication for the third time before returning the medication container to the shelf or discarding it.	11. The label is read three times to prevent medication errors.
12. Crush the tablets into a fine powder with the pestle (Fig. 18–15).	12. Medications in powdered form dissolve more thoroughly than medications in solid form.
13. Pour the powder into a plastic medication cup.	13. The cup is used to dissolve the medication.

▼ *ACTION* _ ▼ *RATIONALE* _ _ _ _ _ _ _ _ _ _ _ _ _ _ _ _

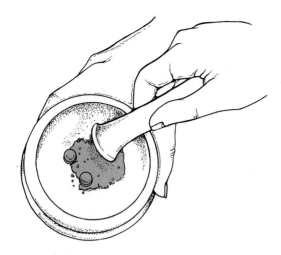

▼ **FIGURE 18–15.** Crushing tablets into a fine powder with a pestle.

14. Add warm water to the powder and mix to dissolve the medication. For the client with a fluid restriction, most medications can be dissolved in 5 to 10 ml of water.

14. Thoroughly dissolving the medication prevents large pieces of medication from obstructing the gastric tube.

15. Carry the medication to the client and introduce yourself.

15. Identifies the caregiver and his or her credentials.

16. Ask the client if he or she has any drug allergies.

16. You should assess the client's chart and medication cards for drug allergies. Asking the client about allergies serves as a final safety check.

17. Verify the client's identity by checking his or her arm band and bed tag and asking the client to state his or her name.

17. Prevents you from administering medications to the wrong client.

18. Elevate the head of the bed 30 to 45 degrees unless elevation is contraindicated by the client's illness.

18. Aids in preventing aspiration.

19. Place a waterproof pad between the nasogastric tube and the client's bed and clothing.

19. Protects the linen and clothing from becoming damp and soiled.

20. Put on examination gloves.

20. Prevents the transmission of microorganisms.

21. Check for the proper position of the nasogastric tube prior to instilling medication.
   a. Use a catheter-tipped syringe to withdraw the gastric contents into the syringe. Return contents to the stomach.
   b. With the catheter-tipped syringe, inject 10 ml of air into the nasogastric tube while listening with a stethoscope over the epigastric area for a swishing sound.

21. Medications or other substances instilled down an improperly positioned tube could be aspirated.
   a. The presence of gastric contents indicates that the tube is in the proper position.

   b. Auscultation of air rushing into the stomach indicates the tip of the tube is in the stomach.

22. Draw up the medication from the cup into the catheter-tipped syringe, clear the syringe of excess air, and inject the medication into the nasogastric tube (Fig. 18–16).

22. Instilling excess air into the stomach may lead to flatus and abdominal discomfort.

▼ *ACTION*   ▼ *RATIONALE*

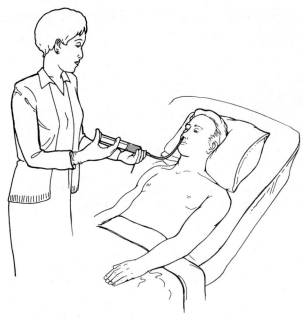

▼ **FIGURE 18–16.** Injecting medication into a nasogastric tube.

23. Administer 30 ml of water into the nasogastric tube after the medication has been injected.

23. The water flushes the medication through the tube into the client's stomach and prevents the tube from becoming obstructed.

24. Clamp the nasogastric tube for 30 minutes.

24. Allows time for the medication to be absorbed.

25. Remove gloves and wash hands.

25. Decreases the transmission of microorganisms.

26. Return the equipment to the medication room.

26. Nondisposable equipment can be used again.

27. Return to the client's room at an appropriate time to assess the effects of the medication.

27. You are responsible for monitoring for the expected effects, potential side effects, and allergic reactions to the medication.

28. Chart the medication given; the time, dose, and route of medication; the position of the nasogastric tube; the client's response to the drug; and any other related information.

28. Communicates to the other members of the health care team and contributes to the legal record by documenting the care given to the client.

Example of Documentation

DATE	TIME	NOTES
1/1/93	0900	Tube placement checked by withdrawing gastric contents. Phenytoin 100 mg given through nasogastric tube.
		H. White, RN

Teaching Tips

Clients often are sent home with nasogastric tubes in place. As you provide care for the client, teach his or her family or other caregiver how to care for the nasogastric tube, how to administer medicines through the tube, and how to prevent complications such as aspiration or obstruction of the tube.

Home Care Variations

Medications can be administered through a nasogastric tube in the client's home using the same technique.

SKILL 18–10   ADMINISTERING SUBLINGUAL MEDICATIONS

Clinical Situations in Which You May Encounter This Skill

Medications are administered by the sublingual route when rapid absorption is necessary. The rapid effect of the medication is from quick absorption of the medication into the bloodstream via the sublingual blood vessels.

Anticipated Responses

▼ The onset of the medication's effect is rapid and produces the expected results.

Adverse Responses

▼ The onset of the medication's effect is delayed and does not produce the expected results.

Materials List

Gather these materials before beginning the skill:

▼ Souffle cup
▼ Correct medication
▼ Chart
▼ Medication tray

▼ ACTION	▼ RATIONALE
1. Obtain a physician's order.	1. The physician is licensed to prescribe medications. You are licensed to administer medications.
2. Verify the correctness of the order and check for drug allergies.	2. You are responsible for all medications administered to the client. A drug allergy is a contraindication to administration of the medication.
3. Wash your hands.	3. Handwashing is the single most effective measure to decrease the transmission of microorganisms from person to person.
4. Concentrate alone.	4. Prevents medication errors from inattention.
5. Select the correct medication and read the label. (This is the first of three times that the label should be read.)	5. The label is read three times to prevent medication errors.
6. Check the expiration date.	6. Expired medications may not give the needed effect.
7. Select the appropriate container with which to administer the medication to the client.	7. A paper souffle cup is used for tablets and capsules.
8. Read the label again.	8. The label is read three times to prevent medication errors.
9. Remove the cap from the medication container or open the unit dose package.	9. Facilitates medication administration.
10. Pour the correct number of tablets into the medication cup and place the cup on the medication tray.	10. You should not touch the medication as you prepare it.
11. Read the label of the medication container for the third time before returning it to the shelf or discarding it.	11. The label is read three times to prevent medication errors.
12. Carry the medication to the client, introduce yourself, and explain your presence.	12. Identifies the caregiver and his or her credentials.

▼ *A C T I O N*   ▼ *R A T I O N A L E*

13. Verify the client's identity by checking his or her arm band and bed tag and by asking the client to state his or her name.

13. Prevents you from administering medications to the wrong client.

14. Ask the client if he or she has any drug allergies.

14. You should read the client's chart and medication cards for drug allergies. Asking the client about allergies serves as a final safety check.

15. Help the client to assume an upright position unless this position is contraindicated by his or her health status.

15. Aids in preventing aspiration of the sublingual tablet.

16. Place the tablet under the client's tongue (Fig. 18–17).

16. The tablet is surrounded by mucous membranes rich with blood vessels for rapid absorption.

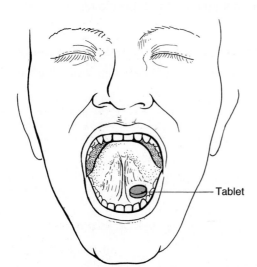

— Tablet

▼ **FIGURE 18–17.** Placing a tablet under the client's tongue.

17. Instruct the client not to swallow.

17. The medication should dissolve and be absorbed through the sublingual mucous membranes.

18. Remain with the client until the tablet is dissolved.

18. Ensures that the client receives the medication.

19. Return the equipment to the medication room.

19. Nondisposable equipment can be used again.

20. Wash your hands.

20. Decreases the transmission of microorganisms.

21. Assess the effects of the drug.

21. You are responsible for monitoring for the expected effect, potential side effects, and allergic reactions to the medication. Because of the rapid absorption of sublingual medications, you will observe effects within minutes of administration.

22. Chart the medication given; the time, dose, and route of medication; the client's response to the drug; and any other pertinent information.

22. Communicates to the other members of the health care team and contributes to the legal record by documenting the care given to the client.

Example of Documentation

DATE	*TIME*	*NOTES*
1/1/93	0915	Client complaining of chest pain. Nitroglycerin gr 1/150 SL administered. Client states chest pain relieved and complaining of mild headache. BP = 110/70, HR = 74, R = 14.
		H. White, RN

Teaching Tips

Teach the client about proper storage of sublingual tablets. Most of these medications should be protected from heat, light, and moisture. The client should know the name of the medication, its purpose, and possible side effects.

PARENTERAL MEDICATIONS

Parenteral medications are given by injection with a needle. Parenteral drugs gain quick access to the circulatory system and cause rapid and powerful effects. Since parenteral medications are absorbed so quickly, they are considered irretrievable. All precautions should be strictly followed to avoid medication errors.

Equipment for Administration of Parenteral Medications

Syringes and Needles

Syringes and needles are used to administer parenteral medications. Syringes may be made of glass or plastic and come in many sizes ranging from 1 ml to 50 ml. Plastic disposable syringes are most commonly used. The syringe may be packaged with a needle attached, or the needle and syringe may be packaged separately.

A syringe (Fig. 18–18) has three parts: the tip, which connects to the needle; the barrel, and the plunger. The tip and shaft of the plunger are considered sterile.

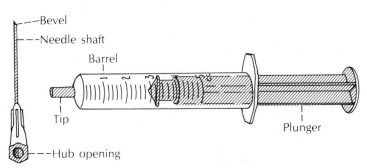

▼ **FIGURE 18–18.** Parts of a syringe.

The three types of syringes are the hypodermic syringe, the insulin syringe, and the tuberculin syringe (Fig. 8–19). Hypodermic syringes usually hold 2, 2.5, or 3 ml of medication and are marked with two scales of measurement, millimeters and minims. Insulin syringes have a nonremovable needle that contains no dead space. The scale of measurement is designed specifically for insulin. For example, U-100 insulin is given with a U-100 insulin syringe. The tuberculin syringe holds 1 ml of medication. It is calibrated with two scales, tenths and hundredths of a milliliter on one scale, and sixteenths of a

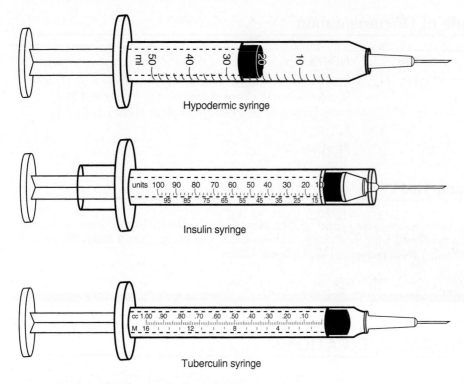

Hypodermic syringe

Insulin syringe

Tuberculin syringe

▼ **FIGURE 18–19.** The three types of syringes.

minim on the other scale. Tuberculin syringes are used to administer tuberculin or other drugs that require very precise measurements (such as pediatric medications).

Needles are made of stainless steel and most are for single use only. The needle has three parts: the hub, which fits over the tip of the syringe; the shaft, or cannula of the needle; and the bevel, or slanted opening at the end of the needle. All parts of the needle are considered sterile. Needles come in various lengths and gauges. The length of needles normally used for injection vary from ⅜ inch to 2 inches. The needle gauge varies from a 26-gauge needle that has a small diameter to an 18-gauge needle that has a larger diameter or bore (Fig. 18–20). Filter needles have a screen device built into the hub that

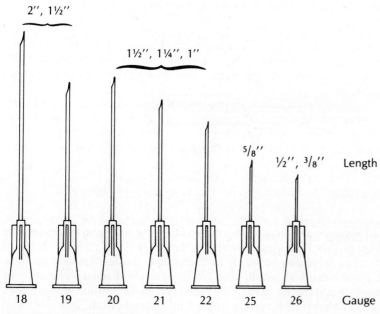

▼ **FIGURE 18–20.** Types of needles.

prevents fine drug particles or glass shards from an ampule from entering the client's circulatory system.

Most medication policies recommend that hypodermic needles not be recapped after use to avoid needlestick injuries. Contaminated needles should be discarded in a designated sharps box (Fig. 18–21).

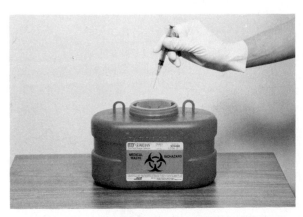

▼ **FIGURE 18–21.** A sharps box.

Ampules, Vials, and Preloaded Medication Systems

Parenteral medications are packaged in ampules, vials, and preloaded medication systems. An ampule (Fig. 18–22*A*) is a glass container of liquid medication intended for

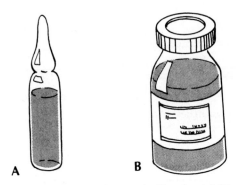

▼ **FIGURE 18–22.** An ampule *(A)* and a vial *(B)*.

use as a single dose. The ampule must be broken open at the neck to withdraw the medication. Once opened, an ampule is an open system and is susceptible to contamination. The medication must be withdrawn immediately into a syringe to maintain sterility. Discard any unused medication.

Vials (see Fig. 18–22*B*) are single-dose or multidose medication containers sealed with a rubber stopper and a metal or plastic cap. The vial may contain medication in a solution or powder that requires reconstitution. Medication is withdrawn from a vial by inserting a needle through the rubber stopper. Refer to Skill 18–11 for further information on withdrawing medications from ampules and vials.

Parenteral medications are also packaged in preloaded medication systems. Fig. 18–23 illustrates a prefilled cartridge system. With this method of medication delivery, a prefilled disposable medication cartridge is loaded into a reusable syringe holder. Figure 18–24 illustrates a closed system device for medication administration. With this system, a prefilled medication cartridge is loaded into a plastic barrel with an attached needle. Many emergency drugs are packaged in this manner.

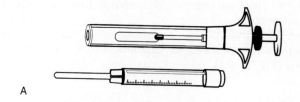

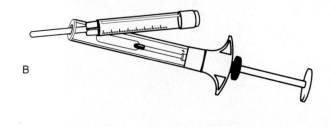

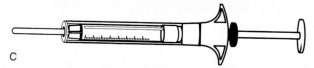

▼ FIGURE 18–23. A prefilled cartridge system.

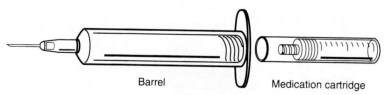

Barrel   Medication cartridge

▼ FIGURE 18–24. A closed system device for medication administration.

SKILL 18–11   WITHDRAWING MEDICATIONS FROM AN AMPULE AND A VIAL

Clinical Situations in Which You May Encounter This Skill

Parenteral medications may be supplied in ampules or vials (see Fig. 18–22). Ampules, which contain a single dose of medication, are small glass bottles with a constricted neck to allow for easy snapping of the ampule into two pieces. The ampule may be scored or a file may be used to partially score the ampule before snapping it.

Vials may contain single or multiple doses of medication. These small glass bottles have rubber stoppers on the top and the needle of the syringe is inserted through the round circle in the top of the rubber stopper for removal of the drug.

Anticipated Responses

▼ The correct amount of medication is withdrawn from the ampule or vial.
▼ No air bubbles remain in the syringe.

Adverse Responses

▼ The incorrect amount of solution is withdrawn.

Materials List

Gather these materials before beginning the skill:

▼ Ampule or vial containing the medication prescribed
▼ Clean gauze or alcohol swab
▼ File (optional)
▼ Syringe with Luer-Lok needle attached
▼ Filter needle (if using an ampule)

▼ *ACTION*	▼ *RATIONALE*
1. Review the physician's order to ensure that you know the right medication, dosage, and time for administration.	1. A physician's order is required for medication administration.
2. Check the label on the ampule or vial to ensure that you have the correct medication.	2. The label should contain the name and concentration of the medicine.
3. Remove the syringe from the paper covering without contaminating the inside of the paper.	3. The inside of the paper covering is sterile and will be needed again if a filter needle is used.
4. Withdraw the medication.	

Withdrawing Medication From an Ampule

a. Unscrew the needle from the barrel of the syringe without contaminating the hub and place the needle on the paper covering from the syringe.	a. The needle will be reapplied to the syringe. The inside of the paper covering is sterile.
b. Connect the filter needle to the barrel of the syringe.	b. The filter needle filters out any glass fragments as the medication is withdrawn from the ampule.
c. Thump the upper portion of the ampule with your finger, or hold the top of the ampule in your hand and rotate the ampule in a large circle.	c. Medication often collects in the top and neck of the ampule. Thumping or rotating the ampule in a large circle forces the liquid into the lower portion of the ampule.
d. If the ampule is not scored, file one side of the neck of the ampule.	d. Facilitates breaking of the ampule's neck.
e. Place a piece of gauze or an alcohol swab around the neck of the ampule.	e. Protects your fingers from being cut when the neck of the ampule is broken.
f. Grasp the neck and body of the ampule and snap the neck of the ampule into two pieces away from you (Fig. 18–25).	f. Breaking the ampule away from you reduces the possibility of getting cut by glass fragments.

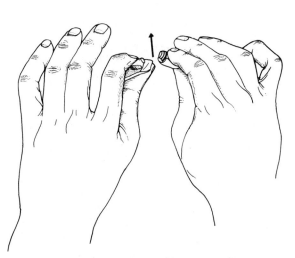

▼ **FIGURE 18–25.** Breaking an ampule.

▼ *ACTION* _ _ _ _ _ _ _ _ _ _ _ _ _ _ _ _ _ _ _

▼ *RATIONALE* _ _ _ _ _ _ _ _ _ _ _ _ _ _ _ _

g. Hold the ampule in one hand and the syringe in the other hand.
h. Insert the needle into the ampule and withdraw all of the medication (Fig. 18–26). (The ampule may need to be slightly tilted and the bevel of the needle may need to be turned downward to withdraw all of the medication (see Fig. 18–26*A*).
OR
Insert the needle into the ampule and invert the ampule to withdraw the medication (see Fig. 18–26*B*).

g. This position gives you control over the ampule and the syringe.
h. If all of the medication is not needed, the excess should be squirted down the sink and not left in the ampule.

The medication does not spill out of the ampule while it is inverted unless air is injected into the ampule while it is inverted.

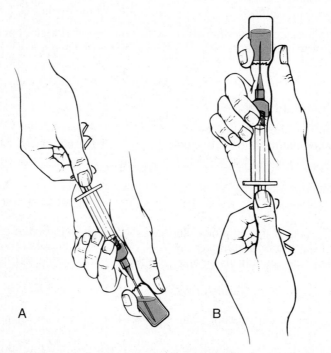

▼ **FIGURE 18–26.** Turning the bevel of the needle downward *(A)* or inserting the needle into the ampule and inverting the ampule to withdraw the medication *(B)*.

i. Discard the ampule in the trash.

j. Remove the filter needle and discard it in the needle container.
k. Reapply the needle. Use sterile technique.

i. Prevents another nurse from possibly getting cut on the broken pieces.
j. Proper needle disposal prevents unnecessary sticks to another nurse.
k. The needle is used to inject the medication.

Withdrawing Medication From a Vial

a. Remove the metal protective covering from the vial. Do not touch the rubber top. If the vial has had medication removed from it previously, swab the top of the vial using a firm and vigorous action.

b. If necessary, reconstitute the medication if it was supplied in a powdered form.
c. Remove the cap from the needle. Use sterile technique.

a. Vials that have not been used have a metal protective covering that is applied at the factory. If you remove the protective covering from the vial immediately prior to withdrawing the medication, swabbing the top of the vial is not necessary because the top is sterile. Friction removes surface microorganisms.
b. Reconstitution is necessary only if the medication was supplied in a powder.
c. Prevents the transfer of microorganisms.

▼ *A C T I O N*   ▼ *R A T I O N A L E*

d. Pull back the plunger on the syringe to equal the amount of medication to be withdrawn from the vial.

e. Insert the needle through the center of the rubber stopper of the vial.

f. Invert the vial so that the needle is above the level of the solution in the vial.

g. Depress the plunger so that the air is injected into the vial (Fig. 18–27A).

d. Air fills as much of the syringe as the amount the plunger is pulled back.

e. The air is injected into the vial.

f. If the needle is in the solution, bubbles may be formed as air is injected.

g. Air creates positive pressure in the vial, thus facilitating the withdrawal of the solution.

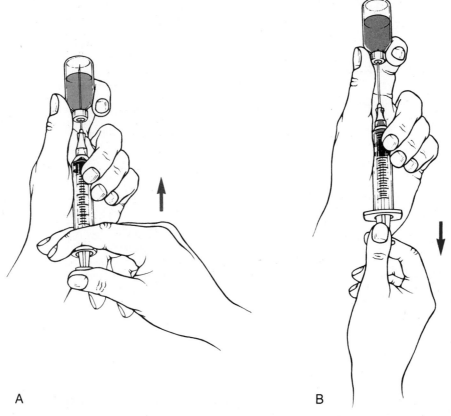

A   B

▼ **FIGURE 18–27.** Pushing air into the vial above the fluid level *(A)* and withdrawing medication *(B)* with a plunger.

h. Withdraw the correct amount of medication by pulling back on the plunger while maintaining the needle so the bevel is within the solution (see Fig. 18–27B).

i. Withdraw the needle from the vial, hold the needle in an upright position, gently tap the syringe with your finger, and push the plunger to expel the air bubbles.

j. Remove the needle from the syringe and discard it.

h. If air is drawn into the syringe, the correct amount of medication is not withdrawn.

i. Holding the syringe and needle upright and tapping the syringe dislodges any air bubbles toward the needle.

j. The bevel of the needle was dulled as it was inserted through the rubber stopper on the vial. Dull needles cause discomfort to the client when the injection is given. The needle used to withdraw the medication contains the medicine in the shaft of the needle. This medication may cause tracking in the client's tissue when it is injected.

▼ *ACTION*

k. Apply a new needle and cap to the syringe. Use sterile technique.
l. If all the medication is not withdrawn (from a multiuse vial), label the vial. Note the reconstitution (dosage per milliliter), date, and time.
m. Check the medication withdrawn from the vial to ensure the correct dosage.

5. Administer the drug. Use correct technique.

6. Record the procedure.

▼ *RATIONALE*

k. Sterile technique prevents the transfer of microorganisms.
l. Ensures that future doses of the medication can be given correctly.

m. Double-checking the dosage helps to prevent errors.

6. Communicates the findings to the other members of the health care team and contributes to the legal record by documenting the care given to the client.

Example of Documentation

DATE	TIME	NOTES
1/1/93	0800	15 units regular insulin SC to right dorsolateral aspect arm.
		C. Lammon, RN

Teaching Tips

The purpose and side effects of the medication should be explained to the client or the client's family. If the medication is to be administered at home, the procedure for administration should be explained to the person who will be administering the medication. It is helpful to write the directions for administration and to allow time for the client or his or her family member to demonstrate the technique.

Home Care Variations

Medications are often administered in the client's home. A container for needle disposal should be taken to the home and removed after the medication has been administered.

SKILL 18–12 ADMINISTERING INTRADERMAL INJECTIONS

Clinical Situations in Which You May Encounter This Skill

An intradermal injection is the administration of medication into the dermis immediately below the epidermal layer. This type of injection is commonly used for allergy testing and for skin tests such as the tuberculin skin test. Injection sites include the arm, the upper anterior chest, and the scapular area (Fig. 18–28). A wheal should be produced as the medication is injected. Absence of a wheal at the injection site, bruising, and bleeding indicate that the injection was administered too deeply.

Anticipated Responses

▼ The client experiences a mild stinging sensation at the site of the injection.
▼ A wheal is seen at the injection site.

Adverse Responses

▼ The medication produces an unwanted reaction.
▼ No wheal is present at the injection site.
▼ There is bruising or bleeding at the injection site.

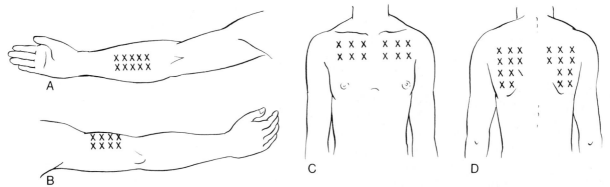

▼ **FIGURE 18–28.** Intradermal injection sites include the arm *(A and B)*, the upper anterior chest *(C)*, and the scapular area *(D)*.

Materials List

Gather these materials before beginning the skill:

- ▼ Correct medication
- ▼ Chart
- ▼ Appropriate needle (usually ³/₈- to ⁵/₈-inch 26- or 27-gauge needle)
- ▼ Tuberculin syringe
- ▼ Alcohol wipes
- ▼ Medication tray
- ▼ Bandage (optional)

▼ ACTION	▼ RATIONALE
1. Obtain a physician's order.	1. The physician is licensed to prescribe medications. You are licensed to administer medications.
2. Verify the correctness of the order and check for drug allergies.	2. You are responsible for all medications administered to the client. A drug allergy is a contraindication to administration of the medication.
3. Wash your hands.	3. Handwashing is the single most effective measure to decrease the transmission of microorganisms from person to person.
4. Concentrate alone.	4. Prevents medication errors from inattention.
5. Select the correct medication and read the label. (This is the first of three times that the label should be read.)	5. The label is read three times to prevent medication errors.
6. Check the expiration date.	6. Expired medications may not give the needed effect.
7. Select the appropriate syringe and needle to administer the medication.	7. Syringe selection depends on the volume of medication to be given and the unit markings required to accurately measure the dose. The needle gauge for intradermal injections is usually a 26 or 27 gauge and the length is ³/₈ to ⁵/₈ inch.
8. Read the label again.	8. The label is read three times to prevent medication errors.
9. Draw up the medication into the syringe and place it on the medication tray. (Refer to Skill 18–11 if needed.)	9. The medication is ready for administration.

▼ _ACTION_

▼ _RATIONALE_

10. Read the label of the medication container for the third time before returning it to the shelf or discarding it.	**10.** The label is read three times to prevent medication errors.
11. Carry the medication to the client and introduce yourself.	**11.** Identifies the caregiver and his or her credentials.
12. Verify the client's identity by checking his or her arm band and bed tag and by asking the client to state his or her name.	**12.** Prevents you from administering medications to the wrong client.
13. Help the client to assume the proper position to receive the injection.	**13.** The area to be injected should be exposed adequately to facilitate location of the injection site landmarks.
14. Cleanse the selected injection site with an alcohol wipe. Use a circular motion from the selected puncture site outward.	**14.** Removes surface contaminants from the injection area.
15. With your nondominant hand, spread the client's skin tautly at the injection site.	**15.** Eases needle insertion.
16. With your dominant hand, grasp the syringe and hold it at a 10-degree angle to the client's skin with the bevel of the needle turned upward.	**16.** If the angle of insertion is any greater the injection will be given too deeply. Administering the injection with the bevel up eases needle insertion.
17. Carefully insert the needle superficially into the client's skin until the bevel opening is occluded by the skin (Fig. 18–29).	**17.** Inserting the full length of the needle results in the injection being given too deeply.

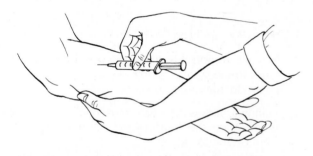

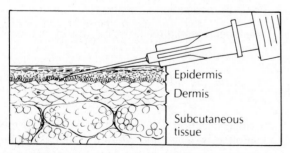

Epidermis

Dermis

Subcutaneous tissue

▼ **FIGURE 18–29.** Angle of needle insertion for administering an intradermal injection.

18. Inject the medication and withdraw the needle. *Do not* aspirate.	**18.** Aspiration is not necessary since an intradermal injection is given superficially where there are no major blood vessels.
19. Observe for the formation of a wheal at the injection site.	**19.** A wheal indicates that the injection was administered correctly. Absence of a wheal indicates that the injection was given too deeply.

▼ *A C T I O N*	▼ *R A T I O N A L E*
1. Obtain a physician's order.	1. The physician is licensed to prescribe medications. You are licensed to administer medications.
2. Verify the correctness of the order and check for drug allergies.	2. You are responsible for all medications administered to the client. A drug allergy is a contraindication to administration of the medication.
3. Assess the proposed injection site.	3. Areas with lesions or trauma; hardened, inflamed, or edematous skin; and underlying nerves, muscles, or blood vessels should be avoided.
4. Wash your hands.	4. Handwashing is the single most effective measure to decrease the transmission of microorganisms from person to person.
5. Concentrate alone.	5. Prevents medication errors from inattention.
6. Select the correct medication and read the label. (This is the first of three times that the label should be read.)	6. The label is read three times to prevent medication errors.
7. Check the expiration date.	7. Expired medications may not give the needed effect.
8. Select the appropriate syringe and needle to administer the medication.	8. Syringe selection depends on the volume of medication to be given and the unit markings required to accurately measure the dose. Needle gauge selection depends on the viscosity of the drug and selection of the needle length depends on the required depth of insertion.
9. Read the label again.	9. The label is read three times to prevent medication errors.
10. Draw up the medication into the syringe and place it on the medication tray. (Refer to Skill 18–11 if needed.)	10. The medication is ready for administration.
11. Read the label of the medication container for the third time before returning it to the shelf or discarding it.	11. The label is read three times to prevent medication errors.
12. Carry the medication to the client and introduce yourself.	12. Identifies the caregiver and his or her credentials.
13. Verify the client's identity by checking his or her arm band and bed tag and asking the client to state his or her name.	13. Prevents you from administering medications to the wrong client.
14. Help the client to assume a proper position to receive the injection.	14. The area to be injected should be exposed adequately to facilitate location of the injection site landmarks.
15. Cleanse the selected injection site with an alcohol wipe. Use a circular motion from the selected puncture site outward.	15. Removes surface contaminants from the injection area.
16. With your nondominant hand, bunch up the client's tissue between your thumb and index finger.	16. Gathers a large area of adipose tissue for the injection of medication.

▼ *ACTION*   ▼ *RATIONALE*

17. With your dominant hand, quickly insert the needle into the injection site. For the average adult, insert the needle at a 45-degree angle for a ½-inch needle and at a 90-degree angle for a ⅜-inch needle (Fig. 18–31). The bevel of the needle should be facing upward.

17. The angle of insertion prevents the injection of medication into the muscle (Fig. 18–32). Inserting the needle quickly with the bevel up eases needle insertion and makes the injection less painful.

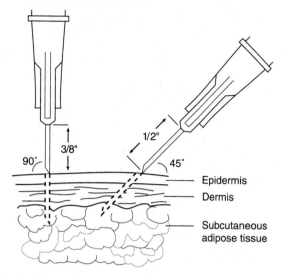

▼ **FIGURE 18–31.** Angle of needle insertion for administering a subcutaneous injection.

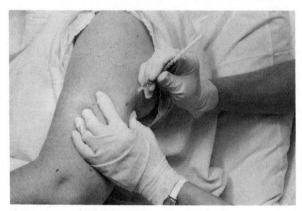

▼ **FIGURE 18–32.** Administering a subcutaneous injection.

> **NOTE:** For an obese client, you may need a longer needle (1 inch) inserted at a 90-degree angle to ensure that the medication is placed in a subcutaneous tissue layer.

18. Aspirate the syringe by pulling back the plunger 0.3 to 0.5 ml.

18. Aspiration is a safety check to ensure that the needle does not lie in a blood vessel.

19. If no blood is detected on aspiration, inject the medication and withdraw the needle.

19. Absence of blood indicates that the needle is not in a blood vessel and that the medication can be administered into the subcutaneous tissue.

> **NOTE:** If blood is detected on aspiration, do not inject the medication. Withdraw the needle and apply pressure to the injection site.
>
> Injection of medication into the blood vessels can cause complications.
>   Pressure is applied to prevent bleeding into the tissues and hematoma formation.

20. Massage the injection area if massage is not contraindicated.

20. Massage increases circulation to the area and enhances absorption of the medication.

21. Place the *uncapped* needle on your medication tray or dispose of it in the needle box at the client's bedside.

21. Needles should not be recapped after use to avoid potential injury and contact with the human immunodeficiency virus, hepatitis B, and other microorganisms.

22. Apply a bandage to the injection site if needed.

22. Protects the site of injection from contamination and aids in stopping bleeding. Bandages should be offered to young children to promote their sense of body integrity.

▼ *ACTION*   ▼ *RATIONALE*

23. Help the client to assume a position of comfort.

24. If there was no needle box in the client's room, dispose of the *uncapped* needle according to the policy of your institution.

25. Return the equipment to the medication room.

26. Wash your hands.

27. Return to the client at the appropriate time to assess the effects of the medication.

28. Chart the medication given; the time, dose, route, and site of the injection; the client's response to the drug; and any other related information.

23. Promotes the client's comfort.

24. Proper disposal decreases the transmission of microorganisms.

25. Nondisposable equipment can be used again.

26. Decreases the transmission of microorganisms.

27. You are responsible for monitoring for the expected effect, potential side effects, and allergic reactions to the medication.

28. Communicates to the other members of the health care team and contributes to the legal record by documenting the care given to the client.

Example of Documentation

DATE	TIME	NOTES
1/1/93	0730	10 units regular insulin administered SQ to right anterior thigh for blood sugar of 210.
		H. White, RN

Teaching Tips

The client should be taught the name of the medication, its purpose, and possible side effects. If the client is learning to self-administer a parenteral medication, the technique should be demonstrated and time should be provided for the client to do a return demonstration.

Home Care Variations

Clients with diabetes mellitus, cancer, vitamin deficiencies, and other conditions may require injections at home. You must assess the client's or caregiver's ability to perform the skill and willingness to learn the procedure. The client or caregiver should learn how to handle the equipment and maintain its sterility, draw up the correct dosage of medication, select and rotate injection sites, and give the injection.

SPECIAL TECHNIQUES FOR HEPARIN

Because of the anticoagulant action of heparin, special administration techniques are necessary to prevent hematoma formation. The abdomen is the site of choice for administration. This subcutaneous site does not overlie major muscles so there is less movement and hematoma formation. A ½-inch 25- to 27-gauge needle should be selected. After drawing up the medication the needle should be changed to avoid depositing any of the medication in the intradermal layers of tissue. Drawing up 0.1 ml of air into the syringe prior to injection also prevents any leakage of heparin into the intradermal tissue. There is controversy regarding aspiration when giving a subcutaneous heparin injection. Some sources recommend not aspirating since needle movement may rupture capillaries and result in bruising and bleeding. You should check your agency policy regarding this maneuver. After injecting the heparin into the abdomen, do not massage the injection site. Finally, heparin injection sites should be rotated to lessen irritation to any one area of abdominal adipose tissue.

SKILL 18–14   MIXING INSULIN IN A SYRINGE

Clinical Situations in Which You May Encounter This Skill

Insulin is a hormone that is given to clients with diabetes mellitus to control their serum blood sugar. Insulin should be mixed from two vials into one syringe when the client is to receive two types (short-acting and long-acting, for example) of insulin at one time. Because long-acting insulin modifies short-acting insulin, the mixture of insulins should be given within 5 minutes of mixing them in the syringe.

Short-acting insulins (regular insulins) are unmodified. When given subcutaneously, regular insulin may be mixed with any other type of insulin. Intermediate-acting and long-acting insulins are modified with protein to slow their absorption rate and are cloudy in appearance. Lente insulins may be mixed with other lente insulins, but may not be mixed with other types of insulin.

Insulin may be stored at room temperature for 30 days. It should not be stored frozen or exposed to direct sunlight. Insulin should be given at room temperature to avoid lipodystrophy (depressed areas of fatty tissue) at the injection sites. The injection sites should be rotated (back of arms, thighs, abdomen, or throughout the abdominal area) to avoid hypertrophied (raised) areas.

A hypoglycemic reaction (sweating, weakness, irritability, malaise) may occur after insulin administration. If the client has a hypoglycemic reaction, an immediate source of sugar must be given to raise the blood sugar. A simple and complex carbohydrate such as saltine crackers and peanut butter followed by milk should also be given. If the client is unconscious, do not try to force oral feedings. Glucagon may be given subcutaneously or dextrose may be given intravenously.

Anticipated Responses

▼ The insulin is mixed into one syringe in the correct dosage.
▼ The client's blood sugar is within normal limits.
▼ The client learns to mix and administer the insulin properly.

Adverse Responses

▼ The insulin lowers the blood sugar too much and the client has a hypoglycemic reaction.
▼ The client does not have the manual dexterity or the mental capability to learn to mix the insulin.

Materials List

Gather these materials before beginning the skill:

▼ Short-acting insulin
▼ Intermediate-acting or long-acting insulin
▼ Insulin syringe with needle
▼ Alcohol swab

▼ ACTION	▼ RATIONALE
1. Check the physician's order for the type of insulin, amount, and frequency of administration.	1. The physician must order the type, amount, and frequency of administration.
2. Ask the client if he or she mixes and self-administers insulin at home.	2. If the client mixes and administers insulin to himself or herself at home, you may ask him or her to demonstrate the technique to you. This allows you to assess the client's technique. If the client's diabetes is newly diagnosed, you can teach the client how to properly mix and administer the insulin.
3. Place the supplies on a clean tabletop.	3. Decreases the possibility of contamination.
4. With an alcohol swab, clean the rubber top on both vials.	4. Removes surface microorganisms.
5. Inject air into the long-acting (cloudy) insulin in an amount equal to the amount of insulin to be withdrawn. Do not let the needle touch the insulin within the vial.	5. Creates positive pressure in the vial to facilitate withdrawal of the insulin. Do not let the insulin contaminate the needle.
6. Withdraw the needle from the vial.	6. Air is injected into the long-acting insulin before it is injected into the short-acting insulin.
7. Inject air into the short-acting clear insulin in an amount equal to the amount of insulin to be withdrawn.	7. Creates positive pressure in the vial to facilitate withdrawal of the insulin.

▼ *A C T I O N*

▼ *R A T I O N A L E*

8. Leave the needle in the second vial of short-acting insulin, invert the vial, and withdraw the amount of insulin prescribed.

8. The short-acting clear insulin is always withdrawn first.

9. Insert the needle of the syringe into the first vial of long-acting cloudy insulin, invert the vial, and withdraw the prescribed amount of insulin (Fig. 18–33).

9. The long-acting cloudy insulin is always withdrawn second.

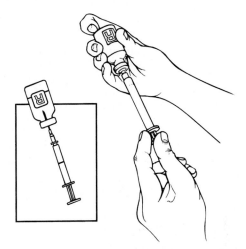

Step C: Withdraw prescribed amount of short-acting (clear) insulin

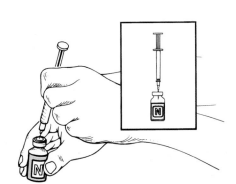

Step A: Inject air into longer-acting (cloudy) insulin

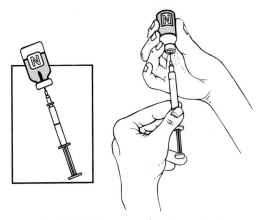

Step D: Withdraw prescribed amount of longer-acting (cloudy) insulin

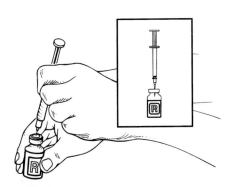

Step B: Inject air into short-acting (clear) insulin

▼ **FIGURE 18–33.** Injecting air into the long-acting (cloudy) insulin in an amount equal to the amount of insulin to be withdrawn. Withdrawing the needle from the vial (A). Injecting air into the short-acting clear insulin in an amount equal to the amount of insulin to be withdrawn (B). Leaving the needle in the second vial of short-acting insulin, inverting the vial, and withdrawing the amount of insulin prescribed (C). Inserting the needle of the syringe into the first vial of long-acting cloudy insulin, inverting the vial, and withdrawing the prescribed amount of insulin (D).

10. Withdraw the needle from the vial and check the total amount of insulin in the syringe.

10. The volume should be equal to the number of units of the short-acting insulin plus the number of units of the long-acting insulin. Checking the volume also serves to double-check the dosage in the syringe.

11. Administer the insulins subcutaneously as prescribed.

11. All insulins other than regular insulins must be administered subcutaneously.

▼ *ACTION*	▼ *RATIONALE*
12. Document on the client's chart the medication given; the time, dose, and route of administration; the client's response to the drug; and any other related information.	**12.** Communicates to the health care team and contributes to the legal record by documenting the care given to the client.

Example of Documentation

DATE	*TIME*	*NOTES*
5/20/93	0800	15 units of isophane and 5 units of regular insulin given subcutaneously in lower right abdomen. Client observed procedure and stated was ready to learn to administer to self.
		S. Williams, RN

Teaching Tips

The client must learn to correctly mix and properly administer insulin. If the client's diabetes is newly diagnosed, you should take the supplies to the client's room so that teaching can begin immediately unless self-administration is contraindicated. If the client's diabetes is not new and he or she has been administering the insulin at home, you must assess the client's ability to properly mix and administer the insulins.

The client must be taught to rotate the injection sites to ensure proper absorption of the insulin. See Figure 18–34 for the usual sites for subcutaneous injections.

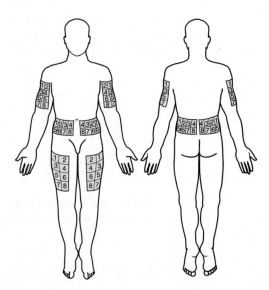

▼ **FIGURE 18–34.** Diagram of usual sites for subcutaneous injections.

If the client is unable (or unwilling) to administer insulin to himself or herself, a family member should be trained to mix and administer the insulin. After you demonstrate the procedure, ask the client or his or her family member to do a return demonstration.

Teach the client the signs and symptoms of hyperglycemia and hypoglycemia and the treatment indicated for both. Also, teach the client how to perform fingersticks to assess his or her blood sugar.

Home Care Variations

Insulin may be premixed and stored for future administration. Since the concentration of mixed insulin changes after 5 minutes, the client should always use premixed insulin instead of freshly mixed insulin. Once the client has been regulated with this concentration, changing the amount of time between mixing and administering the insulin may alter the client's response.

The client may safely reuse disposable syringes at home for as long as 1 week. The client must store the syringes in a clean dry container. Longer than 1 week's use dulls the needles considerably and causes discomfort to the client.

The client and his or her family may be interested in information and services provided by the American Diabetes Association.

SKILL 18–15   ADMINISTERING INTRAMUSCULAR INJECTIONS

Clinical Situations in Which You May Encounter This Skill

Medication is introduced into the muscle by hypodermic injection. The length of the needle varies depending on the injection site selected and the size of the client. If a small muscle such as the deltoid is selected, the needle length may range from ⅝ inch to 1 inch for the average adult. For a large muscle such as the gluteal muscle, the needle length ranges from 1.5 to 2 inches for the average adult. Obese clients require longer needles. Medications intended for intramuscular injection must not be injected into the adipose tissue, as irritation and necrosis may result.

The viscosity of the medication determines the gauge of the needle selected. Aqueous medications can be administered through a 22- to 25-gauge needle. Oily medications require a 21-gauge needle. Very viscous medications such as penicillin G benzathine and penicillin G procaine suspension may require use of an 18-gauge needle. Common intramuscular

injection sites include the dorsogluteal, ventrogluteal, vastus lateralis, and deltoid muscles. Select a muscle site that is free of bruising, nodules, scars, and other abnormalities.

The dorsogluteal site, or gluteus medius muscle, is the desired site for deep intramuscular injections of irritating or viscous medications. You must select the site carefully to avoid damage to the sciatic nerve, gluteal artery, or bone. Hanson's method (Fig. 18–35) is the most accurate method for identifying the injection site. First identify the posterior superior iliac spine. Then draw an imaginary line to the head of the trochanter. The injection is given lateral and superior to this line. The dorsogluteal site is used for adults and children over the age of 3 years. To administer an injection to the dorsogluteal site, have the client lie in the prone position with his or her toes pointing inward (Fig. 18–36). This position relaxes the gluteal muscles. The side-lying position also may be used. Ask the client to flex his or her upper leg at the knee and thigh to relax the gluteal muscles.

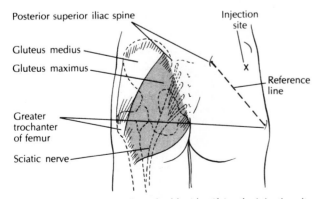

▼ **FIGURE 18–35.** Hanson's method for identifying the injection site.

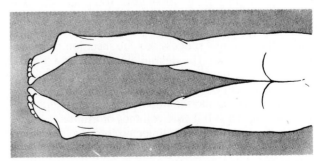

▼ **FIGURE 18–36.** Position for injection into the dorsogluteal site.

The ventrogluteal site, or von Hochstetter's site (Fig. 18–37), is rapidly becoming the preferred gluteal injection site since it is removed from all major nerves and blood vessels and possible fecal contamination. The medication is placed into the gluteus minimus muscle. To locate the client's left ventrogluteal injection site, place the heel of your right palm on the client's greater trochanter of the femur. Place your index finger on the client's anterior superior iliac spine and spread your other fingers posteriorly. The injection is given in the **V** formed between the index finger and the second finger. This site may be used for children and adults. It may be located with the client in the supine or side-lying position.

The vastus lateralis and rectus femoris muscles are other injection sites that are free of major nerves and blood vessels and are safe for use with both adults and children. The sites are located on the anterior and lateral aspects of the thigh. You should divide the area into thirds between the greater trochanter of the femur and the lateral femoral condyle. The injection should be given into the middle third (Fig. 18–38). The client may be in the sitting or supine position.

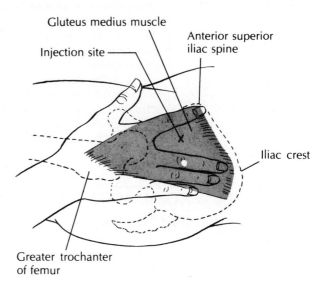

▼ **FIGURE 18–37.** The ventrogluteal site.

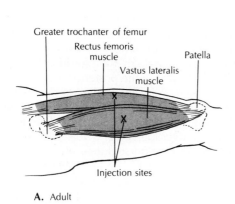

A. Adult

B. Infant

▼ **FIGURE 18–38.** Injection sites for adults *(A)* and infants *(B)* in the anterior and lateral aspects of the thigh.

The deltoid muscle is a small muscle located on the lateral aspect of the upper arm. You must inject the medication into the densest part of the deltoid muscle to avoid the radial nerve and artery. To identify the site, locate the acromial process and the insertion point of the deltoid muscle. The deltoid muscle forms a triangle between these upper and lower boundaries. The injection should be given about 2 inches below the acromial process into the middle third of the deltoid muscle (Fig. 18–39). Large volumes of irritating medications should not be injected into the deltoid muscle.

Anticipated Responses

▼ The client experiences a mild stinging sensation at the site of the injection.

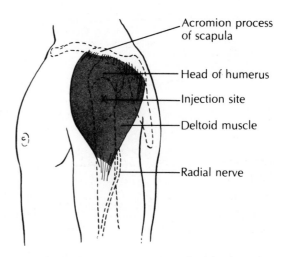

▼ **FIGURE 18–39.** Injection site in the deltoid muscle.

Adverse Responses

▼ The medication produces an unwanted reaction.
▼ The client complains of pain, numbness, or tingling at the injection site.

Materials List

Gather these materials before beginning the skill:

▼ Correct medication
▼ Chart
▼ Appropriate needle (usually 1 to 3 inches, 20 to 25 gauge)
▼ Appropriate syringe
▼ Alcohol wipes
▼ Medication tray
▼ Bandage (optional)

▼ *ACTION*	▼ *RATIONALE*
1. Obtain a physician's order.	**1.** The physician is licensed to prescribe medications. You are licensed to administer medications.
2. Verify the correctness of the order and check for drug allergies.	**2.** You are responsible for all medications administered to the client. A drug allergy is a contraindication to administration of the medication.
3. Wash your hands.	**3.** Handwashing is the single most effective measure to decrease the transmission of microorganisms from person to person.
4. Concentrate alone.	**4.** Prevents medication errors from inattention.
5. Select the correct medication and read the label. (This is the first of three times that the label should be read.)	**5.** The label is read three times to prevent medication errors.
6. Check the expiration date.	**6.** Expired medications may not give the needed effect.
7. Select the appropriate syringe and needle to administer the medication.	**7.** The syringe selection depends on the volume of medication to be given and the unit markings required to accurately measure the dose. Needle gauge selection depends on the viscosity of the drug and the selection of needle length depends on the required depth of insertion.
8. Read the label again.	**8.** The label is read three times to prevent medication errors.
9. Draw up the medication into the syringe and place it on the medication tray. After checking the accuracy of the dosage, draw up an additional 0.2 to 0.5 cc of air in a syringe to provide an air lock (optional).	**9.** The medication is ready for administration. When you administer the injection, the air bubble will float upward toward the plunger and will clear the needle and hub of medication as it is injected through the syringe. The airlock technique seals the medication in muscle and prevents tracking back along the needle path.
10. Read the label of the medication container for the third time before returning it to the shelf or discarding it.	**10.** The label is read three times to prevent medication errors.
11. Carry the medication to the client and introduce yourself.	**11.** Identifies the caregiver and his or her credentials.
12. Verify the client's identity by checking his or her arm band and bed tag and asking the client to state his or her name.	**12.** Prevents you from administering medications to the wrong client.

▼ *ACTION*   ▼ *RATIONALE*

13. Help the client to assume a proper position to receive the injection.

13. The area to be injected should be exposed adequately to facilitate location of the injection site landmarks.

14. Cleanse the selected injection site with an alcohol wipe. Use a circular motion from the selected puncture site outward.

14. Removes surface contaminants from the injection area.

15. Using your nondominant hand, spread the client's tissue between your thumb and index finger.

15. Spreads adipose tissue away from the injection site. Holding the skin tautly decreases the pain of the needle insertion.

16. Hold the syringe in your dominant hand and quickly insert the length of the needle at a 90-degree angle into the injection site (Fig. 18–41).

16. A 90-degree angle is used to inject medications deep into the muscle mass (Fig. 18–40).

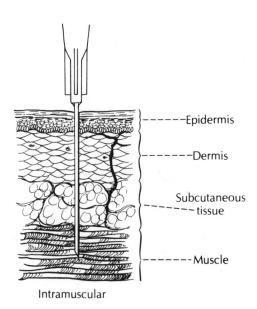

Epidermis

Dermis

Subcutaneous tissue

Muscle

Intramuscular

▼ **FIGURE 18–40.** Angle of needle insertion for administering an intramuscular injection.

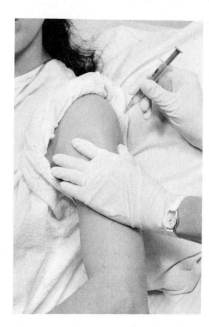

▼ **FIGURE 18–41.** Administering an intramuscular injection.

17. Aspirate the syringe by pulling back on the plunger 0.3 to 0.5 ml.

17. Aspiration is a safety check to ensure that the needle does not lie in a blood vessel.

18. If no blood is detected on aspiration, inject the medication and withdraw the needle.

18. Absence of blood indicates that the needle is not in a blood vessel and that the medication can be administered into the muscle.

NOTE: If blood is detected on aspiration, do not inject the medication. Withdraw the needle and apply pressure to the injection site.

Injection of medication into the blood vessels can cause complications. Pressure is applied to prevent bleeding into the tissues and hematoma formation.

---

19. Massage the injection site if massage is not contraindicated.

19. Massage increases circulation to the area and enhances absorption of the medication.

▼ _ A C T I O N_	▼ _R A T I O N A L E_
20. Place the *uncapped* needle on your medication tray or dispose of it in the needle box at the client's bedside.	**20.** The needle should not be recapped after use to avoid potential injury and contact with human immunodeficiency virus, hepatitis B, and other microorganisms.
21. Apply a bandage to the injection site if needed.	**21.** Protects the site of injection from contamination and aids in stopping bleeding. Bandages should be offered to young chidren to promote their sense of body integrity.
22. Help the client to assume a position of comfort.	**22.** Promotes the client's comfort.
23. If there was no needle box in the client's room, dispose of the *uncapped* needle according to the policy of your institution.	**23.** Proper disposal decreases the transmission of microorganisms.
24. Return the equipment to the medication room.	**24.** Nondisposable equipment can be used again.
25. Wash your hands.	**25.** Decreases the transmission of microorganisms.
26. Return to the client at the appropriate time to assess the effects of the medication.	**26.** You are responsible for monitoring for the expected effect, potential side effects, and allergic reactions to the medication.
27. Chart the medication given; the time, dose, route, and site of injection; the client's response to the drug; and any other related information.	**27.** Communicates to the other members of the health care team and contributes to the legal record by documenting the care given to the client.

SPECIAL TECHNIQUE FOR INTRAMUSCULAR INJECTIONS: THE Z-TRACK TECHNIQUE

The Z-track technique (Fig. 18–42) should be used when the medication to be administered is highly irritating to the subcutaneous tissues. Z tracking creates a zigzag needle path that prevents leakage of medication back into the subcutaneous tissues.

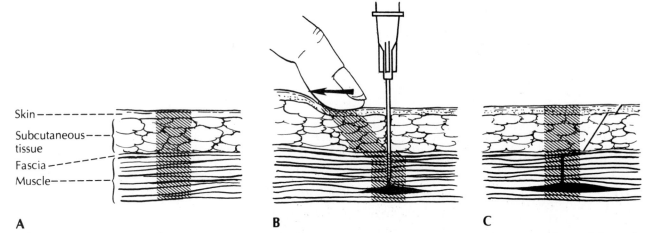

▼ **FIGURE 18–42.** The Z-track technique. Normal tissue before injection *(A)*, altered tissue during injection *(B)*, and normal tissue after injection *(C)*.

▼ *ACTION*   ▼ *RATIONALE*

ACTION	RATIONALE
a. After drawing up the medication, remove the needle and attach a new sterile needle to the syringe.	a. Medications given by the Z-track method are very irritating to the subcutaneous tissue. Changing needles prevents small amounts of the medication that might be present on the needle from being deposited in the subcutaneous tissue during the injection.
b. Draw 0.2 to 0.5 cc of air into the syringe.	b. The bubble creates an air lock that seals the medication into the muscle and prevents tracking of the medication through the subcutaneous tissue as the needle is withdrawn.
c. With your nondominant hand, grasp the client's skin and subcutaneous tissue over the injection site and stretch it to the side 1 to 1½ inches.	c. After giving the injection, this tissue is released to seal the medication into the muscle.
d. With your dominant hand, quickly insert the length of the needle into the injection site at a 90-degree angle.	d. A 90-degree angle is used to inject medications deep into the muscle mass.
e. Without releasing the tightly stretched tissue, use the thumb of your dominant hand to aspirate the syringe by pulling back on the plunger 0.3 to 0.5 ml.	e. Aspiration is a safety check to ensure that the needle does not lie in a blood vessel.
f. If no blood is seen on aspiration, inject the medication while still holding the tissue taut to one side.	f. Absence of blood indicates that the needle is not in a blood vessel and that the medication can be administered into the muscle.

NOTE: If blood is aspirated, withdraw the syringe and apply pressure to the injection site.	Injection of medication into the blood vessels can cause complications. Pressure is applied to prevent bleeding into the tissues and hematoma formation.

g. Maintain traction on the skin for 10 seconds after the injection is given.	g. Allows all the medication to flow into the muscle and be sealed in place with the air lock.
h. Release the traction on the skin slowly as the needle is withdrawn.	h. Allows the subcutaneous tissue to slide over the injection site in a zigzag pattern and prevents the medication from leaking back through the injection tract into the subcutaneous tissue.
i. Do not massage the injection area.	i. Massage may dislodge the medication and allow it to leak back into the subcutaneous tissue.

Example of Documentation

DATE	TIME	NOTES
1/1/93	0830	Meperidine 75 mg IM to right dorsogluteal site for complaints of abdominal pain at surgical incision.
		H. White, RN
	0900	Client states abdominal pain is much less. BP = 122/76, R = 14.
		H. White, RN

Teaching Tips

The client should be taught the name of the medication, its purpose, and its possible side effects. If the client is taught to self-administer a parenteral medication, the technique should be demonstrated and time should be provided for a return demonstration that will enable you to evaluate the client's attainment of this skill.

Home Care Variations

Clients with diabetes mellitus, cancer, vitamin deficiencies, and other conditions may require injections at home. You must assess the client's or caregiver's ability to perform the skill, and willingness to learn the procedure. The client or caregiver should learn how to handle the equipment and maintain its sterility, draw up the correct dosage of medication, select and rotate injection sites, and give the injection.

SKILL 18–16   MIXING MEDICATIONS IN A SYRINGE

Clinical Situations in Which You May Encounter This Skill

Medications can be mixed into one syringe when two medications are ordered to be given intramuscularly and are compatible, and the total dosage to be delivered is less than 2.5 ml. For example, an order may be written for meperidine (25 mg = 1 ml) and promethazine (25 mg = 0.5 ml). Rather than administering two injections, 1 ml of meperidine and a second injection of 0.5 ml of promethazine, the two medications are drawn up into one syringe and administered as one injection.

Prior to mixing medications, you must ensure compatibility. If medications are not compatible, the drugs can precipitate in the syringe or the medications may appear cloudy after they are mixed. If precipitation or cloudiness occurs, discard the syringe containing the medications. Then draw the medications up into two separate syringes and administer them as two injections. Refer to the hospital formulary, a compatibility chart, or a pharmacology reference book to ensure compatibility of medications.

Anticipated Responses

▼ The medications are mixed together in one syringe and administered.

Adverse Responses

▼ The medications are mixed into one syringe and the medications precipitate or become cloudy.

Materials List

Gather these materials before beginning the skill:

▼ Medications to be administered
▼ Alcohol swabs
▼ Syringe

▼ *ACTION*

1. Review the physician's orders for the medications to be administered.

2. Check the labels on the medicines to ensure that you have the correct medications.

3. Ensure that the medications are compatible and that the total dosage will be less than 2.5 ml.

4. Swab the rubber top of the vial or vials with an alcohol swab.

▼ *RATIONALE*

1. Helps to ensure that the correct medicines in the correct dosages are administered.

2. Assists in ensuring that the correct medicines are given.

3. If medications are not compatible, precipitation or cloudiness may occur. The particles that result may not be absorbed.

4. Friction removes surface microorganisms.

▼ A C T I O N	▼ R A T I O N A L E
5. Inject air into the vial or vials in an amount equal to the amount of medication to be withdrawn.	5. If air is not injected into the vial, negative pressure will be created in the vial and will create difficulty in withdrawing the medication.
6. After looking at the label a second time, withdraw the prescribed amount of medication from one vial.	6. Looking at the label a second time helps to prevent errors.
7. After looking at the label a second time, withdraw the drug from the second vial or ampule. Do not allow any of the first medication to enter the second vial as the medication is withdrawn.	7. If the medication is injected into the second (multidose) vial, the vial will not contain the correct medication for subsequent use.
8. Look at the labels a third time to ensure that the correct medications and dosages were withdrawn from the vials.	8. Examining the labels a third time serves as a third check for the prevention errors.
9. Carefully look at the syringe to ensure that precipitation or cloudiness did not occur.	9. Precipitation or cloudiness indicates drug incompatibility and the medication should not be given.
10. Record the medication administration.	10. Communicates to the other members of the health care team and contributes to the legal record by documenting the care given to the client.

Teaching Tips

The purpose of the medicines and any side effects should be explained to the client. The client should also be told that two medications were given in the same syringe. Otherwise the client may not realize that he or she received all the medications ordered.

Home Care Variations

If it is necessary to mix medicines in the client's home, the same procedure can be followed.

SKILL 18–17 ADMINISTERING INTRAVENOUS MEDICATIONS

Clinical Situations in Which You May Encounter This Skill

Medications are given by the intravenous (IV) route when rapid results are needed. The IV route bypasses the absorption phase of the drug and places the medication directly into the bloodstream for distribution to body tissues.

The patency of the IV must be checked before administering IV medications. Some medications are toxic to the tissues if infiltration into the surrounding tissues occurs.

Because of the concentrations of many medications, dilution of the medication (with normal saline or D5W, for example) may be necessary prior to administering the medication intravenously. Refer to the information contained on the package insert, a pharmacology book, or the hospital pharmacy for verification of proper dilution and infusion rates. IV medications are usually administered slowly to avoid discomfort or side effects.

Some medications are incompatible with other solutions or medications. Compatibility must be verified prior to administering any medication through the IV route. If the medication becomes cloudy when injected or precipitates in the tubing, immediately stop the infusion, change the tubing, and verify compatibility. The tubing may need to be flushed prior to and after administering the IV medication. If the client complains of burning as the medication infuses, slow the infusion rate.

Anticipated Responses

▼ No precipitation or cloudiness occurs.
▼ The client has no adverse effects from the medication.

Adverse Responses

▼ The medication precipitates or becomes cloudy as it is administered.
▼ The client complains of burning as the medication is infused.

Materials List

Gather these materials before beginning the skill:

▼ Correct medication
▼ Chart
▼ Alcohol swabs
▼ Medication tray
▼ For push medications, adding medication to a primary bag, and adding medication to a volume administration set chamber
  Syringe with a 21- to 23-gauge needle, label
▼ For piggyback or secondary bag administration:
  Piggyback bag and IV tubing, label, tape, syringe with a 21- to 23-gauge needle
▼ For adding medications through a heparin or saline lock:
  Two syringes with a 21- to 23-gauge needle. Each syringe should be filled with normal saline
  Medication to be injected drawn up in a third syringe with a 21- to 23-gauge needle in place
  Fourth syringe with a heparin flush (if ordered)

▼ **ACTION**	▼ **RATIONALE**
1. Verify the correctness of the medication cards with the physician's order. Check for drug allergies.	1. You are responsible for all medications administered to the client. A drug allergy is a contradiction to administration of the medication.
2. Ask the client if he or she has any drug allergies.	2. Although the chart should indicate drug allergies, it is necessary to double-check to avoid a drug reaction.
3. Verify that the secondary medication is compatible with the primary fluids.	3. Certain medications (phenytoin, for example) are not compatible with other fluids or medications. If incompatible solutions are infused, the two medications or fluids will precipitate.
4. Verify that the IV site is not infiltrated. Observe for redness, pain, swelling, fluids that readily infuse into the vein, and blood return when the IV bag is lower than the IV insertion site.	4. If the IV is infiltrated, pain and local tissue reactions will result as the medication infuses into the surrounding tissue.
5. Select the correct medication and read the label. (This is the first of three times that the label should be read.)	5. The label is read three times to prevent medication errors.
6. Check the expiration date.	6. Expired medications may not give the needed effect.
7. Read the label of the medication for a second time.	7. The label is read a second time to prevent an error.
8. Administer the medication.	

Administering Intravenous Push Medications

a. Select the appropriate syringe and needle to prepare the medication.	a. The needle gauge and length and the size of the syringe depend on the dosage and the medication to be administered.
b. Using sterile technique, reconstitute the medication if necessary and withdraw the medication into the syringe.	b. Sterile technique is required. The medication is administered directly into the client's bloodstream.
c. Recap the needle.	c. Prevents contamination of the needle with microorganisms.

▼ *ACTION* ──────────── ▼ *RATIONALE* ──────────

d. Read the label of the medication for the third time before returning it to storage or discarding it.

e. Verify the client's identity by checking his or her name tag and bed tag and by asking the client to state his or her name.

f. Cleanse the injection port of the IV tubing with an alcohol swab.

g. Using sterile technique, insert the syringe needle into the injection port.

h. Using your fingers, compress the IV tubing above the injection port when injecting the medication. Release the tubing when you are not injecting the medication (Fig. 18–43).

d. The label is read a third time for error prevention.

e. Verification of the correct client is necessary to ensure that the right client is receiving the right drug.

f. Removes surface microorganisms from the insertion port.

g. Reduces the possibility of introducing microorganisms into the client's bloodstream.

h. Prevents the medication from flowing back into the primary bag.

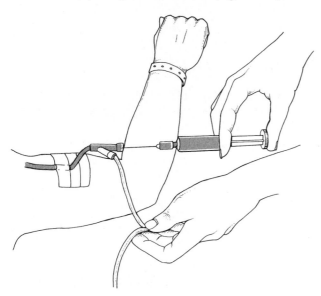

▼ **FIGURE 18–43.** Administering medication through an injection port of IV tubing.

i. Inject the medication at the recommended rate.

i. Some medications must be administered at no more than a milligram per minute. Be sure to check a pharmacologic reference for the recommended rate for the IV push.

Adding Medication to a Primary Bag

a. Select an appropriate syringe and needle to prepare the medication.

b. Using sterile technique, reconstitute the medication if necessary and withdraw the medication into a syringe.

c. Recap the needle.

d. Read the label of the medication for the third time before returning it to storage or discarding it.

e. Cleanse the port of the primary bag with an alcohol swab.

a. The needle gauge and length and the size of the syringe depend on the dosage and the medication to be administered.

b. Sterile technique is required. The medication is administered directly into the client's bloodstream.

c. Prevents contamination of the needle with microorganisms.

e. Removes microorganisms from the port.

▼ *ACTION* _____   ▼ *RATIONALE* _____

f. Insert the needle into the port and inject the medication into the bag of fluid (Fig. 18–44).

f. The medicine is added to the entire bag of fluid. Potassium chloride is often administered in this manner.

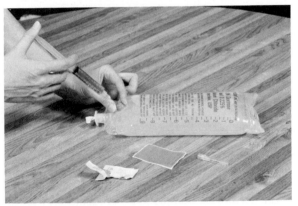

▼ **FIGURE 18–44.** Injecting medication into the bag of fluid.

g. Gently rotate the bag (Fig. 18–45).

h. Prepare a label with the medication added, date, time, and your name and affix it to the primary bag of fluid (Fig. 18–46).

g. Rotating the bag mixes the medication with the fluids.

h. This information is needed for client safety and to determine the next fluids to be hung.

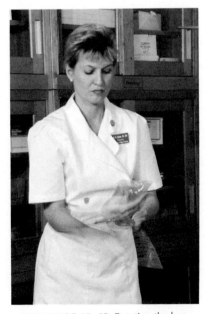

▼ **FIGURE 18–45.** Rotating the bag.

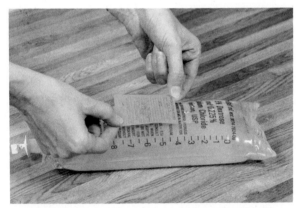

▼ **FIGURE 18–46.** Labelling the primary bag of fluid.

Adding Medications to a Volume Administration Set Chamber

a. Select an appropriate syringe and needle to prepare the medication.

a. The needle gauge and length and the size of the syringe depend on the dosage and the medication to be administered.

▼ _ _A_C_T_I_O_N_ _ _ _ _ _ _ _ _ _ _ _ _ _ _ _ _ _ ▼ _R_A_T_I_O_N_A_L_E_ _ _ _ _ _ _ _ _ _ _ _ _ _ _

b. Using sterile technique, reconstitute the medication if necessary and withdraw the medication into a syringe.

c. Recap the needle.

d. Read the label of the medication for the third time before returning it to storage or discarding it.

e. Verify the client's identity by checking his or her name tag and bed tag and by asking the client to state his or her name.

f. Release the clamp between the main IV bag and the chamber and allow the fluid from the main IV bag to fill the chamber to the required level (usually 50–100 ml).

g. Return the clamp to the closed position.

h. Clean the injection site on the chamber with an alcohol swab.

i. Using sterile technique, inject the medication into the port on the chamber (Fig. 18–47).

b. Sterile technique is required. The medication is administered directly into the client's bloodstream.

c. Prevents contamination of the needle with microorganisms.

d. The label is read a third time for error prevention.

e. Verification of the correct client is necessary to ensure that the right client is receiving the right drug.

f. Allows the fluid into the chamber to dilute the medication to be administered.

g. Prevents the main fluids from continuing to infuse into the volume chamber.

h. Removes surface microorganisms from the chamber port.

i. Prevents the introduction of microorganisms into the client's bloodstream.

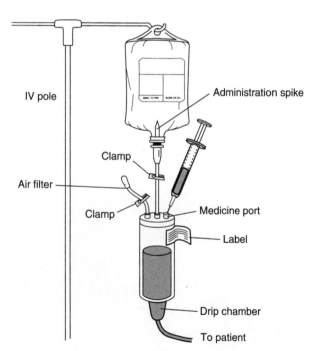

IV pole

Administration spike

Clamp

Air filter

Clamp

Medicine port

Label

Drip chamber

To patient

▼ FIGURE 18–47. Injecting medication into the port on the chamber.

j. Remove the syringe and needle from the port and gently rotate the chamber.

k. Regulate the IV flow rate to administer the medication in the required amount of time, usually 30 to 60 minutes.

l. Label the chamber with the name and amount of medication and the date and time the medication was started.

j. The chamber is rotated to mix the medication and fluid in the chamber.

k. The client does not receive the needed effect from the medicine if it is administered too slowly. If the medicine is administered too rapidly, unwanted side effects could occur.

l. Assists you in determining if the medicine is flowing at the correct rate and alerts others that a medicine is being administered.

▼ _A C T I O N_ ▼ _R A T I O N A L E_ _ _ _ _ _ _ _ _ _ _ _ _ _

m. When the medication has infused, release a small amount of fluid (10–20 ml) into the chamber and allow the fluid to drip through the tubing. Refill the chamber with fluid from the main IV bag and continue the infusion at the rate ordered by the physician.

m. Clears the tubing of any remaining medication.

Administering Medication with a Piggyback/Secondary Bag

a. Remove the plastic protective covering from the bag and discard it.
b. Using an alcohol swab, clean the injection port of the fluid bag.
c. Using sterile technique, inject the medication into the port on the fluid bag.
d. Gently rotate the bag.
e. Place a label on the bag. Write the name and amount of the additive and the time and date when the medication was added to the bag.
f. Obtain a piggyback administration tubing set.

g. Verify the client's identity by checking his or her name tag and bed tag and by asking the client to state his or her name.
h. Uncap the spike of the piggyback administration set and insert it into the appropriate port of the piggyback bag. Use sterile technique.
i. Flush the tubing of the piggyback administration set with fluid from the piggyback bag.
j. Hang the secondary bag on an IV pole. If a hook is provided with the piggyback administration set, use the hook to lower the main IV bag below the level of the secondary bag and hang it on the same pole (Fig. 18–48).

k. Clean the injection port on the main IV tubing and insert the piggyback administration set needle into the port. Use sterile technique.
l. Tape the connection.

m. Regulate the flow of fluids using the roller clamp on the piggyback administration set tubing to administer the medication in the required amount of time (usually 30–60 min).

a. Fluid bags usually are sealed in a protective plastic covering.
b. Prevents microorganisms from entering the fluid.
c. The medicine is administered with the total volume of fluid.
d. Mixes the medication with the solution.
e. Communicates necessary information to others.

f. The secondary bag is piggybacked (connected) into the primary line of IV fluids.

g. Verification of the correct client is necessary to ensure that the right client is receiving the right drug.
h. The piggyback administration set is used to infuse the fluid in the secondary bag.

i. The line is flushed to remove air from the line.

j. Lowering the main IV bag prevents those fluids from entering the IV line and allows the secondary bag infusion to run. Also, by lowering the main bag when the secondary bag infusion is complete, the main infusion begins automatically if the clamp has been left open.
k. Prevents microorganisms from entering the client's bloodstream.

l. Prevents the tubing from becoming disconnected.
m. The client will not receive the needed effect from the medication if it is infused too slowly. An infusion that is too rapid could cause unwanted effects.

Administering Medication Through a Heparin or Saline Infusion Lock

a. Select an appropriate syringe and needle to prepare the medication.

b. Using sterile technique, reconstitute the medication if necessary, withdraw the medication into the syringe, and add medication to the secondary bag.
c. Recap the needle.

a. The needle gauge and length and the size of the syringe depend on the dosage and the medication to be administered.
b. Sterile technique is required. The medication is administered directly into the client's bloodstream.

c. Recapping prevents contamination of the needle with microorganisms.

▼ *A C T I O N*   ▼ *R A T I O N A L E*

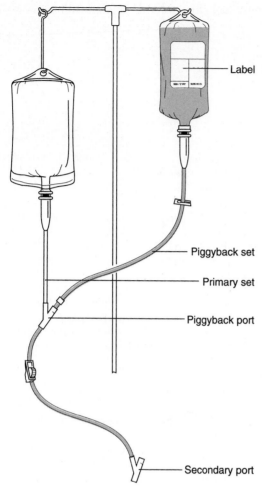

Label

Piggyback set

Primary set

Piggyback port

Secondary port

▼ **FIGURE 18–48.** Piggyback administration set.

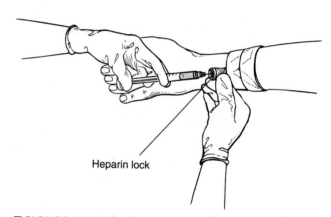

Heparin lock

▼ **FIGURE 18–49.** Blood return upon gentle aspiration verifies correct intravenous placement.

d. Read the label of the medication for the third time before returning it to storage or discarding it.

e. Draw up 2 ml of normal saline into two separate syringes.

f. Verify the client's identity by checking his or her name tag and bed tag and by asking the client to state his or her name.

g. Insert the needle of one of the saline-filled syringes into the port of the intermittent infusion lock and gently pull back on the plunger of the syringe (Fig. 18–49).

h. Slowly inject 2 ml of the saline into the lock (see Fig. 18–50A).

i. Withdraw the needle from the port, hang the bag of medication to be infused, and insert the needle attached to the medication to be infused (see Fig. 18–50B).

j. Release the clamp on the bag and regulate the fluid to infuse in the required length of time, which is usually within 30 to 60 minutes.

d. The label is read a third time for error prevention.

e. The saline is used to flush the intermittent lock before and after medication administration.

f. Verification of the correct client is necessary to ensure that the right client is receiving the right drug.

g. Blood should fill the chamber of the intermittent infusion lock; this verifies that the catheter is placed in the vein and is patent.

h. Clears the solution in the tubing.

i. The medication can be infused once the line has been flushed.

j. The client cannot get the needed effect of the medicine if it infuses too slowly. Infusion that is too rapid can cause unwanted side effects.

▼ *ACTION* ‾ ‾ ‾ ‾ ‾ ‾ ‾ ‾ ‾ ‾ ‾ ‾ ‾ ‾ ▼ *RATIONALE* ‾ ‾ ‾ ‾ ‾ ‾ ‾ ‾ ‾ ‾

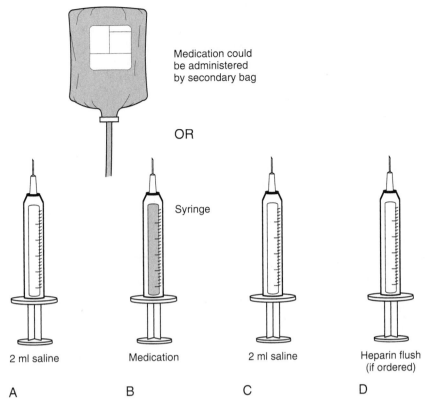

Medication could be administered by secondary bag

OR

Syringe

2 ml saline   Medication   2 ml saline   Heparin flush
                                                              (if ordered)

A   B   C   D

▼ **FIGURE 18–50.** *(A)* First clear blood and heparin solution by injecting 2 ml of saline. *(B)* Then administer the medication. *(C)* Then clear the medication from the lock by injecting 2 ml of saline. *(D)* Refill the lock with dilute heparin solution (if ordered).

k. After infusion is complete, again flush the tubing on the intermittent infusion lock with 2 ml of saline (see Fig. 18–50*C*) and then, if ordered, flush with heparin (see Fig. 18–50*D*).

9. Remain with the client for an appropriate amount of time after administering the medication to observe for effects, side effects, and allergic reactions.

10. Dispose of the used equipment according to your agency guidelines.

11. Wash your hands.

12. Return to the client's room at appropriate intervals to assess the effects of the medication and the accuracy of the flow rate.

13. Record the medication on the drug administration record and any side effects in the nurses' notes.

k. Flushing with saline maintains the patency of the infusion catheter.

9. Helps to provide for the client's safety and also provides data that will be needed for charting.

10. Decreases the transmission of microorganisms.

11. Decreases the transmission of microorganisms.

12. You should observe for both wanted and unwanted effects of the medication. The accuracy of the flow rate can be altered by client movement and other factors.

13. Communicates to the other members of the health care team and contributes to the legal record by documenting the care given to the client.

Example of Documentation

DATE	*TIME*	*NOTES*
9/1/93	0800	500 mg ampicillin IV infused over 30 minutes. IV patent and with no signs of infiltration or phlebitis.
		C. Lammon, RN

Teaching Tips

The purpose and side effects of the medication should be explained to the client. If the client's family will be administering the medicine in the home, the procedure should be explained and demonstrated to the family. Time should also be included for a return demonstration.

Home Care Variations

Medications may be given intravenously in the client's home. You should ensure that a sufficient supply of equipment and medicine is available in the home. You also should assess the means of disposal of the equipment. If the family is administering the medicine, assess their ability as well as their knowledge of the procedure and correct means of disposal.

References

Boortz, M. E. (1994). Administering medications. In V. Bolander (Ed.), *Basic nursing* (3rd ed.). Philadelphia: W. B. Saunders.

deSelva, M. I., et al. (1986). Multidosage medication vials: A study of sterility, use patterns, and cost-effectiveness. *American Journal of Infection Control*, 14 (3), 135–138.

Kasmer, R. J., et al. (1986). Sterility of preloaded insulin syringes. *American Journal of Infection Control*, 14 (4), 180–183.

CHAPTER 19

Administering Intravenous Therapy

Intravenous (IV) therapy involves the administration of fluids into a vein. IV fluids can be administered centrally (into a large vein in close proximity to the heart) or peripherally (into the veins of the extremities or scalp). Physicians typically insert central IV catheters and nurses insert peripheral IV catheters. You will administer IV fluids and care for the client with both types of IV catheters.

IV therapy involves the use of sterile or surgical asepsis since contamination could result in bacteremia and sepsis. Also you should be very careful to use universal blood and body fluid precautions (see front inner cover of this textbook) since you may be exposed to the client's blood as you work with IV devices. Blood spills should be cleaned up promptly and contaminated equipment should be disposed of properly according to your agency's policy.

OVERVIEW OF RELATED RESEARCH

HEPARIN OR SALINE LOCKS

Ashton, J., Gibson, V., and Summers, S. (1990). Effects of heparin versus saline solution on intermittent infusion device irrigation. *Critical Care Technology*, 19 (6), 608–612.

Saline or heparin is used as irrigants to maintain patency of intermittent intravenous devices (IIDs). The authors of this study compared the effectiveness of heparin to the effectiveness of sodium chloride in maintaining patency and reducing phlebitis in patients with IIDs. Thirty-two adult patients participated in the study. Sixteen were randomly assigned to Group A, in which 1 ml of 0.9% of sodium chloride with 1% benzyl alcohol was used as the irrigant. Sixteen patients were assigned to Group B, in which 10 units of heparin in 1 ml of sodium chloride solution with 1% benzyl alcohol was used. Patency was determined by aspirating fluid from the IID and expressing the aspirate onto filter paper for a visual count of clot formation. The findings indicated that there was no significant difference between the two groups. The authors concluded that 1 ml sodium chloride solution is as effective as 10 units of heparin in 1 ml of sodium chloride solution in maintaining the patency of IIDs. The development of phlebitis was not evident in either group.

Jordan, L. (1991). Should saline be used to maintain heparin locks? *Focus on Critical Care*, 18 (2), 144–151.

Many hospitals have changed from the use of heparin to the use of saline solution to maintain patency with intermittent intravenous devices (IIDs), or "heparin locks." Jordan reviewed 28 research studies that had different results about the effectiveness, safety, legality, and economy of saline solution rather than heparin flushes. Jordan concluded that as of 1991, published research studies were flawed and clinical practice should not be changed based on the available research. IV infusion devices should continue to be flushed using a dilute heparin solution and the SASH method (irrigate with saline solution first, administer medication, irrigate again with saline solution, and flush with a heparin solution).

Smith, I, et al. (1990). A randomized study to determine complications associated with duration of insertion of heparin locks. *Research in Nursing and Health*, 13, 367–373.

Hospital policies vary as to the recommended length of time to leave a venous cannula in place to facilitate the injection of intermittent IV medications when continuous infusion of fluids is not indicated. This study was conducted over a 20-month period with a randomized sample of 116 subjects in Group A and 140 subjects in Group B. Subjects in Group A had the venous cannula changed every 72 hours, whereas those in Group B had the cannula left in place up to 168 hours. Patency of the cannula was maintained through the instillation of 10 units of heparin after each instance of cannula use. The findings indicated no differences between the groups in minor complications or incidence of phlebitis. The authors concluded that consideration should be given to extending insertion time to 96 hours and possibly up to 118 hours.

SKILL 19–1 ADMINISTERING AN INTRAVENOUS INFUSION

Clinical Situations in Which You May Encounter This Skill

An over-the-needle intravenous (IV) infusion catheter, through-the-needle infusion catheter, or wing-tipped infusion needle (butterfly) (Fig. 19–1) may be inserted into a client's vein for administration of IV therapy. Figure 19–2 illustrates common peripheral venipuncture sites.

IV therapy may be administered for diagnostic or therapeutic purposes. For diagnostic purposes, an IV may be necessary to infuse dyes or contrast media for radiographic examinations. Therapeutic purposes include the infusion of parenteral medications, blood, or fluids for hydration.

Since the butterfly has a relatively short steel needle, it usually is used for short-term IV infusions. The over-the-needle and through-the-needle catheters are longer and are usually used when IV infusions are administered on a long-term basis.

If the IV infusion slows, quits running, or infiltrates, or the vein shows signs of phlebitis, the butterfly or IV catheter should be removed and restarted. Infiltration involves leaking of fluid into the tissue at the IV site, which causes the surrounding tissue to swell. The skin at the site of the infiltration feels cool to the touch. Phlebitis, an inflammation of the vein, is suspected if there is redness or tenderness above the insertion site, erythema, or warmth. A venous cord may be palpable.

Anticipated Responses

▼ The IV needle is inserted without difficulty into the client's vein.
▼ Fluids enter the vein with little or no discomfort to the client.

Adverse Responses

▼ The IV needle is not inserted into the vein and fluids infiltrate the surrounding tissue.
▼ Phlebitis results from the IV catheter or needle.

Materials List

Gather these materials before beginning the skill:

▼ IV catheter
▼ IV start kit, *or*
▼ Tourniquet
▼ Povidone-iodine pledgets
▼ Alcohol pledgets
▼ Transparent dressing
▼ Tape (1 inch and ¼ inch)

▼ Label
▼ 1% lidocaine (optional)
▼ 25-gauge 1-ml syringe (optional)
▼ Examination gloves
▼ Administration set tubing
▼ Extension tubing
▼ IV fluids
▼ Armboard (optional)
▼ IV pole

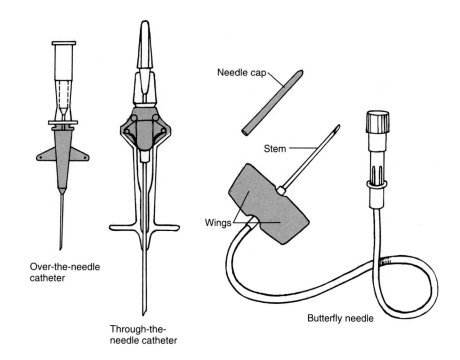

▼ **FIGURE 19–1.** Over-the-needle catheter, through-the-needle catheter, and butterfly needle for IV therapy.

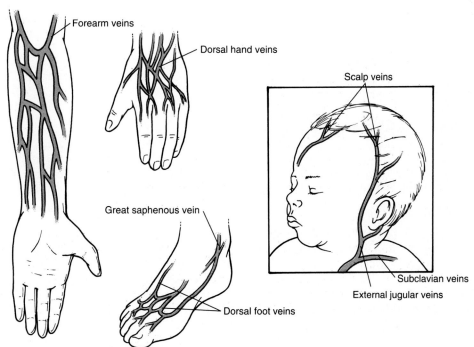

▼ **FIGURE 19–2.** Common peripheral venipuncture sites.

▼ *ACTION* ▼ *RATIONALE*

Preparing the Intravenous Solution

1. Check the physician's order for the type and rate of IV solution to be administered.	1. Types of solutions vary according to the diagnosis of the client's condition and the purpose of the IV. Knowing the required rate, type, and purpose of the infusion helps you to select the correct-sized administration set and needle gauge. For example, blood should be administered through an 18-gauge needle or larger.

2. Calculate the drip rate of IV fluids to be infused:

$$ml/hr = \frac{total\ amount\ of\ fluid\ to\ be\ given\ (in\ ml)}{total\ time\ for\ infusion\ (in\ hr)}$$

$$gtt/min = \frac{total\ volume\ (ml) \times drop\ factor\ (gtt/ml)}{total\ time\ of\ infusion\ (in\ min)}$$

$$gtt/min = \frac{ml/hr}{60\ min/hr} \times \frac{gtt}{ml}$$

2. Drip factors for calculating drip rates vary according to the manufacturer of the administration set for macrodrip sets.
Microdrip administration sets deliver 60 drops/min.

3. Select a catheter or butterfly needle that is large enough to deliver the volume of fluids needed. The usual size for an average-sized adult is 20 gauge. A larger 18-gauge catheter is often selected if it is anticipated that blood may need to be given at a later time. A smaller gauge 21-, 22-, or 23-gauge catheter may be used if the client has very small veins.	3. If a catheter is too large, the blood flow around the cannula will be occluded. The greater the blood flow around the cannula, the quicker the dilution of irritating drugs or solutions.
4. Wash your hands.	4. Decreases the transmission of microorganisms.
5. Visually inspect the IV solution for the expiration date and to ensure that contamination has not occurred. The solution should not be cloudy or contain any particles, the infusion bag should not have any leaks or tears, and the vacuum seal should be intact.	5. Expired IV solutions should not be used. If the solution is cloudy or contains particles or if the bottle does not have the vacuum seal intact, the solution may be contaminated.

> **NOTE:** If any of these problems are present the solution should be discarded and a new solution should be obtained.

6. Using sterile technique, prepare the administration set for insertion of the spiked end into the bag or bottle of IV solution by: a. Opening the IV administration set. b. Sliding the tubing clamp to the distal end of the tubing and closing the clamp.	6. Reduces the possibility of transmission of microorganisms. b. Prevents air from entering the tubing when the spiked end of the tubing is inserted into the solution container.

▼ _ _A C T I O N_ _ _ _ _ _ _ _ _ _ _ _ _ ▼ _ _R A T I O N A L E_ _ _ _ _ _ _ _

7. Insert the spiked end of the tubing into the bottle or bag of IV solution.
   a. For an IV bottle:
      i. Remove the metal disc, maintaining sterility of the rubber stopper on the bottle.

   i. Decreases the transmission of microorganisms.

NOTE: If you accidentally contaminate the rubber stopper, swab the stopper with an antiseptic solution and allow it to dry.

---

      ii. Remove the plastic cap from the IV tubing while maintaining sterility and firmly push the spike through the rubber port on the bottle while listening for a hissing sound.

   ii. Decreases the transmission of microorganisms.
   A hissing sound indicates that the bottle was sealed properly.

NOTE: If you do not hear the hissing of air when the rubber diaphragm is punctured, discard the bottle and get another one.

If no hissing sound is heard, the bottle was probably not sealed and the solution may be contaminated.

---

   b. For an IV bag:
      i. To insert the spike into a bag, invert the bag, insert the spike into the tubing portal, and squeeze the drip chamber.
      ii. Turn the IV bag upright and release the drip chamber.

   i. Prevents air bubbles from entering the IV tubing.

8. Prime the IV tubing by removing the protective cap from the distal end of the tubing, opening the tubing clamp, and allowing the fluid to fill the tubing until the air bubbles are removed from the tubing (Fig. 19–3).

8. Air should be removed from the tubing because the air may act as an embolus in the client's vascular system.

9. Close the clamp on the tubing.

9. Stops the movement of the solution.

10. Replace the protective cap over the end of the IV tubing to maintain the sterility of the tubing.

10. Prevents contamination of the tubing with microorganisms.

11. Place a tape label on the tubing with your initials and the time and date of the attachment of the tubing to the container of IV solution.

11. Tubing should be changed every 24 to 72 hours.

12. Place a label on the container of IV solution with the client's name, room number, any medication added, dosage, drip rate, and the name of the person who prepared the solution (Fig. 19–4).

12. The label provides for easy verification of the fluid when the IV is checked at a later time.

13. Place a time tape on the container of IV solution by:
   a. Hanging the solution upside down;
   b. Placing a strip of adhesive tape beside the milliliter calibration markings;
   c. Writing the time the solution is begun at the top of the container; and

13. The time tape helps you to assess if the correct amount of IV fluid is infusing each hour.

▼ *ACTION* _ _ _ _ _ _ _ _ _ _ _ _ _ _ _ _ ▼ *RATIONALE* _ _ _ _ _ _ _ _ _ _ _ _ _ _ _ _

d. Placing a mark by the milliliter mark where the fluid level should be after 1 hour, 2 hours, 3 hours, etc. until the entire amount infuses.

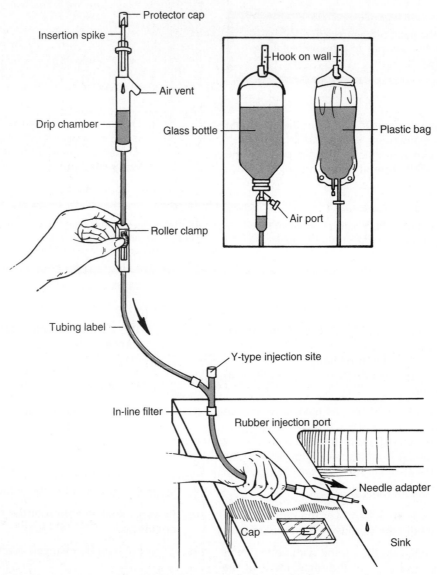

▼ **FIGURE 19–3.** Equipment for IV infusion.

Preparing to Insert an Intravenous Needle

14. a. Ask the client if he or she has ever had an IV before. If not, explain the procedure, including the purpose, what to expect during the insertion of the IV, and the expected duration of the IV.

b. Place a waterproof pad under the extremity in which the IV will be started.

14. a. Simple explanations help to reduce anxiety and apprehension.

b. The waterproof pad helps to protect the bed linen.

▼ *ACTION*   ▼ *RATIONALE*

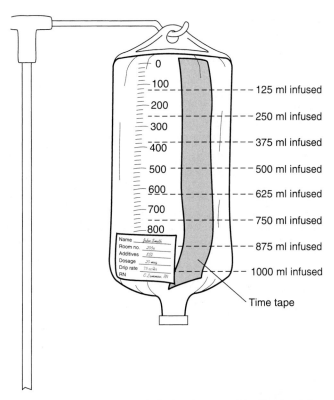

▼ **FIGURE 19–4.** IV bag labelled with patient identification information and time tape.

c. Assess the client's extremities for a site to place
the butterfly or IV catheter by applying a tourniquet or blood pressure cuff securely enough
to impede venous flow. To apply a tourniquet
(Fig. 19–5):

   i. Place the tourniquet approximately 6
inches above the site for IV insertion.

  ii. Secure the tourniquet by crossing the ends
and placing the loop of the tourniquet under the tie.

c. The tourniquet should be tight enough to
impede venous flow and distend veins, but not
so tight as to impede arterial flow.

   i. Promotes venous distention.

  ii. The tourniquet can be removed easily after
insertion of the IV.

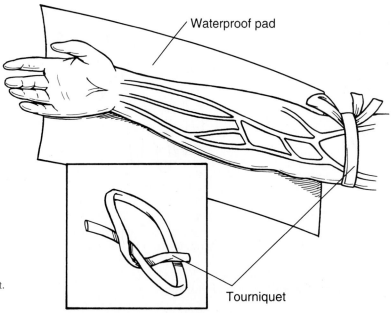

Waterproof pad

Tourniquet

▼ **FIGURE 19–5.** Applying a tourniquet.

▼ *A C T I O N* _____   ▼ *R A T I O N A L E* _____

Instead of a tourniquet, a blood pressure cuff can be placed around the client's arm and inflated enough to impede venous flow and distend the veins (approximately 100 mm mercury).

d. Lower the client's extremity to a dependent position.
e. Select a site at a distal point on a long vein. The client may open and close his or her hand a few times, lower the arm below the level of the heart, or apply warm compresses over the extremity to attain adequate vein distention.

f. Remove the tourniquet or deflate the blood pressure cuff.
g. Shave the IV site if the client has long or thick hair that will be pulled when the tape is removed.
h. Cleanse the IV site with an antiseptic solution. Use a circular motion from the innermost part of the site to the outermost part (Fig. 19–6). (The circle will be several inches in diameter.)

A blood pressure cuff is often more comfortable than a tourniquet because it is wider and the pressure can be adjusted easily.

d. Gravity slows the return of blood and helps to distend the veins for easier insertion of the IV.
e. Selection of an adequate vein is critical to the success of the IV insertion and subsequent maintenance of the IV. Distal points are selected first. If an IV must be replaced, it can be inserted proximal to the original site, unless phlebitis is apparent.
f. Prolonged use of the tourniquet can be uncomfortable to the client.
g. Decreases microorganisms and promotes comfort when the tape is removed.

h. Prevents recontamination of the IV insertion site.

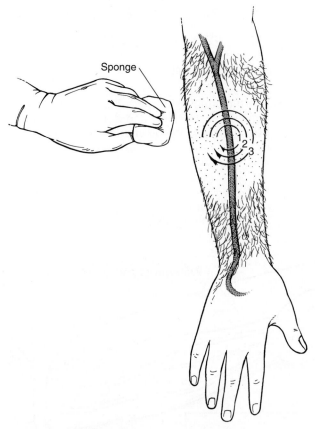

Sponge

▼ **FIGURE 19–6.** Cleansing the IV site.

i. Allow the solution to air-dry.

j. While the solution is drying, tear or cut the tape into the lengths needed.
k. Reapply the tourniquet.
l. Reassess for location of the vein.

i. The solution must be allowed to dry in order to have an antimicrobial effect.
j. The tape will stabilize the IV needle after insertion.

▼ *A C T I O N*   ▼ *R A T I O N A L E*

m. Don examination gloves.

n. Wipe the insertion site with the alcohol pledget to remove excess antiseptic solution.

o. Using sterile technique, remove the protective cover from the butterfly needle or the IV catheter without touching the needle or outside of the catheter.

p. Visually inspect the needle for burrs.

q. With one finger, hold the client's vein taut. If the IV is to be inserted into the hand, slightly bend the client's wrist so that the vein is slightly stretched.

15. Insert the IV needle.

a. To insert a butterfly needle:

   i. Squeeze the butterfly wings together and insert the needle, with bevel up, at a 15- to 45-degree angle, approximately 1 cm below the anticipated site for piercing the vein with the needle until a sudden lack of resistance is felt.

   ii. Decrease the degree of the angle and slowly thread the needle into the vein (Fig. 19–7).

m. Decreases the transmission of microorganisms.

n. Removing the excess antiseptic enables you to see the vein.

o. Decreases the transmission of microorganisms.

p. Occasionally a cannula is defective from the factory. Burrs on the needle cause great discomfort to the client and tear the skin and veins.

q. Securing the client's vein prevents the vein from "rolling."

   i. Resistance is felt as the needle pierces the vein.

   ii. Decreasing the angle helps you to thread the needle and lessens the chance of piercing the other side of the vein.

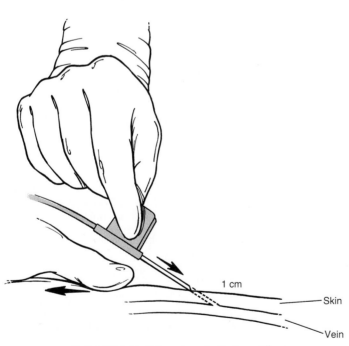

1 cm

Skin

Vein

▼ **FIGURE 19–7.** Inserting a butterfly needle.

b. To insert an over-the-needle catheter:

   i. With the bevel side up, insert the IV catheter directly over the vein and in the direction of the blood flow. Use a 15- to 45-degree angle until a sudden resistance is felt.

   i. Decreases trauma to the vein and allows for backflow of blood into the catheter. Insertion of the catheter at more than a 45-degree angle risks penetration of the vein's posterior wall.

▼ *ACTION* ────────────── ▼ *RATIONALE* ─────────────

   ii. With the needle still in the catheter, advance the catheter approximately halfway and observe for blood in the catheter.

   iii. In one motion, advance the catheter into the vein as you withdraw the needle (Fig. 19–8).

   ii. If the vein has been entered, you will see blood in the catheter.

   iii. There is greater risk of perforation of the posterior vein wall if the needle remains in the catheter as it is advanced.

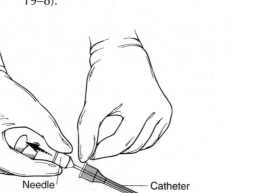

FIGURE 19–8. Inserting an over-the-needle catheter.

16. Remove the tourniquet.

16. If the tourniquet is not removed, it will obstruct the flow of blood.

Attaching the Intravenous Infusion

17. Remove the protective cap from the IV line and attach it to the end of the butterfly needle or catheter. Open the clamp to allow fluids to enter the client's vein.

17. Maintains patency of the butterfly or catheter by establishing a continuous flow of fluid. If the flow of fluid is delayed, the blood in the needle or catheter will clot.

18. Secure the catheter with tape and stabilize the site with an armboard if needed. Figure 19–9 illustrates various methods of securing the IV catheter and butterfly needle.

18. Helps to prevent the tubing from being disconnected.

19. Regulate the drip rate to the amount ordered.

19. Infusion that is too rapid can lead to fluid overload and infusion that is too slow does not allow a sufficient amount of fluid to be infused.

20. Label the site with the date and time of insertion and the type and size of needle or catheter used.

20. Necessary for planning the next dressing or needle change.

Final Activities

21. Dispose of contaminated supplies properly.

21. Prevents transmission of microorganisms and contact with blood-contaminated supplies.

22. Remove gloves and wash hands.

22. Decreases the transmission of microorganisms.

23. Record the procedure. Note the size and type of device inserted, the site, and the type and rate of solution infusing.

23. Communicates to the other members of the health care team and contributes to the legal record by documenting the care given to the client.

24. Observe the infusion frequently for signs of infiltration or phlebitis.

24. Prevents complications of IV therapy.

▼ *ACTION*   ▼ *RATIONALE*

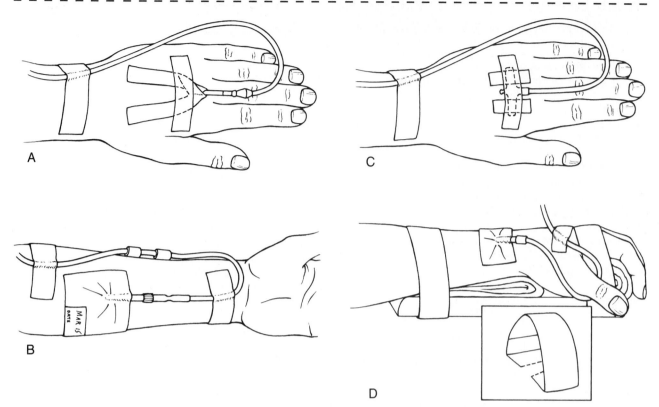

▼ **FIGURE 19–9.** Methods of securing IV catheters and a butterfly needle. Using tape to secure a catheter *(A)*. Using a transparent dressing to secure a catheter *(B)*. Using tape to secure a butterfly needle *(C)*. Using an armboard to secure the catheter near a joint *(D)*. In the inset, tape is placed so that it does not adhere to hair on the arm while the sticky ends of the tape remain free to adhere to the armboard.

Example of Documentation

DATE	*TIME*	*NOTES*
10/18/93	1000	20-gauge catheter inserted into left basilic vein. 1,000 ml D5W at 125 ml per hour.
		S. Williams, RN

Teaching Tips

Teach the client to keep the insertion site clean and dry. The extremity may be wrapped in a plastic bag during tub baths or showers, but the client should prevent water from running directly onto the site. Also, teach the client the signs and symptoms of infiltration or phlebitis and to report them immediately. Encourage the client or the client's family to notify you if the IV stops dripping or the bottle or bag is almost empty.

Home Care Variations

IV lines may be started in the client's home using the same procedure. Place used needles in a clearly marked container and remove it from the home as you leave. IV solutions may be hung on an IV pole if one is available or on a lamp shade, picture hook on the wall, or stepladder placed next to the client's bed or chair.

TROUBLESHOOTING AN INTRAVENOUS LINE

An IV line may slow or stop running completely. Before automatically restarting the IV, assess the complete apparatus.

1. Is the pump plugged in?
2. Is there fluid remaining in the bag or bottle?
3. Are there air bubbles in the IV line?
4. Is the clamp opened?
5. Are there any kinks in the IV line, or is the client lying on the line?
6. Is the IV site swollen, leaking, tender to the touch, or indicative of infiltration or phlebitis?
7. Should you irrigate the IV line? This is not recommended since the chance of a pulmonary embolus from a dislodged clot in the IV catheter is too great to risk. Instead, using aseptic technique, aspirate the clot by attaching a 3-ml (or larger) syringe to the hub of the butterfly needle or catheter. Gently pull back on the plunger. If blood is aspirated, discard about 0.5 to 1.0 ml, flush with 2 to 3 ml of normal saline, reattach the IV fluids, and resume the infusion. If no blood is aspirated, then *gently* flush the catheter with 2 to 3 ml of normal saline. If resistance is felt, *stop immediately and do not proceed with flushing.* The infusion should be restarted in another site. Another alternative is to attain a physician's order for urokinase. Urokinase is a thrombolytic drug that lyses clots that form in IV catheters in about 15 minutes.

SKILL 19–2   INSERTING A HEPARIN OR SALINE LOCK

Clinical Situations in Which You May Encounter This Skill

An intermittent infusion device (heparin or saline lock) may be inserted for therapeutic or diagnostic purposes (Fig. 19–10). For therapeutic purposes, the vein can be kept open for intermittent infusion of pharmacotherapeutic agents without a continuous infusion of IV fluids. A heparin lock may also be inserted for infusion of dyes for diagnostic tests.

An existing IV infusion line can be converted to a heparin or saline lock. However, if the IV site is leaking, the rate of flow has slowed or stopped, or signs of phlebitis are present, discontinue the infusion and insert a new lock.

Anticipated Responses

▼ The IV cannula is inserted into the client's vein without difficulty.
▼ The IV solution infuses without difficulty.

Adverse Responses

▼ The vein develops phlebitis.
▼ The heparin lock becomes occluded.

Materials List

Gather these materials before beginning the skill:

▼ Intermittent infusion adapter (for conversion of an existing IV infusion line to a heparin lock), or a Heparin or saline lock
▼ Tourniquet
▼ Povidone-iodine pledgets
▼ Alcohol pledgets
▼ Transparent dressing
▼ Tape (1 inch and ¼ inch)
▼ Label
▼ Examination gloves
▼ Saline flush (syringe with 2 to 3 cc of normal saline)
▼ 3-ml syringe and 25-gauge needle (1 cc of 1:1,000 heparin flush solution in syringe if heparin is to be used)

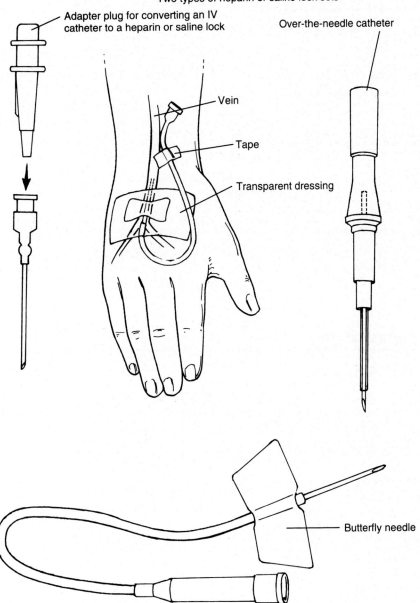

Two types of heparin or saline lock sets

Adapter plug for converting an IV catheter to a heparin or saline lock

Over-the-needle catheter

Vein

Tape

Transparent dressing

Butterfly needle

▼ **FIGURE 19–10.** Heparin or saline lock sets for intermittent infusion.

▼ *A C T I O N*

▼ *R A T I O N A L E*

1. Ascertain if the client has an IV line that can be converted. If not, you should insert an IV catheter (see Skill 19–1).

1. Converting the IV line to a heparin lock is less traumatic to the client than inserting an IV catheter.

2. Wash your hands and put on gloves.

2. Decreases the transmission of microorganisms.

3. To convert an existing IV line:
   a. Stop the IV infusion and disconnect the IV tubing from the catheter or butterfly needle.
   b. Immediately insert the intermittent adapter into the hub of the IV line.

   a. Prevents spillage of the solution. Reduces the leakage of blood from the open hub.

4. To start a new heparin or saline lock, insert a catheter into the client's vein and immediately insert the intermittent adapter plug into the hub of the IV line.

4. Reduces leakage of blood from the open hub.

▼ *ACTION*　　　　　　　　　　　▼ *RATIONALE*

5. Secure the catheter with tape to the client's arm.

6. Cleanse the injection port with an alcohol pledget.

7. Slowly inject the saline flush into the catheter.

8. Slowly inject the heparin flush if heparin is to be used.

9. Label the dressing with your name, the date and time of insertion, and the type of catheter converted.

10. Remove gloves and wash hands.

11. Record the procedure. Note the type and size of the insertion device and the date and time of insertion.

6. Decreases the transmission of microorganisms.

7. Rapid or forceful injection of fluid into the cannula can be uncomfortable to the client. Saline clears the line of accumulated blood and is as effective as heparin in preventing clotting.

8. The heparin flush prevents clotting of the catheter.

9. Provides necessary data for planning the next dressing change.

10. Decreases the transmission of microorganisms.

11. Communicates to the other members of the health care team and contributes to the legal record by documenting the care given to the client.

Example of Documentation

DATE	TIME	NOTES
10/19/93	1300	20-gauge heparin lock inserted into left basilic vein. Flushed with saline and 1 ml of 1:1,000 heparin flush solution.
		S. Williams, RN

Home Care Variations

Teach the client the signs and symptoms of infiltration and phlebitis. Have the client assess the IV site four times per day and report adverse findings immediately. Dispose of the IV needle in a clearly marked container and remove it from the client's home when you leave.

SKILL 19–3　CHANGING INTRAVENOUS TUBING AND AN IN-LINE FILTER

Clinical Situations in Which You May Encounter This Skill

When a client receives continuous IV therapy, the IV tubing and filter should be changed every 24 to 72 hours depending on agency policy. Change the tubing and filter when a new bag or bottle of fluid is hung.

Anticipated Responses

▼ The IV tubing and filter are changed using aseptic technique.

Adverse Responses

▼ Excessive air enters the tubing and the client has an air embolus.
▼ Sepsis occurs from microorganisms entering the bloodstream.

Materials List

Gather these materials before beginning the skill:

▼ IV tubing
▼ IV filter
▼ Examination gloves

▼ *ACTION*

▼ *RATIONALE*

1. Check the date of the last IV tubing change.

1. The tubing should be changed every 24 to 72 hours, depending on agency policy.

2. Explain to the client what you are going to do.

2. Helps to reduce apprehension and anxiety.

3. Wash your hands.

3. Decreases the transmission of microorganisms.

4. Remove the new tubing and filter from their packages without contaminating them.

4. Decreases the transmission of microorganisms.

5. Remove the protective cap from the male end of the IV tubing and the protective cap from the female connector of the IV filter.

5. The male end of the IV tubing is connected to the female end of the filter.

6. Connect the IV tubing to the filter.

7. Close the clamp on the IV tubing of the bottle or bag of fluids.

7. Prevents fluid in the tubing from flowing freely when the tubing is removed from the bag or bottle.

8. Insert the IV tubing into the new bag or bottle of IV fluids. Use sterile technique.

8. Decreases the transmission of microorganisms.

9. Don examination gloves.

9. Decreases the transmission of microorganisms.

10. Remove the transparent covering and tape from the IV site.

10. Facilitates the tubing change.

11. While holding the hub of the catheter securely, gently disconnect the old tubing from the hub.

11. Prevents the catheter from becoming dislodged from the vein.

12. Quickly insert the new IV tubing into the hub.

12. Quickly reestablishing the IV line prevents blood clots from forming in the cannula.

13. Assess the IV site for swelling, erythema, tenderness, leakage of fluid, or warmth.

13. Removal of the tape and protective covering from the IV site provides an excellent opportunity to inspect and palpate the site for adverse responses.

14. Regulate the flow rate as prescribed by the physician's order.

14. Helps to ensure that the client receives the correct amount of fluid.

15. Retape the IV line.

15. Prevents the tubing from becoming disconnected and the catheter from becoming dislodged.

16. Label the new tubing and filter with the date and time.

16. Provides necessary data for planning the next tubing and filter change.

17. Dispose of the old IV tubing according to the agency policy.

17. Decreases the transmission of microorganisms.

18. Assess the IV line for patency and the correct drip rate.

18. Provides for the safety of the client and data necessary for charting.

19. Remove gloves and wash hands.

19. Decreases the transmission of microorganisms.

20. Record the procedure.

20. Communicates to the other members of the health care team and contributes to the legal record by documenting the care given to the client.

Example of Documentation

DATE	TIME	NOTES
10/18/93	1000	IV tubing and filter changed. No swelling, tenderness, or leakage noted at site. 1,000 ml D5W infusing at 125 ml per hour.

S. Williams, RN

Home Care Variations

The duration of time between IV tubing changes varies according to agency policy. Place the old tubing in a disposable container and remove it from the client's home as you leave.

SKILL 19–4 DISCONTINUING AN INTRAVENOUS INFUSION

Clinical Situations in Which You May Encounter This Skill

An IV catheter or needle should be removed using aseptic technique when the IV infiltrates, phlebitis develops, or the IV fluids are no longer necessary.

Anticipated Responses

▾ The IV catheter or needle is removed with no discomfort to the client.
▾ There is little or no bleeding from the IV site.

Adverse Responses

▾ The IV catheter or needle is removed and bleeding from the site continues.

Materials List

Gather these materials before beginning the skill:

▾ Several 4- × 4-inch gauze pads or 2- × 2-inch gauze pads
▾ Small adhesive bandages
▾ Tape
▾ Examination gloves

▾ *A C T I O N*

1. Determine if the IV infusion should be discontinued by:
   a. Checking the physician's order, or

   b. Assessing the IV site for swelling, tenderness, redness, warmth, or excessive coolness.

2. Explain to the client what you are going to do.

3. Wash your hands.

4. Close the clamp.

5. Remove the tape that is securing the IV needle or catheter in place.

6. Don examination gloves.

7. Place a dry 2- × 2-inch piece of gauze on the client's skin over the IV insertion site with your nondominant hand.

▾ *R A T I O N A L E*

a. A physician's order is required to discontinue an IV infusion permanently.
b. If the site is swollen, tender, red, or warm or cool to the touch in comparison to the other extremity, the IV may be infiltrated or the client may have localized phlebitis.

2. Reduces apprehension and anxiety.

3. Decreases the transmission of microorganisms.

4. Prevents the IV fluid from flowing freely when the needle or catheter is removed from the client.

5. Facilitates removal of the IV.

6. Prevents the transmission of microorganisms.

7. Alcohol wipes cause stinging at the site.

▼ *ACTION*   ▼ *RATIONALE*

8. Remove the catheter or needle and immediately apply pressure to the IV site for a minimum of 2 minutes (Fig. 19–11).

8. Applying pressure stops the bleeding.

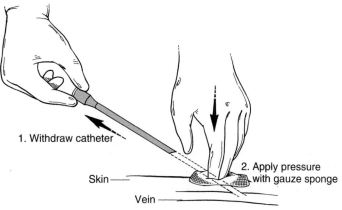

1. Withdraw catheter

Skin

Vein

2. Apply pressure with gauze sponge

▼ **FIGURE 19–11.** Removing the catheter and applying pressure to the IV site with a 4- × 4-inch gauze sponge.

9. Apply a small adhesive bandage to the IV site.

9. The dressing protects the site from the entry of microorganisms.

NOTE: If there is any evidence of bleeding from the site, apply a pressure dressing by folding a clean 4- × 4-inch gauze pad into fourths and taping it securely in place.

---

10. Assess the site for any continued bleeding.

10. If the patient's clotting time is prolonged, pressure may be applied for 5 to 10 more minutes.

11. Dispose of contaminated equipment properly.

11. Reduces the transmission of microorganisms.

12. Remove gloves and wash your hands.

12. Decreases the transmission of microorganisms.

13. Record the procedure. Note that aseptic technique was used.

13. Communicates to the other members of the health care team and contributes to the legal record by documenting the care given to the client.

Example of Documentation

DATE	*TIME*	*NOTES*
12/1/93	0900	IV discontinued. No bleeding, redness, tenderness, or swelling noted at site. Small adhesive bandage applied.
		S. Williams, RN

Teaching Tips

When you remove the IV needle or catheter, teach the client the signs and symptoms of infection that should be reported. Also, follow-up care should be addressed. For example, if the client was taking IV antibiotics and will be taking oral antibiotics, explain the importance of continuing the treatment regimen as prescribed by the physician. If the client was taking IV fluids for rehydration, explain the importance of drinking adequate amounts of fluids.

Home Care Variations

After the IV catheter is removed, place the catheter in a disposable container and remove it from the client's home.

SKILL 19–5   CHANGING THE GOWN OF A CLIENT WITH AN INTRAVENOUS LINE

Clinical Situations in Which You May Encounter This Skill

A client who is receiving IV therapy and has a soiled gown or is being bathed should have the gown changed at least on a daily basis.

Anticipated Responses

▼ The client's gown is changed with no interruption in the flow or integrity of the IV tubing.

Adverse Responses

▼ The client's IV line becomes dislodged.

Materials List

Gather these materials before beginning the skill:

▼ Clean gown
▼ Examination gloves

▼ ACTION	▼ RATIONALE
1. Determine why the client's gown is to be changed.	1. If the client's gown is soiled, you also may need to bathe the client.
2. Wash your hands and put on gloves if the gown is soiled with body secretions.	2. Decreases the transmission of microorganisms.
3. Remove the client's arms from the sleeves of the gown.	3. Facilitates removal of the gown.
4. Place the new gown over the client and put the arm without the IV line into one sleeve.	4. Provides for the client's privacy and comfort.
5. Remove the IV bag or bottle from the IV pole and slip the IV tubing and bag from front to back through the armhole of the soiled gown without dislodging the IV line or disconnecting the tubing (Fig. 19–12A). Discard the soiled gown. If the tubing is connected to a pump, stop the pump and remove the tubing from the pump without disconnecting the tubing and thread the IV bag and tubing through the armhole of the soiled gown.	5. Prevents the gown from becoming tangled in the IV tubing. It is important to maintain the integrity of the IV line and do not disconnect the IV lines while changing the client's gown. If the IV tubing is disconnected, microorganisms can enter the IV tubing. Facilitates changing of the gown. If the tubing is disconnected, microorganisms may enter the tubing.

▼ *ACTION*   ▼ *RATIONALE*

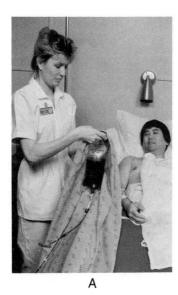
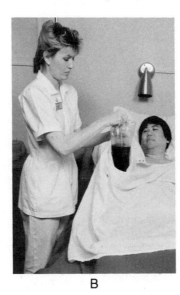
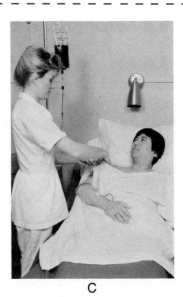

A   B   C

▼ **FIGURE 19–12.** Removing the client's arms from the sleeves of a gown.

6. Thread the IV bag and tubing through the armhole of the new gown from back to front (Fig. 19–12*B*).

6. Threading the tubing through the sleeve in the opposite direction causes it to become tangled in the sleeve. The tubing must be threaded through the sleeve in the same direction in which the client's arm will be placed through it.

7. Hang the IV bag on the IV pole or return the IV to the pump.

7. Reestablishes the flow of IV fluid.

8. Place the client's arm with the IV line through the sleeve of the clean gown (Fig. 19–12*C*).

9. Tie the gown in the back for the client.

9. Prevents the gown from slipping down.

10. Regulate the flow rate of the IV fluid.

10. The flow rate may have slowed or increased during the tubing change.

11. Ensures the patency of the IV tubing and the comfort of the client.

11. Ensures IV is running correctly and client's needs are met.

12. If worn, remove gloves and wash your hands.

12. Decreases the transmission of microorganisms.

Example of Documentation

DATE	TIME	NOTES
12/1/93	0930	A.M. care. IV of D$_5$NS infusing at 75 ml/hour in right forearm.
		S. Williams, RN

SKILL 19–6   USING INFUSION DEVICES

Clinical Situations in Which You May Encounter This Skill

Infusion devices may be used to regulate the flow of IV fluids. There are two types of infusion devices: pumps and controllers.

Pumps (Fig. 19–13A and B) are used to regulate the flow rate of IV fluids and deliver fluids by exerting positive pressure, measured in pounds per square inch (PSI), to force solutions through the IV tubing into the vein. Because pumps do not function by the force of gravity, the pump can be at any height. Infusion pumps maintain an open vein by ensuring a continuous flow rate and overcoming flow resistance. Most infusion pumps are accurate within 2% of the set rate.

Controllers depend on gravity to maintain the flow rate and do not add pressure to the system. The delivery force depends on the height of the container in relation to the IV site. The container must be at least 30 inches above the IV site to deliver IV fluids accurately.

Infusion devices use two types of delivery systems: drop-rate calibration and volume control. The volume control device delivers fluids in milliliters per hour. The drop-rate calibration device controls the rate of the infusion by counting or measuring drops (Fig. 19–13C).

Anticipated Responses

▼ The fluids are delivered at the rate or volume specified in the physician's order.

Adverse Responses

▼ The IV pump malfunctions and the specified rate or volume of fluids is not delivered.

Materials List

Gather these materials before beginning the skill:

▼ IV pump
▼ IV fluids
▼ IV pump tubing for the equipment to be used
▼ IV administration set
▼ Extension tubing
▼ IV pole (if the pump does not have one attached)
▼ Alcohol swabs
▼ Tape
▼ Examination gloves

▼ ACTION

1. Check the physician's order for the type and rate of IV solution to be administered.

2. Wash your hands.

3. Place a time line on the bottle or bag of IV fluids.

   a. Calculate the milliliters per hour of fluid that should infuse.
   b. With the bottle or bag in a hanging position, place a strip of tape next to the numbers on the bottle or bag.
   c. Note the fluid level in the bottle, make a mark on the tape, and write the date and time next to the mark.
   d. Count down the number of milliliters per hour to be infused, mark the tape, and put a time one hour later than the present time.
   e. Continue marking to the bottom of the bottle or bag.

4. Insert the tubing spike into the bag or bottle of IV fluid. Use sterile technique.

5. Fill the drip chamber only one-half to two-thirds full if a drop-rate calibrated infusion device is used, or completely fill the drip chamber if a volume control device is used.

▼ RATIONALE

1. The infusion rate and type of solution vary according to the purpose of the IV line.

2. Reduces the transmission of microorganisms.

3. The time line helps you to estimate whether the IV is infusing at the correct rate.
   a. The bottle or bag are marked according to the milliliters per hour to be infused.
   b. You will need to read the time line when the fluid is hanging.

   c. Provides a starting point.

   d. Provides an estimate of the amount that should infuse by the next hour.

4. Decreases the transmission of microorganisms.

5. If the drip chamber is completely filled on a drop-rate calibrated pump, the drops cannot be accurately counted. Since the volume control device delivers fluids according to milliliters per hour, it is not necessary to count drops.

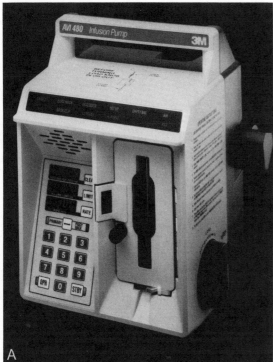

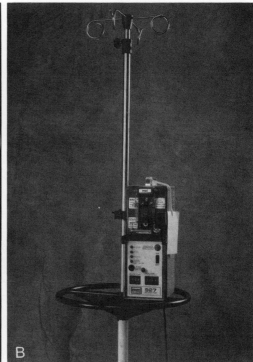

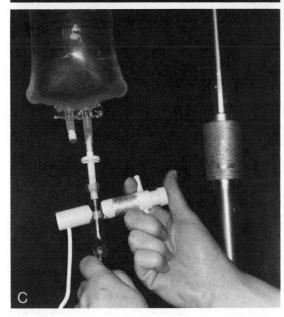

▼ **FIGURE 19–13.** Infusion pumps and sensor. The AVI 480 infusion pump *(A)*. The IMED 927 infusion pump, attached to an IV pole *(B)*. A drop-rate calibration device *(C)*. (Figure 19–14*A* is courtesy of 3M Company, St. Paul, MN).

▼ *ACTION*

6. Close the clamp on the IV tubing.

7. Hang the bag or bottle of IV fluids on the IV pole attached to the machine.

8. Attach and thread the tubing through the machine according to the manufacturer's directions.

9. Insert the plug of the machine into the electrical outlet.

▼ *RATIONALE*

6. Prevents the fluid from being spilled.

7. Facilitates the connection of the IV tubing to the pump.

8. Manufacturers have different instructions for threading the tubing. Read the directions for specific instructions for the model you are using.

9. Although most machines have battery packs, the batteries do not have a long duration. They should be used to allow the client mobility or when the client is being transported to another location. Otherwise, the machine should be plugged into the electrical outlet.

▼ *ACTION*	▼ *RATIONALE*
10. Set the infusion rate or volume on the pump.	**10.** The pump delivers the fluid at that rate or volume.
11. Put on gloves.	**11.** Decreases the transmission of microorganisms.
12. After inserting the IV needle or catheter (see Skill 19–1), attach the IV tubing leading from the machine to the IV catheter.	**12.** Fluid flows from the bottle into the pump and then into the catheter.
13. Open the tubing clamp completely.	**13.** Fluid must flow freely from the bottle into the pump.
14. Turn the machine on by pressing the power button.	**14.** The machine will not operate until the power is on.
15. Count the drops for 1 full minute if a drop-rate pump is used. Observe the pump chamber to see that it is filling and delivering the fluid according to the time line on the bottle of fluid.	**15.** Ensures that the machine is accurately delivering fluids as ordered.
16. Observe the IV site for any early signs of infiltration such as pain, leaking fluid around the insertion site, or swelling.	**16.** If a pressure infusion machine is used, the IV fluid is infused into the tissue even though resistance is encountered.
17. Remove gloves and wash your hands.	**17.** Decreases the transmission of microorganisms.
18. Record the procedure. Note the type of IV pump used.	**18.** Communicates to the other members of the health care team and contributes to the legal record by documenting the care given to the client.

Example of Documentation

DATE	*TIME*	*NOTES*
10/18/93	1200	IV infusion started with 20-gauge catheter in left basilic vein. 1,000 cc D5W at 20 ml per hour per infusion pump.
		S. Williams, RN

SKILL 19–7 PROVIDING SITE CARE FOR A VASCULAR ACCESS DEVICE

Clinical Situations in Which You MAY Encounter This Skill

Vascular access devices (VADs) are inserted into clients for long-term access to a central vein for administering total parenteral nutrition (TPN), drawing or administering blood, or administering drugs such as chemotherapeutic agents or long-term antibiotics. VAD catheters are usually inserted into the subclavian or external jugular vein.

The VAD may be external or internal. The Hickman and Broviac catheters (Fig. 19–14) are external devices. An internal or implantable VAD (Fig. 19–15) consists of an injection port that is surgically implanted under the skin. The port is accessed with a noncoring needle with a Huber bevel.

Site care should be provided every 24 hours for the first week for clients who have a VAD. After this initial period, site care should be done every 3 days or whenever the site becomes soiled or the dressing becomes loose. For the first week a VAD is in place, site care is performed at the insertion site and the exit site using sterile technique as described in the care of a central venous line (see Skill 14–11). After the first week clean technique is used to give site care.

If the client develops fever, hypotension, lethargy, confusion, or other symptoms of sepsis, notify the physician immediately.

Anticipated Responses

▼ The catheter remains patent and the client is free of infection.

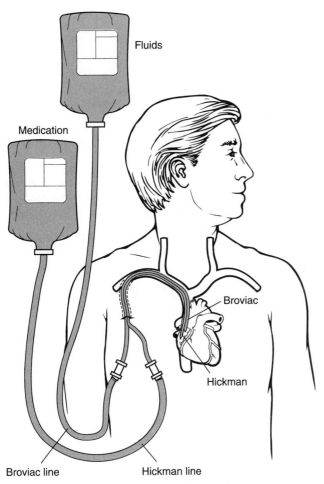

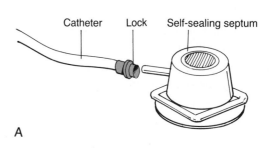

A

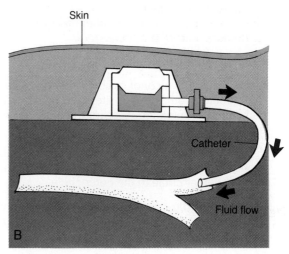

B

▼ **FIGURE 19–14.** Double-lumen Hickman and Broviac catheters.

▼ **FIGURE 19–15.** Implantable vascular access device.

Adverse Responses

▼ The catheter becomes occluded.
▼ The client develops an infection or sepsis.

Materials List

Gather these materials before beginning the skill:

▼ Hydrogen peroxide
▼ Povidone-iodine
▼ Povidone-iodine ointment (optional)
▼ Alcohol swabs
▼ Sterile cotton swabs
▼ Sterile occlusive dressing
▼ Examination gloves
▼ Paper bag

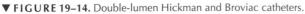

▼ *ACTION*	▼ *RATIONALE*
1. Determine if the site care is to be performed using sterile or clean technique.	1. After 1 week, site care can be performed using clean technique. Check your agency's policy.
2. Open the sterile supplies and place them on the clean overbed table.	2. The equipment should be within easy reach.
3. Help the client to assume a supine or semi-Fowler's position.	3. These positions facilitate site care.
4. Remove the client's gown or lower the client's gown to expose the catheter site.	4. Exposure of the site is necessary for site care.
5. Wash your hands.	5. Decreases the transmission of microorganisms.
6. Don examination gloves.	6. When there is a chance of coming into contact with blood, gloves should be worn to prevent the possible transmission of microorganisms.

▼ *A C T I O N*	▼ *R A T I O N A L E*
7. Remove the dressing on the exit site of the catheter and place it in a paper bag.	7. Decreases the transmission of microorganisms.
8. Observe the exit site for any signs of infection such as redness, swelling, or drainage.	8. Localized infections can be detected early by looking at the site.
9. Remove the gloves and wash your hands.	9. Decreases the transmission of microorganisms and prevents the transmission of microorganisms to and from the client.
10. Moisten sterile swabs with hydrogen peroxide.	10. Hydrogen peroxide is an aerobic cleanser that uses oxygen to inhibit anaerobic microorganism growth and to loosen debris.
11. Cleanse the skin around the exit site. Use a circular motion to move from the inner part of the circle to the outer part of the circle.	11. Moving from the inner circle to the outer circle prevents recontamination of the insertion site with bacteria.
12. Hold the port of the catheter in one hand.	12. Facilitates cleaning of the catheter.
13. Using the sterile alcohol swabs, clean one side of the catheter from the exit site to the port of the catheter in one motion. Discard the alcohol swab after each cleansing action.	13. Alcohol provides bacteriostatic action that inhibits the growth of microorganisms.
14. Cleanse the skin around the exit site in a circular motion with the povidone-iodine swabs. Cleanse from the inner circle to the outer circle.	14. Povidone-iodine is an antiseptic agent that inhibits bacteria and reduces skin infections.
15. Using the sterile cotton swabs, you may apply a small amount of povidone-iodine ointment to the catheter exit site.	15. Povidone-iodine ointment may decrease the chance of infection at the site.
16. Apply a sterile occlusive dressing (see Skill 20–3).	16. Prevents contamination of the exit site with water and bacteria.
17. Place your initials and the date and time of the catheter care on the dressing.	17. Provides an easy means of establishing future dressing changes.
18. Loop the catheter loosely over the dressing and secure it with tape.	18. Prevents accidental pulling on the wound site.
19. Wash your hands.	19. Decreases the transmission of microorganisms.
20. Chart the procedure. Note your observations of the exit site and catheter.	20. Communicates to the other members of the health care team and contributes to the legal record by documenting the care given to the client.

Example of Documentation

DATE	*TIME*	*NOTES*
10/9/93	1300	Catheter site care for VAD using clean technique. Slight redness at exit point. No swelling, drainage, or tenderness noted. Sterile occlusive dressing applied.
		S. Williams, RN

Teaching Tips

Dressing changes provide an opportune time to teach the client how to change dressings using clean technique. Ready-to-use kits are available for the client's use at home. Teach the client the signs and symptoms of infection (redness, swelling, drainage, and tenderness) and to report them. The client's family members should be included in the teaching. The client or family members, or both, should do a return demonstration.

Home Care Variations

The same procedure is used in the client's home. Teach the client to dispose of used supplies in a plastic bag and to remove it from the home.

References

Ashton, J., Gibson, V., and Summers, S. (1990). Effects of heparin versus saline solution on intermittent infusion device irrigation. *Critical Care Technology*, 19 (6), 608–612.

Boortz, M. E. (1994). Administering intravenous therapy. In V. Bolander (Ed.), *Basic nursing* (3rd ed.). Philadelphia: W. B. Saunders.

Jordan, L. (1991). Should saline be used to maintain heparin locks? *Focus on Critical Care*, 18 (2), 144–151.

Smith, I., et al. (1990). A randomized study to determine complications associated with duration of insertion of heparin locks. *Research in Nursing and Health*, 13, 367–373.

CHAPTER 20

Caring for Persons with Wounds

A wound is a disruption in the integrity of the internal or external surfaces of the body. Wounds involving the internal structures of the body are called closed wounds. Wounds involving breaks in the skin are called open wounds. Open wounds are more susceptible to infection than are closed wounds since there is an entry point for microorganisms to invade the body.

When the body is injured, the inflammatory process and the immune system initiate the process of healing. Healing occurs by primary intention or secondary intention. Primary intention wound healing occurs when the edges of the wound are approximated or close together and there is minimal tissue loss. Primary intention healing requires minimal growth of granulation tissue and usually results in a small fine scar. A surgical incision is a wound that usually heals by primary intention.

Wound healing by secondary intention occurs when the wound edges do not approximate and there is tissue loss. Granulation tissue must form to fill in the wound and usually scarring is more extensive than with primary intention healing. Wounds that heal by secondary intention heal from the inside to the outside. The healing time may be prolonged if the size of the wound is extensive and there is risk of infection. A decubitus ulcer is a wound that must heal by secondary intention.

You are responsible for preventing wound infections, managing wound care, and promoting wound healing. This chapter will guide you in many of the skills that accomplish these goals.

OVERVIEW OF RELATED RESEARCH

CARING FOR WOUNDS

Conly, J. M., Grieves, K., and Peters, B. (1989). **A prospective, randomized study comparing transparent and dry gauze dressings for central venous catheters.** *The Journal of Infectious Diseases*, 159 (2), 310–319.

Clients with central venous catheters in place were randomly assigned to receive either a transparent (n = 58) or gauze (n = 57) dressing. The group with transparent dressings had a significantly greater colonization rate than the group with gauze dressings. Furthermore, there were significantly more local catheter-related infections in the clients with transparent dressings. Catheter-related bacteremia occurred in 7 of the patients with transparent dressings. The findings suggest a greater incidence of colonization at the insertion site, local infection, and bacteremia in patients with transparent dressings.

Shivnan, J. C., et al. (1991). **A comparison of transparent adherent and dry sterile gauze dressings for long-term central catheters in patients undergoing bone marrow transplant.** *Oncology Nursing Forum*, 18 (8), 1349–1356.

Clients with long-term central venous catheters were randomly assigned to receive either a transparent adherent (n = 51) or a dry sterile gauze dressing (n = 47). The clients ages ranged from 5 years to 56 years. One client with a transparent adherent dressing developed catheter-related sepsis. No significant differences were found between the transparent adherent and dry sterile gauze dressings in relation to positive skin cultures. The group with dry sterile gauze dressings had significantly more days of skin irritation. These findings indicate that the transparent adherent dressings caused less skin irritation.

Branemark, P. I., and Ekholm, R. (1967). **Tissue injury caused by wound disinfectants.** *The Journal of Bone and Joint Surgery*, 49–A, 48–62.

The findings of a classic study by Branemark and Ekholm suggest that alcohol-containing disinfectants kill tissue. Furthermore, application of hydrogen peroxide interferes with the microvascular system by causing an almost complete blockage. Thus, these solutions impair the ability of tissue to heal. ⬚

PROVIDING CIRCUMCISION CARE

Marchett, L., Main, R., and Redick, E. (1989). **Pain reduction during neonatal circumcision.** *Pediatric Nursing*, 15 (2), 207–210.

Nurses are concerned about the pain suffered by newborn boys during routine unanesthetized circumcision. Forty-eight neonates were randomly assigned to one of three intervention groups: 18 control infants received routine care; music was played for 15 infants; and a tape of intrauterine sounds was played for 15 infants. During circumcision, monitors measured the children's cardiac rate and rhythm, blood pressure, and transcutaneous oxygen. Pain was measured by analysis of videotaped facial expressions with Izard's Maximally Discriminative Facial Movement Coding System. Data indicated that the mean heart rate was above normal limits during all steps of the circumcision for the control group and during some of the steps for the other two groups. The analyzed facial expressions showed that all three groups had pain during the procedure. The authors concluded that the two interventions did not offset the effects of circumcision pain. ⬚

SKILL 20–1 CLEANSING A WOUND

Clinical Situations in Which You May Encounter This Skill

A wound should be cleansed if it is draining, infected, or in the postoperative period until the edges are approximated. Proper cleansing reduces the chance of infection and promotes and enhances the healing of an infected wound. Signs of wound infection may include one or more of the following: an increased body temperature, increased skin temperature at the site of the wound, a bright red appearance, the presence of pus or drainage, and a foul odor.

Anticipated Responses

▼ There are no signs of infection.

▼ The tissue around the client's wound is not inflamed and there are no signs of infection.
▼ There is no wound drainage.

Adverse Responses

▼ The tissue around the client's wound excoriates because of sensitivity of the tissue to the cleansing agent.
▼ The client experiences discomfort as the wound is cleansed.
▼ There are signs of wound infection.

Materials List

Gather these materials before beginning the skill:

▼ Disposable sterile field
▼ Examination gloves
▼ Sterile gloves
▼ Mask (optional)
▼ Cleansing solution (povidone-iodine, sterile saline, or a commercial cleanser as ordered)
▼ Sterile basin (two may be needed if the cleansing solution is to be rinsed off the skin with sterile normal saline)

▼ Sterile 4- × 4-inch gauze pads (1 box)
▼ Sterile pick-up forceps
▼ Tape and dressing materials if the wound is to be redressed after cleansing
▼ Towel or water-resistant pad
▼ Small waterproof disposable bag
▼ Sheet

▼ ACTION	▼ RATIONALE
1. Assess the size and location of the wound to determine if additional supplies will be needed.	1. If the wound is draining excessively, additional supplies may be needed.
2. Tell the client what to expect.	2. Simple explanations help to reduce anxiety and apprehension.
3. Help the client to assume a comfortable position so that the wound is easily accessible.	3. Facilitates cleansing of the wound.
4. Expose the wound area and drape the client with a sheet.	4. Provides access to the wound area and privacy for the client.
5. Place a towel or water-resistant pad under or to the side of the client to absorb excessive cleansing solutions.	5. Solutions may drip onto the client's bed linen. Placing a towel or water-resistant pad under the client prevents the linen from becoming wet.
6. Set up a waterproof disposable bag in a convenient location by: a. Opening the bag. b. Folding the top of the bag down to make a cuff.	6. The cuff provides a means of closing the bag without touching the contents within the bag. Waterproof bag prevents wicking of wound drainage through the bag to the outside by capillary action.
7. Don examination gloves and a mask.	7. Gloves protect you from microorganisms in the wound dressing. The mask protects the wound from contamination with droplet nuclei from your respiratory tract.
8. Remove the dressing and tape, if present. Grasp the edge of the tape, hold the client's skin proximal to the edge of the tape, and gently pull the tape toward the wound.	8. Providing countertraction of the skin as the tape is removed reduces discomfort and promotes skin integrity.
9. Lift the dressing off the wound so the soiled or underside of the dressing is away from the client's face.	9. The appearance of the dressing may be distressing to the client.
10. Dispose of the tape and dressing in a waterproof bag.	10. Decreases the transmission of microorganisms.
11. Remove the disposable gloves inside out and place them in a waterproof bag.	11. Decreases the transmission of microorganisms. By removing the gloves inside out, your hands are not contaminated by the outside of the dirty gloves.
12. Wash your hands.	12. Decreases the transmission of microorganisms.
13. Set up a sterile field on the overbed table. Open all packages of sterile supplies and aseptically place them on the sterile field.	13. The sterile field decreases the chance of contamination of the wound with microorganisms. All sterile supplies must be ready for use. Once you have donned sterile gloves, you cannot touch unsterile objects.
14. Open the bottle of cleansing solution. Place the cap of the bottle upside down on the overbed table.	14. Prevents contamination of the inside of the cap.

▼ *ACTION*

▼ *RATIONALE*

15. This step is optional. If the solution has been opened and used previously, pour approximately 10 to 15 ml into a waterproof bag.

15. Removes microorganisms from the lip of the bottle.

16. Pour the cleansing solution into a sterile basin without wetting the sterile field.

16. Moisture draws microorganisms into the sterile field by capillary action.

17. Apply sterile gloves.

17. Prevents the transmission of microorganisms to the wound.

18. Using sterile forceps, pick up a 4- × 4-inch gauze pad and saturate it with cleansing solution.

18. Use of sterile pick-up forceps lessens the chance of contaminating your sterile gloves as you cleanse the wound.

19. Cleanse the wound with one stroke at a time from the cleanest area to the least clean area (Fig. 20–1). Use one gauze pad for each cleansing action.

19. The wound itself is considered to be the cleanest area. Use of a separate swab for each area prevents recontamination of the wound with organisms from the skin and wound drainage.

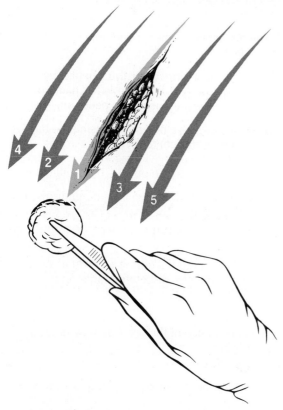

▼ **FIGURE 20–1.** Cleansing a wound.

20. Drop used gauze pads into the bag without touching the inside of the bag with your hand or forceps.

20. The inside of the bag is considered to be contaminated.

21. Using the same action, rinse the area with gauze pads soaked in normal saline. (This step is optional.)

21. Ionized cleansing solutions such as hydrogen peroxide may be irritating to the skin if they are left on the skin surface.

22. Dry the wound area with the dry gauze pads. Use the same one-stroke action.

22. Excessive moisture on the skin promotes the growth of microorganisms.

23. Apply a dressing if ordered or if the wound is draining. Refer to Skill 20–3.

23. Wounds may be left exposed to the air unless they are draining or occur in the immediate postoperative period.

▼ *ACTION*	▼ *RATIONALE*
24. Dispose of the soiled supplies in a bag.	**24.** Prevents transmission of microorganisms and prevents odors in the client's room.
25. Remove gloves and wash your hands.	**25.** Decreases the transmission of microorganisms.
26. Record the procedure. Note your observations of the site.	**26.** Communicates the findings to the other members of the health care team and contributes to the legal record by documenting the care given to the client.

Example of Documentation

DATE	*TIME*	*NOTES*
10/31/93	0900	Abdominal wound cleansed with normal saline. Edges well approximated with no redness, swelling, tenderness, or drainage seen.
		S. Williams, RN

Teaching Tips

While you are cleansing the client's wound, discuss the stages of wound healing that the client can expect as well as precautions that the client should take with the wound.

Home Care Variations

After transporting supplies to the client's home, examine the supplies to ensure that sterility has been maintained. Be sure that packages are intact and have not become moist or contaminated in any way. Examine the seals on caps of solution bottles.

For wound cleansing, place the solutions and supplies on a clean tabletop near the client. Clean the tabletop with an antiseptic solution before placing the supplies on it.

After cleansing the wound, remove the used supplies from the client's home in a waterproof bag.

SKILL 20–2   IRRIGATING AND PACKING A WOUND

Clinical Situations in Which You May Encounter This Skill

A wound should be irrigated and packed if it is open and cannot be sutured, if it is an incision and wound left open to drain, or if it is infected and should heal through granulation from the inside of the body to the outside. Irrigation cleanses the wound and removes the source of infection. Packing the wound prevents the skin from healing and leaving an infected mass of tissue under the surface that results in abscess formation. Solutions for irrigation and schedules for irrigating and packing the wound vary depending on the type of wound and the physician's order.

Anticipated Responses

▼ The client's wound appears clean after irrigation.
▼ The client's wound heals and becomes free of infection and drainage.
▼ The client's skin integrity is maintained.

Adverse Responses

▼ The procedure is extremely painful to the client.
▼ The client's wound opens further.
▼ The client's wound does not heal or the amount of infection increases.

Materials List

Gather these materials before beginning the skill:

▼ Examination gloves
▼ Sterile gloves (2 pairs)
▼ Goggles and gown
▼ Sterile gauze or other packing material as ordered by the physician
▼ Sterile 4- × 4-inch gauze pads (for drying the wound)
▼ Dressing materials (abdominal pad, 4- × 4-inch gauze pads, tape)

▼ Sterile basin
▼ Collecting basin
▼ Normal saline (or other solution as ordered by the physician)
▼ 30-ml Luer-Lok syringe with a large-bore (19-gauge) blunt-tipped needle
▼ Sterile blunt-tipped forceps
▼ Waterproof disposable bag
▼ Waterproof pad

▼ ACTION

▼ RATIONALE

Irrigating the Wound

1. Review the client's record to determine the solution to be used for irrigation.

2. Review the previous wound assessment recorded in the client's chart.

3. Ask the client if he or she has had this procedure before and if the procedure was painful. If the client has not had irrigations before, explain what to expect.

4. Close the door, curtains, and windows in the client's room.

5. Wash your hands.

6. Administer an analgesic if indicated and allow time for it to become effective.

7. Help the client to assume a comfortable position so that the wound is easily accessible.

8. Place a waterproof pad under the client and a collecting basin at the bottom of the wound.

9. Open and set up a disposable waterproof bag in a convenient location. Fold down the top of the bag 1.5 inches to form a cuff.

10. Prepare a sterile field with the following equipment:

    a. Irrigating syringe and needle.
    b. Sterile basin.
    c. Irrigation solution poured in a basin.
    d. Sterile 4- × 4-inch gauze pads.
    e. Sterile dressing materials.
    f. Sterile forceps.
    g. Packing material if the wound is to be packed. See Skill 20–2.

11. Don disposable gloves, goggles, and a gown.

---

1. Solutions vary according to the type of wound and the microorganisms present.

2. Provides baseline data with which to compare your assessment.

3. Simple explanations reduce anxiety and apprehension.

4. Provides for privacy and eliminates drafts.

5. Reduces the transmission of microorganisms.

6. The procedure is often uncomfortable for the client. An oral analgesic becomes effective in 1 hour, and a parenteral analgesic becomes effective in 15 to 20 minutes.

7. Facilitates irrigation and packing of the wound.

8. The pad helps to protect the bed linens and the basin contains used irrigant.

9. The cuff provides a means of closing the bag without touching the contents within the bag. Waterproof bag prevents wicking of wound drainage through the bag to the outside by capillary action.

10. Sterile equipment should be ready to use once the dressing is removed.

11. Prevents the transmission of microorganisms from the dressing to the wound or from the environment to the wound.

▼ *ACTION*   ▼ *RATIONALE*

12. Gently remove the tape from around the dressing. Grasp the edge of the tape, hold the client's skin proximal to the edge of the tape, and gently pull the tape toward the wound.

12. Providing countertraction of the skin as the tape is removed reduces the client's discomfort and preserves skin integrity. If the tape is removed in the direction of the wound there is less tension on the wound.

13. Gently remove the dressing by lifting the dressing up and away from the client's face.

13. The appearance of the dressing may be distressing to the client.

14. Dispose of the dressing in the disposable bag.

14. Decreases the transmission of microorganisms.

15. Remove wound packing, if present.

15. Old packing must be removed to clean the wound.

16. Assess the wound. Note the depth, width, and general appearance of the tissue; redness, tenderness, and exudate; and the presence of necrotic tissue, granulation tissue, and odor.

16. Provides a means of evaluating the healing of the wound.

17. Remove the disposable gloves by turning them inside out and place them in a bag.

17. Your gloves are contaminated with microorganisms from the client's wound.

18. Wash your hands.

18. Decreases the transmission of microorganisms.

19. Don sterile gloves.

19. Prevents contamination of the wound.

20. Withdraw 30 ml of irrigant into the syringe.

20. You will repeat this step several times since 200 ml or more are used to irrigate the wound.

21. Irrigate the wound (Fig. 20–2):
    a. Hold the blunt needle tip 1 to 2 inches above the wound.
    b. Using continuous and gentle pressure, flush the wound from top to bottom. Force should not exceed 8 pounds per square inch.

21. Flushing the wound removes debris. Secondary healing is facilitated. Gentle irrigation of the wound prevents trauma to newly forming granulation tissues.

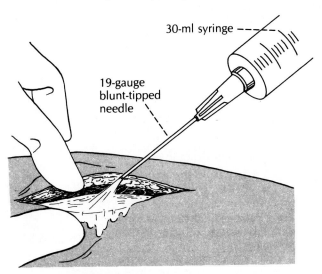

30-ml syringe

19-gauge blunt-tipped needle

▼ FIGURE 20–2. Irrigating a wound.

22. Place several 4- × 4-inch gauze pads in the wound.

22. The pads soak up the irrigating solution.

23. Dry the wound with an additional gauze pad.

23. Moisture promotes the growth of microorganisms. Drying the skin around and in the wound prevents maceration.

▼ _ACTION_   ▼ _RATIONALE_

Packing the Wound

24. Hold the forceps in your dominant hand and gauze or other packing material in your nondominant hand. Use the forceps to guide the gauze loosely into the wound and completely pack the wound (Fig. 20–3).

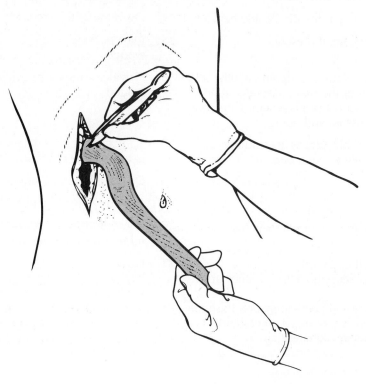

▼ **FIGURE 20–3.** Packing a wound.

25. Place gauze pads on top of the packing.

25. Provides reinforcement for the packing and collects drainage.

26. Place a sterile abdominal pad over the gauze pads covering the wound.

27. Secure the dressing with tape or Montgomery straps.

27. Holds the dressing in place.

28. Remove the waterproof pad from under the client.

29. Help the client to assume a comfortable position.

30. Remove the soiled dressing and supplies from the client's room.

30. Prevents odors and transmission of microorganisms.

31. Remove the sterile gloves and wash your hands.

31. Decreases the transmission of microorganisms.

32. Record the procedure. Note the size of the wound, the general appearance of the tissue, redness, tenderness, exudate, and the presence of necrotic or granulation tissue and odor.

32. Communicates the findings to the other members of the health care team and contributes to the legal record by documenting the care given to the client.

Example of Documentation

DATE	TIME	NOTES
1/8/93	0830	50 mg meperidine IM right gluteal in preparation for wound irrigation and packing.
		S. Williams, RN
1/8/93	0915	Sterile technique used to irrigate and pack abdominal wound. Irrigated with 100 ml of normal saline. Wound 8 cm long, 4 cm wide, and 3 cm deep. Tissue bright pink with foul smelling, yellowish green exudate. Small amount of granulating tissue seen. Wound packed with dry sterile gauze. Complained of moderate pain during irrigation.
		S. Williams, RN

Teaching Tips

Dressing changes provide an opportune time to discuss sterile technique with the client as well as the purpose of wound irrigation and the stages of wound healing. If the client is to continue irrigating the wound after discharge from the hospital, teach the client how to perform the procedure. Have the client or his or her family demonstrate the skill.

Home Care Variations

Assess the client's home to ensure that he or she has adequate lighting and running water. Assess the client's motivation to perform the irrigations and verify that sterile technique is used. Teach the client about adverse responses to report to you or the physician.

SKILL 20–3   APPLYING A DRY STERILE DRESSING

Clinical Situations in Which You May Encounter This Skill

The first time a surgical dressing is changed or any time a wound is draining, a dry sterile dressing should be applied. If the dressing becomes contaminated during the dressing change or if the dressing becomes saturated with blood or drainage, a new sterile dressing should be applied.

If the client has a wound that is draining large amounts of excoriating fluid or the client has skin breakdown from the drainage, an ostomy bag can be applied over the wound to collect all drainage and prevent skin breakdown. See Skill 15–7.

Anticipated Responses

▼ The dry sterile dressing is applied to the client's wound without contamination.

Adverse Responses

▼ The client's dressing becomes contaminated.

Materials List

Gather these materials before beginning the skill:

▼ Examination gloves
▼ Sterile gloves
▼ Mask
▼ Dressing materials (Fig. 20–4):
   Sterile 4- × 4-inch gauze pads
   Sterile 2- × 2-inch gauze pads
   Precut 4- × 4-inch gauze pads (for clients with a Penrose drain or drainage tube)
   Sterile abdominal pad

Gauze roll for head or extremity wounds
Expandable net dressing (to hold dressings on extremities)
Nonadherent absorbent dressing (nonstick dressing)
Tape (1 inch and 2 inches) or Montgomery straps
▼ Disposable sterile field
Disposable waterproof bag
If the wound is to be cleansed, also gather cleansing supplies (see Skill 20–1).

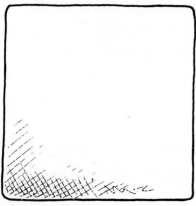

4-x 4-inch gauze pad

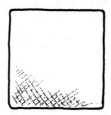

2-x 2-inch gauze pad

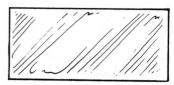

Nonadherent absorbent dressing

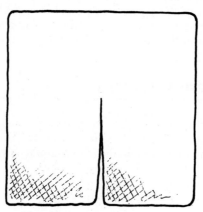

Precut 4-x 4-inch gauze pad

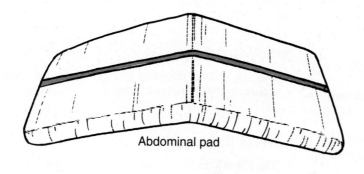

Abdominal pad

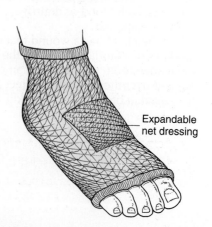

Gauze roll

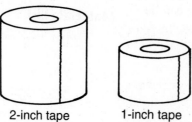

2-inch tape   1-inch tape

Expandable net dressing

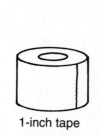

▼ **FIGURE 20–4.** Dressing materials.

▼ *A C T I O N*   ▼ *R A T I O N A L E*

The wound in this skill is an abdominal surgical incision.

1. Review the physician's order to determine if any special procedures should be done during the dressing change (e.g., culture).

2. Wash your hands.

3. Help the client to assume a comfortable position so the wound is easily accessible.

4. If needed, administer an analgesic and allow time for the medication to become effective.

5. Explain the procedure to the client if necessary.

6. Prepare a sterile field with the following equipment:
   a. 4- × 4-inch gauze pads.
   b. Abdominal pad.
   c. If needed, supplies for wound cleansing (see Skill 20–1).

7. Place a waterproof bag nearby with the top folded down 1.5 inches to make a cuff.

8. Don examination gloves and a mask if needed.

9. Gently remove the tape from around the dressing by:
   a. Holding the client's skin proximal to the edge of the tape.

   b. Gently pulling the tape toward the wound.

10. Gently remove the dressing by lifting it up and away from the client's face. If the dressing is stuck to the wound, moisten it with sterile saline before removing it.

11. Dispose of the dressing in the disposable bag.

12. Remove the gloves and place them in the bag. Wash your hands.

13. Don sterile gloves.

14. If needed, cleanse the wound. Use sterile technique.

---

1. If the wound has been draining, a culture may be needed.

2. Decreases the transmission of microorganisms.

3. Makes the dressing change easier.

4. Dressing changes are sometimes uncomfortable for the client. Allow 1 hour for an oral analgesic and 1 to 20 minutes for a parenteral analgesic to become effective before proceeding.

5. Elicits the client's cooperation.

> **NOTE:** See Skill 1–9 for information on preparing and maintaining a sterile field.

7. The cuff allows for closure of the bag without touching the contents. Waterproof bag prevents wicking of wound drainage through the bag to the outside by capillary action.

8. When there is a chance of coming into contact with blood or drainage, gloves should be worn to decrease the transmission of microorganisms. The mask prevents contamination of the wound with droplet nuclei from your respiratory tract.

   a. Providing countertraction of the skin as the tape is removed reduces the client's discomfort and preserves skin integrity.
   b. Pulling the tape in the direction of the wound lessens the tension on the wound.

10. The appearance of the dressing may be distressing to the client. Forceful removal may damage granulation tissue and impair wound healing.

11. Decreases the transmission of microorganisms.

12. Decreases the transmission of microorganisms.

13. The application of the dressing is a sterile procedure.

> **NOTE:** See Skill 20–1.

▼ *ACTION*   ▼ *RATIONALE*

15. Pick up a 4- × 4-inch gauze pad, fold it in half, and apply it lengthwise on the wound.

15. Folding the gauze pad in half adds extra thickness over the wound.

NOTE: Do not touch the wound with your sterile gloves.	The wound is considered to be contaminated and will contaminate your sterile gloves.

16. Continue applying gauze pads until the wound is completely covered. Be sure to consider the direction the drain will flow and apply the gauze pads.

16. Completely covering the wound protects the wound from contamination from airborne microorganisms and collects any drainage from the wound.

17. (This step is optional.) If the client has a drain (Penrose or tube) that is excreting drainage, place precut 4- × 4-inch gauze pads around the tube or drain. Reinforce the precut gauze pads with more gauze pads.

17. The precut gauze pads fit around the drain or tube and protect the client's skin from excoriation from any drainage. Although gauze pads can be cut with sterile scissors, fibers may enter the drain or tube.

18. Apply a sterile abdominal pad on top of the gauze pads.

18. Provides an additional barrier to microorganisms and additional absorption of the drainage.

19. Apply tape so that the dressing is held in place (Fig. 20–5). If the client's skin is irritated, use Montgomery straps instead of tape.

19. Prevents the dressing from becoming dislodged.

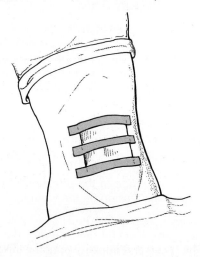

▼ **FIGURE 20–5.** Applying tape to a sterile dressing.

20. Remove the gloves and dispose of them in the bag. Wash your hands.

20. Decreases the transmission of microorganisms.

21. Dispose of the bag of soiled material.

21. Prevents odors and transmission of microorganisms.

22. Record the procedure. Note the condition of the wound (redness, swelling, warmth, approximation of the edges, drainage, or tenderness).

22. Communicates the findings to the other members of the health care team and contributes to the legal record by documenting the care given to the client.

Example of Documentation

DATE	TIME	NOTES
10/30/93	0900	Sterile dressing change at abdominal surgical site. Incision 8 cm long with sutures in place. Incision open 2 mm, red, tender, with moderate amount of serosanguineous drainage.

S. Williams, RN

Teaching Tips

Dressing changes provide opportune times to teach the client about approximate healing times to be expected. Sterile technique can also be discussed and the importance of keeping the dressing dry can be reinforced.

Home Care Variations

Examine the supplies transported to the client's home for any signs of contamination, such as moisture on the package or tears. Teach the client and the client's family about sterile technique as you change the dressing. Tell the client about adverse responses to report immediately to you or the physician.

Place sterile supplies on a tabletop that has been cleaned with an antimicrobial agent. Place all used supplies in a disposable waterproof bag and remove it from the client's home as you leave.

SKILL 20–4   USING MONTGOMERY STRAPS

Clinical Situations in Which You May Encounter This Skill

Montgomery straps are often used if a client has a wound that requires multiple bandage changes. Several strips of wide tape are applied to the skin lateral to the wound with tabs of tape left extending toward the midline. The adhesive sides of the tabs are folded under to prevent them from adhering to the skin and small holes are cut into the tape approximately 1 inch from the end. The tabs are then laced together with gauze or umbilical tape to secure an underlying bandage. Since the tape is unlaced and not removed during dressing changes, the integrity of the skin is maintained.

If the straps become soiled, they may be cleaned with a gentle soap and warm water or replaced. If the client has an allergic reaction to the tape, remove it and secure the dressing with a straight or scultetus binder (see Skill 20–13).

Anticipated Responses

▼ The Montgomery straps are applied securely to the client's skin and they remain in place. The client's skin integrity is maintained.

Adverse Responses

▼ The client has an allergic reaction to the tape and his or her skin becomes excoriated.

Materials List

Gather these materials before beginning the skill:

▼ Prepackaged Montgomery straps, or wide tape (2 or 4 inches wide)
▼ Roll of gauze or umbilical tape
▼ Sterile gloves
▼ Dressing materials including abdominal pad
▼ Scissors

▼ *A C T I O N*

▼ *R A T I O N A L E*

1. Assess the wound to determine if multiple bandage changes over several days are needed.

1. If tape is repeatedly applied and removed, the client's skin integrity is compromised. Montgomery straps remain in place for an extended period of time and thus do not alter skin integrity.

2. Explain to the client what you are going to do.

2. Simple explanations help to reduce anxiety and apprehension.

3. Drape the client and expose only the wound area.

3. Provides for privacy and maintains the client's sense of modesty.

4. Open the package of Montgomery straps or make your own from tape (Fig. 20–6).
   a. Cut or tear the tape into lengths which, when applied to the skin, will overlap the wound by 3 inches (Fig. 20–6A).
   b. Fold one adhesive side of the tape together to make a 3-inch tab and leave approximately 2 inches of the adhesive side unfolded (Fig. 20–6B).
   c. With the scissors, cut a small hole in the middle of the doubled tape tabs (Fig. 20–6C).

   a. Three inches of the tape is folded under to make a tab that is nonadhesive on both sides.

   b. By folding the adhesive sides together, the nonadhesive tabs extend over the dressing and do not adhere to it. The unfolded adhesive side is applied to the client's skin.
   c. The gauze or umbilical tape is threaded through the hole.

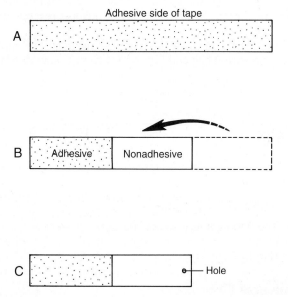

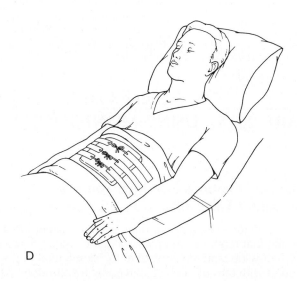

▼ **FIGURE 20–6.** Making Montgomery straps. Cutting or tearing the tape *(A)*. Folding one adhesive side of the tape down *(B)*. Cutting a small hole in the middle of the doubled tape tabs *(C)*. Applying the strips of tape to the client's skin toward the suture line and lacing the straps from the bottom *(D)*.

5. Don sterile gloves.

5. Prevents the transmission of microorganisms.

6. Apply dressing material to the wound. Cover the dressing with an abdominal pad.

6. The abdominal pad helps to hold smaller dressings in place.

7. Remove the gloves and discard them into a receptacle.

7. Prevents the transmission of microorganisms.

8. Apply strips of tape to the client's skin toward the suture line (Fig. 20–6D).

9. With the umbilical tape or roll of gauze, lace the straps from the bottom as though you were lacing a pair of shoes (Fig. 20–6D).

9. The laced gauze or umbilical secures the dressing.

▼ _ACTION_	▼ _RATIONALE_
10. Secure the gauze or tape. Tie the material in a loose knot.	**10.** Keeps the lacing from becoming loose.
11. Wash your hands.	**11.** Decreases the transmission of microorganisms.
12. Record the dressing change. Note that Montgomery straps were applied. Note the condition of the wound or suture line.	**12.** Communicates the findings to the other members of the health care team and contributes to the legal record by documenting the care given to the client.

Example of Documentation

DATE	TIME	NOTES
1/30/93	1030	Montgomery straps with 4-inch adhesive tape applied to wound area. Wound 2 × 8 cm, draining yellow thick pus with foul odor.
		S. Williams, RN

Teaching Tips

Dressing changes provide opportune times to teach the client about sterile technique used with dressing changes. Teaching can also include wound healing and factors that will enhance healing such as good nutrition.

Home Care Variations

When changing dressings in the client's home, have adequate lighting from lamps or sunlight through a window. Dispose of dressing materials in a waterproof bag and place it in a trash receptacle outside the client's home as you leave.

Determine if the client has the materials at home to perform subsequent dressing changes and the knowledge to use and reapply Montgomery straps. The client must know to report the signs of wound infection and allergic reaction to the tape.

SKILL 20–5   APPLYING A WET-TO-DRY DRESSING

Clinical Situations in Which You May Encounter This Skill

Wet-to-dry dressings may be ordered for a client who has an open wound that must be debrided. A wet-to-dry dressing is applied wet and then allowed to dry. When the dry dressing is removed, the wound is debrided.

Open wounds that must be debrided include stasis ulcers, eviscerated wounds, severely infected wounds, or Stage 4 decubitus ulcers. As the tissue is debrided, granulation formation occurs. If the procedure is painful to the client, analgesics may be given prior to applying or removing the dressing.

Anticipated Responses

▼ The wet dressing is applied, allowed to dry, and removed. As the dressing is removed, necrotic tissue is removed and granulation of new tissue is enhanced.

Adverse Responses

▼ The procedure is painful to the client.
▼ Bleeding occurs as the dry dressing is removed.
▼ Maceration of the tissue and infection occur.

Materials List

Gather these materials before beginning the skill:

▼ Examination gloves
▼ Sterile gloves
▼ Fine-mesh gauze or 4- × 4-inch gauze pads without cotton for packing the wound
▼ Extra gauze pads for dressing the wound
▼ Abdominal pad

▼ Normal saline or other solution as ordered by the physician
▼ Sterile basin
▼ Sterile blunt-tipped forceps
▼ 2-inch tape or Montgomery straps
▼ Waterproof bag
▼ Towel or waterproof pad
▼ Sterile field

▼ ACTION	▼ RATIONALE
1. Review the client's chart to determine the solution to be used.	1. Solutions for wet-to-dry dressings vary according to the type of wound and the presence of infection.
2. Examine the wound to determine if additional supplies are needed.	2. Large wounds require additional amounts of gauze.
3. Ask the client if he or she has had this procedure before and if the procedure was painful. If the client has not had wet-to-dry dressings before, explain what to expect.	3. Simple explanations help to reduce anxiety and apprehension.
4. Administer an analgesic if needed and allow time for it to become effective.	4. Oral analgesics require 1 hour to become effective. Parenteral analgesics require 15 to 20 minutes to become effective.
5. Help the client to assume a comfortable position so that the wound is easily accessible.	5. Makes it easier to change the dressing.
6. Close the client's door and the curtains on the windows.	6. Provides privacy for the client.
7. Expose the wound area and drape the client.	7. Provides access to the wound area and provides privacy for the client.
8. Place a towel or waterproof pad in a dependent position under the client to absorb fluids or drainage.	8. Helps protect the client's bed sheets.
9. Open and set up a disposable waterproof bag in a convenient location. Fold the top down 1.5 inches to make a cuff.	9. The cuff provides a means of closing the bag without touching the contents within the bag. Waterproof bag prevents wicking of wound drainage through the bag to the outside by capillary action.
10. Don examination gloves.	10. Prevents the transmission of microorganisms from the dressing on the wound.
11. Gently remove the tape around the dressing by: a. Grasping the edge of the tape. b. Holding the client's skin proximal to the edge of the tape. c. Gently pulling the tape toward the wound.	11. Providing countertraction of the client's skin as the tape is removed reduces the client's discomfort and promotes preservation of skin integrity.
12. Gently remove the dressing by lifting it up at a 90-degree angle from the wound. Hold the inside of the dressing away from the client's face. Remove packing.	12. Lifting the dressing up at a 90-degree angle removes loose tissue and exudate from the wound. The appearance of the dressing may be distressing to the client.

NOTE: Do not moisten the dressing to remove it.

| 13. Dispose of the dressing in the disposable bag. | 13. Decreases the transmission of microorganisms. |

▼ *A C T I O N*   ▼ *R A T I O N A L E*

14. Assess the wound. Note the depth, width, and general appearance of the tissue; redness, tenderness, and exudate; and the presence of necrotic tissue and granulation tissue.

14. Provides data for further comparison of the stages of healing.

15. Remove the examination gloves by turning them inside out and place them in a disposable bag.

15. The gloves are contaminated from the client's wound.

16. Wash your hands.

16. Decreases the transmission of microorganisms.

17. Set up a sterile field with:
  a. A basin.
  b. Two packages of 4- × 4-inch gauze pads added to the basin.
  c. Solution poured on the sterile gauze in the basin.
  d. Four packages of 4- × 4-inch gauze pads within the sterile field.
  e. Sterile forceps.
  f. An abdominal pad.

17. The procedure is sterile to decrease the transmission of microorganisms.

18. Don sterile gloves.

18. Decreases the transmission of microorganisms into the client's wound.

19. Pick up the soaked gauze and gently squeeze it to remove the excess solution (the gauze should not drip with the solution).

19. If the dressing is excessively moist, the client's tissue may remain too moist and tissue maceration may result because of delayed drying.

20. Open the wet gauze completely.

20. Makes insertion of the gauze easier.

21. Hold the forceps in your dominant hand and gauze in your nondominant hand. Guide the gauze into the client's wound until all inner surfaces are covered.

21. The forceps make insertion of the gauze easier.

22. Place a dry 4- × 4-inch gauze covering over the moistened dressing.

22. The dry gauze aids in the transfer of moisture from the wound.

23. Place an abdominal pad over the wound and dressings.

23. The pad protects the wound from microorganisms while allowing air to enter the wound.

24. Secure the dressing edges with tape or Montgomery straps (see Skill 20–4). Do not cover the top of the dressing to form an occlusive dressing.

24. An occlusive dressing inhibits the drying of the gauze and defeats the debridement purpose of the wet-to-dry dressing.

25. Remove gloves and wash your hands.

25. Decreases the transmission of microorganisms.

26. Record the procedure. Note the condition of the wound and the type of solution used.

26. Communicates the findings to the other members of the health care team and contributes to the legal record by documenting the care given to the client.

Example of Documentation

DATE	*TIME*	*NOTES*
11/30/93	1030	Wet-to-dry dressing change of sacral area with sterile normal saline. Yellowish green drainage on dry dressing removed. Wound 2 cm wide × 5 cm long × 2 cm deep. Patchy areas of granulating tissue present throughout area. Bright pink tissue present on edges. Client complained of slight discomfort during dressing change.

S. Williams, RN

Teaching Tips

Dressing changes provide opportune times to discuss the appropriate stages of healing with the client. Signs of poor wound healing should be discussed. If the client is to have wet-to-dry dressings at home, the family should be included in the person's care and encouraged to change the dressing under supervision prior to discharge. Encourage the client not to apply pressure to the wound area and to lie in a position (prone, side-lying, etc.) that avoids wound pressure.

Discuss appropriate nutrition to encourage wound healing. A dietary consultation may be necessary. Encourage the daily intake of protein and vitamins in the diet.

Home Care Variations

Teach the client or his or her family member the procedure for wet-to-dry dressings. Have them demonstrate the skill. Ensure that the client or his or her family knows how often to change the dressing and about appropriate disposal of soiled dressings.

SKILL 20–6 APPLYING A TRANSPARENT DRESSING

Clinical Situations in Which You May Encounter This Skill

An occlusive transparent dressing may be applied to any surgical, intravenous, or wound site. These dressings offer several advantages including easy visibility of the wound, prevention of infection, and promotion of healing by retention of serous exudates that enhance epithelial growth. Transparent dressings do not require frequent dressing changes and the dressing does not adhere to the wound. The dressings are elastic and therefore lend themselves to applications over joints. A client can shower or bathe without removing a transparent dressing.

Allergic reactions to the dressing material are possible, and require that the dressing be removed.

Anticipated Responses

▼ The transparent dressing is applied to the site and visibility is possible for assessment of wound healing and any signs of infection.

▼ The client's wound heals without aerobic bacterial growth.

Adverse Responses

▼ The client has an allergic reaction to the transparent dressing. The signs of the reaction are bullae formation, itching, or urticaria of the surrounding skin.

Materials List

Gather these materials before beginning the skill:

▼ Transparent dressing
▼ Examination gloves
▼ Sterile gloves
▼ 1-inch tape
▼ Disposable bag

▼ ACTION	▼ RATIONALE
1. Check the client's chart for a previous description of the client's skin condition.	1. Provides data with which to make a comparison.
2. Don examination gloves.	2. Decreases the transmission of microorganisms.
3. Remove the old dressing by: a. Holding the client's skin taut under the edge of the existing dressing. b. Lifting the edge of the dressing. c. Pulling the dressing off in the direction of the person's hair growth.	3. Holding the person's skin taut and pulling the dressing in the direction of hair growth lessens the client's discomfort and helps to maintain skin integrity.

▼ *ACTION*

▼ *RATIONALE*

4. Discard the dressing in a disposable bag.

4. Decreases the transmission of microorganisms.

5. Assess the wound site for approximation of the edges, edema, redness, warmth, and drainage.

5. Provides data for further comparison of the stages of healing.

6. Provide wound care, if ordered.

6. Decreases the chance of infection if there is an open wound.

7. Remove your gloves and discard them in a disposable bag.

7. Decreases the transmission of microorganisms.

8. Wash your hands.

8. Decreases the transmission of microorganisms.

9. Open the package containing the transparent dressing.

9. Allows easy access to dressing after you apply sterile gloves.

10. Don sterile gloves.

10. Decreases the transmission of microorganisms.

11. Grasp the backing tab on the underside of the dressing (the tab is nonadhesive) and separate the backing approximately 1 inch from the transparent dressing.

11. Applying a small portion at a time allows for better control and makes it easier to apply a smooth, wrinkle-free dressing.

12. Place a 1-inch section of adhesive transparent dressing directly above the area to be covered.

12. Position the dressing above the arm before application since you cannot move the dressing once it comes in contact with the skin.

13. While holding the dressing in place with one hand, peel the backing away from the dressing as you slowly smooth and apply the dressing to the site (Fig. 20–7).

13. Wrinkles are more likely when the backing is peeled away entirely before application. Wrinkles can lead to skin breakdown.

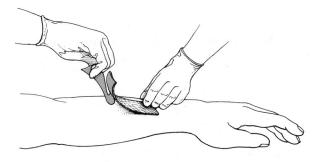

▼ FIGURE 20–7. Applying a transparent dressing.

14. Reinforce the edges of the dressing and tape if needed.

14. Holds the dressing securely in space.

15. Place the date and time and your initials on the dressing.

15. Provides a reference for future dressing changes.

16. Remove gloves and wash your hands.

16. Decreases the transmission of microorganisms.

17. Record the procedure. Note your observations about the wound and type of dressing.

17. Communicates the findings to the other members of the health care team and contributes to the legal record by documenting the care given to the client.

Example of Documentation

DATE	TIME	NOTES
12/3/93	0800	Transparent dressing change to incision site on right forearm. No redness, edema, drainage, pain, or warmth noted. Edges approximated. Granulation tissue present.
		S. Williams, RN

Teaching Tips

Teach the client the signs and symptoms of infection to report and the stages of healing to expect. Encourage the client to keep the dressing dry.

Home Care Variations

Teach the client and his or her family member to apply the dressing. Have then demonstrate the skill. Dressing changes at home can be performed using clean technique (handwashing and no use of gloves). Dressings that are removed should be placed in a plastic bag and removed from the client's home as you leave.

SKILL 20–7 MANAGING WOUND DRAINS AND WOUND SUCTION DEVICES

Clinical Situations in Which You May Encounter This Skill

Drains are inserted to take away excessive serosanguineous exudate or purulent exudate from an incision or a wound. Failure to remove this drainage could result in abscess formation and the failure of underlying tissues to heal. There are two basic types of drains that may be inserted: the Penrose drain and a closed wound drainage system. Both devices are usually inserted during surgery.

The Penrose drain (Fig. 20–8) is a piece of flat latex tubing that is inserted into the wound via a separate incision called a stab wound. The drain is located a few inches from the main incision to prevent contamination of the incision with wound drainage.

Penrose drains vary in length and width depending on their location. As the wound heals, the drain is usually pulled out or shortened 1 to 2 inches per day until it is completely removed. The physician may perform this procedure or may leave orders for you to shorten the drain. The drain is usually shortened when the dressing is changed.

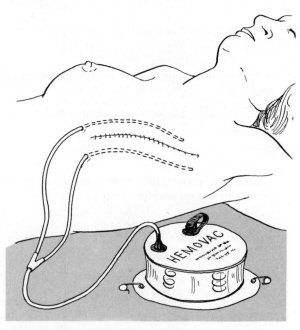

▼ **FIGURE 20–9.** The Hemovac system.

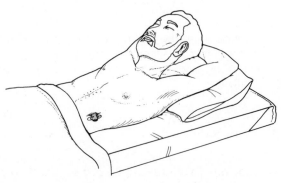

▼ **FIGURE 20–8.** The Penrose drain.

A closed drainage system includes a round plastic drainage tube connected to a suction device. The suction device may be electric or may be a manual compression device that works on the principle of creating a vacuum. The Hemovac (Fig. 20–9) and Jackson-Pratt (Fig. 20–10) systems are manual compression closed drainage systems.

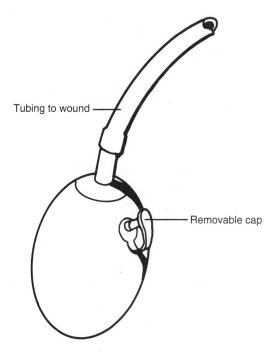

Tubing to wound

Removable cap

▼ **FIGURE 20–10.** The Jackson-Pratt manual compression closed drainage system.

Anticipated Responses

▼ The drain site remains free of infection.
▼ The drain remains patent.

Adverse Responses

▼ Infection develops at the drain site.
▼ The drain becomes obstructed.
▼ The drain is accidentally dislodged or removed.

Materials List

Gather these materials before beginning the skill:

▼ For cleaning and dressing a wound drain and shortening a Penrose drain:
  Waterproof disposable bag
  Examination gloves
  Sterile gloves
  Mask
  Sterile hemostat
  Sterile forceps
  Sterile cotton-tipped applicators
  Sterile 4- × 4-inch gauze pads
  Sterile precut 4- × 4-inch gauze pads
  Abdominal pads
  Tape
  Sterile normal saline
  Suture removal kit (for the first time you shorten drain only)
  Sterile scissors
  Sterile safety pin
▼ To empty a closed wound drainage system and reestablish suction:
  Examination gloves
  Graduated container to hold drainage

▼ *ACTION*

Cleaning and Dressing a Drain Site and Shortening a Penrose Drain

1. Check the client's record to verify the physician's order regarding shortening the Penrose drain.

2. Refer to Skill 20–1 to cleanse the incision site.

3. Cleanse the drain site (Fig. 20–11). With the hemostat in your nondominant hand, lift up the drain. Using forceps in your dominant hand, cleanse around the drain site with a saline-soaked gauze pad or a cotton-tipped applicator. Cleanse in a circular pattern from the drain site outward.

4. To shorten the Penrose drain for the first time, use the suture removal kit to release the suture holding the drain in place.

5. Using sterile forceps, grasp the Penrose drain across its entire width close to the client's skin.

▼ *RATIONALE*

1. The physician determines when the drain is to be shortened and the length it is to be shortened.

2. The incision is considered to be cleaner than the drain site and therefore is cleansed first.

3. Cleansing in a circular pattern prevents you from pulling microorganisms from the client's skin into the drain stab wound.

4. The drain is initially sutured in place to prevent it from moving.

5. Provides even traction and prevents you from tearing the drain.

▼ _A C T I O N_   ▼ _R A T I O N A L E_ _ _ _ _ _ _ _ _ _ _ _ _ _ _ _ _ _

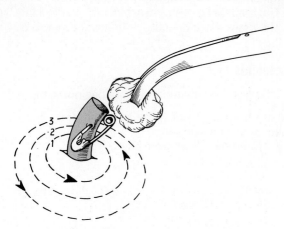

▼ **FIGURE 20–11.** Cleansing the drain site.

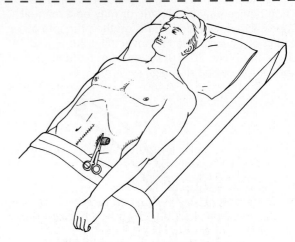

▼ **FIGURE 20–12.** Pulling the drain out.

6. Pull the drain out the ordered number of inches (Fig. 20–12).

7. Insert a sterile safety pin through the drain as close to the client's skin as is possible (Fig. 20–13).

7. The pin replaces the suture and prevents the drain from slipping into the client's body through the stab wound.

8. Use sterile scissors to cut off the excess drain. Leave 2 inches remaining above the skin (Fig. 20–14). Discard the cut-off drain in a bag for disposal.

8. Reduces the transmission of microorganisms.

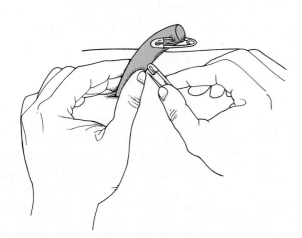

▼ **FIGURE 20–13.** Inserting a sterile safety pin through the drain.

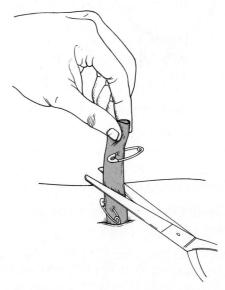

▼ **FIGURE 20–14.** Cutting off the excess drain.

9. Reapply dressings to the wound and drain site as described in Skill 20–3 (Fig. 20–15).

9. Dressings absorb drainage and protect the wound from airborne microorganisms.

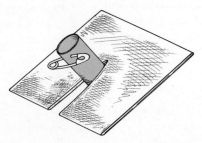

▼ **FIGURE 20–15.** Reapplying dressings to the wound and drain site.

▼ _ACTION_	▼ _RATIONALE_
10. Document the procedure.	**10.** Communicates with the other members of the health care team and contributes to the legal record by documenting the care given to the client.

Emptying a Closed Wound Drainage System and Reestablishing Suction

1. Put on examination gloves.	**1.** Protects you from contact with body fluids.
2. Open the drain plug and invert the drainage evacuation receptacle. Drain the contents into a graduated collection container.	**2.** Facilitates measurement and assessment of the drainage.
3. Place a Hemovac evacuation receptacle on a firm flat surface. Hold a Jackson-Pratt evacuation receptacle in your hand.	**3.** Prepares the device for reestablishing suction.
4. Compress the evacuation receptacle and close the drain plug while still compressing the device (Figs. 20–16 and 20–17).	**4.** Establishes a vacuum that provides suction.

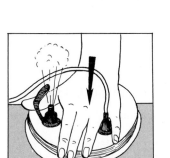

▼ **FIGURE 20–16.** Compressing the Hemovac and closing the drain plug.

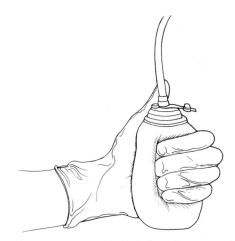

▼ **FIGURE 20–17.** Compressing the Jackson-Pratt evacuation receptacle and closing the drain plug.

5. Remove the gloves and wash your hands.	**5.** Reduces the transmission of microorganisms.
6. Document the procedure.	**6.** Communicates the findings to the other members of the health care team and contributes to the legal record by documenting the care given to the client.

Example of Documentation

DATE	TIME	NOTES
1/1/94	0900	Abdominal incision and drain site cleansed. No redness or edema noted. Yellow serous drainage noted from Penrose drain. Drain shortened 1 inch and sterile dressings reapplied.
		S. Smith, RN
1/1/94	1000	Hemovac emptied of 50 ml brownish red drainage. Vacuum reestablished and effective suction seen through drain.
		S. Woods, RN

Teaching Tips

When caring for wounds, you can discuss with the client wound healing and the client's progress toward wound resolution.

Home Care Variations

These same procedures can be instituted in the client's home. Place contaminated dressings in a plastic red bag and dispose of them according to your agency policy. Drainage should be flushed down the toilet.

SKILL 20–8   REMOVING SUTURES

Clinical Situations in Which You May Encounter This Skill

Sutures are usually removed 7 to 10 days after surgery and with a physician's order. Retention sutures, which are large surgical wound sutures, may be left in place for 14 to 21 days. Sutures may adhere to the skin if they are left in place for too long. If adherence occurs, apply hydrogen peroxide to the site with a cotton-tipped applicator or soak the area with gauze saturated with normal saline to loosen any encrustations or dried exudate before suture removal. Figure 20–18 illustrates various types of suture stitches.

Anticipated Responses

▼ The sutures are removed and the edges of the client's wound remain well approximated.
▼ Wound healing is promoted and no infection occurs.

Adverse Responses

▼ The sutures adhere to the client's skin.
▼ The edges of the wound are not well approximated and dehiscence or evisceration occurs.
▼ The wound becomes infected.

Materials List

Gather these materials before beginning the skill:

▼ Suture removal kit,
or
▼ Sterile forceps and sterile suture removal scissors
▼ Gauze 4- × 4-inch squares
▼ Waterproof disposable bag
▼ Sterile saline and gauze 4- × 4-inch pads for cleansing or prepackaged antiseptic swabs
▼ Sterile gloves
▼ Examination gloves
▼ Adhesive strips or butterfly adhesive tape (optional)

▼ *ACTION*	▼ *RATIONALE*
1. Assess the wound to determine whether the edges are well approximated and healing of the suture line has occurred.	1. Physicians often have standing orders for sutures to be removed at a specified date. If the wound is not well healed, the sutures should be left in place longer.
2. Ask the client if he or she has had sutures removed before. If not, explain the procedure.	2. Simple explanations reduce anxiety and apprehension.
3. Close the door and close the curtains around the client's bed.	3. Provides for privacy.
4. Help the client to assume a position of comfort with easy access and visibility of the suture line.	4. Facilitates removal of the sutures.
5. Drape the client so that only the suture area is exposed.	5. Provides for privacy and protects the modesty of the client.
6. Open the suture removal kit, or assemble supplies within easy access on a clean surface.	

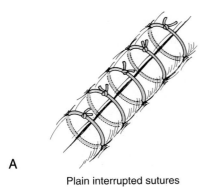

A

Plain interrupted sutures

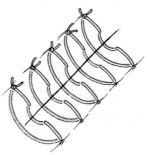

B

Mattress interrupted sutures

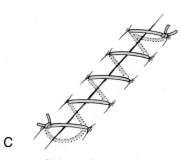

C

Plain continuous sutures

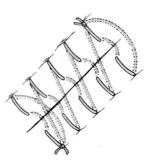

D

Mattress continuous sutures

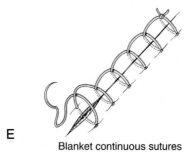

E

Blanket continuous sutures

▼ **FIGURE 20–18.** Types of suture stitches.

▼ *A C T I O N* _____   ▼ *R A T I O N A L E* _____

7. Don examination gloves. Remove the old dressing and put it in a disposable bag.

7. Protects the client from the transmission of microorganisms.

8. Remove examination gloves and wash your hands.

8. Decreases the transmission of microorganisms.

9. Don sterile gloves and cleanse the incision with saline-soaked gauze pads or antiseptic swabs.

9. Removes microorganisms from the incision.

10. To remove an interrupted suture, hold forceps in your nondominant hand and grasp the suture near the knot.

10. Pulls the suture up and away from the person's skin.

11. Place the curved edge of the scissors under the suture at or near the knot.

11. Facilitates clipping of the suture.

12. Cut the suture and pull it to remove it in one piece (Fig. 20–19).

12. Facilitates suture removal.

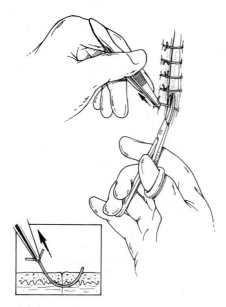

▼ **FIGURE 20–19.** Cutting and removing the suture.

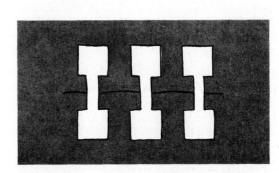

▼ **FIGURE 20–20.** Butterfly tape adhesive strips.

13. If the client has a continuous suture, cut both the first and second suture before removing them.

13. Facilitates removal of the suture without traumatizing the incision line.

14. Remove every other suture. Assess the suture line to ensure that the edges remain approximated.

14. Any dehiscence can be detected early, and every other suture can be left in place.

15. Discard the sutures onto the gauze squares as they are removed. Place the gauze squares in the disposable bag when all of the sutures have been removed.

15. Decreases the transmission of microorganisms.

16. (This step is optional.) Apply adhesive strips or butterfly tape adhesive strips (Fig. 20–20) across the suture line to secure the edges. Depending on the length of the suture line, adhesive skin closures may be placed 1 inch apart or closer together.

16. If the suture line pulls apart a little after the sutures are removed, adhesive skin closures can be used to reinforce the suture line.

17. Dispose of the soiled equipment.

17. Reduces odors in the client's room and prevents the transmission of microorganisms.

18. Remove gloves and wash your hands.

18. Decreases the transmission of microorganisms.

▼ *A C T I O N*	▼ *R A T I O N A L E*
19. Record the procedure. Note the appearance of the suture line, including redness, exudate, swelling, and approximation of the edges.	19. Communicates the findings to the other members of the health care team and contributes to the legal record by documenting the care given to the client.

Example of Documentation

DATE	TIME	NOTES
1/10/93	1100	Sutures removed. Suture line pink. No swelling or exudate present. Edges well approximated. Adhesive tape strips applied.
		S. Williams, RN

Teaching Tips

While you remove the sutures, teach the client about complications to report. For example, the client should report any drainage or separation of the edges of the suture line. If the wound is well healed, the client can use clean technique while performing dressing changes at home. Have the client and his or her family demonstrate the skill.

SKILL 20–9   REMOVING STAPLES

Clinical Situations in Which You May Encounter This Skill

Staples are used to close a wound after surgery. They are usually removed after 7 to 10 days, although variation occurs because of individual healing differences and physicians' preferences. Rarely does a wound dehisce after the staples are removed. If dehiscence occurs, cover the wound immediately with a sterile towel or dressing moistened with warm normal saline and notify the physician.

Anticipated Responses

▼ The staples are removed and the edges of the wound remain well approximated.
▼ Wound healing is promoted and no infection occurs.

Adverse Responses

▼ The edges of the wound are not well approximated and dehiscence or evisceration occurs.
▼ Signs and symptoms of infection occur.

Materials List

Gather these materials before beginning the skill:

▼ Staple extractor
▼ Gauze squares
▼ Examination gloves
▼ Sterile gloves
▼ Adhesive skin closure strips (optional)
▼ Butterfly adhesive tape (optional)
▼ Waterproof disposable bag
▼ Sterile saline and gauze 4- × 4-inch pads for cleansing or prepackaged antiseptic swabs

▼ *A C T I O N*	▼ *R A T I O N A L E*
1. Assess the wound to determine whether the edges are well approximated and healing of the suture line has occurred.	1. Physicians often have standing orders for staples to be removed at a specified date. If the wound is not healed well, the staples may need to remain in place longer.
2. Ask the client if he or she has had staples removed before. If not, explain the procedure.	2. Simple explanations reduce anxiety and apprehension.

▼ *A C T I O N*	▼ *R A T I O N A L E*
3. Close the door and the curtains around the client's bed.	**3.** Provides for privacy.
4. Help the client to assume a position of comfort with easy access and visibility of the suture line.	**4.** Facilitates removal of the staples.
5. Drape the client so that only the suture area is exposed.	**5.** Provides for privacy and protects the modesty of the client.
6. Remove the staple extractor from the covering and place it within easy access on a clean surface.	
7. Open a package of gauze pads and place it within easy reach.	**7.** The staples are placed on the gauze pads after removal.
8. Don examination gloves. Remove the old dressing and place it in a disposable bag.	**8.** Protects the client from the transmission of micro-organisms.
9. Remove examination gloves and wash hands.	**9.** Decreases the transmission of microorganisms.
10. Put on sterile gloves and cleanse the incision with saline-soaked gauze pads or antiseptic swabs (see Skill 20–1).	**10.** Removes microorganisms from the incision line.
11. Place the lower edge of the staple extractor under the first staple.	**11.** Staples are removed one at a time.
12. Press the handles of the staple extractor together and lift the staple out of the client's skin (Fig. 20–21).	**12.** The staple is depressed in the center and the staple edges lift upward out of the client's skin.

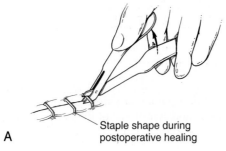

A — Staple shape during postoperative healing

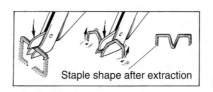

Staple shape after extraction   B

▼ **FIGURE 20–21.** Removing staples.

13. Leave the handles pressed together and move the staple over to the gauze square. Release the handles.	**13.** Releasing the handles allows the staple to drop onto the gauze square.
14. Continue the process, removing every other staple.	**14.** Any dehiscence can be detected and the remaining staples can be left in place.
15. Assess the suture line to ensure that the edges remain well approximated.	**15.** If the edges are not well approximated, adhesive skin closure strips may need to be applied or the remaining staples may be left in place.
16. Continue to remove all of the sutures if the suture line appears well healed.	**16.** All sutures should be removed after the wound has healed.
17. (This step is optional.) If needed, apply adhesive skin closure strips or butterfly adhesive strips (see Fig. 20–20) across the suture line to secure the edges. Depending on the length of the suture line, adhesive skin closure strips may be placed 1 inch apart or closer together.	**17.** Adhesive skin closure strips help to keep skin edges approximated after sutures are removed.

▼ A C T I O N	▼ R A T I O N A L E
18. Dispose of soiled equipment.	18. Reduces the transmission of microorganisms.
19. Remove gloves and wash your hands.	19. Decreases the transmission of microorganisms.
20. Record the procedure. Note the appearance of the suture line, including redness, exudate, swelling, and approximation of the edges.	20. Communicates the findings to the other members of the health care team and contributes to the legal record by documenting the care given to the client.

Example of Documentation

DATE	TIME	NOTES
8/10/94	1000	Staples removed. Suture line pink. No swelling or exudate present. Edges well approximated. Adhesive skin closure strips applied.
		S. Williams, RN

Teaching Tips

While you remove the staples, teach the client about complications to report. For example, the client should report any drainage or separation of the edges of the suture line. If the wound is closed, the client should use clean technique while performing dressing changes at home. Have the client and his or her family demonstrate the skill.

SKILL 20–10   PROVIDING UMBILICAL CORD CARE FOR AN INFANT

Clinical Situations in Which You May Encounter This Skill

Umbilical cord care is necessary for every newborn infant. The umbilical cord is clamped or tied with umbilical tape and cut immediately after delivery.

Anticipated Responses

▼ The umbilical cord dries, shrivels, becomes black, and falls off within 2 to 3 weeks of birth.

Adverse Responses

▼ Bleeding occurs from the umbilical cord.
▼ Healing is delayed.

▼ Redness, swelling, and tenderness of the skin around the umbilical stump indicate that the cord has become infected.

Materials List

Gather these materials before beginning the skill:

▼ Triple-dye antimicrobial solution
▼ Alcohol
▼ Cotton balls
▼ Examination gloves

▼ A C T I O N	▼ R A T I O N A L E
1. Check the hospital policy for cord care.	1. Hospital policies vary.
2. When the infant arrives in the nursery, inspect the vessels in the cord.	2. There should be two arteries and one vein. The presence of only one artery may indicate congenital anomalies. The umbilical cord should be white and gelatinous.
3. Don examination gloves.	3. Prevents the transmission of microorganisms.

▼ *ACTION*   ▼ *RATIONALE*

Providing Initial Umbilical Cord Care

4. Open the container of triple-dye solution.	**4.** The solution is applied to the cord stump to prevent infection.
5. Gently pull the stump upward to raise it off the baby's abdomen.	**5.** Exposes the entire stump, including the base of the stump.
6. Swab the stump with triple-dye solution, proceeding from the clamp to the base of the stump on the baby's abdomen.	**6.** Triple-dye solution is a broad-spectrum antimicrobial agent used to prevent infections of the umbilical stump.
7. Swab 1 inch around the stump in a circular motion, starting adjacent to the base of the stump and moving outward.	**7.** Prevents contamination of the umbilical cord stump.
8. Remove the gloves and wash your hands.	**8.** After the gloves are removed, wash your hands to prevent the possible transmission of microorganisms.
9. Assess the parents' knowledge and ability to care for the cord following discharge.	**9.** The parents may require information.
10. Record the procedure. Note the number of vessels and the type of solution used on the umbilical cord.	**10.** Communicates the findings to the other members of the health care team and contributes to the legal record by documenting the care given to the client.

Providing Subsequent Cord Care

11. Don examination gloves.	**11.** Prevents the transmission of microorganisms.
12. At each diaper change, gently raise the umbilical stump up off the baby's abdomen.	**12.** Exposes the entire umbilical stump.
13. Swab the umbilical cord stump and base with alcohol-soaked cotton balls.	**13.** Promotes drying of the stump. If the stump is moist, healing is delayed.
14. Immediately before discharge, or at 2 days of age, remove the umbilical clamp.	**14.** The arteries and vein are closed and the danger of hemorrhage has passed.
15. Remove the gloves and wash your hands.	**15.** After the gloves are removed, wash your hands to prevent the possible transmission of microorganisms.
16. Record the procedure. Note the condition of the cord.	**16.** Communicates the findings to the other members of the health care team and contributes to the legal record by documenting the care given to the client.

Example of Documentation

DATE	TIME	NOTES
10/19/93	1000	Umbilical clamp removed. Cord dry, shriveled. No odor noted. Mother instructed as to home cord care. Return demonstration by mother.
		S. Williams, RN

Home Care Variations

Teach the mother or the primary caretaker to lift the baby's umbilical cord and apply alcohol at each diaper change. The infant should not be submerged in a full tub bath until the cord has fallen off. Whenever the cord becomes wet, soak the cord with alcohol.

SKILL 20–11   PROVIDING CIRCUMCISION CARE

Clinical Situations in Which You May Encounter This Skill

Male infants may have a surgical procedure to remove the prepuce, or foreskin, from the glans of the penis before discharge from the newborn nursery. Parents may request that a circumcision be performed because of personal preferences (e.g., they may want the infant to look like the father or brother), hygienic purposes, or religious preferences. The foreskin may be removed with a Gomco clamp or a Plastibell.

Anticipated Responses

▼ The glans of the infant's penis appears very red for 24 to 36 hours.
▼ The circumcision site heals without evidence of hemorrhage or infection.
▼ The infant is able to void without difficulty.

Adverse Responses

▼ The circumcision site hemorrhages or becomes infected.
▼ The infant has difficulty voiding because of trauma and edema.

Materials List

Gather these materials before beginning the skill:

▼ Circumcision board
▼ Gomco clamp or Plastibell
▼ Petroleum jelly gauze
▼ Sterile gloves

▼ ACTION	▼ RATIONALE
1. Make sure that the consent form has been signed by the parents.	1. Parents must be informed of the risks associated with circumcision.
2. Determine if the parents have further questions about the circumcision.	2. Provides an opportunity for education.
3. Remove the infant's diaper.	3. Exposes the penis.
4. Restrain the infant on the circumcision board.	4. Prevents movement of the infant.
5. Administer analgesics as ordered by the physician.	5. Reduces the pain from the procedure.
6. During the circumcision, assess the infant's response.	6. The infant may experience pain.
7. If the infant cries in pain, gently stroke his forehead and talk in a calm and soothing voice.	7. May calm the infant and distract his attention from the pain.
8. Following the procedure, put on sterile gloves and apply petroleum jelly gauze to the circumcision site.	8. Controls bleeding and prevents the diaper from adhering to the area.
9. Assess the circumcision site for bleeding. If bleeding occurs, report it to the physician.	9. The circumcised area oozes blood, but no frank bleeding should occur.
10. Position the infant on his side with the diaper loosely attached.	10. A side-lying position and a loose diaper prevent pressure on the circumcision area.
11. Remove gloves and wash your hands.	11. Decreases the transmission of microorganisms.

▼ *ACTION*	▼ *RATIONALE*
12. Watch the infant void to assess for the adequacy of the stream, amount, and the presence of blood.	**12.** Trauma and edema should be reported to the physician.
13. Teach the parents to assess for signs and symptoms of infection (foul smelling discharge, swelling) and to report them to the clinician immediately. If a Plastibell is used, teach the parents that the bell will fall off within 3 to 4 days.	**13.** Infections should be treated. Client education helps the parents to adequately care for the infant.
14. Record the procedure. Note the amount of bleeding and edema and the pattern of voiding.	**14.** Communicates the findings to the other members of the health care team and contributes to the legal record by documenting the care given to the client.

Example of Documentation

DATE	TIME	NOTES
10/19/93	0900	Circumcision using Gomco per Dr. Jones. Petroleum jelly gauze applied. No bleeding or edema noted. Parents taught to cleanse circumcision site with warm water after each bowel movement. Mother repeated instructions.
		S. Williams, RN

SKILL 20–12   APPLYING BANDAGE WRAPS

Clinical Situations in Which You May Encounter This Skill

Bandages may be applied to any body part. A variety of bandage materials and techniques may be used to immobilize a joint, secure a dressing or piece of equipment (such as Bucks traction) in place, position an extremity, provide comfort and warmth, facilitate deep respirations or coughing, reduce swelling, maintain or improve circulation, or provide general support to an area of the body.

The type and size of the bandage used depend on its purpose and the body part bandaged. Bandages are made of cotton materials such as lightweight porous gauze, elastic materials, muslin, or flannel.

The technique used to apply a bandage varies according to the body part to be covered and the purpose of the bandage. Circular turns are used for bandaging digits or the wrists. Using spiral turns to apply a bandage is appropriate if the bandage is to cover cylindrical body parts such as slender wrists or forearms that do not vary significantly in contour. Spiral reverse turns may be used to bandage a part of the body that forms an inverted cone, such as a larger forearm or the calf of the leg. Figure-of-eight turns effectively cover and immobilize joints. Recurrent turns may be used to bandage the head like a cap or to bandage an amputated limb.

Gauze bandages allow circulation of air and are used only once. Gauze is available in ½-inch to 6-inch widths. The narrow gauze is used on small body parts such as fingers or toes. The wider gauze is used to cover larger surfaces.

Elastic wraps are available in 1- to 6-inch widths for use on small children or adults. The elastic bandage assumes the shape of the body part covered and may be used multiple times to secure dressings on amputated limbs, extremities, a hand, or a foot. The elastic bandage is lightly stretched with even pressure around the body part.

Flannel and muslin bandages provide support, strength, and warmth to a body part. Triangular slings of muslin provide support for an upper extremity or lower extremity in traction. Slings may be used to immobilize a fracture of the humerus, radius, or ulna.

Anticipated Responses

▼ The bandage is applied in a smooth manner with even pressure to the body part.
▼ The client is comfortable and does not have signs of nervous impairment such as pain, numbness, or tingling of the bandaged area or areas distal to the bandage.

▼ The client's circulation is not impaired. His or her extremities remain warm and pink in color and have palpable pulses equal in comparison to the other extremity and good capillary refill. If a breast binder is used, chest expansion is not impeded.

Adverse Responses

▼ Venous stasis occurs. The bandage is applied too tightly and impaired circulation results. Impaired circulation is determined by pallor or cyanosis, cool skin, or weak or absent pulses distal to the bandage. The client may complain of pain, numbness, or tingling in the bandaged area. If this occurs, the bandage should be removed, the area should be reassessed, and the physician should be notified (depending on the assessment).

▼ The joint is positioned incorrectly and a contracture results. The bandage is not applied in a smooth manner with even pressure and skin breakdown occurs under the bandage.

Materials List

Gather these materials before beginning the skill:

▼ Clips, safety pin, or tape to secure the bandage in place

▼ Bandage material as needed for the type of bandage to be used:
For an arm sling:
   Triangular muslin cloth
   Safety pin
For a circular wrap:
   1-inch-wide roll of gauze
   Scissors
   1/4-inch tape
For a spiral wrap:
   1-inch-wide roll of gauze or elastic bandage
   Scissors
   1/4-inch tape
For a spiral reverse wrap:
   1-inch-wide roll of gauze or elastic bandage
   Scissors
   1/4-inch tape
For a figure-of-eight wrap:
   Elastic bandage
   1/4-inch tape
For a recurrent wrap:
   1-inch-wide roll of gauze
   1/4-inch tape

▼ ACTION	▼ RATIONALE
1. Introduce yourself to the client and explain the procedure.	1. Simple explanations reduce anxiety and apprehension.
2. Assess the area to be bandaged to determine the bandaging materials needed.	2. The material required varies according to the area to be covered and the purpose of the bandage.
3. Assess the skin to be bandaged for broken areas, redness, or swelling.	3. Provides a means of comparison when the bandage is removed.
4. Apply the bandage.	

Applying an Arm Sling

a. Place the open sling across the client's chest with the apex of the triangle extending beyond the client's elbow on the affected side (Fig. 20–22A).	a. Facilitates application of the sling.
b. Place the upper point of the triangle across the client's clavicle on the unaffected side and behind the client's neck (Fig. 20–22B).	b. The lower point of the sling is brought up and around on the affected side to tie the sling at the back of the client's neck.
c. Help the client to position his or her arm at an 80-degree or lower angle.	c. This angle prevents dependent edema in the hands and fingers.
d. Bring the sling over the client's forearm and hand.	d. The sling provides support for the forearm and hand.
e. Extend the lower point of the sling around the client's neck on the affected side.	e. Allows the sling to be tied around the client's neck.
f. Reassess the angle of the client's arm.	f. Adjustments in the angle of the arm may need to be made.
g. Secure the sling with a square knot or safety pin at a point on the client's upper anterior chest wall.	g. Keeps the sling from becoming loose. This knot placement prevents pressure and discomfort at the person's neck.

▼ *A C T I O N*　　　　　　　　　　　　▼ *R A T I O N A L E*

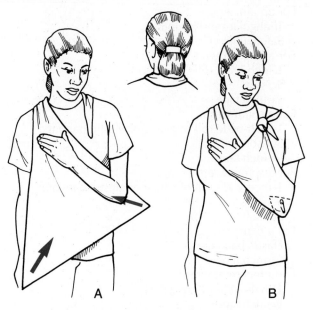

▼ **FIGURE 20–22.** Applying an arm sling.

h. Fold the remaining cloth extending from the client's elbow and secure it with a safety pin.	h. Encloses the client's elbow with the extra material.
i. Place padding under the knot if needed.	i. Promotes comfort.
j. Inspect the clavicle area and check the angle of the client's arm.	j. Ensures that the sling is providing support to the arm and prevents pressure on the clavicle.

Applying a Bandage Using Circular Turns

a. Hold the roll of gauze in your dominant hand.	a. This hand is used to apply the gauze.
b. Place the flat surface of gauze on the anterior surface to be bandaged.	b. Allows the gauze to be applied smoothly.
c. Unroll the gauze. Overlap and circle it two times around the digit or wrist being bandaged (Fig. 20–23).	c. Provides even pressure to the body part being bandaged.

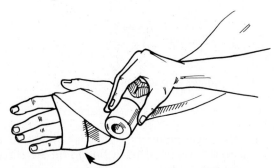

▼ **FIGURE 20–23.** Applying a bandage using circular turns.

d. Cut the gauze with scissors.	d. Since only a portion of the gauze is usually used, it can be cut and the rest can be saved.
e. Fold the end under.	e. Gauze ravels if the edges are exposed.
f. Secure the end of the gauze with tape.	f. Helps to keep the gauze from unrolling.

▼ ACTION

Applying a Bandage Using Spiral Turns

   a. Circle the bandage two times around the distal end of the body part being bandaged.

   b. Apply the dressing from the distal to the proximal border by overlapping the previous turn one-half to three-quarters the width of the bandage (Fig. 20–24).

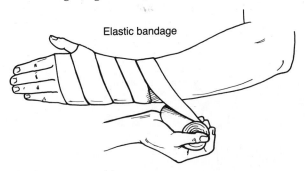

▼ FIGURE 20–24. Applying a bandage using spiral turns.

   c. Cut the end of the bandage with scissors.

   d. Secure the dressing with tape.

Applying a Bandage Using Spiral Reverse Turns

   a. Circle the bandage two times around the distal end of the body part being covered.

   b. Apply the bandage from the distal border to the proximal border at a 30-degree angle (Fig. 20–25) by:

     i. Placing your thumb on the anterior surface of the bandage.

     ii. Folding the bandage onto itself so the folded edges form an inverted "V."

     iii. Wrapping the bandage around the posterior aspect of the body part.

   c. Repeat Steps 27 through 28 until the entire area to be covered is bandaged.

   d. Complete the bandaging with two circular turns.

   e. Secure the dressing with tape.

▼ RATIONALE

   a. Secures the bandage in place.

   b. Allows the entire area to be covered.

   c. Any excess bandage material should be removed. Excess bandage material can cause uneven pressure.

   d. Keeps the bandage from unrolling.

   a. This turn anchors the bandage.

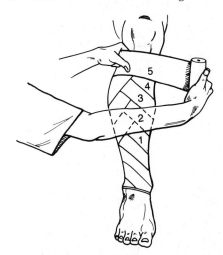

▼ FIGURE 20–25. Applying a bandage using spiral reverse turns.

     i. Holds the bandage in place.

     ii. This turn forms the "reverse" spiral portion of the dressing.

     iii. Covers the posterior part of the body part.

   d. Secures the bandage.

   e. Tape keeps the bandage from unrolling.

▼ *ACTION*   ▼ *RATIONALE*

Applying a Bandage Using a Figure-of-Eight Turn

a. Circle the bandage two times around the distal end of the body part being bandaged.

b. Advance the bandage above the joint and circle it around the posterior aspect of the limb.

c. Bring the bandage down. Cross over the anterior aspect of the joint.

d. Continue wrapping the bandage above and below the person's joint to form the figure-of-eight turns until the joint is completely wrapped (Fig. 20–26).

a. Secures the bandage.

b. Forms the top of the figure of eight.

c. Forms the bottom of the figure of eight.

d. The entire joint is covered for support.

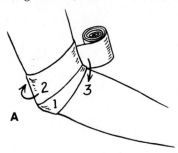 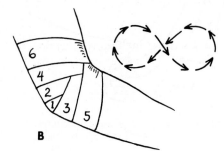

▼ **FIGURE 20–26.** Applying a bandage using a figure-of-eight turn.

e. Complete the bandaging with two circular turns.

f. Secure the dressing with tape.

e. Secures the bandage in place.

f. Helps to keep the dressing from loosening.

Applying a Bandage Using Recurrent Turns

a. Wrap the bandage around the proximal area in two circular turns.

b. In the center front, make a reverse turn and advance the gauze toward the back of the body part being covered and end in the center back.

c. Reverse the turn in the back and advance the gauze over the body part being covered, ending in the center front.

d. Continue the reverse turns until the entire body part is covered (Fig. 20–27).

a. Secures the bandage in place.

b. Allows the head to be covered evenly and smoothly.

Recurrent bandage used on head

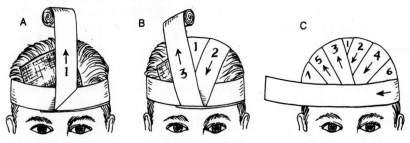

Recurrent bandage used on leg stump

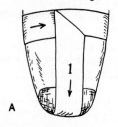 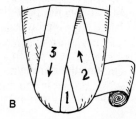 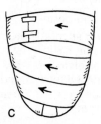

▼ **FIGURE 20–27.** Applying a bandage using recurrent turns.

▼ *ACTION*

▼ *RATIONALE*

    e. Complete the bandaging with two circular turns.

    f. Secure the dressing with tape.

    e. Secures the bandage.

    f. Helps keep the bandage from loosening.

NOTE: When changing a bandage:
    a. Assess the skin integrity, color, and temperature.
    b. Assess the client's level of comfort and ability to conduct activities of daily living.

Provides continuing data for evaluating and comparing the client's health status.

---

5. Record the procedure and include your evaluation of the client.

5. Communicates the findings to the other members of the health care team and contributes to the legal record by documenting the care given to the client.

Example of Documentation

DATE	TIME	NOTES
2/5/94	0930	Changed dressing on forearm using spiral bandaging. Wound 2 cm × 4 cm. No redness, swelling, or exudate present.
		S. Williams, RN

Teaching Tips

Dressing changes provide opportunities to teach the client and his or her family how to apply the bandage and to assess their ability to apply the dressing. Have the client and his or her caregiver demonstrate the skill.

Home Care Variations

Assess the client's environment to determine his or her safety and mobility with a bandage in place. Assess the client's dexterity and his or her motivation and ability to apply and wear the bandage as recommended by the primary health care provider.

SKILL 20–13 APPLYING BINDERS

Clinical Situations in Which You May Encounter This Skill

Breast and abdominal binders are used for support and protection. Breast binders may be a rectangular-shaped piece of muslin cloth with or without Velcro, or a vest-style binder. The breast binder may be used to apply pressure to the breast tissue and thus suppress lactation after childbirth or to provide support after breast surgery. The breast binder is applied snugly to the chest wall, but it must not impede respiration.

Abdominal binders (straight and scultetus) provide protection and support to the abdomen and protect suture lines from tension or stress. The straight binder has a long extension on each side to surround, protect, and support the abdomen. The scultetus binder has many tails that are wrapped around the abdomen to provide suppport.

T-binders are used to secure bandages if a client has had perineal or anal surgery. The single T-binder is used for female clients, and the double T-binder is used for male clients.

Anticipated Responses

▼ The binder is applied in a smooth manner with even pressure to the person's body part.
▼ The client is comfortable and chest expansion is not impeded.

Adverse Responses

▼ The breast or abdominal binder is applied too tightly and the client's chest expansion is impaired.

▼ The binder is not applied in a smooth and even manner and skin breakdown occurs under the bandage.

Materials List

Gather these materials before beginning the skill:

▼ Select the correct binder:
Breast binder
Abdominal, straight, or scultetus binder
T-binder or double T-binder
▼ Safety pins

▼ ACTION

1. Assess the area to be bandaged to determine the bandaging materials needed.

2. Assess the skin to be bandaged for broken areas, redness, or swelling.

3. Help the client to assume a supine position.

4. Apply the binder.

Applying a Breast Binder

   a. Remove the client's gown from his or her upper torso and drape the client. Expose only the person's chest area.
   b. Place a muslin rectangular cloth behind the client's chest.
   c. Bring the binder edges around to the client's anterior chest (Fig. 20–28) by
     i. Having the client inhale deeply.

     ii. Overlapping the edges of the binder.
     iii. Placing your fingers under the binder at the nipple line and next to the client's skin.
     iv. Pinning the edges of the binder together starting at the nipple line and moving up and down the edges of the binder.
   d. For a vest-style binder, put the vest on the client and follow the above procedure for closure.

▼ RATIONALE

1. The material required varies according to the area to be covered and the purpose of the bandage.

2. Provides a means of evaluation when the bandage is removed.

3. A comfortable position facilitates application of the binder.

   a. Protects the client's privacy.

   b. The binder is applied from back to front.

     i. Prevents excessive constriction of the client's chest wall.

     iii. Prevents the pins from sticking to the client's skin.
     iv. Secures the binder ends.

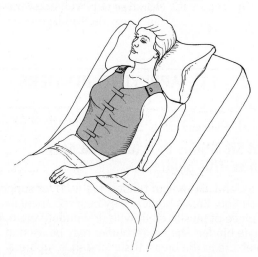

▼ **FIGURE 20–28.** A breast binder.

▼ _A C T I O N_   ▼ _R A T I O N A L E_

Applying Straight and Scultetus Abdominal Binders

a. Fanfold half of the binder lengthwise.

b. Raise the side rail opposite you.
c. Help the client to roll onto his or her side facing the raised side rail.
d. Place a folded binder under the client and have the client roll back onto the binder and to the other side. Pull the remainder of the binder from under the client.
e. Help the client to assume a supine position with his or her head slightly elevated and knees slightly bent.
f. Apply the binder. To apply a straight abdominal binder (Fig. 20–29):
   i. Pull the sides of the binder together to meet vertically in the middle.

> **NOTE:** The binder should be between the client's symphysis pubis and the lower rib cage.

a. Makes placement of the binder under the client easier.
b. Prevents the client from falling off the bed.
c. Helps you to place the binder under the client.

d. Conserves your energy and facilitates application of the binder.

e. Reduces tension and stress on the abdominal suture line.

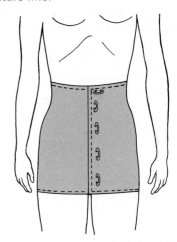

▼ **FIGURE 20–29.** A straight abdominal binder.

   ii. Secure the binder with Velcro or with safety pins.

To apply a scultetus abdominal binder (Fig. 20–30):
   i. Starting at the left bottom tail of the binder, pull the tail to the midline. Maintain tension and overlap the tail with the bottom right tail.
   ii. Continue overlapping each pair of tails with tension until all are secured in the middle.
   iii. Secure the top set of tails with a safety pin.

   ii. Maintains continuous and even support to the abdominal wall and suture line.

   i. Maintains continuous and even support to the abdominal wall and suture line.

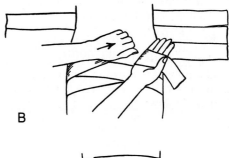

B

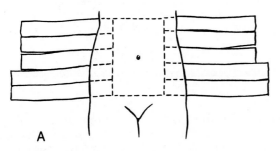

A

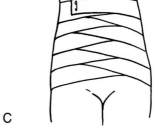

C

▼ **FIGURE 20–30.** A scultetus abdominal binder.

▼ *ACTION* _____   ▼ *RATIONALE* _____

Applying T-Binders and Double T-Binders

a. Help the client to bend his or her knees and slightly raise his or her buttocks.

b. Place the binder under the client with the horizontal bands under his or her waist and the bottom portions of the T-binder under the client's gluteal folds.

c. Overlap the horizontal band around the client's waist (above the iliac crest).

d. Secure the bands in the middle of the client's waist with a safety pin placed horizontally.

e. Secure the binder.

   i. For a T-binder (Fig. 20–31*A*):

   • Bring the bottom portion of the T-binder up between the client's legs, over the perineum, and under the waistband.

a. Reduces tension on the client's abdominal wall and suture line.

b. The horizontal bands are secured around the client's waist to anchor the binder in place. The bottom of the T-binder comes between the client's legs and is anchored in the front at the waist.

c. Secures the binder around the waist.

d. Allows for comfort when the client bends at the waist.

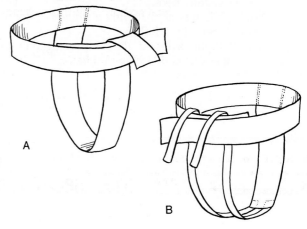

▼ **FIGURE 20–31.** T-binder *(A)* used for women and double T-binder *(B)* used for men.

   • Fold the flap over the waistband and secure it with a horizontally placed safety pin.

   ii. For a double T-binder (Fig. 20–31*B*):

   • Bring the bottom portions of the T-binder between the client's legs, over the scrotal and perineal areas, and to either side of the penis.

   • Fold the flaps over the waistband and secure them with horizontally placed safety pins.

   • Provides for comfort as the client bends at the waist and maintains pressure on the perineal area.

   • Provides support to the perineum and avoids undue pressure on the penis.

   • Allows for comfort as the client bends.

NOTE: When changing the bandage:
   a. Assess the skin integrity, color, and temperature.
   b. Assess the client's level of comfort and ability to deep breathe and conduct activities of daily living.

This information should be recorded in the client's chart. It assesses the safety of the binder application.

---

5. Record the procedure and include your evaluation of the client.

5. Communicates the findings to the other members of the health care team and contributes to the legal record by documenting the care given to the client.

Example of Documentation

DATE	TIME	NOTES
1/23/94	0800	Breasts engorged and leaking milk. Skin smooth and shiny. Client complaining of breast discomfort. Breast binder applied smoothly with even pressure. Client states that she feels more comfortable with binder in place.

S. Williams, RN

Home Care Variations

Assess the client's or his or her family member's ability to apply the binder correctly and comply with the procedure.

Teaching Tips

Teach the client to remove the T-binder before urinating or defecating and how to reapply the binder. With any binder, clients should be taught to report any increased pain, drainage, or numbness.

SKILL 20–14   APPLYING A SPLINT

Clinical Situations in Which You May Encounter This Skill

Clients who require immobilization of a body part may need a splint. The body part may be fractured or sprained, or its movement may impede other treatments such as intravenous infusions.

Anticipated Responses

▼ The body part immobilized by the splint is in correct alignment.
▼ Circulation in the body area distal to the immobilized area is uncompromised.
▼ The client's pain is decreased.
▼ The client does not complain of numbness or any signs of increased swelling.

Adverse Responses

▼ The body part immobilized by the splint is out of alignment.
▼ Circulation in the body area distal to the splinted area is compromised.
▼ The client complains of numbness, increased pain, or swelling in the splinted part.

Materials List

Gather these materials before beginning the skill:

▼ Splint (the type [Fig. 20–32] depends on the body part to be immobilized)

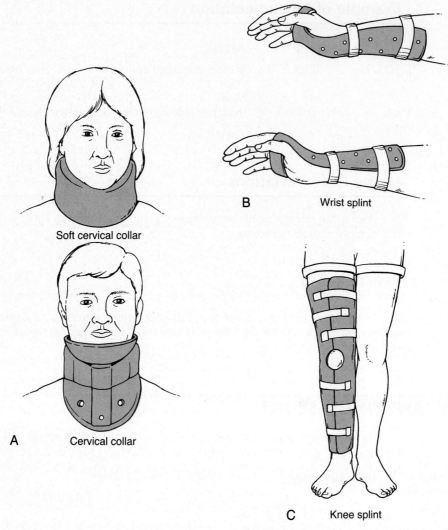

Soft cervical collar

B   Wrist splint

A   Cervical collar

C   Knee splint

▼ **FIGURE 20–32.** Types of splints.

▼ *A C T I O N*

1. Determine the area that needs to be immobilized and the reason for immobilization.

2. Assess circulation in the body area at and distal to the injured area. Observe the area for color, moisture, temperature, swelling, edema, pulses, capillary refill, intact skin, and whether or not the client has any pain or numbness.

3. Allow the client to talk about what happened to him or her.

4. Choose a splint that will immobilize the area.

5. Place the splint on the client's body so that it will support the area and inhibit movement of that area.

6. Assess the circulation of the body area distal to the splint.

7. Wash your hands.

▼ *R A T I O N A L E*

1. Assists you in deciding what needs to be done and which materials are needed.

2. Provides baseline data.

3. The client may be upset about the cause and extent of the injury. Talking helps to allay anxiety.

4. An appropriate splint provides support and immobilization to the area.

5. The purpose of a splint is to provide support and limit mobility.

6. The splint should provide support, but venous return should not be compromised.

7. Decreases the transmission of microorganisms.

▼ _A C T I O N_	▼ _R A T I O N A L E_
8. Record the procedure.	**8.** Communicates the findings to the other members of the health care team and contributes to the legal record by documenting the care given to the client.
9. Periodically evaluate whether or not the splint is providing immobilization as needed.	**9.** Determines the effectiveness of the splint.
10. Assess the circulation in the body parts distal to the splint, as well as the client's comfort.	**10.** Determines the effectiveness of the splint.

Example of Documentation

DATE	TIME	NOTES
1/23/93	1138	Immobilizing splint applied to client's left hand and forearm. Hand distal to splint is pink, warm, and dry. No swelling noted, and skin is intact. Radial pulse is 2+. Capillary refill time is <1 second. Client denies numbness in affected extremity.
		S. Williams, RN

Teaching Tips

Explain the purpose of the splint to the client. Instruct the client to seek medical help if the distal portion of the extremity that is splinted becomes cool or numb or has decreased movement. The client should also seek medical care if the skin under the splint becomes irritated or develops a rash.

Home Care Variations

Temporary splints can be applied in the client's home using a sturdy object such as a tongue blade or board and tape.

SKILL 20–15   DRESSING AN AMPUTATED LIMB

Clinical Situations in Which You May Encounter This Skill

A residual limb (stump) must be carefully wrapped in the postoperative period to shrink and shape the stump into a conical form in preparation for application of a prosthesis. Wrapping the stump supports the soft tissue, facilitates venous return, prevents swelling, and shapes the stump into a cone. The bandage is applied so that remaining muscles needed to operate the prosthesis are as firm as possible, and those muscles no longer useful will atrophy.

In the immediate postoperative period, hemorrhage is the most common complication. Thus, a tourniquet is needed at the client's bedside.

The client should be placed in the prone position for several hours each day following the amputation of a lower extremity. This position extends the amputated limb and prevents a flexion contracture at the remaining joint.

Anticipated Responses

▼ The stump is wrapped in an elastic Ace bandage in a smooth and even manner.

▼ The stump assumes a firm cone shape.
▼ Venous return is promoted and there is no edema in the stump.
▼ Range of motion of the extremity is maintained.
▼ The client does not complain of pain, numbness, or tingling in the stump area.
▼ The skin is intact, pink, and warm.

Adverse Responses

▼ The client develops circulatory problems or a poorly shaped stump that does not fit well into the prosthesis.

▼ The client complains of tingling or numbness in the wrapped area.
▼ The extremity becomes cool, cyanotic, or blanched.

Materials List

Gather these materials before beginning the skill:

▼ 3- to 4-inch Ace elastic bandage (or smaller for an upper extremity or child)
▼ Metal clips or tape
▼ 4- × 4-inch gauze pads (optional)
▼ Sterile gloves (optional)

▼ ACTION	▼ RATIONALE
1. Check the client's chart for the date of surgery and the surgical procedure.	1. The stage of wound healing depends on the date of surgery. The type of bandage depends on the type of surgery.
2. Ask the client if he or she has a preference for the type of bandaging technique to be used.	2. The client may be aware of a bandaging technique that has been effective and provided comfort to him or her in the past.
3. Close the door and draw the curtains around the client's bed. (Steps 4–11 apply to clients in the immediate postoperative period if the suture line is not healed.)	3. Provides for privacy.
4. Help the client to assume a supine position.	4. A supine position facilitates visibility of the stump and the subsequent bandage change.
5. Drape the client, exposing only the stump area.	5. Provides for privacy and prevents exposure of the client.
6. Remove the bandage presently on the stump.	6. Allows for visibility of the stump.
7. Assess the stump for size and stage of healing.	7. The size of the stump determines the size of the elastic bandage needed. The stage of healing dictates the type of dressing material to be applied directly to the suture line. Assessing the stump alerts you to whether or not the stump is healing properly.
8. Don sterile gloves.	8. Prevents the transmission of microorganisms.
9. Clean the suture line, if needed, according to your agency procedure.	9. If the suture line is not completely healed, exudate may need to be removed.
10. Place unfolded 4- × 4-inch gauze pads on the suture line of the amputated limb.	10. The sterile 4- × 4-inch gauze pads absorb drainage and protect the incision from microorganisms that may cause infection.
11. Remove and discard your gloves in a proper receptacle.	11. Proper disposal decreases the transmission of microorganisms.
12. Help the client to assume a semi-Fowler's position in bed or a sitting position on the side of the bed.	12. This position facilitates dressing the amputated stump.
13. Hold the elastic wrap in your dominant hand with the roll facing upward.	13. Facilitates unrolling the bandage and application in a smooth and even manner.
14. Figure-eight dressing (for above-the-knee amputation): a. Beginning on the client's anterior thigh, wrap the bandage at an oblique angle toward the distal end of the client's stump (Fig. 20–33A).	

▼ *ACTION*   ▼ *RATIONALE*

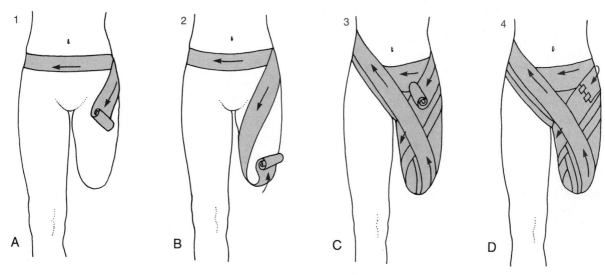

▼ **FIGURE 20–33.** Figure-eight dressing, above the knee amputation.

b. Continue wrapping the bandage around the medial and lateral aspects of the client's stump (Fig. 20–33*B*).
c. Continue wrapping the bandage around to the anterior aspect of the stump, forming a figure eight.
d. Circle the bandage up and around the client's hips.
e. Continue wrapping the bandage up the client's stump, overlapping the previous figure-eight turns (Fig. 20–33*C*).
f. Anchor the bandage with tape or metal clips that are provided with the bandaging material (Fig. 20–33*D*).

    d. Circling the bandage around the client's hips secures the bandage in place.
    e. Completely covers the area.

    f. Tapes or clips secure the bandage and help keep it from becoming loose.

15. Recurrent bandage for above- or below-the-knee residual limb or amputation below the elbow:
    a. Anchor the bandage at the proximal end of the stump toward the client's body with two circular turns.
    b. Cover the entire stump with recurrent turns (see Skill 20–12).
    c. Wrap the bandage with two circular turns at the proximal site.
    d. Secure the dressing with tape or metal clips.

    a. Prevents bandage from slipping.

    b. Assists with shaping the stump into a cone form.
    c. Helps prevent the dressing from dislodging.

    d. Prevents the dressing from becoming loose.

16. Figure-eight bandage of above-the-elbow residual limb:
    a. Cover the end of the amputated limb with two recurrent turns.
    b. Wrap the stump with figure-eight turns using even and smooth pressure.
    c. Wrap the dressing around the client's back and shoulders.
    d. Secure the dressing with metal clips.

    a. Anchors the dressing in place.

    b. If the bandage is not smooth, skin breakdown can occur.
    c. Prevents the dressing from sliding off the limb.

    d. Prevents the dressing from becoming loose.

17. Spiral bandage of amputated limb:
    a. Cover the distal end of the stump with recurrent turns (anterior to posterior) to cover the incision line.

    a. Protects the incision line from friction and exposure.

▼ ACTION	▼ RATIONALE
b. Cover the remaining stump (from distal to proximal toward the client's body) with spiral turns using smooth and even pressure.	b. Assists with shaping the stump into a cone form.
c. Wrap the bandage around the client's hips.	c. Secures the dressing and prevents the bandage from falling down.
d. Secure the dressing with tape or metal clips.	d. Prevents the dressing from becoming loose.
18. Evaluate the client's level of comfort.	**18.** If the bandage is applied too tightly or with uneven pressure, the client may have discomfort or pressure sores may develop.
19. Evaluate the movement of the client's proximal joints.	**19.** The client should be able to move the proximal joints to prevent flexion contractures.
20. Record the procedure. Note the appearance, healing, and shape of the stump.	**20.** Communicates the findings to the other members of the health care team and contributes to the legal record by documenting the care given to the client.

Example of Documentation

DATE	TIME	NOTES
2/3/94	0800	Dressing on left above-the-knee stump changed. Sterile dressing applied. Entire stump dressed with Ace bandage using figure-eight technique.
		S. Williams, RN

Home Care Variations

The client will need continued support and guidance at home. Assess the client's home environment for safety and the client's mobility. Help the client to arrange transportation for health care appointments.

During visits to the home, assess the client's physiologic and psychologic adjustment to the amputation. The client may want to attend support groups in the local area to share problems, solutions, and resources. If the client is elderly, it may be necessary to secure additional assistance in the home.

Teaching Tips

The client should be taught to properly bandage the residual lower limb. (A residual arm should be dressed by another person.) Demonstrate the technique to the client or caregiver and assess learning through the client's or caregiver's return demonstration.

If the client is to have a prosthesis, referral to the prosthetist is necessary. After complete healing of the suture line, the residual limb will need to be "toughened" in preparation for the prosthesis. Activities to accomplish this goal may begin by having the client push the residual limb into a soft pillow and then progress to a firm surface. The client must massage the residual limb to soften and mobilize the scar, decrease tenderness, and improve circulation. Teach the client preventative skin care.

SKILL 20–16   APPLYING A PRESSURE DRESSING

Clinical Situations in Which You May Encounter This Skill

A pressure dressing is used to prevent bleeding or to control sudden and unexpected bleeding. The wound may be from a traumatic injury, suicide attempt, arterial puncture site, or postoperative debridement of a wound. A pressure dressing is applied to prevent hemorrhage at a puncture site if a client has a bleeding disorder (such as hemophilia) or is undergoing anticoagulant therapy. Control of the bleeding requires quick assessment and action.

Anticipated Responses

▼ The bleeding is controlled, circulation to the extremity is maintained, and circulating fluid volume is maintained.

Adverse Responses

▼ The bleeding is not controlled. Circulation to the extremities is not maintained and the client has resulting necrotic tissue that may require amputation. A thrombus forms at the site of bleeding and results in a pulmonary embolus. The client has a large fluid loss and suffers from hypovolemic shock.

Materials List

Gather these materials before beginning the skill:

▼ 4 to 6 sterile gauze compresses
▼ Sterile gloves (2 pairs)
▼ Roll of gauze
▼ Tape or Ace bandages
▼ Stethoscope
▼ Sphygmomanometer
▼ Scissors

▼ ACTION

(If treatment is for *prevention* of bleeding, go to Step 7.)

First Nurse

1. Quickly assess the wound to determine the site of the hemorrhage.

2. Call for assistance.

3. Put on sterile gloves and apply pressure directly to the site of hemorrhage.

4. Elevate the extremity.

Second Nurse

5. Don sterile gloves.

6. Quickly apply sterile compresses to the hemorrhage site as the first nurse lifts his or her fingers from the site. Be sure to have the first nurse maintain pressure between applications of the compresses.

7. Apply gauze around the extremity, completely covering the dressing and wound. Have the first nurse maintain pressure, only quickly lifting his or her fingers as you wrap each layer of the roller bandage.

▼ RATIONALE

1. Large volumes of blood can be lost rapidly from arterial sites.

2. If the hemorrhage is unexpected, a second nurse should gather supplies. A client who has a life-threatening condition will need continuous assessment and support and should never be left alone.

3. Gloves decrease transmission of microorganisms. Firm pressure occludes the site of hemorrhage.

4. Helps to reduce blood flow to the area.

5. Decreases the transmission of microorganisms.

6. Sterile compresses are used so as not to introduce microorganisms into the open wound. However, hemorrhage is a life-threatening condition that requires immediate action. If no sterile supplies are available, use any type of clean compress to temporarily control the bleeding.

7. The gauze bandage secures the compresses and helps maintain pressure on the site.

▼ *ACTION*	▼ *RATIONALE*
8. Tear or cut the tape into strips that will completely cover the dressing over the site of the hemorrhage.	
9. Apply the tape to the dressing to form an occlusive dressing. Each strip should overlap the other strip.	**9.** The tape aids in the control of the bleeding.
10. (Optional.) If an Ace or elastic bandage is used over the sterile compresses, snugly wrap the elastic bandage in a figure eight. Completely cover the wound and dressing.	**10.** The elastic bandage applies pressure to the wound and secures the compresses in place.
11. Remove the gloves and wash your hands.	**11.** Decreases the transmission of microorganisms.
12. Assess the client's pulse and blood pressure.	**12.** Provides an indication of early stages of hypovolemic shock.
13. Assess the pulses distal to the wound.	**13.** Arterial blood flow should not be completely occluded. Oxygen deprivation of tissue distal to the wound results in tissue necrosis.
14. Assess the extremity for color, warmth, sensation, and capillary refill.	**14.** Provides an indication of the circulatory status to the extremity.
15. If the hemorrhage was sudden or unexpected, a. Notify the physician. b. Start intravenous infusions (requires a physician's order). c. Continue to monitor the client's vital signs every 15 minutes until they are stable for 1 hour.	a. Specific treatment measures should be implemented. b. An intravenous line should be started to replace the circulating blood volume. c. Vital signs are monitored to detect shock.
16. Record the intervention. Note the amount of blood loss, vital signs, and the color, warmth, sensitivity, and capillary refill of the extremities, as well as follow-up interventions.	**16.** Communicates the findings to the other members of the health care team and contributes to the legal record by documenting the care given to the client.

Example of Documentation

DATE	TIME	NOTES
1/9/94	1300	Arrived per stretcher via ambulance. 4- × 2-cm deep wound on right inner wrist. Large amount of blood noted on clothing. Pressure dressing applied. Dr. Smith notified. Lactated Ringer's started to infuse per 18 gauze angiocath at 200 cc/hr. VS: BP=100/60; P=120; R=28. Awake and complaining of pain. Typed and crossmatched for 2 units of blood. Family with client at present. *S. Williams, RN*

Teaching Tips

Clients who are at risk for hemorrhage (e.g., clients with hemophilia) should be taught the difference between arterial bleeding and venous bleeding. Arterial bleeding is bright red and pulsates. Venous bleeding is darker red and does not pulsate. Capillary bleeding oozes from the wound. Demonstrate application of pressure dressings for the client and family members and confirm learning through a return demonstration. Discuss use of gloves as a barrier to prevent blood contact.

Home Care Variations

Clients may use clean linens or towels to temporarily control bleeding. The client should know that he or she should elevate the extremity and notify a physician. The emergency number for the area (911) or the local emergency room or ambulance service number should be posted near the telephone.

SKILL 20–17   APPLYING A HYDROCOLLOID DRESSING

Clinical Situations in Which You May Encounter This Skill

Hydrocolloid dressings are composed of a nonpermeable outer layer made of polyurethane and an inner layer composed of a gumlike material such as karaya, gelatin, or pectin. These occlusive dressings provide a sterile, moist environment that encourages wound healing through rapid epithelialization of the wound surface and mild debridement of necrotic tissue.

The dressing that remains in place for 2 to 7 days also protects the wound from mechanical injury and contamination. Another advantage of hydrocolloid dressings is their flexibility. They can be shaped to conform to curved body structures such as heels, elbows, knees, and the sacrum. A disadvantage of the dressing is its opaque nature that prevents observation of the wound without removal of the dressing. Hydrocolloid dressings should not be used with infected wounds or third-degree burns.

Anticipated Responses

▼ The wound appears to increase in size and depth during initial use of the dressing due to the debriding action of the dressing.
▼ The wound has a pronounced odor when the dressing is first removed. Cleansing the wound of the gel-like dissolved inner dressing alleviates this problem.
▼ Wound healing occurs.

Adverse Responses

▼ The wound becomes infected.
▼ The wound does not heal.

Materials List

Gather these materials before beginning the skill:

▼ Hydrocolloid dressing of the correct size (the dressing should extend 1.5 inches beyond the wound margin on all sides)
▼ Sterile scissors (optional, used to cut the dressing to size)
▼ Absorptive granules or paste (optional)
▼ Sterile isotonic saline
▼ Wound irrigation set (contains a 30-ml syringe and a 19-gauge blunt-tipped needle)
▼ Sterile 4- × 4-inch gauze pads
▼ Examination gloves
▼ Sterile gloves
▼ Tape
▼ Sterile basin
▼ Waterproof bag for used dressing
▼ Plastic red bag for nondisposable contaminated items

▼ *A C T I O N*	▼ *R A T I O N A L E*
1. Assess the need for a dressing change.	1. Hydrocolloid dressings are left in place for 2 to 7 days. When the dressing becomes loose or is leaking, it should be changed.
2. Check the client's chart for the physician's orders relative to the dressing change.	2. Orders may contain specific details of how the dressing should be changed or specific products to use such as absorptive paste or granules.
3. Explain the procedure to the client.	3. Prepares the client and elicits cooperation.
4. Provide privacy by closing the door, pulling the bed curtains, and draping the client appropriately. Raise the bed to a working height.	4. Protects the client's modesty and dignity. Raising the bed protects your back from injury.

▼ *ACTION*   ▼ *RATIONALE*

5. Wash your hands.

5. Reduces the transmission of microorganisms.

6. Put on examination gloves to remove the old dressing.

6. Protects you from contact with the client's blood and body fluids and microorganisms.

7. Remove the old dressing. Press down in the client's skin around the wound with one hand while gently lifting the edge of the dressing toward the wound with your other hand. Loosen the dressing on all sides, then lift it carefully from the wound (Fig. 20–34).

7. Removing the dressing in this manner prevents trauma to new cell growth in the wound.

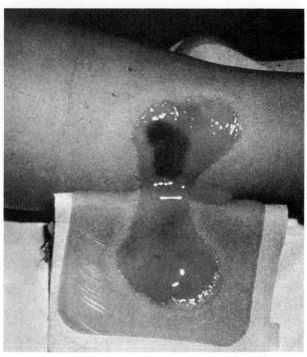

▼ **FIGURE 20–34.** Appearance of wound when hydrocolloid dressing is removed.

8. Discard the old dressing and examination gloves into a waterproof bag for proper disposal.

8. Sealing the gloves and old dressing in a bag for removal from the room reduces the chance of contact with contaminated articles and also reduces odors in the client's room.

9. Wash your hands.

9. Reduces the transmission of microorganisms.

10. Open a sterile irrigation set and sterile basin, using the inner wrap to create a sterile field. Open the 4- × 4-inch gauze pads and place them on the sterile field. Open the dressing and place it on the sterile field. Pour sterile saline into the basin. Peel back the corner of the backing paper on the granule packet (if it is to be used). Do not place it on the sterile field, but within easy reach.

10. You must set up your sterile field before putting on sterile gloves. See Skill 1–9 on setting up a sterile field if necessary.

11. Put on sterile gloves.

11. Sterile gloves protect the wound from contamination with microorganisms from your hands. Gloves also protect you from contact with the client's body fluids.

▼ _ACTION_ | ▼ _RATIONALE_

12. Irrigate the wound with isotonic saline using the 30-ml syringe with a 19-gauge blunt-tipped needle at 8 PSI pressure.

12. Irrigation with isotonic saline at 8 PSI pressure removes liquefied wound dressing and wound drainage without damaging new granulation tissue. Irrigation also provides a mild debriding effect on loosely connected necrotic tissue in the wound.

13. Using sterile 4- × 4-inch gauze pads, dry the skin surrounding the wound. Work from the wound margin toward the periphery.

13. Drying the skin prevents maceration and enhances adhesion of the dressing to the skin.

14. Assess the appearance of the clean wound for erythema, unusual odor, drainage, necrotic tissue, or change in size or depth of wound.

14. Since hydrocolloid dressings debride wounds autolytically, the wound may increase in size and depth during the first few dressing changes. This growth will be followed by formation of new granulation tissue and wound healing. If the wound develops an uncharacteristic odor, change in appearance of drainage, fever, tenderness, or erythema, the presence of infection should be suspected and reported to the physician. Hydrocolloid dressings should not be applied to an infected wound.

15. Apply granules or paste if ordered. These products are usually used if the wound is 1 cm or more in diameter and extends into the subcutaneous tissue. Fill the wound with granules or paste no higher than skin level.

15. Granules or paste are used to fill dead space in the wound to prevent fluid collection and abscess formation. These products also absorb excess drainage, preventing leakage around the dressing.

> **NOTE:** Your gloves are no longer sterile after touching the packet containing the paste or granules.

16. Peel back the inner covering of the hydrocolloid dressing and discard it. Apply the dressing directly over the wound, rolling it from one side to the other. Smooth the dressing into place. Do not stretch the dressing.

16. Take your time in securing the dressing in place, and avoid wrinkles. Body heat will increase the adhesion of the dressing.

> **NOTE:** The dressing can be cut with sterile scissors to fit a variety of body surfaces.

17. Remove the gloves and discard them.

18. Tape the edges of the dressing in place on all sides (Fig. 20–35).

18. Taping secures the dressing and helps prevent leaking.

19. Place the client in a position of comfort and replace the bed covers. Lower the bed to the lowest position.

19. Promotes the client's comfort and safety.

20. Remove all used equipment. Discard disposable equipment. Place nondisposable equipment in a red bag and return it to the appropriate area for cleaning and sterilization.

20. Proper handling of contaminated equipment prevents the spread of microorganisms.

▼ *ACTION* _ _ _ _ _ _ _ _ _ _ _ _ _ ▼ *RATIONALE* _ _ _ _ _ _ _

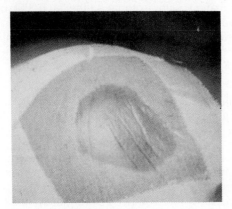

▼ **FIGURE 20–35.** Hydrocolloid dressing in place.

21.	Wash your hands.	**21.** Reduces the transmission of microorganisms.
22.	Record the procedure. Note the appearance of the wound and how the client tolerated the dressing change.	**22.** Communicates the findings to the other members of the health care team and contributes to the legal record by documenting the care given to the client.

Example of Documentation

DATE	TIME	NOTES
05/05/94	1300	Hydrocolloid dressing changed on sacral ulcer. Ulcer irrigated with normal saline. Ulcer measures 2 cm in diameter and is shallow. Pink granulation tissue evident in wound bed. No skin breakdown around wound. No wound drainage, erythema, or fever noted. Client tolerated dressing change well. Voices no complaints at this time. C. Lammon, RN

Teaching Tips

Explain how the hydrocolloid dressing works and what to expect in the initial period of use (i.e., an increase in the size and depth of the wound and the presence of an unpleasant odor and drainage when the dressing is first removed). Teach the client the signs of infection and that these should be reported immediately.

Home Care Variations

The same technique for applying hydrocolloid dressings can be used in the home. Remove contaminated items from the home after the dressing change, and dispose of them according to your agency policy.

References

Branemark, P. I., and Ekholm, R. (1967). Tissue injury caused by wound disinfectants. *The Journal of Bone and Joint Surgery*, 49–A, 48–62.

Conly, J. M., Grieves, K., and Peters, B. (1989). A prospective, randomized study comparing transparent and dry gauze dressings for central venous catheters. *The Journal of Infectious Diseases*, 159 (2), 310–319.

Harkreader, H., and Morse, C. (1994). Providing physical protection and bodily support. In V. Bolander (Ed.), *Basic nursing* (3rd ed.). Philadelphia: W. B. Saunders.

Marchett, L., Main, R., and Redick, E. (1989). Pain reduction during neonatal circumcision. *Pediatric Nursing*, 15 (2), 207–210.

Shannon, M. L. (1994). Caring for persons with wounds. In V. Bolander (Ed.), *Basic nursing* (3rd ed.). Philadelphia: W. B. Saunders.

Shivnan, J. C., et al. (1991). A comparison of transparent adherent and dry sterile gauze dressings for long-term central catheters in patients undergoing bone marrow transplant. *Oncology Nursing Forum*, 18 (8), 1349–1356.

CHAPTER 21

Postmortem Care

After an individual dies, the nurse performs postmortem care. The components of postmortem care vary relative to the cause of the client's illness and death, but may include:

▼ Preparation of the body for viewing by the family and significant others.
▼ Obtaining consent for an autopsy from the client's next of kin.
▼ Obtaining consent from the next of kin for harvesting tissues or organs, or both, for transplant.
▼ Performing any procedures necessary to preserve organs and tissues before their retrieval for transplant. Nonvital tissues such as corneas, skin, long bones, and middle-ear bones can be removed after death. Vital organs such as the heart, liver, lungs, kidneys, and pancreas must be removed after the person is clinically dead but while the body is still receiving circulatory and ventilatory support to maintain organ perfusion.

In most states, a nurse or physician is required by law to request permission from the next of kin for organ and tissue donation when a client dies. The family also must be informed of their right to refuse organ donation.

Legal requirements surrounding death, autopsy, and organ donation vary from state to state. The physician or coroner usually certifies the person's death and completes the death certificate. The death certificate then is filed with the state department of health and the family is given a copy.

The physician may request permission from the family to perform an autopsy. This postmortem examination is used to confirm a diagnosis, determine the cause of death, or gather information on a disease process and its response to treatment. Autopsies may be limited to certain body areas such as the trunk only or may entail examination of the entire body. The immediate next of kin must sign a consent form that gives permission for the autopsy to be performed. In cases of unexpected death or death due to a violent crime, an autopsy is required by law. Each state has regulations that define circumstances under which an autopsy must be performed. Once the autopsy has been completed, the body is released to the mortuary for burial. It is essential that you protect the dignity of the deceased and provide support for the family and significant others during this period of loss.

SKILL 21–1   POSTMORTEM CARE

Clinical Situations in Which You May Encounter This Skill

Postmortem care is provided whenever a client dies.

Anticipated Responses

▼ The family receives support as they experience and express grief.
▼ The hospital staff complies with legal requirements regarding completion of the death certificate, consent forms for autopsy, and request for organ donation.
▼ The client's body is protected from skin damage or other injury post mortem.

Adverse Responses

▼ Family members are unable to express grief.
▼ Skin surfaces are damaged during preparation and positioning of the body.
▼ You have difficulty locating the next of kin for legal decisions regarding organ donation, permission for autopsy, or location and name of the mortuary to which the body is to be sent.

Materials List

Gather these materials before beginning the skill:

▼ Washbasin with water
▼ Washcloth
▼ Towel
▼ Examination gloves
▼ Disposable pads to protect bed
▼ Paper or plastic bag (for personal items)
▼ Valuables list and envelope
▼ Dressing materials such as gauze and tape
▼ Small pillow or folded towel
▼ Abdominal pads
▼ Gown
▼ Aromatic spirits of ammonia
▼ Body bag with two identification tags or a shroud kit (contains sheeting to wrap the body, gauze ties, and two identification tags)
▼ Stretcher
▼ Tape or gauze if not using shroud kit

▼ ACTION

1. Escort the family to a private area before they are informed of the person's death.

2. After the family has been notified of the person's death, offer them the opportunity to view the body. Explain that it will take a short period of time to prepare the body for viewing.

3. Determine the client's religious and cultural heritage. Ask the family if they wish a priest, minister, or other religious person to be present.

4. Check the client's chart to determine the presence of any infectious disease that would require isolation precautions.

5. If the deceased person occupied a semiprivate room, make arrangements for the remaining client and visitors to leave the room.

6. Wash your hands.

7. Put on examination gloves.

8. Identify the body by checking the arm band and bed tag. Remove the arm band.

▼ RATIONALE

1. Providing privacy facilitates the family's expressions of grief and loss.

2. The physician usually notifies the family of a client's death. The nurse supports the family and provides postmortem care for the body.

3. Various cultures and religions require specific ceremonies at the time of death.

4. Even after the client's death, universal precautions must be taken to prevent the spread of infection.

5. Decreases the remaining client's anxiety and provides privacy for the grieving family to view the body.

6. Decreases the transmission of microorganisms.

7. Protects you from contact with bodily secretions as you cleanse the body and remove intravenous, nasogastric, urinary drainage, or other tubes.

8. Enables you to complete body tags and forms correctly. Removing the arm band prevents tissue injury.

▼ *A C T I O N*

▼ *R A T I O N A L E*

9. Position the body in the supine position with the arms at the sides and the palms down.

9. Places the body in alignment and facilitates a natural appearance.

10. Place the person's head on a small pillow. Do not use a thick pillow. A small folded towel may be used if the pillow is too large.

10. Elevates the head slightly to prevent facial discoloration due to pooling blood. A large pillow flexes the neck and makes the person appear uncomfortable.

11. If necessary, use your fingertips to gently close the eyes and hold them closed for a few seconds.

11. Creates a natural sleeping appearance.

12. Provide grooming and hygiene to the person's face and hair by:
    a. Washing any secretions from the face.
    b. Combing the hair in a neat style.
    c. Removing any hair clips or pins.

    d. Inserting clean dentures into the mouth. A rolled towel may be placed under the chin to hold the mouth closed.

12. Cleansing and grooming the body provides support to the family.

    c. Hard hair ornaments can damage the person's skin.
    d. Insertion of dentures is more difficult after rigor mortis occurs. Dentures give the face a more natural appearance.

13. Provide hygiene and grooming to the body by:
    a. Disconnecting all bags, bottles, and collection devices from tubes exiting the body.
    b. Removing tubes unless an autopsy is to be performed (usually tubes are clamped and left in place if an autopsy is needed).
    c. Washing soiled body parts.

    d. Placing an absorbent disposable pad under the buttocks.
    e. Placing a clean gown on the body and covering the body with a sheet or blanket. Leave the person's head and upper shoulders exposed.

13. Provides support to the family.
    a. Collection devices are not needed for an autopsy.
    b. Facilitates a natural appearance. Agencies have specific guidelines for handling of tubes if an autopsy is needed.
    c. A complete bath will be given by the mortician. Removing secretions decreases odors, reduces the spread of microorganisms, and prepares the body for viewing.
    d. Absorbs any feces or urine that may be excreted due to relaxation of the sphincters.
    e. Prepares the body for viewing and prevents exposure of the body.

14. Fill out two identification tags and attach one to the ankle or great toe and the other to the outer cover of the shroud.

14. Provides for accurate identification of the body.

15. Collect the client's clothing and other nonvaluable items and place them in a bag to be returned to the family.

15. You are responsible for ensuring the safekeeping of the client's belongings.

16. Gather all of the client's valuables, including jewelry. Use the valuables list to account for all items. Return these belongings to the most immediate next of kin and obtain a signature that indicates receipt of the valuables.

16. You are responsible for ensuring the safekeeping of all of the client's valuables.

> **NOTE:** The family may request that the person's wedding ring be left in place. If so, secure it to the finger with a small piece of tape.

▼ _ACTION_	▼ _RATIONALE_
17. Prepare the room by providing soft lighting and chairs.	**17.** Provides quiet and comfort for the grieving family.
18. Obtain aromatic spirits of ammonia.	**18.** Members of the person's family may faint when viewing the body. Aromatic spirits of ammonia helps to revive a family member that has fainted.
19. Escort the family to the client's bedside and remain with them for a short period of time to respond to any questions or requests they may have. Then allow the family private time with the deceased.	**19.** Families need time to express grief and loss privately.
20. After the family leaves, wrap abdominal pads around the ankles and tie them together with a strip of gauze.	**20.** Prevents tissue injury from the ties.
21. Place the body in a body bag or wrap the body in shroud sheeting (Fig. 21–1) and attach an identification tag to the outside of the bag. If the patient's head was shaved, be sure to send hair with client's body.	**21.** The tag will identify the body. The hair may be used by the mortician in preparing the body for viewing.

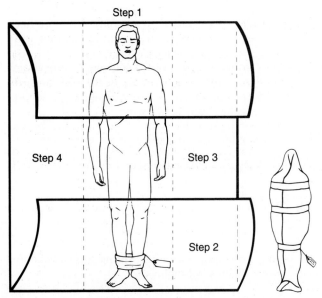

▼ **FIGURE 21–1.** Wrapping the body in a shroud.

22. Clear the hallways of visitors and clients and close the doors to other client rooms.	**22.** It may be upsetting to other clients and family members to see the body.
23. Place body on stretcher and take the body to the morgue.	**23.** The body will be kept in the morgue until the funeral service claims the body.
24. Remove gloves and wash your hands.	**24.** Decreases the transmission of microorganisms.
25. Record the procedure. Note the time of death, events surrounding the death, time of notification of the family, postmortem care delivered, disposition of clothing and valuables, any permits obtained, and the time the body was delivered to the morgue.	**25.** Communicates the procedure to other members of the health care team and contributes to the legal record by documenting the care given to the client.

Example of Documentation

DATE	*TIME*	*NOTES*
5/10/93	0910	No respirations, pulse, or blood pressure present. Do not resuscitate order noted. Code not initiated. Dr. Petry notified.
		H. White, RN
	0915	Dr. Petry in to see client. Time of death 0915. Wife notified of death. Client placed in supine position. Hygienic care given. Dentures placed in mouth. IV removed. Morgue and mortuary notified of death.
		H. White, RN
	0945	Wife in to see client. Clothing and jewelry given to wife.
		H. White, RN
	1015	Body prepared and sent to morgue with identification tag on right great toe and outside of body bag.
		H. White, RN

Home Care Variations

Often clients with terminal illnesses such as cancer wish to remain at home to die without medical intervention. The home care nurse can support the family in this endeavor. When the client dies, the nurse can assist the family in providing care for the body as described in this procedure.

References

Maliski, S. (1994). Coping with loss and grief. In V. Bolander (Ed.), *Basic nursing* (3rd ed.). Philadelphia: W. B. Saunders.

APPENDIX

Guidelines for Health History and Physical Assessment

Health assessment is an increasingly important part of nursing practice. It is an activity shared with other health professionals. Although the processes are similar, each professional uses health assessment with a differing focus. For nurses, health assessment is an examination of a person's state of health rather than diagnosis of disease. It enables you to view the person holistically.

The ability to perform a health assessment can be a very exciting and challenging aspect of the learning process. As your knowledge increases regarding health assessment, so will your ability to make clinical judgments.

This chapter is an overview of health assessment skills as they relate to establishing a nursing data base. Health assessment can be performed in other settings besides the hospital unit: clinics, health fairs, physician's offices, and the home.

The person requiring health care is central to all assessment processes. It is this person alone who experiences both symptoms and assessment processes. It is this person who interacts with the people performing these processes and whose life, mind, and body are affected by them.

Health assessment, which includes the health history and the physical assessment, is a holistic assessment of an individual that identifies normal physical and psychosocial functioning and highlights deviations from normal. It also identifies individual health risks and points to preventive measures.

While assessment skills are described, it is important to remember that supervised practice is essential if you are to be accomplished. Do not perform activities for which you are not fully prepared and authorized. It is assumed that you already know basic normal human physical structure and functions.

It is important for you to understand the difference between signs and symptoms. A **sign** is an objective observation made by physical assessment. A **symptom** is a person's subjective experience that something is abnormal, e.g., pain, dizziness, nausea, fatigue, and anxiety.

GUIDELINE A-1   TAKING A HEALTH HISTORY

Careful history-taking can provide useful information about an individual.

Principles of History-Taking

History-taking is obtaining information in an organized manner. Communication skills and interviewing techniques are used to elicit pertinent information from the individual. As one prepares to obtain the client health history, communication principles must be considered. It is important to conduct the interview in a setting that will ensure the individual's privacy. If the individual is in a private room, be sure to close the door. If the individual is in a semiprivate room, be sure to draw the drapes between the beds. Try to interview the individual during a time when daily activities are at a minimum.

Be sure to obtain only information needed to support the health history. Inform the individual that all information provided will remain confidential within the health care team. The individual has the right not to answer a question if deemed inappropriate. Be sure to discuss this freedom with the individual. Offer to show the individual what is being written on the health history form.

Set a time frame for obtaining the client health history. This will allow the individual to be aware of how long the interview will take, and it will assure you of obtaining any and all needed information.

The tone of an interview is important. The first 5 minutes are probably most important in setting the tone. It is important that the person experience the interviewer as genuinely concerned, attentive, trustworthy, and skilled.

Consider what a person is concealing as well as revealing. Omissions in history are not necessarily intentional. Some details are simply forgotten. A skilled interviewer notices and assesses obvious omissions, sudden shifts of subject matter, shying away from topics, and nonverbal cues, e.g., facial expression, gestures, tone of voice.

A person's account of one's own history and symptoms is affected by (a) hopes and fears, (b) confidence in and reactions to the interviewer, (c) mental competence, (d) view of what actually is a reportable health disorder, and (e) ability to observe and describe life events (past experiences).

Try to assess a person's reliability in history reporting. This is important not only in interpreting information but also in considering how an individual may cooperate with treatment.

In addition to discussing an individual's present problem, it is also important to obtain information about the person's lifestyle, family history, and history of previous health problems. Finally, a thorough "systems review" (discussed later) is conducted to identify abnormalities in the various body systems.

Major Components of a Health History

Chief Complaint

The **chief complaint** is a person's description of the major problem he or she is experiencing. It is written in the person's own words and is contained within direct quotes. Help the person be specific. A person's main concerns are often a change in usual condition or the presence of pain or dysfunction. The chief complaint provides a broad beginning for assessment. It usually consists of one statement, containing one to two symptoms and the duration. Examples of a chief complaint are "I've been having chest pain for the last 2 days" or "I've been short of breath for 3 to 4 weeks."

Present Illness

The present illness is derived from the chief complaint. It details the course of the illness or the sequence of events leading up to the present illness. The history of the present illness usually identifies major disease mechanisms and may even establish the diagnosis when symptoms are precise.

To reconstruct the events leading up to the present illness, you must acquaint yourself with the seven variables central to obtaining pertinent information from the person:

Body Location. Pinpoint the body system or organs involved. A question you may ask is "Where does it hurt?"

Quality. Usually a person will equate a symptom with an analogy, by stating it is "like" something. For example, "My chest pain feels like a knife is being thrust in my chest."

Quantity. You need to quantify the symptom according to the level of intensity, how it affects activities of daily living, frequency, volume, number, and size or extent of the symptom. For example, ask the person, "On a scale of one to ten with ten most severe, what is your level of pain?"

Chronology. You need to consider the symptom in relation to time. For example, when did the symptom first appear? Does the symptom begin gradually or suddenly? Does it stay the same in quality and intensity? How often does it occur? Does it wake the person from sleep?

Setting. Consider where and what the person was doing when the symptom occurred.

Aggravating or Alleviating Factors. Identify what worsens (aggravates) or relieves (alleviates) the symptom. For example, does the chest pain increase during physical activity? Does it require rest? Does emotional upset make the symptom worse?

Associated Factors. Assess the associated factors or symptoms. Some disorders produce symptoms in various body parts. For example, a person with congestive heart failure may have swollen ankles and abdomen and may experience shortness of breath. Exploration of associated factors may reveal useful information. For example, an acutely ill child may have eaten a poisonous substance, or a desperately ill adult might have been traveling recently and developed malaria or some other regional disorder.

Past Health History

The past health history reflects a chronologic review of previous disorders and contacts with health professionals. The first information you will need to obtain is a description of the person's general health immediately prior to the present illness. You may ask the person to describe health prior to this particular illness. The following are areas to be included in the past health history:

▼ Pediatric and adult illness: Inquire whether the person has ever had measles, mumps, chickenpox, hypertension, polio, hepatitis, pneumonia, diabetes, cancer, mental illness, scarlet fever, anemia, rheumatic fever, seizures, chronic bronchitis, heart disease, whooping cough, stroke, diphtheria, or malaria. If the person answers yes to any of these illnesses, question the person concerning the time frame and any complications resulting from the illness.

▼ Previous hospitalizations: Obtain the date, physician, disorder, and hospital location.

▼ Operations and injuries without hospitalization

▼ Immunizations

▼ Allergies or sensitivities, e.g., asthma, hayfever, food, skin, drugs (note drug allergies or sensitivities and manifestations)

▼ Transfusions

▼ Current medications: This should include medications prior to and during hospitalization. Remember to include prescription as well as over-the-counter medications.

▼ Current treatments, e.g., physical or occupational therapy, respiratory therapy

Family Health History

The family health history is a past medical history of relatives. You will need to assess the person's family history with respect to the present illness and future health risks. The following are areas to be included in the family health history:

▼ Present status of parents and siblings: Question the person concerning the age and health status of the mother, father, and each of the siblings, or the age at death and cause.

▼ Medical problems: Question the person concerning the family history of disorders that may be influenced by heredity (familial disorders) or contact. Also ask about family allergies, deformities, or serious illnesses. Include the following: diabetes, hypertension, heart disease, renal disease, cancer, tuberculosis, stroke, deafness, anemia, gout, arthritis, mental illness, alcoholism, seizures, obesity.

▼ Similar illness or symptoms in family: Is anyone in the family experiencing an illness or symptoms resembling a person's present illness?

Personal and Social History

The personal and social history pertains to information concerning the person's personality and lifestyle. Some of the information may be emotionally charged and difficult for the person to describe. Question the person concerning the following areas (only information needed to care for the person should be obtained):

▼ Marital status
▼ Number of dependent children
▼ Other people in the household
▼ Religion
▼ Occupation
▼ Military service
▼ Daily routines, e.g., food intake, elimination, sleep pattern, exercise
▼ Habits, e.g., tobacco, caffeine, alcohol, drugs
▼ Pets
▼ Housing and living arrangements
▼ Family responsibilities
▼ Interests
▼ Daily activity, e.g., description of an average day
▼ Source of income
▼ Health insurance
▼ Travel
▼ Past development, e.g. childhood and adolescence, educational experiences, occupational experiences
▼ Patterns of interaction and communication, e.g., sexual relations, personality (mood, feelings, temperament, and general attitudes)

Systems Review

A review of systems is included in the client health history. You will be questioning the person about the structure and function of the body systems in order to identify symptoms that the person may not have previously reported. Some of the terms used will be new to you, but they are common medical terms you will have to know in your role as a nurse. You are urged to look them up and become familiar with them. Remember to communicate in terms that the individual providing the information can understand. The following systems should be addressed:

▼ Integument: color change, pruritus, nevi, infections, inflammations, rash, tumor, hair changes, nail changes, excessive bruising, cuts failing to heal
▼ Eyes: visual acuity, glasses/contact lenses, blurring, diplopia, pain, inflammation, excessive tearing, visual defects, date of last eye examination
▼ Ears: hearing loss, tinnitus, discharge, hearing aid, earache, vertigo, infection

▼ Nose and sinuses: frequent colds, sinusitis, epistaxis, discharge, obstruction, postnasal drip, pain
▼ Mouth and throat: gums, teeth, partial/full dentures, sore tongue, sore throat, difficulty swallowing, hoarseness, voice change, goiter, bleeding gums, date of last dental examination
▼ Neck: pain, thyroid or lymph node enlargement, limitation of motion
▼ Respiratory: cough, sputum, hemoptysis, wheezing, dyspnea, recurrent respiratory tract infections, night sweats, recent chest x-ray, pain, positive tuberculin test (date)
▼ Cardiovascular: chest pain, dyspnea, orthopnea, palpitations, murmur, hypertension, syncope, anemia, edema, varicosities, thrombophlebitis, claudication, pain
▼ Gastrointestinal: appetite changes, dysphagia, eructation, nausea, vomiting, hematemesis, pain, gas, indigestion, jaundice, change in bowel habits, food intolerance, constipation, diarrhea, stools (color, character), hemorrhoids, hernia, melena, use of laxatives, weight change, rectal itching
▼ Genitourinary/reproductive: frequency, nocturia, urgency, dysuria, incontinence, albuminuria, flank pain, venereal disease, discharge, lesions, contraception, hesitancy, hematuria, pyuria, infections, stones, glycosuria, infertility, libido, testicular mass or pain, impotence, menarche, LMP (last menstrual period), cycle, duration, regularity, dysmenorrhea, gravida, para, abortions, spotting, leukorrhea, pruritus, last pelvic examination, last Pap smear, menopause, complications
▼ Musculoskeletal: myalgia, weakness, pain, swelling, heat, limitation of motion, stiffness, redness
▼ Endocrine: sensitivity to environmental temperature, change in body configuration, changes in scalp or hair, body weight in relation to appetite, sweating, polyuria, postural hypotension, change in voice, polydipsia, polyphagia
▼ Neurologic: headache, syncope, convulsions, seizures, vertigo, diplopia, paralysis, paresis, spasm, muscle weakness, paresthesia, tremor, ataxia, memory change, unconsciousness, speech problems, coordination
▼ Psychologic: nervousness, insomnia, depression, nightmares, indecisiveness, hyperventilation, work difficulty, mood, emotional difficulty, sense of failure, social withdrawal, memory loss

A variety of printed forms are available for recording the client's health history. It is important to remember that a client health history is privileged information. Information should not be sought unless it will be used in a professional, confidential manner.

GUIDELINE A-2 PREPARING FOR PHYSICAL ASSESSMENT

Purpose

Physical assessment is a component of the first step of the nursing process, Assessment. Data are objective because you are obtaining pertinent information from the client through the use of the senses: sight, hearing, smell, and touch. The purpose of physical assessment is to identify normal and deviations from normal. Nurses use it to identify deviations in health patterns, and they derive nursing diagnosis upon which planning, nursing interventions, and evaluation are based. Physical assessment is the key means of collecting baseline data and establishing a need for continued focused assessment. Physical assessment is done for people who are experiencing symptoms and as a health maintenance procedure for people who are well. Physical assessment often offers opportunity for health teaching—for example, breast and testicular self-examination.

Accurate assessment requires knowledge of body structure and function (anatomy and physiology), as well as pathologic changes or abnormalities. Skilled physical assessment depends on thoughtful practice and accumulated experience.

Equipment Needed

When performing a physical assessment, you will rely heavily on your senses, but in order to complete aspects of the assessment, you must use certain equipment (Fig. A-1). This equipment is, in a sense, an extension of your senses.

▼ Stethoscope: An instrument with two earpieces connected by flexible tubing to a cone or bell, used to listen to and amplify sounds produced by internal organs, e.g., lungs, heart, intestine.
▼ Scopes: Instruments for looking inside structures; e.g., an ophthalmoscope is an instrument used to examine the interior of the eye, obtaining information about not only the eye but also the central nervous system and blood vessels; an otoscope is an instrument used to examine the external ear canal and eardrum.
▼ Speculums: Instruments used to distend or open a body orifice or cavity, permitting visual inspection of the interior. Examples include a nasal speculum and a vaginal speculum.
▼ Tuning fork: An instrument to test air and bone conduction, auditory nerve function, and vibration sensation.
▼ Percussion hammer (reflex hammer): An instrument used to test superficial, deep tendon, and pathologic reflexes.
▼ Snellen chart: A chart used to test a person's visual acuity.
▼ Tongue depressor: A wooden stick used to aid in viewing the pharynx and stimulating the gag reflex.

▼ Safety pins and cotton swabs: Accessories used to test a person's ability to differentiate dull and sharp pain and sensitivities of touch.
▼ Penlight: An instrument used to illuminate areas for better viewing and to test pupil constriction.
▼ Instruments of measurement: examples are a scale to measure weight and a height measurement rod (often attached to the scale) to measure height. A blood pressure cuff attached to a sphygmomanometer measures blood pressure, and a thermometer measures body temperature. Pulse and respirations are counted, using a watch with a secondhand. A tape measure and small ruler may be used to make linear and circumference measurements. A special marking pen (surgical marker) may be used to mark areas on the body that require measurements.

Neurologic Assessment

Additional items are required for *neurologic* assessment.

▼ Audiometer, watch, or some other item for assessing hearing
▼ Containers of sugar and salt for testing taste
▼ Dry cotton balls for testing corneal reflex
▼ Test tubes (two) filled with cold and hot water for testing temperature sensation
▼ Vials (closed) containing fresh materials with easily recognizable odors, e.g., onion, orange extract, peanut butter, vanilla
▼ Various objects of differing, easily recognizable textures and shapes (key, paper clip, coin) for testing texture discrimination and stereognosis (ability to recognize an object by feeling it) while the individual's eyes are closed

Techniques

Inspection, palpation, percussion, and auscultation are basic maneuvers used during physical assessment. The sense of smell is also used. Figure A-2 shows how the body can be divided into planes and subdivided for descriptions of the parts assessed. Figure A-3 shows how various instruments and techniques are applied to common head-to-toe assessments.

A systematic approach to physical assessment is important to prevent omissions. The usual sequence of assessment activities is to (1) look (inspect), (2) feel (palpate), (3) tap or thump (percuss), and (4) listen (auscultate).

This sequence is not used to assess the abdomen. Instead the sequence is inspection, auscultation, percussion, and palpation. Palpation is performed last in this instance, because feeling a sensitive abdomen may produce additional symptoms—for example, suppress early bowel sounds, trigger painful spasms.

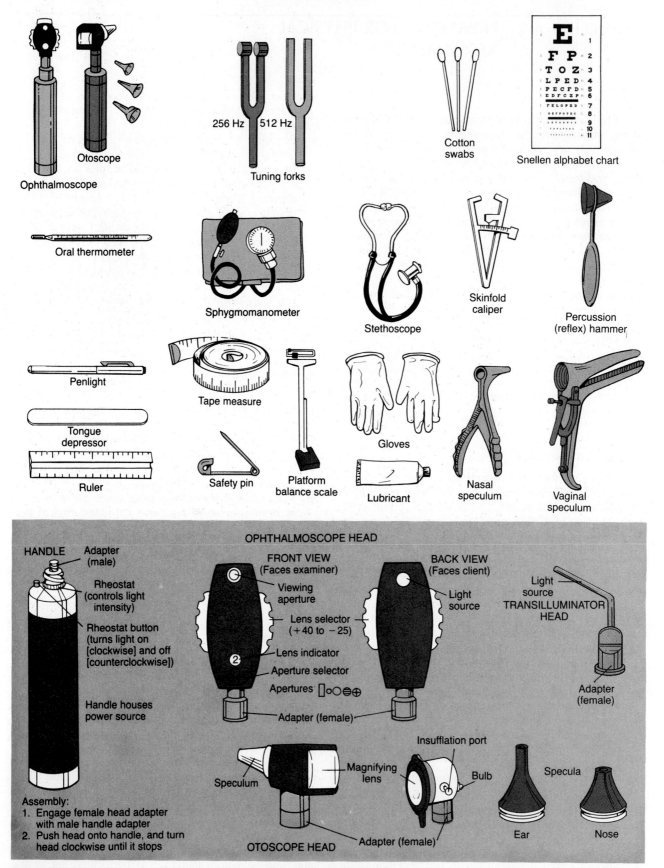

▼ **FIGURE A–1.** Equipment used by the nurse. (Modified from Black, J.M., & Matassarin-Jacobs, E. [1993]. Luckmann and Sorensen's Medical-Surgical Nursing: A Psychophysiologic Approach [4th ed]. Philadelphia: W.B. Saunders.)

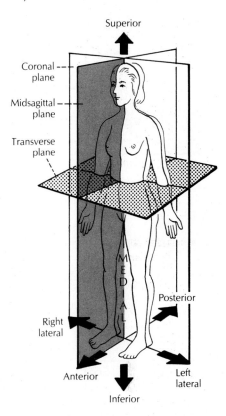

▼ **FIGURE A–2.** Anatomic section and position reference terms. (Modified from Jacob, S.W., & Francone, C.A. [1989]. Elements of anatomy and physiology [2nd ed.]. Philadelphia: W.B. Saunders.)

Inspection

Inspection is an assessment technique in which the examiner observes the body surface. As you inspect an area, try to develop a *visual description* of what you are seeing in your mind. Observe events (e.g., movements), colors, contours, and symmetry or asymmetry. Good lighting and adequate (but not excessive) exposure of the appropriate area facilitate proper inspection.

You must expose that which you wish to look at. You cannot inspect that which is not visible.

Whenever possible, take *measurements* (with a soft tape measure or small ruler) to quantify observations. This provides a baseline for future measurements and allows comparison with established normal ranges. Measurements are commonly made of height, weight, body temperature, and vital signs (i.e., pulse, respirations, blood pressure). Other measurements include head and limb circumference or the diameter of a lesion.

Palpation

Technique of Palpation. Palpation is an assessment technique in which the examiner feels with his or her fingers and one or both hands. Skill and gentleness are important. The degree of pressure applied during palpation varies, depending on, for example, the tenderness of the area and the depth of palpation required. Light or deep palpation (Figs. A-4 and A-5) may be used when palpating the abdomen. Palpation is difficult to do on people who are anxious or tense, experiencing physical discomfort, obese, or ticklish. With ticklish or tense people, place the person's hands beneath your hands during the initial palpation. It is best to examine tender areas last and to observe the individual's face for nonverbal responses such as grimacing or smiling during the examination. During palpation, encourage the person to report feelings of discomfort (e.g., pressure, fullness, tenderness) or pain when you touch certain places.

Purpose of Palpation. Palpation confirms data gathered by inspection and helps provide information about structure or function. Numerous characteristics may be assessed by touching an individual's body with different parts of the examiner's hand and by exerting varying amounts of pressure. For example:

▼ *Temperature changes* can be detected by running the backs of the fingers or the dorsum of the hand over the skin. Cool areas may indicate reduced blood flow, and warmth may indicate inflammation.

▼ *Moisture* may be felt while lightly stroking the skin.

▼ *Events* (vibrations, such as fremitus and thrills, crepitus, pulsations, spasticity, rigidity, elasticity, or other movements or qualities of movements occurring under the examiner's hand) can be detected by using the fingers and entire palm. Vibrations are best felt with the palm or ulnar side of the hand.

▼ *Textures* (e.g., unevenness) can be noted using fingertips. Fingertips have many nerve endings and are therefore very sensitive to touch.

▼ *Locations and dimensions or contours* are assessed by using several fingers or one or both entire hands, depending upon the size of the body part being examined. For example, swelling may be felt and organ sizes and locations assessed. Firm deep pressure is required to palpate deep organs such as the kidneys, spleen, or liver. Light touch is used to palpate the eye.

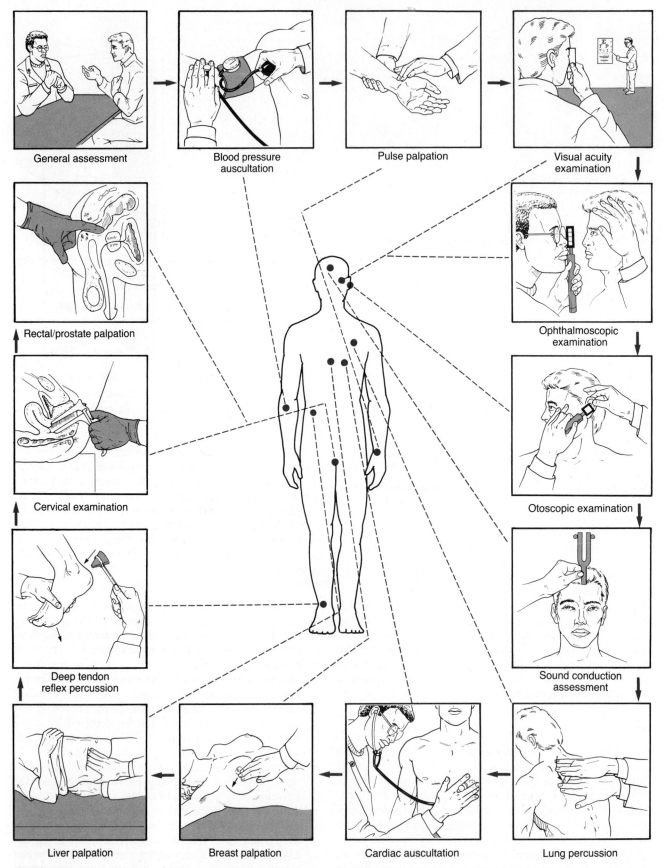

General assessment

Blood pressure auscultation

Pulse palpation

Visual acuity examination

Ophthalmoscopic examination

Rectal/prostate palpation

Cervical examination

Otoscopic examination

Deep tendon reflex percussion

Sound conduction assessment

Liver palpation

Breast palpation

Cardiac auscultation

Lung percussion

▼ **FIGURE A–3.** Common head-to-toe screening physical assessments. Note that the examiner wears gloves for the pelvic, rectal, and prostate examinations.

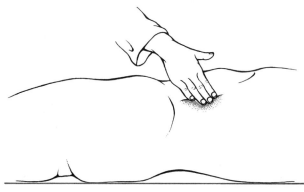

▼ FIGURE A–4. Position of the hand during light palpation.

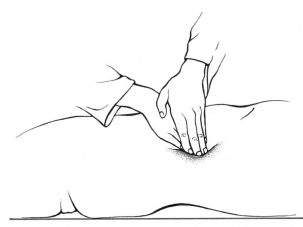

▼ FIGURE A–5. Position of hands during deep palpation.

▼ *Consistencies* (hard, soft, rubbery, flaccid, tense) are determined by the fingertips.

Palpation is commonly used to take a pulse (to feel blood pulsating through arteries) and during breast examination. However, all accessible body parts may be examined by palpation, e.g., blood vessels, organs, skin, muscles, bones, glands. It is also possible to feel the vibrations of some body sounds, e.g., thrills, tactile fremitus.

Types of Palpation. Firm pressure reduces the sensitivity in an examiner's fingers, as in palpation of deep organs. To counteract this problem, use both hands when applying pressure (Fig. A-5). Keep the lower hand (touching the individual) relaxed. Apply pressure by placing the other hand on top of the resting hand. The upper hand also directs exploratory movements of the relaxed lower hand on the person's body. Palpation of deep organs should be performed only in the presence of a qualified examiner, since injury can occur as a result of prolonged pressure.

Percussion

Techniques of Percussion. Percussion is an assessment technique in which the examiner "thumps" or "taps" a body surface with a percussion hammer or the hand or fingers. Percussion assesses *density* (relative solidness, hardness, or fullness) of a cavity or organ. The location and size of underlying organs can also be determined. Diagnostic deductions can be made from the sound produced by the thumping.

Sounds of Percussion. Percussed sounds differ in various body areas, depending in part upon the density of underlying structures. The sounds produced by percussion over solid structures differ from those over hollow structures. Sounds range from *flat* (nonresonant) to *dull, resonant, hyperresonant,* and *tympanic.* Tympanic sounds occur over hollow or gas-filled organs. Flat sounds are heard over muscle, whereas dull sounds are heard over solid organs such as the liver. It is possible, for example, to differentiate between normal air-filled lung tissue and diseased solidified lung tissue. Nurses often percuss the abdomen to identify distention, and the urinary bladder to assess the amount of urine it contains.

Types of Percussion. Percussion may be direct or indirect. *Direct percussion* is done by the examiner's striking the fingers directly against the person's skin. With *indirect percussion,* the examiner places the first phalanx (i.e., terminal phalanx) of the middle finger of one hand (the nondominant hand) firmly against the person's skin and then strikes the phalanx (just behind the fingernail bed) with the end of the middle finger of the dominant hand (Fig. A-6). Remember:

▼ Do not allow other fingers of the nondominant hand to touch the person (this will damp or suppress the percussed sound).
▼ Hold the forearm of the dominant arm steady and use a quick, flicking wrist action from a flexed wrist for the striking force.
▼ Quickly withdraw the striking finger to avoid damping the percussed sound.
▼ Strive for a brief, intense tap.

▼ FIGURE A–6. Percussion. *A,* First phalanx of middle finger of nondominant hand is placed firmly on person's skin. *B,* Phalanx on skin is struck with end of middle finger of dominant hand.

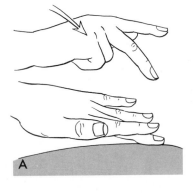

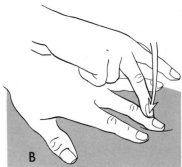

Auscultation

Technique of Auscultation. Auscultation is an assessment technique in which the examiner listens to and assesses the sound produced by various body organs and tissues such as heart, lung, or bowel. Auscultation of the lungs and heart is routinely performed not only as a preliminary scanning procedure but also for ongoing assessment of a person receiving treatment. Auscultation of the abdomen and peripheral blood vessels is also useful. Blood vessels in the neck and head are auscultated at times—for example, if a brain aneurysm is suspected.

Sounds of Auscultation. The following are assessed by auscultation:

▼ *Frequency:* high pitch, low pitch
▼ *Intensity:* loud sounds, soft sounds
▼ *Quality:* differences between two sounds of equal pitch and intensity coming from differing sources, as the lungs and bowels
▼ *Duration* or length of the sound

Types of Auscultation. Auscultation can be performed either directly or indirectly. *Direct auscultation* (immediate auscultation) is less commonly used. The examiner places his or her ear directly against the person's body. This method is limited because the sounds are too diffuse and too soft, especially with obese people. The *indirect method* (most common) is done with a stethoscope.

A quality stethoscope (Fig. A-7) having both a bell and a flat diaphragm is recommended. When gently placed against a person, the bell collects low-frequency sound while permitting high-frequency sound to escape. The *flat diaphragm*, when firmly placed, excludes low-frequency sounds and picks up high-frequency sounds.

Ear pieces should fit comfortably without totally occluding the ear canals. Ear pieces should be clean to maintain unobstructed openings. The tubing should be about one foot long and free of leaks. The tubing should fit tightly on both the ear pieces and the head of the stethoscope. During auscultation, nothing should touch the tubing (otherwise, distracting noises are produced). Tell the person to remain silent unless following directions from the examiner to speak, cough, or breathe deeply through the open mouth. Ask the person to turn the head away from the examiner's face and cover the mouth when coughing and deep breathing. Give the person a tissue. As with other assessment techniques, auscultation is performed systematically.

Olfaction

Olfaction (sense of smell) may help in the diagnosis of many disorders, some of which are serious. Table A-1 lists some characteristic odors and their possible causes.

Promoting Client Comfort During Physical Assessment

A nurse's primary responsibility is to the person receiving care. This includes observing the person care-

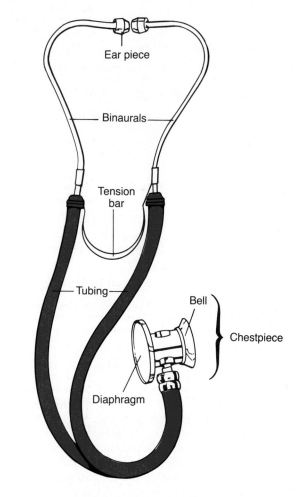

▼**FIGURE A-7.** Stethoscope. The *bell* is used for low-pitched sounds such as bruits. The *diaphragm* is used to assess high-pitched sounds such as lung sounds and blood pressure. See text for further discussion.

fully and making sure comfort is maintained. The person is usually anxious, which is uncomfortable for the person and can distort assessment findings.

Explain the assessment process to the person and the reasons it is being performed. Assure the person that appropriate draping will be provided so that there will be no unnecessary exposure of the person's body.

Before beginning the physical assessment, suggest the person go to the toilet. This helps the person relax and facilitates examination of the abdomen, male genitals or vagina, and rectum. If a urine or stool specimen is needed, you may assist the person in collecting the specimen. Promptly label the specimen with the date and time and your initials after it is collected.

Additional guidelines for promoting client comfort during the physical assessment are as follows:

▼ Keep necessary instruments and equipment assembled, close at hand, and ready for use.
▼ Keep examining area comfortable and private.
▼ Keep personal exposure to a minimum; expose only the area being examined and for only as long as necessary.
▼ Keep the person warm. Elderly, anxious, or ill people chill easily. Provide a lightweight blanket as needed and prevent drafts.

TABLE A–1. Characteristic Odors Detectable During Physical Assessment and Their Possible Causes

Characteristic Odor	Possible Cause
Alcohol, liquefied Sterno, lighter fluid	Intake of these substances
Ammoniac urine (ammonia-like odor)	Urinary tract infection with urea-splitting bacteria
Bitter almond odor	Cyanide poisoning
Body odor (general)	Poor hygiene; excessive perspiration (hyperhidrosis), foul-smelling perspiration (bromhidrosis)
Burnt rope odor	Marijuana
Camphor odor	Mothball ingestion
Fecal odor (in older person)	Wound infection; abscess
Feculent odor	*Bacteroides* abscess
Fetid breath	Lung abscess
Foul-smelling stools (infant)	Malabsorption syndrome, e.g., cystic fibrosis
Garlic odor	Arsenic poisoning
Halitosis ("bad breath")	Poor dental and oral hygiene
"Horsey" or musty odor (infant)	Phenylketonuria (PKU)
Ketone, acetone, sickening sweet odor	Diabetic acidosis
Musty "new-mown clover" odor (fetor hepaticus)	Liver disease, hepatic coma
Nasal malodor (foul odor from nose)	Foreign body in nose; pharyngitis; chronic postnasal drip; nasal crusts; allergic, atrophic, or chronic rhinitis
Paraldehyde odor	Acute poisoning
Stale urine odor	Uremic acidosis
Sweet, heavy, thick odor	*Pseudomonas* infection
Vaginal odor	Fungal infection; poor hygiene

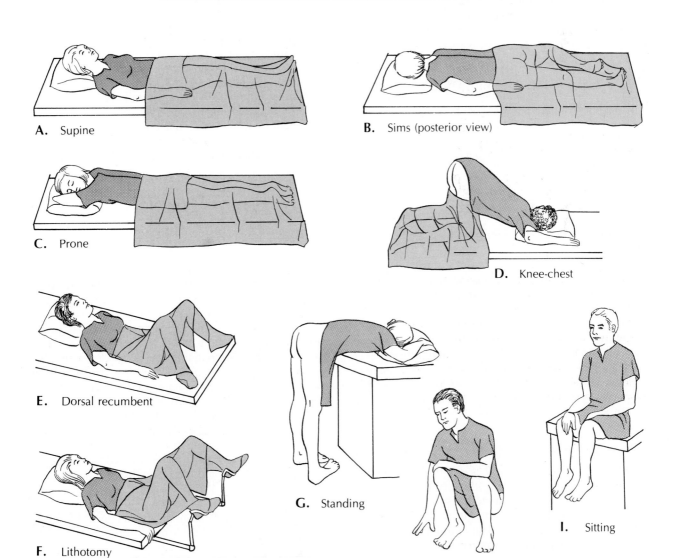

A. Supine

B. Sims (posterior view)

C. Prone

D. Knee-chest

E. Dorsal recumbent

F. Lithotomy

G. Standing

H. Squatting

I. Sitting

▼ **FIGURE A–8.** Common examination positions.

▼ Examiner's hands should be warm, smooth, and clean.
▼ Keep your fingernails clean, short, and smooth. Wash hands just before beginning and immediately after assessment process in the presence of the person.
▼ Warm instruments; for example, warm the bell of a stethoscope by rubbing it between your hands before placing it on a person.
▼ Talk with the person throughout so that activities are not unexpected. "I'm going to listen to your chest now." Give the person clear instructions: "Breathe in and out slowly and deeply through your mouth."

▼ Avoid undesirable nonverbal communication (such as frowning, looks of concern).
▼ A relaxed, friendly, yet professional attitude on the examiner's part helps put a person at ease.
▼ Help the person into required positions (Fig. A-8). Some positions, such as lithotomy and knee-chest, are embarrassing and uncomfortable. Keep a person in these positions no longer than necessary.
▼ Initiate physical contact in nonthreatening ways.

GUIDELINE A-3   ASSESSING GENERAL APPEARANCE

The following areas are to be considered when assessing a person's general appearance (you may have obtained some of this information when taking the client history):

▼ Age: A person's age may influence the physical characteristics observed by the nurse. For example, an elderly person may exhibit the normal physiologic changes of aging, such as loose, wrinkled skin, kyphosis (stooped posture), and a slowed, stiff gait.
▼ Race and sex: The sex of a person can influence the type of examination being performed. Sex and race can influence different physical characteristics observed by the nurse.
▼ Body type, posture, and gait: Assessment of body type, posture, and gait can provide data related to a person's general level of health. Observe a person's build as thin, average, or obese. Note whether the person assumes an erect, bent, or slouched posture. Observe the person's style of walking for smoothness and coordination.
▼ Nutritional status: A person's nutritional state can reflect the level of general health. It can also affect physical characteristics observed by the nurse.

GUIDELINE A-4   ASSESSING MENTAL STATUS AND SPEECH

The assessment of a person's mental status and speech can begin during the client health history. As you collect information concerning the history, observations can be made regarding grooming, dress, and hygiene as well as the person's judgment, orientation, memory, affect, consciousness, and speech. To obtain a complete and detailed assessment of mental status, it will be helpful for you to remember the acronym J-O-M-A-C-S (judgment, orientation, memory, affect, consciousness, speech).

Grooming, Dress, and Hygiene

During the mental status assessment, you will be making observations regarding the person's grooming, type of dress, and hygiene. Some questions you may ask yourself are is the person clean and well-kept? Are the person's hair, skin, and nails clean and well-groomed? Is the clothing appropriate for the present weather conditions and season?

When making these observations, you must also consider the person's lifestyle, cultural orientation, peer group interaction, socioeconomic group, and age. A person may appear to have poor hygiene and grooming habits as a result of pain and weakness that may prevent normal activities of daily living, poor self-esteem, depression, or organic brain syndrome; or poor hygiene may be a result of peer group norms. Elderly individuals will wear extra clothing related to sensitivity changes in body temperature.

Judgment

A person's judgment can be affected by the level of intelligence, educational level, socioeconomic level, and cultural orientation. When assessing this area you may ask the person, "What do you do at a stop sign?" "What do you wear when it is raining?" or "Who will be taking care of your children while you are in the hospital?" You can assess the person's judgment by noting the responses given to each of these questions.

To assess abstract thinking, you may ask the person

to interpret a proverb. Some proverbs you might use are "Don't look a gift horse in the mouth," "A rolling stone gathers no moss," or "A stitch in time saves nine." The person who can correctly explain the meaning of "Don't look a gift horse in the mouth," for example, is capable of abstract thought. However, a person who interprets this proverb by saying "Don't look in a horse's mouth if it is a gift" is thinking on a concrete level. You need to remember that persons for whom English is a second language may translate the proverb literally and may not comprehend the abstract meaning of the proverb.

Orientation

An assessment is made of a person's orientation to person, place, and time. To assess "person," you may ask the individual, "What is your name?" To assess "place," you may ask the person, "Where are you?" or "Where do you live?" To assess "time," you may ask the person, "What time of day is it?" "What day of the week is it?" or "What is the date and year?"

Memory

When assessing memory, you need to test the person's immediate, recent, and remote memory. Immediate memory is tested by reciting a series of seven digits and asking the person to repeat the digits back to you. Normally, a person should be able to repeat seven digits without great difficulty. Choose digits such as zip codes or telephone numbers. Make sure the digits are not in consecutive order.

Recent memory is tested by asking questions that apply to events of the day. Questions may be asked concerning what the person ate for breakfast, weather conditions of the day, and what types of tests the person had during the day. Be sure that you know the answers to each of these questions in order to check the accuracy of the person's memory.

Remote memory is tested by inquiring about past events, such as types of employment, mother's maiden name, birthday and anniversary dates, and social security number. Again, you must be sure of the accuracy of the information the person is giving you to arrive at an accurate assessment.

Affect

Affect is an emotional state, such as fear, anger, depression, elation, and frustration. As you observe the person, note the lack of emotional response or the presence of outward manifestations that may suggest emotion. Does the person smile, frown, exhibit anger, or cry appropriately according to the situation being discussed? Keep in mind that cultural norms may dictate one's affect.

Consciousness

The assessment of consciousness begins with noting whether the client is awake and alert. While communicating, note whether the person is able to answer your questions appropriately and within a reasonably quick time frame. If the person has an altered level of consciousness, assess whether the person is demonstrating obtundation, stupor, or coma.

Speech

Throughout the client health history and physical examination, you need to note the characteristics of the person's speech. Speech is assessed for quantity (talkative or silent), rate (fast or slow), loudness, and enunciation.

GUIDELINE A-5   ASSESSING THE SKIN

The integumentary system serves as a source of protection for the body from the environment, as a body temperature regulator, and as a sensor for temperature, pain, and touch. The layers of the skin tissue are the epidermis, dermis, and subcutaneous tissue. When assessing the skin, you may choose to assess the entire skin surface at one time or as a part of each body system. The assessment techniques used with the integumentary system are inspection, palpation, and olfaction.

Areas to consider when assessing the skin are color, temperature, texture, mobility, lesions, and vascularity. Prior to beginning your assessment, make sure that you have a good light source. Have a pair of sterile gloves ready in case you encounter a draining skin lesion, for it will require palpation. Skin odors, if any, usually will be detected in skin folds or in the axillary area.

Color

Inspect the skin for generalized color. Skin color will vary according to body part. A person's race will also affect skin color. The color of the skin will range from light to dark pink, light to dark brown, or yellow to olive. Assess those areas of least pigmentation for any possible color changes such as the palms, soles, sclera, and nails.

Abnormal changes in skin color include cyanosis, jaundice, and pallor. **Cyanosis,** a bluish mottled discoloration of the skin, nailbeds, and mucous membranes, caused by decreased oxygenation of the blood, can best be assessed in the legs, buccal mucosa, and tongue. In persons with darker skin tones, cyanosis may be detected better in the palms, soles, palpebral conjunctiva, and nails. **Jaundice,** a yellow discoloration of the skin resulting from an increase in bilirubin, may be assessed in the bulbar and palpebral conjunctiva, lips, hard palate, posterior aspect of the tongue, and the skin itself. **Pallor** is an absence of color in the skin, which appears whitish-gray in a light-skinned person and ashen gray or as a loss of red glow tones in a person with dark skin. Pallor is best assessed in the fingernails, lips, mucous membranes, and palpebral conjunctiva.

Temperature and Moisture

Skin temperature should remain relatively the same over the entire body. When there is a change in temperature over a body area, it is an indication of a change in blood circulation to that part of the body. Palpation is the technique used in assessing skin temperature. Temperature is best assessed using the dorsum or back of the hand. Normally, the skin temperature is warm. Excessive coolness or warmth indicates a deviation from normal.

Skin moisture is assessed by inspection and palpation. Normally, the skin should be dry to touch with the exception of skin folds and the axilla, which normally are moist. Moisture refers to wetness and oiliness. Palpate the skin for temperature and moisture. Compare similar body parts in relation to temperature and moisture.

Texture

The skin's texture should be smooth, soft, and flexible over the majority of the body. Normally, some areas such as the palms and the soles possess a thicker texture. The skin should be palpated to assess texture. Note the location of areas where there are irregularities in texture.

Turgor and Mobility

Skin turgor is an indication of hydration status, assessed by pinching up the skin and releasing it. It de-

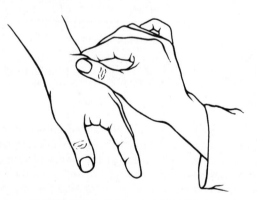

▼ **FIGURE A-9.** Assessing skin turgor.

notes the skin's elasticity. To assess skin turgor, pinch up the skin on the forehead, sternum, dorsum of the hand, or forearm, and release. You should note the speed at which the skin returns to its former state. Normally, the skin returns to its original position quickly (Fig. A-9). Skin turgor is classified as poor when it takes 3 seconds or longer for the skin to return to its original position.

As a result of age, the elderly person loses skin elasticity. You may note upon examination that the skin turgor of an elderly person will show a delayed response. Skin turgor and mobility will be diminished when edema is present.

Lesions

Normally, the skin should be free of lesions. Primary lesions arise from normal skin tissue. Secondary lesions occur as a result of changes in the primary lesion. If you observe a lesion on the skin, note the size in centimeters, location, distribution (localized or generalized), pattern (linear, clustered, or annular), color, and type. Palpate the lesion to denote mobility (fixed or mobile), contour (flat or raised), and consistency (soft or hard). Be sure to wear sterile gloves when palpating draining lesions. Table A-2 summarizes some common skin lesions.

Vascularity

Vascularity involves the blood circulation of the skin and the appearance of superficial blood vessels. **Petechiae** (minute hemorrhages under the skin) and ecchymosis can result from abnormal vascularity. Petechiae are tiny purple or red spots on the skin. **Ecchymosis** (bruising) is a discoloration of an area of the skin. **Edema** is an accumulation of excessive fluid in the interstitial spaces. The area will appear swollen, shiny, and taut. On inspection, you should note the location and the appearance. During palpation, you should note mobility, consistency, and tenderness.

As tissue fluid increases, pitting edema will occur. Upon palpation, you will note that your finger leaves an indentation in the edematous area. To test for the degree of pitting edema, press your finger into the edematous area for 2 to 3 seconds and note the depth of the indentation. Pitting edema is described on a scale from 1+ to 4+. Table A-3 demonstrates the degrees of edema. A measuring tape may also be used to measure edema. You would indicate the exact measure of one body part and compare it with the other body part. Both measurements would be charted.

TABLE A-2. Skin Lesions

Lesion	Characteristics	Example

Primary Lesions

	Macule	Small, up to 1 cm	Freckle, petechia
	Patch	Larger than 1 cm	Vitiligo
	Papule	Up to 0.5 cm	Elevated nevus
	Plaque	Flat, uneven surface larger than 0.5 cm	Coalescence of papules
	Nodule	0.5 cm to 1–2 cm, deeper and firmer than a papule	Wart

Table continued on following page

TABLE A–2. Skin Lesions Continued

Lesion	Characteristics	Example

Primary Lesions

Tumor — Elevated and deep, larger than 1–2 cm — Epithelioma

Wheal — Area of localized skin edema — Insect bite

Vesicle — Contains serous fluid up to 0.5 cm — Blister

Bulla — Contains serous fluid greater than 0.5 cm — Second-degree burn

Pustule — Filled with pus — Acne

Secondary Lesions

Ulcer — Deep loss of skin surface — Venous stasis ulcer

TABLE A–2. Skin Lesions Continued

Lesion		Characteristics	Example
Primary Lesions			
	Fissure	Linear crack in the skin	Athlete's foot
	Crust	Dried residue of serum, pus, or blood	Impetigo
	Scale	Thin flake of exfoliated epidermis	Dandruff, dry skin

TABLE A–3. Grades of Edema

	Grade	Characteristics
	1+	Slight pit, normal contour
	2+	Deeper pit, fairly normal contour
	3+	Puffy appearance, deeper pit
	4+	Extremely deep pit, definitively swollen

Illustrations from Judge, R., et al. (1982). Clinical diagnosis (4th ed.). Boston: Little, Brown.

GUIDELINE A-6   ASSESSING THE HAIR AND SCALP

When assessing the head, you will be inspecting and palpating the hair, scalp, skull, and face. You will begin your assessment by asking if the person has noted any changes in relation to the hair and scalp.

Hair. Inspect the hair for quality, quantity, and distribution. The quality of the hair refers to the texture and color of the hair. Terms used to describe the texture are "coarse" and "fine". A sudden change in texture, such as dryness, brittleness, or fragility, may indicate a bodily dysfunction. An increase in dryness and coarseness of the hair may indicate hypothyroidism, whereas an increase in silkiness and fineness may indicate hyperthyroidism. You will need to observe for nits, which are tiny, white, ovoid eggs of lice. The color of a person's hair will be significant only when there has been a sudden change in it. This may indicate nerve injury involvement.

The quantity and distribution of a person's hair will vary with age. You will need to inspect for any areas of alopecia (partial or complete loss of hair). This can be a result of normal aging, an endocrine disorder, a drug reaction, or skin disease. Also, observe for any abnormal facial hair.

Scalp and Skull. When inspecting and palpating the scalp and skull, it is important to separate the hair and take a thorough look at the skin underlying the hair. You will be observing for areas of inflammation, cysts, warts, moles, insect bites, flaking, and scaliness. If you observe any masses, be sure to describe the size, shape, consistency, and location.

Palpation of the scalp and skull involves using a rotary motion with the pads of your fingers. You will begin with the frontal region (forehead) and palpate over the entire skull to the occipital region. This includes palpating the temporal and parietal regions. You will be inspecting and palpating the skull for size, shape, symmetry, and tenderness.

GUIDELINE A-7   ASSESSING THE FACE AND CRANIAL NERVES

Cranial Nerves

The assessment of the cranial nerves is a crucial aspect of the neurologic system assessment. The cranial nerves originate from the brain stem with the exception of the olfactory nerve, which is located in the temporal lobe, and the optic nerve, which is located in the occipital lobe. Since many of the tests for cranial nerve function also measure various structures and muscles within the head and neck, assessment of cranial nerves is included in the section on head and neck.

To learn and remember the cranial nerves, you may associate the name and type of nerve with several phrases.

To remember the name of each cranial nerve, learn the following sentence: "On old Olympus' towering tops, a Finn and German viewed some hops." The first letter in each word is the same as the first letter in each of the cranial nerves. To remember the type (sensory, motor, or both) of each cranial nerve, learn the following phrase: "Some say marry money but my brother says bad business marry money." The first letter of each word represents sensory, motor, or both types. Each word corresponds to one cranial nerve. For example, "Some" represents the sensory function of the olfactory nerve. Table A-4 summarizes the functions of the cranial nerves.

Face

Inspect the face for size, shape, symmetry, and any tics or abnormal movements. A good reference point for asymmetry of the face is the palpebral fissures of the eyes and the nasolabial folds. The palpebral fissures are the spaces between the upper and lower eyelids (Fig. A-10). They should be equal in size when comparing the right and left fissure. The nasolabial folds are creases that

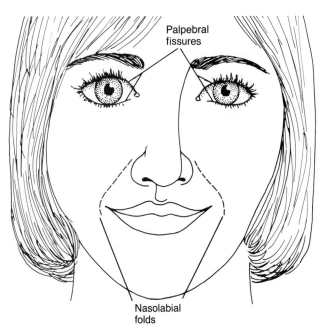

▼ **FIGURE A–10.** To assess facial symmetry, observe the palpebral fissures and nasolabial folds. They should be equal bilaterally.

TABLE A–4. Cranial Nerve Functions

Cranial Nerve Number	Name	Type	Function
I	Olfactory	Sensory	Smell
II	Optic	Sensory	Visual fields
			Visual acuity
			Color discrimination
			Vision
III	Oculomotor	Motor	Pupil constriction and dilation
			Convergence
			Extraocular movement
IV	Trochlear	Motor	Extraocular movement
V	Trigeminal	Sensory and motor	Corneal sensitivity
			Sensation to skin of face
			Motor nerve to masseter and temporal muscles
VI	Abducens	Motor	Extraocular movement
VII	Facial	Sensory and motor	Facial expression
			Taste (anterior tongue)
VIII	Auditory	Sensory	Hearing
IX	Glossopharyngeal	Sensory and motor	Gag reflex
			Taste (posterior tongue)
X	Vagus	Sensory and motor	Sensation of the pharynx
			Swallowing ability
			Vocal cord movement
XI	Spinal Accessory	Motor	Head and shoulder movement
XII	Hypoglossal	Motor	Tongue movement

extend from the angle of the nose to the corner of the mouth. They should be bilaterally symmetrical.

During the inspection and palpation of the face, test the function of the trigeminal and facial cranial nerves.

Trigeminal Nerve. The trigeminal nerve (CN V) has a motor and sensory function. The motor function of the trigeminal nerve is to innervate the muscles used in chewing. To test this function, ask the person to clench the teeth while you palpate the temporal muscles (temporal area) and the masseter muscles (jaw area). Note the strength of muscle contraction. A weakness or absence on one side may indicate a trigeminal nerve lesion.

The trigeminal nerve also innervates the nasal and oral mucosa, facial skin, and corneal reflex through its sensory branches. To test the sensory function, instruct the person to close the eyes. With a safety pin, touch the forehead, cheeks, and jaw area with the point of the safety pin, intermittently substituting the blunt end of the pin. Have the person tell you whether it is sharp or dull. Be sure to compare each side of the face. The sensory function related to the corneas will be discussed when examination of the eyes is described.

Facial Nerve. The facial nerve has sensory and motor functions. The sensory function will be discussed in relation to the mouth. To test the motor function, ask the person to smile, frown, raise the eyebrows, close the eyes tightly, and puff out the cheeks. Observe for asymmetry and weakness.

GUIDELINE A-8   ASSESSING THE EYES

Inspection and palpation are used to assess the eyes (Fig. A-11). Areas to be assessed are the position and alignment of the eyes, eyebrows, eyelids, lacrimal apparatus, conjunctiva and sclera, pupils, and cranial nerves (occulomotor, trochlear, abducens, trigeminal, and optic). The desirable position for a person during the examination is sitting, if possible, looking straight ahead unless otherwise noted.

Position and Alignment

When inspecting the eyes for position and alignment, ask yourself: Are the eyes in line with the top of the ears? When you and the person look at each other, is the person's gaze focused directly on yours and do the eyes look alike? Normally, the upper quadrant of the iris cannot be seen when you are facing the person because the eyelid covers it. Any abnormal protrusion of the eyes is called exophthalmos.

Eyebrows

Inspect the quantity and distribution of the eyebrows. Ask the person if the eyebrows have been plucked. Observe for scarring, lesions, and hair loss. Hair loss may indicate a fungal infection.

Bulbar conjunctiva

Sclera

Palpebral conjunctiva

Upper eyelid

Cornea

Pupil

Iris

Lens

Retina

Lower eyelid

▼ **FIGURE A–11.** Eye structures.

Eyelids

Inspect the eyelids for symmetry, position in relation to the eyeballs, inflammation, lesions (chalazion, sty), edema, and **ptosis** (drooping of the eyelid). Drooping of the eyelid may indicate oculomotor damage because the oculomotor nerve (CN III) innervates the upper lid to open and remain open. Inspect the eyelashes, which should be full and extend outward along the entire eyelid. Crusting, scaling, and hair loss are signs of infection.

Lacrimal Apparatus

The lacrimal apparatus comprises the lacrimal gland, sacs, ducts, and the nasolacrimal ducts (Fig. A-12). The puncta are openings located in the inner canthus of the upper and lower eyelid. The major function of this apparatus is to create tears. Tears keep the eyes moist and clean. Upon inspection, note any excessive dryness or tearing of the eye. Gently palpate the inner canthus and observe the fluid from the puncta. A purulent fluid indicates infection.

Conjunctivae and Sclerae

The conjunctiva is a membrane that protects the outer surface of the sclera and the inner surface of the eyelids. The conjunctiva that covers the sclera is called bulbar. Palpebral conjunctiva covers the inner surfaces of the upper and lower eyelids. Inspect the palpebral conjunctiva and sclera by pulling down the lower lid while instructing the person to look up. Inspect for lesions, inflammation, and swelling. Normally, the palpebral conjunctiva is reddish in color due to tiny blood vessels. Anemia is suspected when the palpebral conjunctiva is pale. Bulbar conjunctiva is clear but appears white due to the sclera being located beneath it. When the bulbar

conjunctiva is yellow, it is indicative of jaundice. The sclera is white. You will note a yellowish color to the sclera in dark-skinned people. Because of this, you will need to ask the person if a change has been observed in the color of the sclera.

The palpebral conjunctiva of the upper eyelid is inspected when a foreign body is suspected. This requires eversion of the upper eyelid, which is an advanced skill. Therefore, it will not be discussed in this appendix.

Pupils

Inspect the pupils for equality, size, shape, reaction to light, and accommodation. The oculomotor (CN III), trochlear (CN IV), and abducens (CN VI) nerves are tested at this time because they innervate pupillary constriction. Pupillary reaction to light and accommodation test these three cranial nerves.

Normal pupillary function is documented as "PERRLA": Pupils Equal, Round, React to Light and Accommodation.

Pupillary Reaction. Pupillary reaction to light is assessed by the direct and consensual light reflex. A pen-

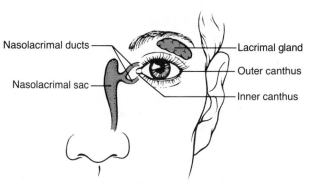

Nasolacrimal ducts

Nasolacrimal sac

Lacrimal gland

Outer canthus

Inner canthus

▼ **FIGURE A–12.** The lacrimal apparatus.

light is used to assess this reflex. Instruct the person to focus on a distant object. This is important so that the pupils do not constrict in an attempt to focus on something close or because they are looking at you. Shine the penlight into the pupil of one eye (about 8 inches away from the eye). Observe the reaction to the light in both eyes. Normally, the illuminated pupil constricts (direct light) and the other pupil constricts simultaneously (consensual response). Test both pupils. If you should have difficulty assessing pupillary constriction, darken the room and use a bright light before making the judgment that pupillary reaction is absent. Intracranial pressure can affect the pupil's reaction to light.

Accommodation. Accommodation (eye's adaptation for near vision) is tested by asking the person to focus on a distant object, then on a near object. You may use your finger, a pencil, or an unlit penlight, holding it 8 to 12 inches from the bridge of the nose. Instruct the person alternately to look at the object and then into the distance. Normally, the pupils should converge and constrict symmetrically as the eyes focus on a near object.

Oculomotor, Trochlear, Abducens Nerves

In addition to innervating pupillary constriction (see pupils), the oculomotor, trochlear, and abducens nerves control the horizontal, vertical, and diagonal movements of the eyes. The cardinal positions test, cover-uncover test, and the corneal light reflex test are used to assess extraocular movements of the eye.

Cardinal Positions Test. To perform the cardinal positions test, hold your finger or a pencil about 6 to 12 inches from the person's eyes. Instruct the person to follow it with the eyes while keeping the head still. Take the person through the six cardinal positions of gaze (Fig. A-13). Pause at each position in order to detect nystagmus (abnormal rhythmic oscillations of the eyes).

Cover-Uncover Test. To perform the cover-uncover test, instruct the person to stare directly at an object with both eyes. Take a card and cover one eye for 10 seconds, remove it, and observe any movement in the once-covered eye as it attempts to refocus on the designated object. Repeat on the opposite eye. Normally, no movement will be noted. If movement is observed, this signifies a muscle imbalance (strabismus).

Corneal Light Reflex Test. To test for the corneal light reflex, stand about 2 feet directly in front of the person. Shine your penlight at the bridge of the nose and inspect the reflections in the person's corneas. The cornea should reflect the light in exactly the same place

in both eyes. An asymmetrical reflex indicates strabismus.

Trigeminal Nerve

To assess another aspect of the sensory function of the trigeminal nerve (CN V), you will assess the corneal reflex. This is a higher level assessment skill and should not be attempted without supervision. Be sure to explain the procedure to the person before proceeding. Using a small piece of cotton, gently stroke the cornea of the eye. The normal reaction should be a blink. Test both eyes. Remember to use a separate piece of cotton for each eye to avoid cross-contamination. If the person does not have a normal response, a trigeminal lesion is suspected.

Optic Nerve

To assess the optic nerve (CN II), the person is tested for visual fields, visual acuity, color discrimination, and abnormalities of the inner eye structures (ophthalmoscopic examination).

A person's visual field is the entire area seen by the eye when it is focused on a designated point. Instruct the person to sit 2 feet in front of you. Your eyes should be at the same level as those of the person being tested. Have the person cover one eye and stare at your eye directly opposite. Close your other eye. You may use a pencil or your fingers to test the person. Instruct the person to answer when the pencil or finger is first seen. Then move the object into the person's field of vision from each direction. You and the person should see the object at the same time. You may note that the temporal visual field of both you and the person will extend beyond your testing hand. You will need to start by placing the object behind the person and out of the visual field when testing the temporal area. This test identifies marked restriction of peripheral vision. Normally, the object should be seen within 50 degrees superiorly, 60 degrees nasally, 70 degrees inferiorly, and 90 degrees temporally.

Distance Visual Acuity

A Snellen chart is a chart used to test a person's visual acuity (see Fig. A-1). The Snellen chart has numbers at the end of each line of letters. The numerator is always 20, which is the distance in feet between the chart and the person being examined. The denominator is the distance at which a person with normal vision can read a particular line. For example, 20/30 means that a person stood 20 feet away to read a line that a person with normal vision can read at 30 feet away. As the denominator increases, the distance vision decreases. Test each eye separately by covering the other eye with the person's hand or card. Then test both eyes uncovered. If the person wears corrective lenses, the lenses may be worn for the test. Standing 20 feet away, the person is instructed to read the smallest, clearest line. A person must be able to read a line correctly with no more than two errors. The line read then indicates the person's distance visual acuity.

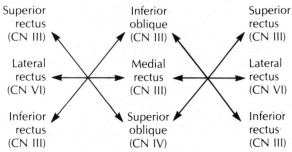

▼ **FIGURE A–13.** Six cardinal positions of gaze.

Near Visual Acuity

When testing near visual acuity, a newspaper with various sizes of print may be used. Hold the newspaper 6 to 12 inches from the face. Instruct the person to read several lines. Test each eye separately and then together.

Color Discrimination

To test color discrimination, have the person distinguish colors, usually red and green. You may use the Snellen chart for this test since it has various colors on it.

Ophthalmoscopic Examination

To perform the ophthalmoscopic examination, the room must be darkened. Instruct the person to stare at a designated spot. Standing in front of the person, about 18 inches away and 15 degrees to the right of the person's line of vision, shine the light of the ophthalmoscope on the pupil. To steady yourself, it might help to place your opposite hand on the person's forehead.

The ophthalmoscope should be set at 0 diopters, and your index finger should be placed on the lens selector. As the light of the ophthalmoscope enters the pupil, move the lens selector until you have the various structures in focus. Try to keep both your eyes open, as this decreases the blurriness experienced.

You should observe the following: (1) red reflex, which indicates that the lens is free of opacity (cataract) and clouding; and (2) retinal structures, which include the retinal vessels, retinal background, optic disk, and macula (Fig. A-14). If you have difficulty finding the optic disk, look for a retinal blood vessel and follow the

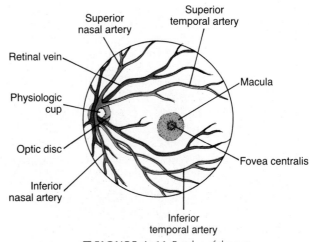

▼ FIGURE A–14. Fundus of the eye.

vessel nasally. The vessels become larger in diameter as they enter the optic disk. Evaluate the size, shape, and arteriovenous crossing of the blood vessels. Normal arteries will not displace or indent veins. The arteries will be a light red, and the veins will be larger and darker in color. The ratio of arteries to veins is 4:5. The optic disk is a round, yellowish orange to creamy pink structure. It should be lighter than the retinal background. The macula should be examined last since it is the area of the retina with the greatest visual acuity and sensitivity to light. It is located temporal to the optic disk. When inspecting the retinal background and structures, assess any areas of hemorrhage, cotton wool patch, arteriovenous nicking, and papilledema.

GUIDELINE A-9   ASSESSING THE EARS

Inspection and palpation are the techniques used to examine the ear. Areas to be assessed are the external ear (auricle) and ear canal, internal ear canal and tympanic membrane (by performing an otoscopic examination), and the acoustic nerve (Fig. A-15).

Auricles

Inspect the auricle for color, size, configuration, location, and angle of attachment to the head (Fig. A-16). The color of the ear should be the same as that of the person's skin, and the size should be in proportion to the head. The auricle should be at a level equal to the outer canthus of the eye. Inspect the external ear canal for intactness, general hygiene, a buildup of cerumen (ear wax), discharge, redness, and swelling. The normal ear canal should be clean, dry, free of lesions, and with a minimal amount of cerumen. If discharge is observed, note the color, amount, consistency, and clarity.

Palpate the external ear for nodules and tenderness. The mastoid process is also palpated for tenderness. If the person complains of pain when the auricle is moved up and down, it is indicative of an external ear infection. If palpation elicits pain in the mastoid process, otitis media is a possibility.

Otoscopic Examination

To inspect the internal ear canal and tympanic membrane, an otoscope must be used. With your dominant hand, hold the otoscope upside down and prop your hand against the person's head. This will prevent any injury to the ear canal in case the person makes a sudden move. Use a speculum large enough to fit the ear comfortably. Instruct the person to tilt the head to the opposite shoulder. With the nondominant hand, pull the auricle up and back to straighten the ear canal. Insert the speculum slowly and cautiously.

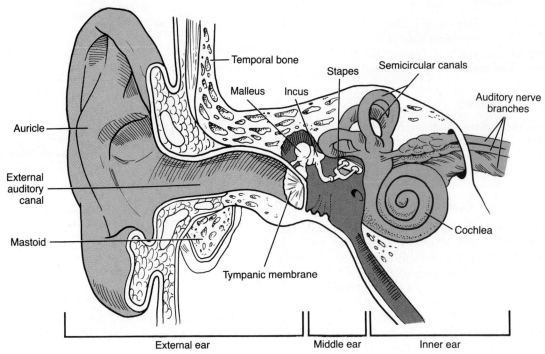

▼ **FIGURE A–15.** The external, middle, and inner ear structures.

Inspect the internal ear canal for impacted cerumen, foreign bodies, discharge, masses, redness, and swelling. Normally, you will view some cerumen, which varies in color (yellow, brown) and consistency (flaky, sticky). Inspect the tympanic membrane (Fig. A-17), which is usually a shiny pearly gray or light pink. Note the landmarks, which include the handle and short process of the malleus, pars flaccida, pars tensa, and cone of light. The cone of light will be located at five o'clock in the right ear and seven o'clock in the left ear. Observe for perforations, altered or absent landmarks, distorted or absent cone of light, abnormal color, bulging or retraction, discharge, fluid or air bubbles behind the tympanic membrane, absence of normal movement, and scars.

Acoustic Nerve

The acoustic nerve is assessed by auditory acuity, Weber lateralization test, Rinne air and bone conduction test, and Schwabach test. Auditory acuity is assessed by the watch and whisper test. The watch test screens high-

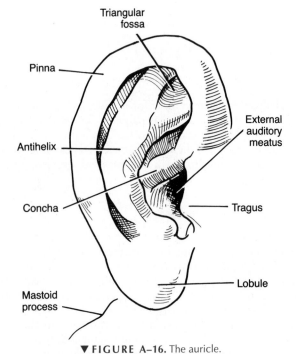

▼ **FIGURE A–16.** The auricle.

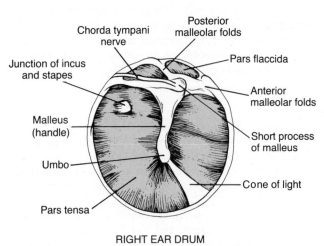

RIGHT EAR DRUM

▼ **FIGURE A–17.** A normal tympanic membrane.

frequency impairment. Instruct the person to occlude one ear. Move a watch toward the person's unoccluded ear and determine the distance at which the person hears the watch. Test both ears. The whisper test is performed by having the person occlude one ear. You will stand 1 to 2 feet away from the person and whisper a two-digit number with your mouth covered. Note the person's ability to hear you. Test both ears. If abnormalities are detected, further testing is needed using an audiometer.

Weber Lateralization Test. To perform the Weber lateralization test, place the stem of a vibrating tuning fork in the center of the forehead (Fig. A-18). Ask the person where the sound is heard best. Normally, sound is heard equally well in both ears as it is conducted through the bones. Note any lateralization of sound (sound heard better in one ear than the other). A person with a unilateral conductive hearing loss will hear the sound best in the impaired ear. This can occur with otitis media, perforation, or an obstruction. Sound is heard best in the good ear with a unilateral sensorineural hearing loss.

Rinne Air and Bone Conduction Test. The Rinne air and bone conduction test compares bone-conducted sound with air-conducted sound in one ear at a time (Fig. A-19). Place the stem of the vibrating tuning fork on the mastoid process behind the ear. Quickly move the fork beside the ear canal as soon as the person says the sound is gone from contact with the mastoid bone. Placement beside the ear tests air conduction. With a normal (positive) Rinne test, sound is heard twice as long by air conduction as by bone conduction. This finding is documented as AC > BC. You should time the length using a watch.

Schwabach Test. The Schwabach test compares the person's bone conduction with yours. Place the vibrating

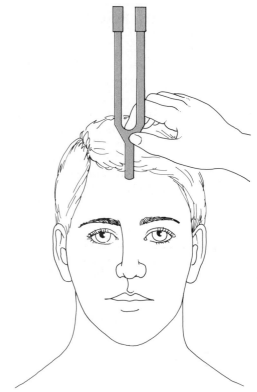

▼ **FIGURE A–18.** Weber lateralization test.

tuning fork on the person's mastoid process and then on your mastoid process. Continue to move the tuning fork back and forth until the sound is diminished. Normally, the bone conduction should be approximately equal between you and the person being examined.

▼ **FIGURE A–19.** Rinne air and bone conduction test.

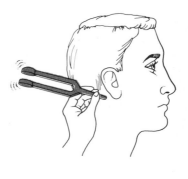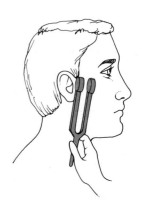

GUIDELINE A-10   ASSESSING THE NOSE AND SINUSES

The nose is assessed by inspection and palpation. Inspect the external surface of the nose for symmetry in color, shape, and size. It is common for one ala nasi to be slightly larger than the other. Inspect the external septum for symmetry and any signs of deviation. The septum should separate the nares in a straight line. Palpate the external nares for tenderness. To assess the patency, ask the person to occlude one ala nasi while breathing through the other.

Nasal Cavity

When inspecting the nasal cavity, you may use a penlight. A nasal speculum can also be used but only by a more experienced examiner. Instruct the person to tilt the head back, then shine the penlight into the nasal cavity. Inspect the mucosa. It should be moist and pink. Note any swelling, lesions, or drainage. Inspect the middle and inferior turbinates. They should be the same color as the adjacent nasal mucosa. Note any pallor, redness, swelling, or polyps.

Frontal and Maxillary Sinuses

The frontal and maxillary sinuses are palpated for tenderness, swelling, thickening, or secretions (Fig. A-20). Palpate the frontal sinuses by pressing up on the skull on either side of the nose under the eyebrows. Do not press on the eyes. Palpate the maxillary sinuses by pressing up over the lower part of the cheekbones on either side of the nose.

Olfactory Nerve

To assess the sensory function of the olfactory nerve (CN I), instruct the person to close the eyes and occlude one ala nasi. Provide a familiar scent such as coffee or cinnamon for the person to smell. Test both nares. An absence of the sense of smell may result from excessive smoking, cocaine use, or a sinus condition.

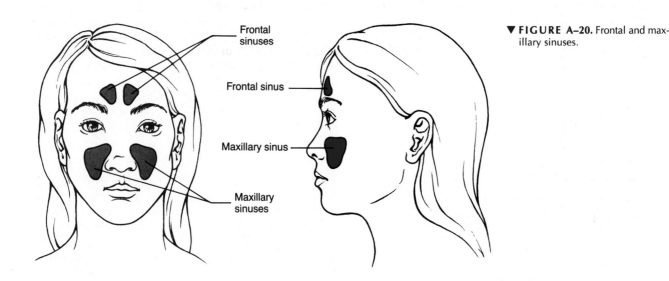

▼ **FIGURE A–20.** Frontal and maxillary sinuses.

Frontal sinuses

Frontal sinus

Maxillary sinus

Maxillary sinuses

GUIDELINE A-11 ASSESSING THE MOUTH AND PHARYNX

The mouth and pharynx are assessed through inspection and palpation. Areas to be examined include the lips, buccal mucosa, gums and teeth, tongue, soft and hard palate, pharynx, and glossopharyngeal, vagus, facial, and hypoglossal nerves. A penlight, tongue blade, gauze, and a pair of gloves will be needed to complete the assessment. Remember to wear the gloves when assessing the mucosa of the mouth (Fig. A-21).

Lips

Inspect the lips for symmetry, color, edema, and any surface abnormalities. Note that the lips are more pigmented than the facial skin. The most common lesions associated with the lips are fissures, commonly seen with chapped lips and herpes simplex (cold sores). Using a gloved hand, palpate the lips for moistness, induration, intactness, and lesions.

Gums and Teeth

Inspect the gums by placing your gloved hand on the lower lip and gently pulling it down to expose the gums. Repeat the procedure on the upper lip. Normally, the gums are pink in color and free of lesions, inflammation, and bleeding. Palpate the gums for retraction away from the teeth, lesions, swelling, and hypertrophy. If the person wears dentures, provide a paper towel and tissues for denture removal.

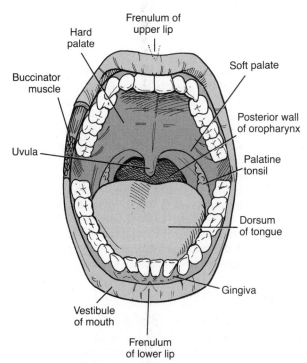

Hard palate
Frenulum of upper lip
Buccinator muscle
Soft palate
Posterior wall of oropharynx
Uvula
Palatine tonsil
Dorsum of tongue
Gingiva
Vestibule of mouth
Frenulum of lower lip

▼ **FIGURE A–21.** Structures of the mouth.

The teeth should be clean, white, straight, firm, evenly spaced, and free of obvious decay. Normally, there are 32 teeth. Inspect for caries, plaque, missing or loose teeth, dentures (note the fit of the denture), and color. Inspection of the teeth can also provide information regarding the person's attitude toward general hygiene.

Buccal Mucosa

When inspecting the buccal mucosa, you will need a tongue blade to displace the cheeks to the side in order to view the mucous membranes with a penlight. Be sure to inspect both cheeks, because diseases of the mouth are not always manifested symmetrically. Inspect the mucosa for color, pigmentation, ulcers, white patches, and nodules. Normally, the mucosa will be pink, smooth, moist, and free of lesions. In a dark-skinned person, the mucosa will have a patchy brown pigmentation, which is normal.

Tongue

Inspect and palpate the tongue, using a gloved hand and a piece of gauze. Note the symmetry, movement, and color of the tongue. Normally, it should be pink, moist, and smooth, with papillae and fissures present. Ask the person to extend the tongue so that you may palpate it from front to back. Wrap a piece of gauze around the tongue during palpation. Note any masses. Instruct the person to touch the tip of the tongue to the top of the mouth, so that you may examine the floor of the mouth for cyanosis, pallor, and any lesions or nodules. The floor of the mouth is a common site for oral cancer.

Soft and Hard Palates

The hard palate is located in the anterior roof of the mouth. It is white or pale pink in color and firm in nature. The hard palate is where jaundice can be readily detected. The soft palate is located posteriorly and is pink in color, with a spongy texture. Inspect the hard and soft palate for lesions and asymmetry. Also, inspect for absence of elevation in the soft palate when the client says "Ah."

Pharynx

Inspect the posterior wall of the mouth with your penlight by asking the person to extend the tongue. A tongue blade may be used to press against the person's tongue for better viewing. Normally, it should be pink and free of drainage. The pharynx of a smoker will appear yellowish red with small nodules present. If drainage is observed, note the amount, color, and consistency. Unless they have been surgically removed, inspect the tonsils, which are small, pink surface growths. Note any enlargement of the tonsils with exudate present. Inspect the uvula, which should be located in the midline. Note any deviation from the midline.

Glossopharyngeal and Vagus Nerves

These two cranial nerves are usually tested together because they innervate many of the same structures. Instruct the person to extend the tongue and say "Ah." Note the uvula and soft palate. Both structures should rise up. There should be no deviation to the side by the uvula. Next, take your tongue blade and touch the back of the throat gently. A gag reflex should be elicited. A lesion of the glossopharyngeal or vagus nerve is suspected when there is an absent gag reflex. Be sure to warn the person when you are going to test the gag reflex.

To test the sensory portion of the glossopharyngeal nerve, place a taste, such as sugar, salt, or lemon juice,

on the posterior one third of the tongue. With closed eyes, the person should be able to identify the taste. When applying different tastes to the tongue, use separate cotton-tipped applicators. Allow the person to drink water between tastes.

Facial Nerve

The sensory portion of the facial nerve is tested by applying a taste on the anterior two thirds of the tongue. With eyes closed, a person should readily identify the taste.

Hypoglossal Nerve

To test the motor function of the hypoglossal nerve (CN XII), observe the tongue for position (midline) and movement (smooth, no tremors). Instruct the person to move the tongue from side to side and touch the roof of the mouth. Observe for symmetry of movement.

GUIDELINE A-12   ASSESSING THE NECK

Assessment of the neck is performed using the techniques of inspection and palpation. Upon examination, the person should be in an upright position to facilitate extension and rotation of the neck. Inspect the neck for color, symmetry, masses, enlargement of the thyroid or lymph nodes, abnormal pulsations, impaired range of motion, lesions, and scars. Palpate the neck for skin temperature and texture. Instruct the person to move the neck carefully through the entire range of motion, which includes right and left lateral, right and left rotation, flexion, extension, and hyperextension. The neck should move easily without any discomfort. The elderly person may experience some discomfort from neck movement, because of a decrease in range of motion.

Lymph Nodes

Palpate the lymph nodes, using the pads of your index and middle fingers. Instead of moving your fingertips over the skin surface, move the skin over the node area. Gently palpate in sequence bilaterally the preauricular, posterior auricular, occipital, tonsillar, submaxillary, submental, anterior cervical, posterior cervical, supraclavicular, and infraclavicular lymph nodes (Fig. A-22).

If a node is palpated, note the location, size (in centimeters), shape (usually round), mobility (movable or fixed), consistency (soft, hard, firm), tenderness, and delimitation (discrete or matted together). If you have difficulty distinguishing an enlarged node from other structures of the neck, remember that a lymph node is able to roll up and down and side to side.

Thyroid

Inspect and palpate the thyroid gland for size, shape, symmetry, and any masses by instructing the person to swallow water while extending the neck (Fig. A-23). Normally, the thyroid gland and the thyroid and cricoid cartilage will rise as the person swallows. An en-

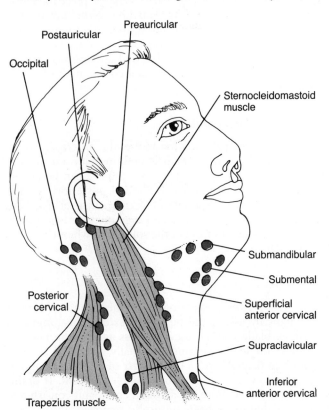

▼ FIGURE A–22. Lymph nodes of the neck.

Sternocleidomastoid muscle

Thyroid cartilage

Trachea

Thyroid gland

LATERAL VIEW

Anterior triangle

Sternocleidomastoid muscle

Internal carotid artery

Posterior triangle

Trapezius muscle

Clavicle

Thyroid cartilage

Cricoid cartilage

Thyroid gland lobe and isthmus

Trachea

ANTERIOR VIEW

▼ FIGURE A–23. The thyroid and surrounding neck structures.

larged thyroid gland is called a **goiter.** You may palpate the thyroid gland by standing in front of or behind the person. Instruct the person to extend the neck as you place your fingers just below the cricoid cartilage. Ask the person to swallow. You will be able to feel the thyroid isthmus rise beneath your fingers.

Trachea

Inspect and palpate the trachea for any deviation from the midline by placing two fingers over the trachea at the suprasternal notch. Place one finger laterally to the left while placing another finger laterally to the right. Deviation of the trachea from the midline may indicate a mass or respiratory problems such as atelectasis and pneumothorax (Fig. A-23).

Carotid Arteries

Inspect and palpate the carotid arteries to assess symmetry, amplitude, and rate and rhythm of the pulsations (Fig. A-23). Palpate only one carotid artery at a time, remembering that these arteries supply essential blood to the brain. Do not press the carotid sinus (near the jaw angle) as this can cause a sudden drop in the pulse or blood pressure. Note any diminished, absent, expansile, or abnormally forceful pulsations. Auscultate the carotid artery by using the bell of the stethoscope, beginning at the base of the artery and moving up toward the chin. It will be helpful if you instruct the person to hold the breath as you auscultate. Note any **bruits,** a blowing sound that indicates a distortion of a blood vessel that could interfere with blood flow.

Spinal Accessory Nerve

The spinal accessory nerve (CN XI) innervates the major neck muscles (trapezius and sternocleidomastoid)

(Fig. A-23). Assess this nerve and muscle strength by asking the person to shrug the shoulders against the resistance of your hands and to turn the head from one side to the other as you try to resist these movements.

External Jugular Veins

Inspect the jugular veins for abnormal or unusual distention. The jugular veins are not normally distended when the person sits or stands upright. However, when the person is supine and relaxed, jugular filling occurs, and the veins appear distended (not bulged) from the clavicle to the jaw's angle (Fig. A-24).

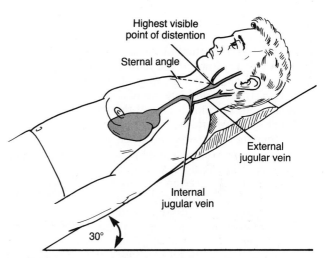

Highest visible point of distention

Sternal angle

External jugular vein

Internal jugular vein

30°

▼ FIGURE A–24. Assessment of the external jugular vein.

GUIDELINE A-13   ASSESSING THE CHEST AND LUNGS

Examination of the chest involves assessment of the respiratory system (lungs) and the cardiovascular system (heart). The primary function of the respiratory system is to maintain ventilation (the exchange of oxygen and carbon dioxide in the lungs and tissue) and regulate the acid-base balance. Any changes or abnormalities within the respiratory system will affect other body systems. The cardiovascular system's primary organ is the heart. The heart acts as a pump that moves the blood throughout the body, thereby transporting oxygen and nutrients to the cells of the body and transporting and removing carbon dioxide from the lungs and the body cells. The lungs and heart work so closely together that it is difficult to assess them separately.

A thorough examination of the chest requires you to use the techniques of inspection, palpation, percussion, and auscultation. The posterior chest is examined first, with the person in a sitting position. The anterior chest is examined with the person in either a sitting or supine position, and the examination of the heart is performed with the person in a supine position. Good lighting is imperative to assess the chest area, and the person will need to undress to the waist.

During the assessment of the thorax, bear in mind the thoracic reference lines (Fig. A-25) and familiar landmarks—for example, ribs, sternal angle (angle of Louis), costal angle, suprasternal notch, and vertebra prominens. These make possible (a) accurate documentation of the location of findings, and (b) accurate mental visualization of underlying thoracic structures, such as lobes of lungs.

Posterior Chest

Inspection

The posterior chest is inspected for any skeletal deformities that could affect the status of the respiratory system. Some common abnormalities are **kyphosis** (an exaggerated curvature of the thoracic vertebrae), **scoliosis** (a lateral curvature of the spine), and **lordosis** (an exaggerated curvature of the lumbar vertebrae) (Fig. A-26). Further inspection involves observing the slope of the ribs, retraction and bulging of the intercostal spaces, local lag, and rate and rhythm of the respirations.

The ribs are attached to the spine at a 45-degree angle (oblique). A horizontal slope of the ribs will be assessed on a person with emphysema. Note any retractions of the intercostal spaces on inspiration and bulging of the intercostal spaces on expiration. This abnormality may be the result of asthma, emphysema, pleural effusion, or tension pneumothorax. Unilateral local lag indicates respiratory movement impairment. When assessing for local lag, ask yourself these questions: "Does the chest move synchronously?" "Does the chest expand equally?"

The rate and rhythm of the respirations should be assessed at this time. Some abnormal respiratory patterns you may assess are tachypnea, bradypnea, apnea, hyperpnea, hyperventilation, Cheyne-Stokes, Biot's, and Kussmaul's.

Palpation

The posterior chest is palpated for tenderness, masses, and sinus tracts. Palpate with the palmar surface of the hand, assessing the chest and comparing the right side to the left (Fig. A-27). Respiratory excursion is assessed by placing your thumbs parallel to the 10th ribs and grasping the lateral rib cage. Instruct the person to inhale deeply as you note the chest move upward and outward, and your thumbs should move apart. As the person exhales, your thumbs should return to the midline.

Fremitus is a vibration transmitted through the chest wall as the person speaks. To palpate the vibration with the palmar surface or ulnar side of the hand, ask the person to repeat the words *ninety-nine* or *one-one-one*. Use only one hand to palpate fremitus to avoid any discrepancies as a result of differing sensitivity between the hands. You will cover the entire chest, moving back and forth from one side to the other, making sure to assess the upper and lower lobes of the lungs. Expect to feel an increase in fremitus over the main stem bronchi and upper lobes, where there is increased airflow. Also note an increase in fremitus during an inflammatory process such as pneumonia and in the presence of a mass. A decrease in fremitus will be assessed with an obstructed bronchus, pleural effusion, and pneumothorax. The level of the diaphragm is estimated in the area where fremitus is no longer felt.

Percussion

The posterior chest is percussed to determine whether the underlying tissue is air filled, fluid filled, or solid (Fig. A-28). The normal lung should be air filled, producing a resonance sound that is low pitched, of loud intensity, and of long duration. Table A-5 illustrates other percussion sounds in relation to pitch, intensity, and duration. It is important for you to be able to identify the five percussion sounds in order to distinguish normal from abnormal (Fig. A-29). Following the posterior chest sequence, percuss the chest for any abnormal percussion sound. A lung mass will elicit a flat sound, whereas a hyperinflated lung elicits a hyperresonant sound. Normally, when resonance changes to dullness, you are at the estimated level of the diaphragm (usually at the T10 level).

Diaphragmatic excursion is movement of the diaphragm as it descends on inspiration and rises on expi-

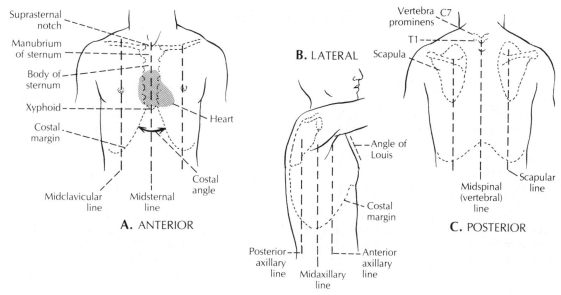

▼ **FIGURE A–25.** Landmarks and reference lines on the thorax.

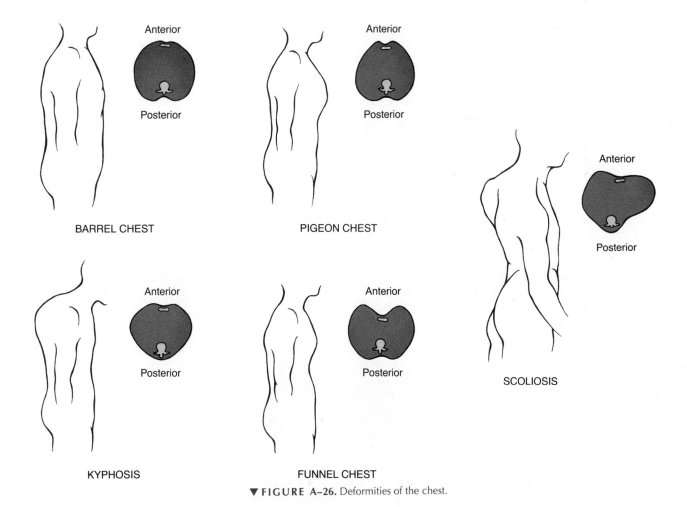

▼ **FIGURE A–26.** Deformities of the chest.

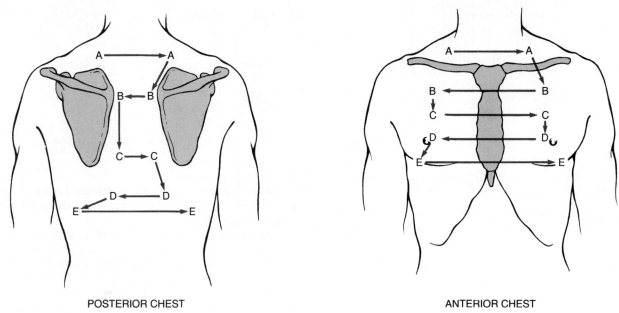

POSTERIOR CHEST

ANTERIOR CHEST

▼ **FIGURE A–27.** Sequence for thoracic palpation.

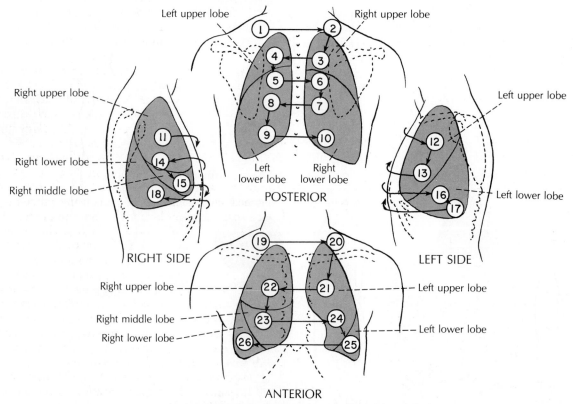

▼ **FIGURE A–28.** Sequence for thoracic percussion and auscultation.

TABLE A–5. Percussion Sounds

Sound	Intensity	Pitch	Percussion Example
Flatness	Soft	High	Thigh, muscle
Dullness (Thudlike)	Medium	Moderate	Liver
Resonance (Hollow)	Loud	Low	Normal lung
Hyperresonance (Booming)	Very loud	Lower	Emphysematous lung
Tympany (Drumlike)	Loud	Higher	Puffed-out cheek Gastric air bubble

ration. Diaphragmatic excursion is assessed by performing the following steps:

1.   Instruct the person to inhale and to hold the breath.
2.   Percuss downward from the bottom of the scapulae at the midscapular line.
3.   When you note the percussion sound change from resonance to dullness, mark it with your special marking pen.
4.   Instruct the person to exhale and to hold it.
5.   Percuss upward (beginning at your pen marking) until the percussion sound changes from dullness to resonance. Mark it with your marking pen.

The distance between the points is measured and the procedure is then repeated on the opposite side. Normally, the range in measurement is 3 to 6 cm.

Auscultation

Auscultation is useful in assessing airflow; the presence of fluid, mucus, or obstruction; and the surrounding lung and pleural spaces. When auscultating, instruct the

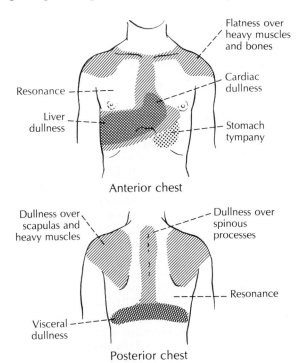

▼ FIGURE A–29. Percussion tones.

person to take deep breaths through the mouth. Be sure to use the diaphragm of the stethoscope. Listen at least one full breath in each location following the percussion sequence (see Fig. A-28).

Normal Breath Sounds. Normal breath sounds are vesicular, bronchial, and bronchovesicular. **Vesicular breath sounds** are soft, low-pitched, fine rustling sounds located over the periphery of the lung. If vesicular sounds are decreased over the periphery, this may indicate pneumonia, emphysema, pleural effusion, or atelectasis. Bronchial breath sounds are loud, high-pitched "tubular" sounds located over the trachea and major bronchi. **Bronchial or tracheal breath sounds** are loud, high-pitched tubular sounds located over the trachea and major bronchi that are heard louder and longer during expiration. Bronchial sounds auscultated over the periphery of the lungs may indicate consolidation or atelectasis. **Bronchovesicular breath sounds** are moderately pitched sounds located between the scapulae posteriorly and on either side of the sternum at the first and second intercostal spaces anteriorly. Bronchovesicular breath sounds auscultated over the periphery of the lung may indicate consolidation. Symbols for documentation of normal breath sounds are illustrated in Table A-6.

Adventitious Breath Sounds. Adventitious breath sounds are abnormal breath sounds such as crackles, wheezes, rhonchi, and friction rubs. **Crackles** (formerly known as rales) are noises created when air is traveling through vessels containing abnormal moisture. They are more pronounced on inspiration. Crackles are divided into fine and coarse. Fine crackles are soft and high pitched and sound like two hairs being rubbed together. Coarse crackles are louder and lower in pitch and have a bubbling quality. **Wheezes** are high-pitched sounds produced as air passes through a narrowed or defective vessel. They may occur during inspiration, expiration, or both. The cause may be a mucous plug, bronchospasms, or tumor. **Rhonchi** (gurgles) are coarse rattling sounds, louder and lower in pitch than crackles, caused by narrowed airways. Rhonchi are more pronounced on expiration. **Friction rubs** are crackling, grating sounds produced when two roughened or inflamed pleural spaces rub across each other during respiration. They are heard on inspiration and expiration. Note the location and the relationship in the respiratory cycle of the adventitious sounds (Table A-7).

Spoken and Whispered Sounds. Spoken and whispered sounds are based on the principle that sound car-

TABLE A–6. Documentation Symbols of Normal Breath Sounds

Breath Sound	Symbol/Description

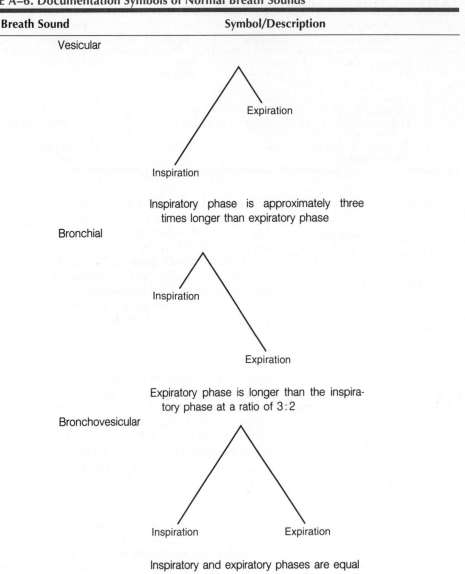

Vesicular

Inspiratory phase is approximately three times longer than expiratory phase

Bronchial

Expiratory phase is longer than the inspiratory phase at a ratio of 3:2

Bronchovesicular

Inspiratory and expiratory phases are equal

ries best through a solid, not as well through fluid, and poorly through air. Instruct the person to say "ninety-nine" while you auscultate the posterior chest. Normally, the sound should be muffled and indistinct. If the sound is clear, it is called bronchophony. Instruct the person to say "ee" while you auscultate the posterior chest. Normally the sound should be muffled and indistinct. If the sound is heard as "ay," it is called egophony. Instruct the person to whisper "ninety-nine" while you auscultate. Normally, the sound is very faint and indistinct. If the sound is louder and clear, it is called whispered pectoriloquy.

Anterior Chest

Inspection

The anterior chest is inspected for any skeletal deformities. Some common abnormalities are barrel chest, pectus carinatum, and pectus excavatum. The **barrel chest** is a thoracic abnormality characterized by horizontal ribs, slight kyphosis, and a prominent sternal angle. The chest appears to be in a continuous inspiration. **Pectus carinatum** (**pigeon chest**) is a thoracic abnormality characterized by the forward projection of the sternum. **Pectus excavatum** (**funnel chest**) is a thoracic abnormality characterized by the sternum pointing posteriorly, which may cause pressure on the heart. Inspection is also performed regarding the slope of the ribs, retraction and bulging of the intercostal spaces, and local lag, as discussed in the section on the posterior chest. Some areas are inspected on the anterior chest only; this includes the anteroposterior (AP) diameter, costal angle, and use of the accessory muscles.

In a normal adult, the ratio of anteroposterior (AP) to lateral diameter is about 1:2. In an elderly person, you will observe an increase in the AP diameter, which is normal. A barrel chest and pectus carinatum will result

TABLE A–7. Documentation Symbols of Abnormal Breath Sounds

Abnormal Breath Sounds	Symbol/Description
Crackles (formerly rales)	Inspiration Expiration More pronounced during inspiratory phase
Wheezes	Inspiration Expiration May be auscultated during inspiratory or expiratory phases or both
Rhonchi (gurgles)	Inspiration Expiration More pronounced on expiration
Friction rubs	Inspiration Expiration Auscultated during inspiratory and expiratory phases

in an increase in the AP diameter. The costal angle should be less than 90 degrees. The accessory muscles are composed of the sternocleidomastoid, trapezius, and abdominal muscles. Inspect the use of these muscles to aid in ventilation. You will observe the muscles contracting.

Palpation

The anterior chest is palpated for areas of tenderness, respiratory excursion, and fremitus (see Fig. A-27). To assess respiratory excursion, place your thumbs along the costal margins, grasping the lateral rib cage with your hands. Slide your thumbs toward each other to raise a skin fold between the thumbs. Instruct the person to inhale deeply as you observe the divergence of the thumbs and assess the symmetry of respiratory movement.

The assessment of fremitus differs anteriorly owing to the decreased or absent vibration over the precordium (the area of the chest overlying the heart). In a woman, you will be unable to feel the vibration through breast tissue. You may have to displace the breast to complete the assessment of fremitus.

Percussion

Percuss the anterior and lateral chest (see Fig. A-28). Normally, resonance is percussed over the entire lung area. You will percuss dullness to the left of the sternum at the third to fifth intercostal spaces as a result of the heart's presence. The liver and stomach will produce dull and tympanic sounds, respectively. Be sure that you are familiar with the location of these structures.

Auscultation

The anterior chest is auscultated using the percussion sequence (see Fig. A-28). Auscultate for vesicular, bronchial, and bronchovesicular breath sounds. Note any adventitious sounds heard, as discussed in the section on posterior chest.

GUIDELINE A-14   ASSESSING THE HEART

Inspection, percussion, palpation, and auscultation are the techniques used in the examination of the heart. To identify the precordial points, you must be familiar with the landmarks (Fig. A-30). The angle of Louis is palpated as a prominence on the upper third of the sternum. Palpate this area and move the fingers laterally to identify the second intercostal space. The aortic area is located at the second intercostal space to the right sternal border. The pulmonic area is located at the second intercostal space to the left sternal border. Erb's point is located at the third intercostal space to the left sternal border. The tricuspid area is located at the fourth or fifth intercostal space to the left sternal border. The mitral (apical) area is located at the fifth intercostal space medial to the midclavicular line. The epigastric area is the area overlying the xiphoid process.

Inspection

Before beginning the assessment, position the person in a supine position or lying with the head of the bed at a 30- to 45-degree angle. The latter position will

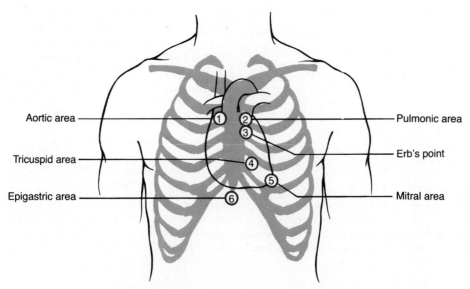

▼ **FIGURE A–30.** Precordial points of the heart.

facilitate breathing for the person with heart or respiratory problems. Stand at the person's right side. This will assist you in viewing any pulsations.

Inspect the precordial points of the chest for any abnormal pulsations or lift-heaves and the apical impulse. An example of an abnormal pulsation you might observe is a pulsation located at the pulmonic area, or Erb's point, resulting from an abnormally sharp closure of the pulmonic value associated with pulmonary hypertension. Normally the only pulsation observable on the chest wall is the apical impulse. The **apical impulse** (point of maximal impulse) is a pulsation located over the apex of the heart, at the fifth intercostal space medial to the midclavicular line. If the heart is displaced or enlarged, the apical impulse may be located lateral to the midclavicular line. If this is the case, position the person in a left lateral horizontal position to observe the apical impulse.

The heart's pumping action may be so forceful that you observe the chest lift or heave. A lift is a slight movement, while a heave is a more vigorous movement. Each is the result of forceful cardiac action and is considered abnormal.

Palpation

The precordial points of the chest are palpated for any abnormal pulsations, thrills, lift-heaves, apical impulses, and aortic pulsations. You may decide to palpate as you inspect each area. A **thrill** is a palpable cardiac murmur. It feels similar to the neck of a purring cat and is considered abnormal. You should not be able to palpate any pulsations at any of the precordial points except for the mitral area. To palpate the apical impulse, place the heel of the hand on the sternum with your fingers stretched across the chest, just under the breast area. After you have located the apical impulse, palpate it with your fingertips. When palpating for lifts and heaves, observe in the area at or near the sternum (right ventricular heave) and at or near the apex (left ventricular heave). The aortic pulse is palpated in the epigastric area.

Percussion

Cardiac dullness is located in the third to fifth intercostal spaces. Since chest x-ray films are much more practical and efficient in determining the size of the heart, percussion is no longer used in the assessment of the heart.

Auscultation

The auscultation technique assesses the normal heart sounds (S_1 and S_2), extra heart sounds (S_3, S_4, split S_1, and split S_2), and murmurs. Auscultate over the precordial areas (Fig. A-30) with both the stethoscope's diaphragm and bell. Listen at each area through several breaths in and out. Instruct the person to breathe through the nose to decrease the interference of breath sounds as you are listening. Press the diaphragm firmly against the chest wall, but when auscultating with the bell hold it lightly. Describe the heart sounds according to their pitch, loudness, and timing in the cardiac cycle. Low-pitched sounds are best heard with the stethoscope bell and higher, louder sounds with the diaphragm.

First Heart Sound. The first heart sound (S_1) is produced by the closure of the mitral and tricuspid heart valves. It is best heard at the apex of the heart.

Second Heart Sound. The second heart sound (S_2) is produced by the closure of the aortic and pulmonic heart valves. It is best heard at the base of the heart (aortic area). Remember that the heart is upside down, with its apex located at the fifth intercostal space medial to the midclavicular line, and its right and left bases located at the second intercostal space, along the sternal borders. S_1 and S_2 are both high-pitched sounds, so use the stethoscope's diaphragm to listen. When auscultating, listen to S_1 and S_2 at each site (mitral and aortic), and note the time between S_1 and S_2 (systole) and between S_2 and S_1 (diastole).

Third Heart Sound. The third heart sound, S_3 (ventricular gallop), is a low-pitched sound heard in the cardiac cycle immediately after S_2 (diastole). It is normal in children and young adults. It is considered abnormal in adults over 30 years of age. It is best heard in the mitral area with the person in a left lateral horizontal position, using the bell of the stethoscope. It represents an enlarged ventricle or overly rapid ventricular filling, a sign of left ventricular failure.

Fourth Heart Sound. The fourth heart sound, S_4 (atrial gallop), is a low-pitched sound heard in the cardiac cycle just before S_1. Using the bell of the stethoscope, auscultate for S_4 in the mitral area with the person in a left lateral horizontal position. It is considered abnormal in most adults and is associated with ischemia, coronary artery disease, and aortic stenosis.

Split First Heart Sound. A split first heart sound (split S_1) occurs when the mitral and tricuspid heart valves are not closing together. It is a high-pitched sound heard best in the tricuspid area using the stethoscope's diaphragm. It is associated with a right bundle branch block.

Split Second Heart Sound. A split second heart sound (split S_2) occurs when the aortic and pulmonic heart valves are not closing together. It is a high-pitched sound heard best in the pulmonic area with the stethoscope's bell. It is more common in children. If you auscultate a split S_2, note whether the split occurs on inspiration or expiration. A split S_2 on expiration may indicate right or left bundle branch block, atrial septal defect, or valvular problems.

Heart Murmur. A **heart murmur** is a harsh, rumbling, blowing sound caused by blood flow across a defective valve, or the shunting of blood through an abnormal passage. A heart murmur is assessed for timing, location, radiation, intensity, quality, and pitch. Timing involves determining whether the murmur occurs during diastole (between S_2 and S_1) or systole (between S_1 and S_2). Describe the location according to the precordial areas and note whether the murmur radiates. Intensity of a murmur refers to the loudness and is graded on the following scale:

Grade I	very faint
Grade II	quiet but audible
Grade III	moderately loud
Grade IV	loud
Grade V	very loud
Grade VI	very loud; may be audible with the stethoscope completely off the chest wall

---

GUIDELINE A-15   ASSESSING THE BREASTS

Inspection and palpation are performed during the assessment of the breasts. It is important to remember that assessment of the breasts includes not only women but also men. During breast assessment, help women and men learn to perform breast self-examination and encourage the use of this valuable health maintenance practice (Fig. A-31).

The female breast is composed of glandular tissue, fibrous tissue, and fat. It is located between the second and sixth ribs, between the sternal edge and the midaxillary line. It may feel soft and granular, nodular, or lumpy. Nodularity may increase prior to the menstrual period each month. This is why female breasts are examined following a menstrual period rather than just prior to one.

The male breasts should be flat, smooth, nontender, and bilaterally symmetrical in appearance. The nipple and areolae should be inspected and palpated for nodules, swelling, and edema. If you observe breast enlargement, distinguish it from obesity (soft enlargement) and gynecomastia (firm enlargement) through palpation.

Inspection

Several positions are assumed when inspecting the breasts: sitting, arms at the sides; sitting, arms raised over the head (the person may rest the arms on top of the head); leaning forward (breasts hanging down) while sitting or standing; and the hands pressed firmly on the hips or palms pressed firmly together.

The assessment begins with the person sitting and the arms at the sides. The chest area must be completely exposed in order to inspect the breast for size and symmetry, contour, and appearance of the skin. The nipples are also inspected for size, shape, rashes, ulcerations, and discharge.

When observing the breasts for size and symmetry, you may observe a slight difference in each. This is considered normal. You should not note a difference in the breasts as a result of movement, rest, or over a period of time. This is a good time to ask the person if any changes have been noticed. Comparing one breast with the other, inspect the contour, which should be smooth and convex. Observe for any masses, flattening, or dimpling of the breasts. Dimpling may be particularly evident when the person presses the hands on the hips. The skin is inspected for color, thickening or edema, and venous pattern. The skin should be intact, movable, and smooth (possibly slightly wrinkled or with striae). Redness and inflammation may indicate infection or carcinoma. Thickening or edema may be produced by lymphatic blockage. The skin that resembles an orange peel (thickened skin and large pores) suggests cancer of the breast. An increased prominence of venous pattern is also suggestive of breast cancer.

When inspecting the nipples, note that size and color may vary. Nipple inversion is considered a normal variation if it has been long-standing. Inversion occurring in a previously erect nipple is suggestive of malignancy. The nipples should point outward and downward. Note any deviation from this, since a malignancy can deviate the direction in which the nipple points. Observe for any rashes, ulcerations, or discharge. It is normal for a discharge to occur during the lactation phase of pregnancy. If discharge is present, note the odor and type of drainage (purulent, serous, or sanguineous).

Examine a large breast bimanually, with one hand under the breast to support it (Fig. A-32). Carefully assess axillary skin folds and under pendulous breasts.

Palpation

The person should be in a supine position with a pillow under the scapula of the side being examined. The arm should be raised above the head of the side being examined. To describe any findings, the breast should be divided into four quadrants: right upper, right lower, left upper, and left lower; or the breast should be viewed as the face of a clock (Fig. A-33). Any abnormality will be located by the time—for example, nine o'clock—and by the distance (centimeters) from the nipple.

Palpate all four quadrants, both areolae, tails of breasts, and axillae for lumps or nodules. To palpate the breast, gently use the finger pads in a rotating movement, progressing slowly across the breast tissue until the total breast is examined (Fig. A-34). Maintain continuous finger contact with the tissue rather than lifting the fingers up and down to change sites. If the person reports a lump, palpate the breast without the lump first, thus becoming familiar with the person's "normal" breast tissue before assessing the deviation from normal. If a nodule is detected, note the location (as described earlier), size (centimeters), shape (round, disk-shaped, oblong, tubular), consistency (soft, hard, firm), mobility (mobile, fixed), and borders (well-defined, poorly demarcated). Compress the areola and nipple of each breast

▪ WHY DO THE BREAST SELF-EXAM?

There are many good reasons for doing a breast self-exam each month. One reason is that it is easy to do and the more you do it, the better you will get at it. When you get to know how your breasts normally feel, you will quickly be able to feel any change, and early detection is the key to successful treatment and cure.

Remember: A breast self-exam could save your breast—and save your life. Most breast lumps are found by women themselves, but, in fact, most lumps in the breast are not cancer. Be safe, be sure.

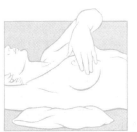 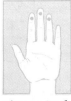

Finger Pads

▪ WHEN TO DO BREAST SELF-EXAM

The best time to do breast self-exam is right after your period, when breasts are not tender or swollen. If you do not have regular periods or sometimes skip a month, do it on the same day every month.

▪ NOW, HOW TO DO BREAST SELF-EXAM

1. Lie down and put a pillow under your right shoulder. Place your right arm behind your head.

2. Use the finger pads of your three middle fingers on your left hand to feel for lumps or thickening. Your finger pads are the top third of each finger.

3. Press firmly enough to know how your breast feels. If you're not sure how hard to press, ask your health care provider. Or try to copy the way your health care provider uses the finger pads during a breast exam. Learn what your breast feels like most of the time. A firm ridge in the lower curve of each breast is normal.

4. Move around the breast in a set way. You can choose either the circle (A), the up and down line (B), or the wedge (C). Do it the same way every time. It will help you to make sure that you've gone over the entire breast area, and to remember how your breast feels.

5. Now examine your left breast using right hand finger pads.

6. If you find any changes, see your doctor right away.

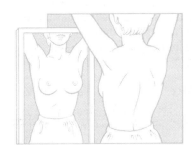

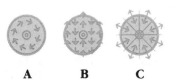

A   **B**   **C**

▪ FOR ADDED SAFETY:

You should also check your breasts while standing in front of a mirror right after you do your breast self-exam each month. See if there are any changes in the way your breasts look: dimpling of the skin, changes in the nipple, or redness or swelling.

You might also want to do a breast self-exam while you're in the shower. Your soapy hands will glide over the wet skin making it easy to check how your breasts feel.

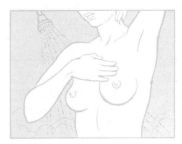

▼ **FIGURE A–31.** A technique for self-examination of the breast. (How to Do Breast Self-Examination. Used with permission. American Cancer Society, Inc., 1992.)

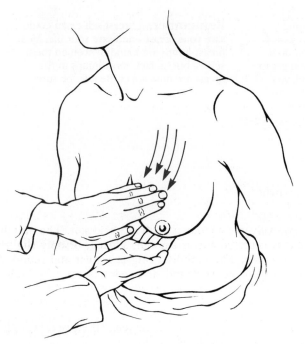

▼ **FIGURE A–32.** Bimanual breast palpation.

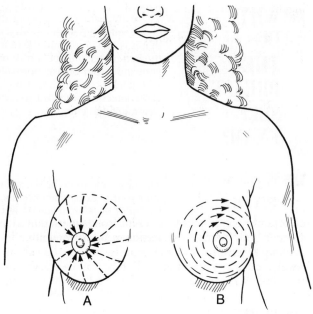

▼ **FIGURE A–34.** Patterns of breast palpation.

with the thumb and index finger to denote any discharge. Note the amount, color, consistency, and location.

Cancerous lesions are hard, fixed, nontender, and irregular in shape.

Axillae

Inspection and palpation are used to assess the axillary area with the person in a sitting position.

Inspection

Inspect each axilla for rashes, redness, infection, and unusual pigmentation. Redness and infection may originate from the sweat glands. A change in pigmentation may suggest an underlying malignancy.

Palpation

When performing palpation of the axilla, place your fingers into the apex of the axilla with the person's arm down and the wrist resting in your hand. Bring your

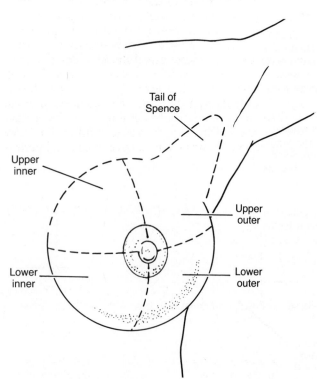

▼ **FIGURE A–33.** Breast quadrants used for assessment.

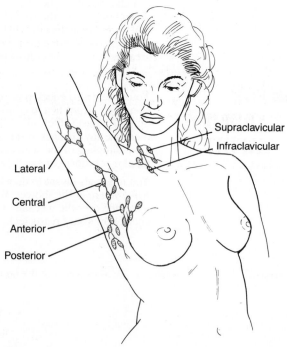

▼ **FIGURE A–35.** Lymph nodes of the breast and axillary area.

fingers down over the surface of the ribs, compressing the nodes against the chest. Lymph nodes associated with breast lymphatic drainage are normally not palpable. Some tenderness occurs high in the axilla during palpation for lymph nodes. Assess the supraclavicular, infraclavicular, central and lateral axillary, central axillary, and pectoral lymph nodes (Fig. A-35).

GUIDELINE A-16   ASSESSING THE ABDOMEN

Assessment of the abdomen involves inspection, auscultation, percussion, and palpation. It will also include the assessment of abdominal reflexes. Remember, the order of techniques is different from the examination of other body parts. Auscultation is performed after inspection to ensure that the motility of the bowel and bowel sounds are not altered. Before you can begin the abdominal assessment, you need to be familiar with the quadrants or regions of the abdomen. The abdomen is divided into four quadrants, right upper, right lower, left upper, and left lower (Fig. A-36). The abdomen may also be divided into nine regions. Figure A-36 illustrates the regions of the abdomen. It is also important to know the underlying organs located in each quadrant (Fig. A-37).

Prior to the examination, ask the person to empty the bladder. The person will assume a supine position with the arms at the side or draped across the chest. Instruct the person to flex the knees slightly. This position aids in relaxation of the abdomen. Expose the abdomen from the epigastric area to the symphysis pubis. Be sure to drape the female chest. The equipment needed for the examination will include a small ruler, marking pen, and stethoscope.

Inspection

When inspecting the abdomen, stand on the person's right side. Be sure that you have good lighting. Inspect the contour and symmetry, skin, umbilicus, and assess for peristalsis and pulsations.

Observe the contour of the abdomen. Is it flat, sunken, or protruding? Are all four quadrants equal in size, or is there asymmetry between the quadrants? Observe the skin for any scars, striae, or lesions. Note the contour, location, and any signs of inflammation or herniation of the umbilicus. Looking across the person's abdomen, observe for peristalsis and any pulsations. Normally, the abdomen is smooth and soft. The umbilicus is centered and is smooth, sunken, or only slightly protruding. The umbilical ring is regular and round. A fine venous network and silver-white striae may be apparent. The abdominal contour is evenly rounded or flat. Peristalsis is usually not visible except in very thin people. The aortic pulsation may be observed in the epigastric area. Remember, pregnancy can affect the contour and symmetry of the abdomen. The abdomen will protrude and appear asymmetric. Disease processes may also cause protrusion of the abdomen. If pathology is suspected, measure the abdominal girth. Dehydration may cause the abdomen to appear sunken, whereas distention, obesity, or tumors may cause a protrusion of the abdomen. Fluid (ascites), masses, or an intestinal obstruction may cause asymmetry of the abdomen.

Auscultation

The abdomen is auscultated for bowel sounds, bruits, friction rubs, and venous hums. Prior to beginning, be sure to warm the stethoscope's diaphragm with your hands. A cold diaphragm may cause the person to tense the abdominal muscles. Bowel sounds are created by peristalsis and indicate bowel motility. Bowel sounds are high pitched, gurgling sounds estimated at 5 to 35 per minute, and they occur every 5 to 15 seconds. Bowel sounds within the range of 5 to 35 per minute are normal bowel sounds. Hypoactive bowel sounds are fewer than 5 per minute and indicate decreased motility. This may be seen in bowel obstruction, paralytic ileus, and perito-

▼ **FIGURE A–36.** Terminology used with reference to abdominal anatomy.

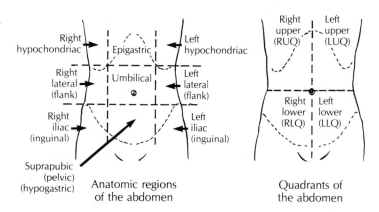

Right hypochondriac
Epigastric
Left hypochondriac
Right lateral (flank)
Umbilical
Left lateral (flank)
Right iliac (inguinal)
Left iliac (inguinal)
Suprapubic (pelvic) (hypogastric)
Anatomic regions of the abdomen

Right upper (RUQ)
Left upper (LUQ)
Right lower (RLQ)
Left lower (LLQ)
Quadrants of the abdomen

ORGANS FOUND IN EACH ABDOMINAL QUADRANT	
Right Upper Quadrant (RUQ)	**Left Upper Quadrant (LUQ)**
Adrenal gland (right)	Adrenal gland (left)
Colon (hepatic flexure and portions of ascending and transverse)	Colon (splenic flexure and portions of transverse and descending)
Duodenum	Kidney (portion of left)
Kidney (portion of right)	Liver (left lobe)
Liver	Pancreas (body)
Gallbladder	Spleen
Pancreas (head)	Stomach
Pylorus	
Loops of small intestine in all quadrants	
Right Lower Quadrant (RLQ)	**Left Lower Quadrant (LLQ)**
Appendix	Bladder (if distended)
Bladder (if distended)	Colon (sigmoid and portion of descending)
Cecum	Kidney (lower pole of left)
Colon (portion of ascending)	Ovary (left)
Kidney (lower pole of right)	Salpinx (uterine tube; left)
Ovary (right)	Spermatic cord (left)
Salpinx (uterine tube; right)	Ureter (left)
Spermatic cord (right)	Uterus (if enlarged)
Ureter (right)	
Uterus (if enlarged)	

▼ **FIGURE A–37.** Organs found in each abdominal quadrant.

nitis. Hyperactive bowel sounds are greater than 35 per minute and indicate an increase in bowel motility, as seen in gastroenteritis and intestinal obstruction.

Auscultate each quadrant for bowel sounds; be sure to listen at least 5 minutes before concluding they are absent. Absent bowel sounds may indicate paralytic ileus, peritonitis, or complete obstruction. Note any abnormal sounds. A high-pitched, tinkling sound may indicate fluid, whereas a rush of high-pitched sounds coinciding with an abdominal cramp may indicate an obstruction. The abdominal aorta and renal, iliac, and femoral arteries are auscultated for bruits. The aorta and renal arteries are located in the epigastric area, while the iliac arteries are located in the lower umbilical area. The femoral arteries are located in the groin area. Remember, a bruit is a low-pitched, purring sound that must be auscultated using the stethoscope bell for detection. Auscultate over the liver and spleen area for any possible friction rub. This abnormal, rough, grating sound is present during infection, malignancy, or infarction. A venous hum may be auscultated in the epigastric and umbilical area. It is an abnormal, continuous, medium-pitched sound that suggests hepatic cirrhosis.

Percussion

The percussion notes of the abdomen are dullness and tympany. Dullness is percussed over solid structures (abdominal organs), whereas tympany is percussed over air-filled areas. Prior to beginning, ask the person whether any abdominal pain is present and if so, where. Percuss this area last. Percuss all four quadrants of the abdomen, noting the change in percussion notes.

To percuss the liver borders (Fig. A-38), start at the nipple in the midclavicular line and percuss downward from resonance to dullness. Using your marking pen, mark the area where dullness begins. This is the upper liver border. Then begin percussion at the level of the umbilicus, midclavicular line, and percuss upward from tympany to dullness. Mark the area where dullness begins. This is the lower liver border. The distance between the two markings should be 6 to 12 cm in an adult. Using the same procedure, percuss along the mid-

sternal line. The distance at the midsternal line should be 4 to 8 cm.

The spleen is percussed at the lowest interspace in the left anterior axillary line. When the spleen is of normal size, you should elicit a tympanic note in this area. If the spleen is enlarged, tympany will be replaced by dullness. The gastric air bubble will be located between the sixth and seventh ribs on the person's left side. You will have a tympanic percussion note from this area.

Palpation

Light and deep palpation are used to examine the abdomen. Light palpation is used to assess tenderness, muscle tone, abdominal stiffening, and superficial masses. Deep palpation is used to distinguish masses, organs, and deep pain. Begin with light palpation, using the palmar surfaces of the fingertips. Depress the abdomen about 1 cm. Be sure to assess all abdominal quadrants. If the person demonstrates voluntary guarding (muscle rigidity), this usually means the person is not relaxed. Ask the person to take some deep breaths through the mouth and exhale through the nose. Involuntary guarding may indicate acute appendicitis, pelvic inflammatory disease, or acute cholecystitis. After the completion of light pal-

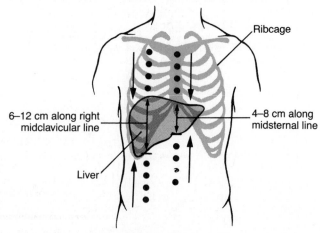

▼ **FIGURE A–38.** Assessment of liver borders using percussion.

pation, you may deeply palpate all quadrants. Deep palpation requires more pressure than light palpation. Therefore, you will need to proceed cautiously and with supervision when performing this form of palpation. It is sometimes easier to place one hand on top of the other. If any masses are palpated, note the size, location, contour, mobility, consistency, and tenderness.

To palpate the liver deeply, place your fingertips below the lower border of liver dullness. Ask the person to take a deep breath as you gently push inward and upward. You should be able to palpate the edge of the liver as the person inhales. The liver should feel smooth, firm, and sharp. If the liver feels hard, this may indicate cirrhosis.

The spleen is generally not palpable in an adult unless it is enlarged. To palpate, place the right hand below the left costal margin and palpate in toward the spleen.

The kidneys are usually not palpable, but you may be able to feel the lower pole of the right kidney in a thin adult. To palpate the right kidney, place your left hand on the person's back just below and parallel to the 12th rib. Place your right hand in the right upper quadrant, parallel to the rectus muscle. Instruct the person to take a deep breath. With your left hand, push the kidney upward. With your right hand push downward. You should have the kidney between your hands. Ask the person to exhale as you slowly release your right hand. If you are able to palpate, note the size, contour, and any tenderness. The left kidney is palpated by standing on the person's left side using the opposite hands while following the same procedure as for the right kidney.

The aorta is palpated by pressing firmly into the epigastric area slightly left of the midline with your fingertips. Identify the aortic pulsation. A prominent pulsation with lateral expansion may indicate an aortic aneurysm.

Abdominal Reflex Assessment

A reflex assessment tests both sensory input and motor response. A **reflex** is an involuntary body response mediated by the spinal cord. The pathway of the reflex arc is the coordinated functioning of the horn cells at each segment of the spinal cord. Initiation of reflexes may be obtained by stimulating the skin (superficial or cutaneous reflexes) or by stimulating the tendon by tapping a tendon, bone, or muscle (deep tendon reflexes). Table A-8 describes the procedure for eliciting the upper and lower abdominal reflexes and the cremasteric reflex.

When documenting reflexes, use a comparison chart. This may be a simple stick figure drawing with the degree of reflex activity recorded on the right and left sides, using a scale of 1+ to 4+ (Table A-8). An alternative method is to use a simple chart such as that shown in Figure A-39.

REFLEX	RIGHT	LEFT
Lower abdominal	2+	2+
Cremasteric	2+	2+

▼ **FIGURE A–39.** A simple method for charting client reflexes.

TABLE A–8. Reflex Assessment*

Reflex	Type	Procedure	Normal Response
Upper and lower abdominal	Superficial (cutaneous)	Stroke each side of abdomen above and below the level of the umbilicus, using the pointed end of the reflex hammer. Stroke toward the umbilicus	Abdominal muscle contraction and umbilicus deviation toward stimulus
Cremasteric	Superficial (cutaneous)	Stroke the inner thigh of men with the pointed end of the reflex hammer	Testes rise in the scrotum
Biceps	Deep tendon	Person's arm should be flexed with the palm down. Examiner's thumb should be placed on the biceps tendon at the antecubital space. Strike the thumb with the reflex hammer	Flexion of the elbow and contraction of the biceps muscle
Triceps	Deep tendon	Person's arm should be flexed and placed across the chest. Strike the triceps tendon directly above the elbow with the reflex hammer	Elbow extension and contraction of the triceps muscle
Supinator or brachioradialis	Deep tendon	Person's arm should rest on the abdomen with the palm down. Strike the brachioradialis tendon approximately 2 inches proximal to the wrist over the radius with the reflex hammer	Forearm supination
Knee (patellar)	Deep tendon	Person should sit with knees bent and legs hanging freely. Strike the patellar tendon with the reflex hammer	Quadriceps contraction and extension of the leg
Ankle (Achilles)	Deep tendon	Dorsiflex the person's foot at the ankle. Strike the Achilles tendon with the reflex hammer	Plantar flexion
Plantar (Babinski)	Superficial (cutaneous)	Stroke the sole of the foot from the heel to the ball, curving across the ball of the foot. Use the pointed end of the reflex hammer	Flexion of the toes

Normal reflexes are categorized as superficial or cutaneous (elicited by stimulating the skin) and deep tendon (elicited by tapping a tendon). Reflexes are graded on a 4-point scale: 0, no response; 1+, slightly diminished; 2+, normal; 3+, brisker than normal; 4+, brisk, hyperactive. Remember to compare one side of the body with the other.

GUIDELINE A-17   PREPARING TO EXAMINE THE GENITALS AND RECTUM

The genital and rectal areas are examined using inspection and palpation. Genital and rectal examinations often are anxiety-provoking for the men and women being examined. Help the person feel more comfortable by maintaining a relaxed but competent attitude. Keep the person informed of your actions. Do not make quick movements. Avoid any actions or statements that the person can interpret as sexually provocative. It may be helpful to have another health professional present during the genital/rectal examinations. Use firm touch rather than gentle stroking. If the person does become sexually stimulated, alter the examination sequence if

necessary, but continue the examination in a professional manner. Enhance comfort during the genital examinations by also:

▼ providing privacy and preventing exposure, e.g., screen, door shut, drapes;
▼ not prolonging the examination unduly;
▼ warming instruments, such as vaginal speculum;
▼ using lubricants when possible to minimize discomfort during insertion, as of gloves or speculum.

Remember to wear gloves during the genital and rectal examinations.

GUIDELINE A-18   ASSESSING THE MALE GENITALIA

Inspection and palpation of the *male genitalia* are performed with the person in a supine position and then in a standing position.

Inspection

Inspection of the male genitalia (Fig. A-40) includes the penis, scrotum, and inguinal ring and canal. To assess secondary sex characteristics, observe the penis and testes for size and shape, color and texture of the scrotal skin, and distribution of the pubic hair. Observe for the presence of lice or nits attached to the pubic hair.

Inspect the skin, prepuce (foreskin) if present, and the glans of the penis. Observe for any lesions, odor, discharge, or inflammation. Normally, the area should be clean. The urethra should open in the center of the glans tip. The prepuce should be retracted to observe for chancres or carcinomas. Smegma (cheesy white material) may be observed under the foreskin. This is considered normal. The urethral meatus should be observed for discharge by compressing the glans between your index finger and thumb. Inspect the scrotal skin and contours for any sores, rashes, swelling, lumps, or veins. Also inspect for any groin masses by asking the person to cough

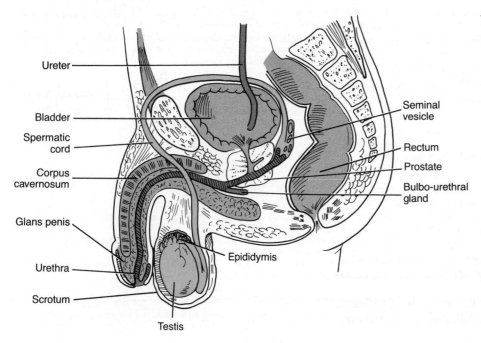

▼ **FIGURE A–40.** Structures of the male urogenital tract.

while you observe for any bulging that may indicate an inguinal hernia.

Palpation

Palpate the penis using your thumb and first two fingers. Note any tenderness or induration. The testes and epididymis of the scrotum are palpated using the thumb and first two fingers. Note size, shape, and con- sistency, and any tenderness or nodules. Normally, the testes feel firm (not hard), possibly spongy. Each testicle is egg (oval)-shaped, about 4 cm long and 2 to 2.5 cm wide. The testicle is descended in each side of the scro- tum, with the left testicle lower than the right. The epididymis is located behind the testicles and is soft (spongy). The spermatic cords are palpated for nodules and swelling. They should be firm, smooth, and tubular. Each structure in the scrotum should be bilaterally similar.

GUIDELINE A-19   ASSESSING THE FEMALE GENITALIA

Inspection and palpation are the techniques used to examine the female genitalia. As stated earlier, the stu- dent as well as the person being examined may experi- ence anxiety and embarrassment thinking about the prospect of examining the genitalia as well as having one's genitalia examined. It is important for you to main- tain a professional manner and be attuned to the person's fears and behaviors. Prior to beginning the examination, instruct the person to empty the bladder. If a urine spec- imen is needed, have the person save one at this time. The female genitalia is examined with the person in a lithotomy position. In the lithotomy position, the person is lying on the back on an examining table with the knees flexed and the feet in stirrups. Elevate the person's head slightly, as this aids in relaxing the abdominal muscles. A drape should cover the person's thighs and knees.

Be sure to explain each step of the examination. Upon palpation, touch the person's thigh prior to contact with the genitalia and avoid any sudden or unexpected movements. The equipment used during this examina- tion includes a gooseneck lamp, vaginal speculum, water- soluble lubricant, disposable gloves, glass slides, wooden spatulas, and a specimen bottle with fixative solution. Be sure that all equipment is assembled before beginning the examination. A female student may perform the ex- amination alone or may have another female health professional present. A male student will need to have a female present in the room during the examination.

Inspection and Palpation

External Inspection. Inspect the external genitalia (Fig. A-41) (mons pubis, labia, and perineum). Note the character and distribution of the pubic hair. Separate the labia and inspect the labia minora, clitoris, urethral ori- fice, and the introitus (vaginal opening). Observe for inflammation, discharge, ulceration, and nodules. If you observe any swelling, inspect and palpate Bartholin's glands by palpating the posterior area of the labia majora with the thumb and index finger (placed near the poste- rior end of the introitus).

The pubic hair should be normally distributed. There should be no odor and minimal, clear discharge.

No lesions should be observed. The vulva should be more darkly pigmented than the other skin. Before menopause, the labia majora are filled out and well formed. After menopause, the labia majora are thinned and eventually become atrophied. The size of the clitoris is variable, usually 3 to 4 mm. The labia minora are thinner than the labia majora and tend to lie open in women who have experienced childbirth. In a virgin, the labia minora will lie close together. The urethral orifice is located between the clitoris and the introitus. There should be no discharge from this area.

Internal Inspection. The inspection of the internal

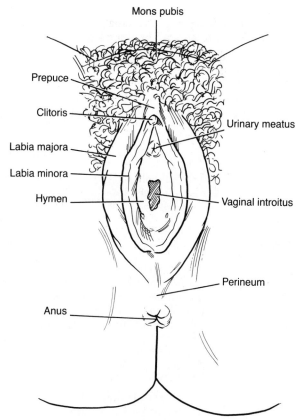

▼ **FIGURE A-41.** External female genitalia.

genitalia is considered an advanced assessment skill. Beginning students usually do not perform this aspect of the examination. Therefore, it will be discussed briefly.

Insert your gloved index finger (lubricated with water only) into the vagina and locate the cervix. Assess the size of the introitus. This will help in deciding the size speculum you will wish to use. Next, with the labia separated, instruct the person to strain down. Observe for any bulging of the vaginal walls.

The internal genitalia (cervix and vagina) are inspected using a speculum. The speculum should be warm and lubricated with water prior to insertion. Do not use a water-soluble lubricant on the speculum because it may distort examination of the cytologic specimen. Inform the person that you are going to perform the speculum examination. Using your left index and middle fingers, depress the perineum. With your right hand, insert the speculum at an oblique angle into the introitus, passing over your left fingers. Be sure that you do not introduce the speculum vertically, as this could injure the urethral orifice and the urethra. When the speculum is completely inserted, rotate it to a transverse position and open slowly. The handle of the speculum should be pointed downward. Tighten the set screw in order to keep the speculum open. You should be able to visualize the cervix.

Inspect the cervix and os for color, position, and surface characteristics. Normally, the cervix is round, pink, and smooth. Note any ulcerations, nodules, masses, bleeding, or discharge. A cervical discharge is normally present and varies from thin and clear to thick, white, and stringy. It depends on the menstrual cycle. An endocervical swab is obtained using a cotton-tipped applicator that is inserted into the cervix and rotated. It is then removed and smeared gently on a glass slide. The slide is then placed in a fixative or sprayed with a fixative. A cervical scrape is also obtained using a wooden spatula inserted into the os. The spatula is turned and scraped in a full circle and then the specimen is placed on a second glass slide. The vaginal mucosa is inspected as the speculum is withdrawn. Observe the color of the mucosa and any inflammation, discharge, ulcerations, or masses. Normally, the vaginal mucosa is moist and pink.

A bimanual examination is performed next by placing your lubricated, gloved index and middle fingers into the vagina. Palpate the perineum for tenderness and nodules. This includes the region of the bladder and urethra, anteriorly. Palpate the cervix for position, size, mobility, and tenderness. Next, place your other hand on the abdomen slightly above the symphysis pubis. Push upward on the cervix as you push downward on the abdominal wall. Attempt to grasp the uterus between your two hands, palpating the size, shape, consistency, and mobility. Note any tenderness on palpation. The adnexa (ovaries and fallopian tubes) are examined next by moving your outside hand to the right lower quadrant of the abdomen and your inside hand to the right lateral fornix. Press in the abdomen, trying to identify the right ovary. Note the size, shape, consistency, mobility, and tenderness. To palpate the left ovary, perform the procedure on the left side.

During palpation, the normal cervix can be gently moved sideways without pain. It feels smooth and firm and lies midline usually on the anterior wall. The cervix points away from the fundus of the uterus. The uterus is usually in an anterior position but can be retroverted in some women. The rectovaginal wall is smooth, firm, and resilient when palpated. The normal ovary (4 to 6 cm) is slightly tender when palpated but should be smooth, firm, and oval. The fallopian tubes cannot be palpated.

GUIDELINE A-20   ASSESSING THE RECTUM

Inspection and digital palpation are performed with the person in a left lateral (Sims') position. Females may be in the lithotomy position.

Inspection

The anal area is inspected by gently spreading the buttocks to expose the anus. The rectal skin should be darker than the surrounding skin. The anal and perianal surfaces should be clear and moist without hairs. Observe the anal area for hemorrhoids, rashes, inflammation, and ulcers.

Digital Palpation

Instruct the person to strain down (Valsalva maneuver). Using a gloved finger and lubricant, palpate the anus with your finger tip. When the anus is relaxed, gently insert your well-lubricated finger by turning the finger and pushing toward the person's umbilicus. Tell the person when you are going to insert your finger. Ask the person to tighten the anus around your finger. Rotate your finger to palpate all surfaces and muscles. Palpate to a depth of 6 to 10 cm. In a male, examine the prostate, feeling each lobe (Fig. A-42). Note size, shape, nodules, consistency, and tenderness. A prostate that is tender, enlarged, soft, or hard is abnormal. Examine the stool (taken from the glove) for blood or pus. A Hemoccult test may be performed as a screening for colorectal cancer. In a woman, a vaginal/rectal palpation will be performed. This is another higher-level assessment skill that requires supervision.

Normally, the anal sphincter tone should be strong. The rectal mucosa should be smooth, without any masses. The prostate should be palpable anteriorly. The rectal-vaginal septum should be firm and smooth, and the muscles should be firm. Finally, the stool should be brown and soft.

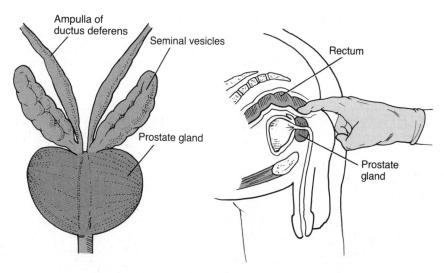

▼ **FIGURE A–42.** Examining the prostate gland using palpation technique.

GUIDELINE A-21   ASSESSING THE UPPER EXTREMITIES

The upper extremities are inspected beginning at the fingertips and moving toward the shoulder. The person should be in a sitting position. Observe size and symmetry, color and texture of the skin and nailbeds, venous pattern, and any edema. The nail base should be firm, with a 160-degree angle between the fingernail and the nail base (Fig. A-43). When assessing the nailbeds, observe for any **clubbing,** an abnormality of the nail in which the nailbed appears springy (early clubbing) or swollen (late clubbing) and the angle of the nail is 180 degrees or greater. Clubbing may suggest hypoxia or lung cancer. Blanch the nailbed and note the amount of time required for capillary refill. A capillary refill occurring in less than 3 seconds is considered normal, between 3 to 4 seconds is sluggish, and greater than 4 seconds is abnormal. A prominence in venous pattern and edema may suggest a venous obstruction.

The brachial, radial, and ulnar pulses are palpated for rate, rhythm, and quality (force) (Table A-9). Remember to compare the volume of the pulses on each arm. Attempt to palpate the epitrochlear lymph node. It is located by having the person flex the elbow to 90 degrees while you palpate the depression between the biceps and triceps muscle. Normally it is very difficult to

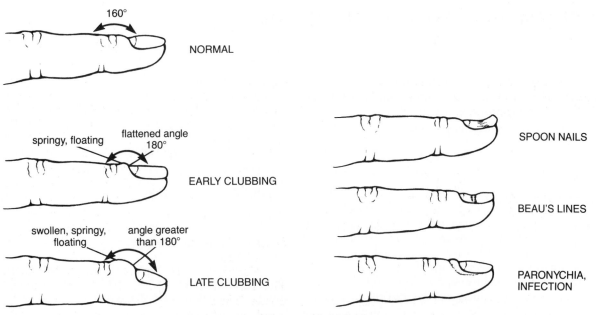

▼ **FIGURE A–43.** Nail abnormalities.

palpate, but if present, note its size, consistency, and any tenderness.

Auscultate the brachial, radial, and ulnar pulses for bruits. Remember to use the stethoscope bell because bruits are low-pitched blowing sounds. The biceps, triceps, and supinator (brachioradialis) reflexes are assessed at this time. The procedure for performing these reflexes and their normal responses are presented in Table A-8.

GUIDELINE A-22   ASSESSING THE LOWER EXTREMITIES

The lower extremities are examined with the person in a supine position, external genital area draped, and legs exposed. Inspection begins at the groin and buttock area and extends to the toes. Observe for size and symmetry, venous pattern, color and texture of the skin and nailbeds, hair distribution on lower legs, feet and toes, pigmentation, rashes, scars, ulcers, and edema. Test the toenails for capillary refill. A person experiencing arterial insufficiency will experience pain, decreased peripheral pulses, pale skin color, cool skin temperature, mild edema, thin, shiny skin, loss of hair over the feet and toes, and thickened nails. Ulcers may or may not be present.

Palpation begins by examining the superficial inguinal lymph nodes. These nodes are located horizon-tally and vertically to the inguinal area. Normally, you may palpate a nontender node in this area up to 2 cm in diameter. Palpate the femoral, popliteal, dorsalis pedis, and posterior tibialis pulses, comparing the volume of each pulse on each leg (Table A-9). Test for **Homan's sign,** an indicator of deep phlebitis, in which pain and soreness are present in the calf area when the foot is dorsiflexed. The person's flexed leg is supported by the calf with your nondominant hand while you dorsiflex the foot with your dominant hand. Note any pain or soreness in the calf area. If present, this would be a positive Homan's sign, indicating the possible presence of phlebitis. The patellar, ankle, and plantar reflexes are assessed at this time in the examination.

TABLE A–9. Grading Pulse Quality and Symmetry*

Pulse Grade	Characteristics
0	Absent pulse
1$^+$	Weak, thready pulse
2$^+$	Normal pulse, easy to palpate
3$^+$	Bounding pulse

*To compare symmetry, record both the right and left pulse quality. Example: 1$^+$/2$^+$.

GUIDELINE A-23   ASSESSING THE MOTOR SYSTEM

Inspect the voluntary muscles for atrophy, **fasciculations** (uncontrollable twitching), and involuntary movements. In addition, you will need to assess gait, Romberg's sign, muscle strength, and coordination.

Gait

Gait is a person's style of walking. To assess gait, instruct the person to walk across the room, turn, and walk back toward you. Observe the person's balance and posture. Normally, the arms are swinging at the sides of the body and balance is easily maintained. Movements such as turns should be smooth. Next, instruct the person to walk in a straight line, heel to toe (tandem walking). Inability to do tandem walking can reveal a condition known as ataxia. **Ataxia** is an uncoordinated gait that results from cerebellar disease or intoxication.

Romberg's Test

Romberg's test is a test of sensory equilibrium. Instruct the person to stand with the feet together and eyes open. Note the person's balance. Then have the person close the eyes. Normally, you will observe minimal swaying. Stay close to the person during this test. If the person should lose balance, this is considered a "positive Romberg" and may suggest cerebellar ataxia.

Tests of Muscle Strength

Muscle strength is assessed by having the person move against your resistance. All major muscle groups should be tested. Muscle strength is graded on a scale of 0 to 5.

Flexion and extension of the elbow are tested by having

the person pull and push against your hand. *Extension of the wrist* is tested by trying to pull the person's formed fist in a downward motion. *Finger abduction* is tested by instructing the person to spread the fingers while you try to force them back together. *Thumb opposition* is tested by instructing the person to touch the thumb to the little finger while you apply resistance to the thumb. *Hip flexion* is tested by applying your hand to the person's thigh and instructing the person to raise the leg against your resistance. *Abduction of the hip* is tested by placing your hand on the outside of the legs at the knee level and instructing the person to spread both legs against your resistance. *Hip adduction* is tested by placing your hands on the inside of the person's legs (knee level) and instructing the person to bring the legs together. *Knee flexion* is tested by placing one hand on the person's slightly flexed knee and your other hand behind the ankle with the person's foot resting on the examination table. Instruct the person to flex the knee against your resistance, without moving the foot. *Ankle dorsiflexion* and *plantar flexion* are tested by asking the person to pull up and push down the foot against your hand.

Tests of Coordination

Coordination is assessed using rapid alternating movements (RAM) and point-to-point testing. The person is instructed to pat the leg with the hand as rapidly as possible, to turn the hand over and back as quickly as possible, and to touch each finger with the thumb as rapidly as possible. Test each hand separately. Note smooth quick movements. Movements that are slowed and uncoordinated may indicate cerebellar dysfunction. The finger-to-nose test is performed with the person in a sitting position and the arms extended forward. Instruct the person to touch the nose with the forefinger, then return the arm to the extended position. Perform this with alternating hands. Test the person first with the eyes open and then with the eyes closed. Observe for smooth movements and maintenance of proper body posture. Cerebellar dysfunction is indicated when the person fails to perform this task.

GUIDELINE A-24   ASSESSING THE SENSORY SYSTEM

The sensory system is examined through the assessment of pain, temperature, light touch, vibration, and position. The sensations are relayed through different pathways. Sensory discrimination tests, which include stereognosis, number identification, two-point discrimination, point localization, and extinction, are considered components of the sensory system. These test the ability of the cortex to analyze and interpret sensations. Prior to beginning the assessment, ask the person about any areas of numbness or unusual sensation. In each test, the person's eyes should be closed. Remember, you will be comparing both sides of the body, including arms, legs, and trunk. Note any numbness or tingling and the degree of stimulation necessary to elicit a response.

Light Touch/Superficial Pain

Using a wisp of cotton and a safety pin, alternately touch the distal and proximal portions of the upper and lower extremities. Ask the person to identify the location and the type of sensation (soft or sharp). If the person exhibits an abnormal pain sensation, test the temperature sensation.

Temperature

The temperature test should be performed only when the person's perception of pain is abnormal. Fill two test tubes with water, one hot and the other cold. Touch all medial and lateral limb surfaces, while alter-nating symmetrical areas. Instruct the person to identify whether the sensation is hot or cold.

Vibration

Vibration is assessed by tapping a tuning fork and placing it firmly on the person's interphalangeal joint of the finger and great toe. Ask the person to describe the sensation (pressure or vibration) and to identify when the sensation ends. Other areas to assess are the forehead, bridge of nose, elbow, wrists, knees, and ankles. Proceed from distal to proximal areas.

Position (Proprioception)

Position is assessed by holding one of the person's fingertips between your thumb and forefinger. Slowly flex and extend the finger. Also perform the test on the great toe. Instruct the person to identify when the finger is moving and in which direction. If the person demonstrates difficulty in identifying position, proceed to the next joint and repeat the procedure.

Stereognosis

Stereognosis is the act of recognizing objects on the basis of touching and manipulating them. Place a familiar object, such as a key, paper clip, or pencil, in the person's hand and have them identify the object. The person should be able to perform this test without difficulty. If an abnormality exists, perform the number identification test.

Number Identification (Graphesthesia)

Trace several numbers on each of the person's palms with the blunt end of a pen or pencil. The person should be able to identify the numbers.

Two-Point Discrimination

When assessing two-point discrimination, touch the person alternately with one or two safety pins on a particular body part, such as the fingerpads. Ask the person if one or two sensations are felt. Find the minimal distance the person can discriminate one from two sensa-

tions. For sensitive fingerpads, the average distance is less than 5 mm.

Point Localization

This is assessed by touching various parts of the person's body with a wisp of cotton. The person is instructed to open the eyes after having felt the touch and point to the area.

Extinction

Extinction is assessed by touching the person's skin simultaneously on opposite sides of the body with safety pins and asking the person to identify whether one sensation or two were felt. Repeat the procedure several times on different symmetric areas. Occasionally, apply only one stimulus to test the person's reliability.

GUIDELINE A-25   CONCLUDING THE PHYSICAL ASSESSMENT

When the physical assessment is over, remove the drape (without exposing the individual) and help the person with clothing (and bed linens if the person is in bed). Clean rectal and perineal areas to remove lubricant or body secretions. Be sure the person is safe and comfortable. Deal with linens, pads, and equipment as appropriate and leave the examining area in order.

Documentation. Various *forms* are available for *documentation* of a client health history and a total physical assessment, or findings may be written out in a narrative, outline format. Also document the following: time of examination, name of examiner, observations made that may contribute to planning nursing care, specimens collected and their disposition (for example, "sent to laboratory").

Bibliography

1. Bates, B. (1991). *A guide to physical examination and history taking* (*5th ed.*). Philadelphia: J.B. Lippincott.
2. Becker, K., & Stevens, S. (1988). Performing in-depth abdominal assessment. *Nursing*, 18, 59–63.
3. Boyd-Monk, H. (1990). Assessing acquired ocular disease. Nursing Clinics of North America, 25(4), 811–822.
4. Bravermun, B. (1990). Eliciting assessment data from the patient who is difficult to interview. *Nursing Clinics of North America, 25*(4), 743–750.
5. Dennison, R. (1986). Cardiopulmonary assessment: How to do it better in 15 easy steps. *Nursing*, 16, 34–40.
6. Judge, R., et al. (1982). *Clinical diagnosis (4th ed.)*. Boston: Little, Brown.
7. Kaufman, J. (1990). Assessing the twelve cranial nerves. *Nursing*, 20, 56–58.
8. Malasanos, L., et al. (1991). *Health assessment*. St. Louis: C.V. Mosby.
9. McConnell, E. (1988). Getting the feel of the lymph node assessment. *Nursing*, 18, 55–57.
10. Morgan, W.L., & Engel, G.L. (1969). *The clinical approach to the patient*. Philadelphia: W.B. Saunders.
11. Morton, P. (1990). *Health assessment*. Springhouse, PA: Springhouse Corporation.
12. O'Toole, M. (1990). Advanced assessment of the abdomen and gastrointestinal problems. *Nursing Clinics of North America*, 25(4), 771–776.
13. Roach, L. (1977). Color changes in dark skin. *Nursing*, 7(1), 48–51.
14. Seidel, H., et al. (1991). *Mosby's guide to physical examination*. St. Louis: C.V. Mosby.
15. Stevens, S., & Becker, K. (1988). How to perform picture-perfect respiratory assessment. *Nursing*, 18, 57–63.
16. Sullivan, J. (1990). Neurologic assessment. *Nursing Clinics of North America*, 25(4), 795–809.
17. Swartz, M. (1989). *Textbook of physical diagnosis: History and examination*. Philadelphia: W.B. Saunders.
18. Willard, M., et al. (1986). The educational pelvic examination: women's responses to a new approach. *JOGNN*, 15, 135–140.

INDEX

Note: Page numbers in *italics* refer to illustrations; page numbers followed by t refer to tables.